Designed for the maintenance of good nutrition of practically all healthy people in the United States

Water-Soluble Vitamins							Minerals						
Vitamin C (mg)	Thiamin (mg)	Riboflavin (mg)	Niacin (mg NE)[f]	Vitamin B6 (mg)	Folate (μg)	Vitamin B12 (μg)	Calcium (mg)	Phosphorus (mg)	Magnesium (mg)	Iron (mg)	Zinc (mg)	Iodine (μg)	Selenium (μg)
30	0.3	0.4	5	0.3	25	0.3	400	300	40	6	5	40	10
35	0.4	0.5	6	0.6	35	0.5	600	500	60	10	5	50	15
40	0.7	0.9	9	1.0	50	0.7	800	800	80	10	10	70	20
45	0.9	1.1	12	1.1	75	1.0	800	800	120	10	10	90	20
45	1.0	1.2	13	1.4	100	1.4	800	800	170	10	10	120	30
50	1.3	1.5	17	1.7	150	2.0	1,200	1,200	270	12	15	150	40
60	1.5	1.8	20	2.0	200	2.0	1,200	1,200	400	12	15	150	50
60	1.5	1.7	19	2.0	200	2.0	1,200	1,200	350	10	15	150	70
60	1.5	1.7	19	2.0	200	2.0	800	800	350	10	15	150	70
60	1.2	1.4	15	2.0	200	2.0	800	800	350	10	15	150	70
50	1.1	1.3	15	1.4	150	2.0	1,200	1,200	280	15	12	150	45
60	1.1	1.3	15	1.5	180	2.0	1,200	1,200	300	15	12	150	50
60	1.1	1.3	15	1.6	180	2.0	1,200	1,200	280	15	12	150	55
60	1.1	1.3	15	1.6	180	2.0	800	800	280	15	12	150	55
60	1.0	1.2	13	1.6	180	2.0	800	800	280	10	12	150	55
70	1.5	1.6	17	2.2	400	2.2	1,200	1,200	300	30	15	175	65
95	1.6	1.8	20	2.1	280	2.6	1,200	1,200	355	15	19	200	75
90	1.6	1.7	20	2.1	260	2.6	1,200	1,200	340	15	16	200	75

[f]NE (niacin equivalent) is equal to 1 mg of niacin or 60 mg of dietary tryptophan.

Estimated Safe and Adequate Daily Dietary Intakes of Selected Vitamins and Minerals[a]

Category	Age (Years)	Vitamins	
		Biotin (μg)	Pantothenic Acid (mg)
Infants	0.0–0.5	10	2
	0.5–1.0	15	3
Children and adolescents	1–3	20	3
	4–6	25	3–4
	7–10	30	4–5
	11+	30–100	4–7
Adults		30–100	4–7

Category	Age (Years)	Trace Elements[b]				
		Copper (mg)	Manganese (mg)	Fluoride (mg)	Chromium (μg)	Molybdenum (μg)
Infants	0.0–0.5	0.4–0.6	0.3–0.6	0.1–0.5	10–40	15–30
	0.5–1.0	0.6–0.7	0.6–1.0	0.2–1.0	20–60	20–40
Children and adolescents	1–3	0.7–1.0	1.0–1.5	0.5–1.5	20–80	25–50
	4–6	1.0–1.5	1.5–2.0	1.0–2.5	30–120	30–75
	7–10	1.0–2.0	2.0–3.0	1.5–2.5	50–200	50–150
	11+	1.5–2.5	2.0–5.0	1.5–2.5	50–200	75–250
Adults		1.5–3.0	2.0–5.0	1.5–4.0	50–200	75–250

[a]Because there is less information on which to base allowances, these figures are not given in the main table of RDAs and are provided here in the form of ranges of recommended intakes.

[b]Since the toxic levels for many trace elements may be only several times usual intakes, the upper levels for the trace elements given in this table should not be habitually exceeded.

FOOD AND NUTRITION BOARD, INSTITUTE OF MEDICINE—NATIONAL ACADEMY OF SCIENCES

DIETARY REFERENCE INTAKES: RECOMMENDED LEVELS FOR INDIVIDUAL INTAKE

Life-Stage Group	Calcium (mg/d)	Phosphorus (mg/d)	Magnesium (mg/d)	D (µg/d)†‡	Fluoride (mg/d)	Thiamin (mg/d)	Riboflavin (mg/d)	Niacin (mg/d)§	B_6 (mg/d)	Folate (µg/d)‖	B_{12} (µg/d)	Pantothenic Acid (mg/d)	Biotin (µg/d)	Choline# (mg/d)
Infants														
0–5 mo	210*	100*	30*	5*	0.01*	0.2*	0.3*	2*	0.1*	65*	0.4*	1.7*	5*	125*
6–11 mo	270*	275*	75*	5*	0.5*	0.3*	0.4*	4*	0.3*	80*	0.5*	1.8*	6*	150*
Children														
1–3 yr	500*	460	80	5*	0.7*	0.5	0.5	6	0.5	150	0.9	2*	8*	200*
4–8 yr	800*	500	130	5*	1*	0.6	0.6	8	0.6	200	1.2	3*	12*	250*
Males														
9–13 yr	1300*	1250	240	5*	2*	0.9	0.9	12	1.0	300	1.8	4*	20*	375*
14–18 yr	1300*	1250	410	5*	3*	1.2	1.3	16	1.3	400	2.4	5*	25*	550*
19–30 yr	1000*	700	400	5*	4*	1.2	1.3	16	1.3	400	2.4	5*	30*	550*
31–50 yr	1000*	700	420	5*	4*	1.2	1.3	16	1.3	400	2.4	5*	30*	550*
51–70 yr	1200*	700	420	10*	4*	1.2	1.3	16	1.7	400	2.4**	5*	30*	550*
>70 yr	1200*	700	420	15*	4*	1.2	1.3	16	1.7	400	2.4**	5*	30*	550*
Females														
9–13 yr	1300*	1250	240	5*	2*	0.9	0.9	12	1.0	300	1.8	4*	20*	375*
14–18 yr	1300*	1250	360	5*	3*	1.0	1.0	14	1.2	400††	2.4	5*	25*	400*
19–30 yr	1000*	700	310	5*	3*	1.1	1.1	14	1.3	400††	2.4	5*	30*	425*
31–50 yr	1000*	700	320	5*	3*	1.1	1.1	14	1.3	400††	2.4	5*	30*	425*
51–70 yr	1200*	700	320	10*	3*	1.1	1.1	14	1.5	400	2.4**	5*	30*	425*
>70 yr	1200*	700	320	15*	3*	1.1	1.1	14	1.5	400	2.4**	5*	30*	425*
Pregnancy														
≤18 yr	1,300*	1250	400	5*	3*	1.4	1.4	18	1.9	600‡‡	2.6	6*	30*	450*
19–30 yr	1,000*	700	350	5*	3*	1.4	1.4	18	1.9	600‡‡	2.6	6*	30*	450*
31–50 yr	1,000*	700	360	5*	3*	1.4	1.4	18	1.9	600‡‡	2.6	6*	30*	450*
Lactation														
≤18 yr	1,300*	1250	360	5*	3*	1.5	1.6	17	2.0	500	2.8	7*	35*	550*
19–30 yr	1,000*	700	310	5*	3*	1.5	1.6	17	2.0	500	2.8	7*	35*	550*
31–50 yr	1,000*	700	320	5*	3*	1.5	1.6	17	2.0	500	2.8	7*	35*	550*

µg = microgram; mg = milligram

NOTE: This table presents Recommended Dietary Allowances (RDAs) and Adequate Intakes (AIs) followed by an asterisk (*). RDAs and AIs may both be used as goals for individual intake. RDAs are set to meet the needs of almost all (97% to 98%) individuals in a group. For healthy breastfed infants, the AI is the mean intake. The AI for other life stage groups is believed to cover the needs of all individuals in the group, but lack of data or uncertainty in the data prevent clear specification of this coverage.

† As cholecalciferol. 1 µg cholecalciferol = 40 IU vitamin D.

‡ In the absence of adequate exposure to sunlight.

§ As niacin equivalents. 1 mg of niacin = 60 mg of tryptophan; 0–5 months = preformed niacin (not mg NE).

‖ As dietary folate equivalents (DFE). 1 DFE = 1 µg food folate = 0.6 µg of folic acid (from fortified food or supplement) consumed with food = 0.5 µg of synthetic (supplemental) folic acid taken on an empty stomach.

Although AIs have been set for choline, there are few data to assess whether a dietary supply of choline is needed at all stages of the life cycle, and it may be that the choline requirement can be met by endogenous synthesis at some of these stages.

** Since 10% to 30% of older people may malabsorb food-bound B_{12}, it is advisable for those older than 50 years to meet their RDA mainly by consuming foods fortified with B_{12} or a B_{12}-containing supplement.

†† In view of evidence linking folate intake with neural tube defects in the fetus, it is recommended that all women capable of becoming pregnant consume 400 µg of synthetic folic acid from fortified foods and/or supplements in addition to intake of food folate from a varied diet.

‡‡ It is assumed that women will continue taking 400 µg of folic acid until their pregnancy is confirmed and they enter prenatal care, which ordinarily occurs after the end of the periconceptional period—the critical time for formation of the neural tube.

Reprinted with permission from *Dietary Reference Intakes*. Copyright 1999 by the National Academy of Sciences. Courtesy of the National Academy Press, Washington, D.C.

NUTRITION THROUGHOUT THE LIFE CYCLE

Edited by

BONNIE S. WORTHINGTON-ROBERTS, M.S., Ph.D.

Professor, Nutritional Sciences Program (retired)
School of Public Health, University of Washington

SUE RODWELL WILLIAMS, R.D., M.P.H., Ph.D.

President, SRW Productions, Inc. Clinical Nutrition Consultant
Davis, California

Contributors

DONNA B. JOHNSON, R.D., Ph.D.

Acting Assistant Professor, Nutritional Sciences, University of Washington
Nutritionist, Pediatric Pulmonary Center, University of Washington

CRISTINE M. TRAHMS, R.D., Ph.D., F.A.D.A.

Head, Nutrition, Center on Human Development and Disability
Lecturer, Department of Pediatrics
Core Faculty, Nutritional Sciences
University of Washington

BONNIE A. SPEAR, R.D., Ph.D.

Assistant Professor, Pediatrics
University of Alabama at Birmingham

ELEANOR D. SCHLENKER, R.D., Ph.D.

Professor, Human Nutrition, Foods, and Exercise
College of Human Resources and Education
Virginia Polytechnic Institute and State University

DIANNE NEUMARK-SZTAINER, R.D., M.P.H., Ph.D.

School of Public Health, Division of Epidemiology
University of Minnesota

With Assistance of

JILLIAN K. MOE, R.D., M.S., M.P.H.

Research Assistant, School of Public Health, Division of Epidemiology
University of Minnesota

FOURTH EDITION
With 92 illustrations

Boston   Burr Ridge, IL   Dubuque, IA   Madison, WI   New York   San Francisco   St. Louis
Bangkok   Bogotá   Caracas   Lisbon   London   Madrid
Mexico City   Milan   New Delhi   Seoul   Singapore   Sydney   Taipei   Toronto

McGraw-Hill Higher Education

A Division of The McGraw-Hill Companies

NUTRITION THROUGHOUT THE LIFE CYCLE, FOURTH EDITION

1 2 3 4 5 6 7 8 9 0 QPD/QPD 0 9 8 7 6 5 4 3 2 1 0

ISBN 0–07–292732–1

Vice president and editorial director: *Kevin T. Kane*
Publisher: *Colin H. Wheatley*
Senior development editor: *Lynne M. Meyers*
Senior marketing manager: *Pamela S. Cooper*
Project manager: *Joyce M. Berendes*
Senior production supervisor: *Mary E. Haas*
Coordinator of freelance design: *Rick Noel*
Photo research coordinator: *John C. Leland*
Compositor: *Carlisle Communications, Ltd.*
Typeface: *10/11.5 Galliard*
Printer: *Quebecor Printing Book Group/Dubuque, IA*

Cover designer: *Mary Sailer*
Interior designer: *Kathy Theis*
Cover image: © *The Image Bank—Family at Breakfast / L. D. Gordon*

Library of Congress Cataloging-in-Publication Data

Nutrition throughout the life cycle / [edited by] Bonnie Worthington-
    Roberts. — 4th ed.
        p.   cm.
    Includes index.
    ISBN 0–07–292732–1
    1. Nutrition   I. Worthington-Roberts, Bonnie S., 1943–
TX354.N87   2000
613.2—dc21   99–26466
                                              CIP

www.mhhe.com

CONTENTS

PREFACE

The fourth edition of NUTRITION THROUGHOUT THE LIFE CYCLE is designed to provide students, teachers, and practitioners with a unified view of the life cycle as a whole, with each life cycle stage supported by the nutrition foundations that are essential for positive development. While many aspects in the development and aging of the human being are genetically programmed, environmental factors are now recognized as highly significant in the manifestation of human characteristics. Nutrition is one of these influential pieces of lifestyle that impact the developmental process at every stage from conception to death. Attention to this detail can make a tremendous difference in the overall quality of life.

OBJECTIVES OF THE BOOK ≋

This text is designed to meet the needs of a broad spectrum of students with varying levels of exposure to the concepts of basic nutrition. It is appropriately used in courses focusing on life cycle nutrition, with the intent of contributing to the preparation of professionals who work in both individual and community health programs. Nutritional needs are presented on the basis of both physical growth and psychosocial development. The basic message is that nutrition choices and practices contribute significantly to health at all ages.

Material is presented in this text in the order that seems logical for best learning. After a review of basic nutrition concepts and terminology, the life cycle information is presented from the time of the embryo through the period preceding death in old age. The authors developing the synopses of each period of the life cycle are known experts in their fields. Reference to scientific research is found throughout, along with practical suggestions for translating scientific evidence into clinical application.

NEW TO THE FOURTH EDITION ≋

It is with delight that we include several new contributors to this text. Drs. Neumark-Sztainer and Spear bring their expertise in adolescent nutrition. Dr. Johnson updates the original work of Peggy Pipes covering infant nutrition. Cris Trahms (first author of the text NUTRITION IN INFANCY AND CHILDHOOD) updates the area of childhood nutrition. Other contributors remain the same, each bringing into their discussions the most recent developments in their fields.

The material in this edition has been divided into more chapters. While the length of the text remains about the same, fourteen chapters are now provided. Efforts have been made to avoid duplication among chapters. All chapters include figures and tables, as well as offsets entitled ONE STEP FURTHER. Additional offsets entitled STRATEGIES IN NUTRITION EDUCATION are included where applicable. These offsets break up the solid print while addressing new or interesting asides related to the accompanying text.

Useful features remaining from the previous edition include *marginal definitions, case studies, chapter summaries, review questions, cited references,* and *appendices*. The inside covers also provide useful reference tables related to recommended dietary intakes and height/weight standards. The advent of Dietary Reference Intakes has been addressed. Internet sources of nutrition information are also identified.

NUTRITION THROUGHOUT THE LIFE CYCLE

1

INTRODUCTION TO THE LIFE CYCLE: THE ROLE OF NUTRITION

Bonnie S. Worthington-Roberts

≈≈ ≈≈ ≈≈ ≈≈ ≈≈ ≈≈ ≈≈ ≈≈ ≈≈

Basic Concepts

❑ *An integral component of health promotion for all persons throughout the life cycle is optimal personal and community nutrition.*

❑ *Each stage of the life cycle is associated with a distinct set of nutritional priorities.*

❑ *All persons throughout life need the same nutrients but in varying amounts.*

❑ *Through their specific and interdependent physiologic roles, certain nutrients in the food we eat are essential to life, health, and well-being.*

❑ *Changing nutrient needs throughout the life cycle relate to normal growth and development and resulting changes in body composition.*

❑ *Health promotion and disease prevention are underlying lifetime goals.*

❑ *At times, especially in the later years, disease management may impact significantly on dietary planning.*

*F*rom beginning to end, the human life cycle is a fascinating sequence of events. From the moment of fertilization through the stages of growth, development, maturation, and aging, the interaction between genes and environment determines the details of the process. The importance of the genetic base cannot be ignored, but it is clear that an assortment of environmental factors has the potential of significantly modifying the course of events. Nutrition is one of those influential factors demanding special attention.

This text considers in some depth the contributions that diet and nutrition make to support the growth and developmental process throughout the life cycle. Each chapter illustrates that in this health promotion process our food and its nutrients are essential to preventing deviations from the normal state or the establishment of acute or chronic disease.

NUTRITION AND THE NUTRIENTS: A BRIEF REMINDER ≈≈

Nutrition is the study of how foods and their individual parts affect the survival and health of living things. Human beings require many nutrients. A *nutrient* is a chemical substance (present in foods, powders, or pills) that is used by the body for growth, reproduction, and maintenance of health. Most nutritional needs are met by eating a variety of foods. However, today's technology allows for the production of "artificial" nutrient sources, such as pills, powders, and liquid supplements; these are taken by mouth. It is also possible to get all the necessary nutrients through liquid preparations that can be placed directly

TABLE 1-1 *Essential Nutrients in the Human Diet*

	Energy Nutrients				
Carbohydrates	Fats (Lipid)	Proteins (Amino Acids)	Vitamins	Minerals	Water
Glucose (or a carbohydrate that yields glucose)	Linoleic acid (omega-6) α-Linolenic acid (omega-3)	Histidine Isoleucine Leucine Lysine Methionine Phenylalanine Threonine Tryptophan Valine	A D E K Thiamin Riboflavin Niacin Pantothenic acid Biotin B-6 B-12 Folate C	Arsenic Boron Calcium Chloride Chromium Cobalt Copper Fluoride Iodide Iron Magnesium Manganese Molybdenum Nickel Phosphorus Potassium Selenium Silicon Sodium Sulfur Zinc	Water

into the body through the blood vessels. This latter strategy is used only in situations where normal eating is impossible or insufficient.

Nutrients are classified into six categories (table 1-1), including the energy-yielding **macronutrients** (carbohydrates, fats, and proteins), the **micronutrients** (vitamins and minerals), and water. Their basic features include the following:

1. *Carbohydrates* contain carbon, hydrogen, and oxygen combined in small molecules called sugars and large molecules represented mainly by starch.
2. *Lipids* (fats and oils) contain carbon, hydrogen, and oxygen, as do carbohydrates, but in lipids the amount of oxygen is much less. **Triglyceride** is the main form of food fat.
3. *Proteins* contain carbon, hydrogen, and oxygen, plus nitrogen and sometimes sulfur atoms arranged in small compounds called **amino acids.** Chains of amino acids make up dietary proteins.
4. *Vitamins* are organic compounds that catalyze or support a number of biochemical reactions in the body.
5. *Minerals* are inorganic elements or compounds that play important roles in metabolic reactions and serve as structural components in body tissues, such as bone.
6. *Water* is vital to the body as a solvent and lubricant and as a medium for transporting nutrients and waste.

Nutrients are carried into the body, usually in foods, and are released from these foods through a process of digestion. This begins in the mouth by the action of chewing and the chemical activity of enzymes in the saliva. Further digestion takes place in the stomach and the small intestine. Nutrients are then absorbed from the inside of the small intestine into the bloodstream and are carried to the sites in the body where they are needed. There a

Triglyceride
(Gr *treis*, three; L *glycerinum*, glycerol) Chemical name for fat; a compound of three fatty acids esterified to glycerol base. A neutral fat, synthesized from carbohydrate, stored in adipose tissue. It releases free fatty acids into the blood when hydrolyzed by enzymes.

Amino acids
(*amino,* the monovalent chemical group NH_2) Carriers of essential element nitrogen; structural units of protein; specific amino acids being linked in specific sequence by peptide chains to form specific proteins.

number of chemical reactions take place that assure the growth and maintenance of body structures and functions. The parts of foods that are not absorbed continue to move down the intestinal tract and are largely excreted from the body as feces.

Energy

Carbohydrates: basic fuel source. All three of the macronutrients in our food—carbohydrates, fat, and protein—can be **metabolized** to yield body **energy.** However, the body uses carbohydrates as its basic fuel supply, along with fat, and reserves protein mainly for its unique tissue-building role. In the human energy system, this major carbohydrate fuel comes from the two forms of carbohydrate foods we eat—starches and sugars. To produce energy from a basic fuel supply, a successful energy system must be able to do three things: 1) change the basic "raw" fuel to a refined fuel form that the system is designed to use, 2) carry this refined fuel to the places that need it, and 3) burn this refined fuel at these energy production sites in the special equipment set up there to do it. Far more efficient than any machine, the body easily does these three things. It digests its basic food fuel, carbohydrates, changing it to the refined fuel **glucose,** then absorbs this refined fuel and transports it through blood circulation to the cells that constantly need it. There glucose is broken down in the cell's highly specific equipment, releasing energy through its intricate biochemical pathways, **glycolysis** and the **citric acid cycle,** of cell metabolism. In this overall process, glucose is broken down to its basic carbon and hydrogen atoms and is combined with oxygen, yielding energy as the cell's energy currency compound **adenosine triphosphate (ATP),** with its high-energy phosphate bonds, and releasing carbon dioxide and water as end products.

The classes of food carbohydrates vary from simple to complex structures and, thus, differ in the speed with which they yield energy (table 1-2). **Simple carbohydrates**—sugars—made up of only one or two sugar (saccharide) units are broken down easily, releasing energy quickly. On the other hand, **complex carbohydrates**—polysaccharides—are

Metabolism

(Gr *metaballein,* to change) Sum of all the various biochemical and physiologic processes by which the body grows and maintains itself (anabolism) and reshapes tissues (catabolism), transforming energy to do its work.

Glycolysis

Initial energy production pathway by which 6-carbon glucose is changed to active 3-carbon fragments of acetyl CoA, the fuel ready for final energy production.

Citric acid cycle

Final energy production pathway in the cell mitochondria that transforms the ultimate fuel acetyl CoA from carbohydrates and fat, capturing energy for cell metabolism in high-energy phosphate bonds.

Adenosine triphosphate (ATP)

The energy currency of the cell, binding energy in its high-energy phosphate bonds for release as these bonds are split.

Complex carbohydrates

Main dietary carbohydrates, the polysaccharide starch in varied foods, such as legumes, grains, breads, cereals, and potatoes.

TABLE 1-2 *Summary of Carbohydrate Classes*

Chemical Class Names	Class Members	Sources
Polysaccharides Multiple sugars, complex carbohydrates	Starch	Grains and grain products Cereal, bread, crackers, and other baked goods Pasta Rice, corn, bulgar Legumes Potatoes and other vegetables
	Glycogen	Animal tissues, liver, and muscle meats
	Dietary fiber	Whole grains Fruits Vegetables Seeds, nuts, skins
Disaccharides Double sugars, simple carbohydrates	Sucrose	"Table" sugar: sugar cane, sugar beets Molasses
	Lactose	Milk
	Maltose	Starch digestion, intermediate Sweetener in food products
Monosaccharides Single sugars, simple carbohydrates	Glucose (dextrose)	Starch digestion, final Corn syrup (large use in processed foods)
	Fructose	Fruits, honey
	Galactose	Lactose (milk)

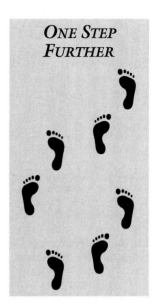

ONE STEP FURTHER

Do Dairy Products "Disagree" with You?

Some people find it difficult to consume milk and other dairy products because of the intestinal symptoms they experience. These symptoms include bloating, distention, cramps, flatulence (gas), and diarrhea. The basis for these unpleasant reactions to dairy products is an inherited trait: they have relatively low levels of the intestinal enzyme lactase, which is responsible for digestion of the milk sugar lactose.

The discomforts associated with dairy product intake can begin in early childhood, but they may not manifest until later in life. Whenever they occur, limitation in milk consumption is an understandable reaction. However, many "lactose intolerant" people handle moderate amounts of dairy foods without difficulty. For those with more serious responses, many low-lactose (or lactose-hydrolyzed) products are now available.

Lee, M., and S. Krasinski. 1998. Human adult onset lactase decline: An update. *Nutr Rev* 56:1.
McBean, L.D., and G.D. Miller. 1998. Allaying fears and fallacies about lactose intolerance. *J Am Diet Assoc* 98:671.

TABLE 1-3   *Summary of Dietary Fiber Classes*

Classes	Sources	Functions
Cellulose	Main cell wall constituent of plants	Holds water; reduces elevated colonic intraluminal pressure; binds zinc
Noncellulose polysaccharides		Slows gastric emptying; provides fermentable material for colonic bacteria with production of gas and volatile fatty acids; binds bile acids and cholesterol
Gums	Secretions of plants	
Mucilages	Plant secretions and seeds	
Algal polysaccharides	Algae, seaweeds	
Pectin substances	Intercellular cement plant material	
Hemicellulose	Cell wall plant material	Holds water and increases stool bulk; reduces elevated colonic pressure; binds bile acids
Lignin	Woody part of plants	Is an antioxidant; binds bile acids, cholesterol, and metals

large, complex compounds of many saccharide units. For example, starch, the most significant polysaccharide in human nutrition, is made up of both straight-chained coiled structure (amylose, 15% to 20% of the molecule) and many branching chains (amylopectin, 80% to 85% of the moelcule). Each of the multiple branching chains is composed of 24 to 30 sugar units of glucose, which are gradually split off in digestion to supply a steady source of energy over a period of time. **Glycogen,** the body's small amount of stored carbohydrates, sometimes called *animal starch,* has a similar, large "tree-like" structure and sustains energy during brief fasting periods, such as sleep hours.

Certain other carbohydrate compounds, fibrous polysaccharides, are nondigestible, because humans lack the necessary enzymes to split their particular saccharide links.[1] However, these compounds, especially those that are water-soluble, contribute valuable **dietary fiber** essential to health (tables 1-3 and 1-4). A list of some major food sources of dietary fiber is provided in appendix K.

Fats: concentrated energy. Fats supply a concentrated fuel source for the body's energy system, yielding over twice the energy value of carbohydrates. Because the body can

Glycogen
Briefly stored form of carbohydrates in the body cells, available for energy fuel during fasting periods of sleep; built up in larger amounts by high-starch meals prior to endurance athletic events for sustained energy.

Dietary fiber
Nondigestible form of carbohydrate; of nutritional importance in gastrointestinal disease, such as diverticulosis, and management of serum lipid and glucose levels in risk reduction related to chronic conditions, such as heart disease and diabetes.

TABLE 1-4 *Summary of Soluble and Insoluble Fibers in Total Dietary Fiber*

Insoluble	Soluble
Cellulose	Gums
Most hemicelluloses	Mucilages
Lignin	Algal polysaccharides
	Most pectins

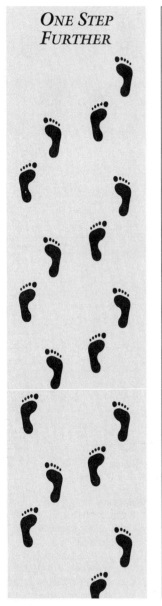

ONE STEP FURTHER

Nutritive and Nonnutritive Sweeteners: Many Alternatives

Originally developed for use by diabetics, alternative sweeteners are now available in most parts of the world. Those used in the United States have been rigorously tested and "deemed safe" by the Food and Drug Administration (FDA); other countries use their own regulatory agencies to assign designations of safety.

The grouping of sweeteners into nutritive and nonnutritive categories recognizes their differences in energy value. Nutritive sweeteners include sugar sweeteners (e.g., refined sugars, high-fructose corn syrups, crystalline fructose, glucose, dextrose, corn sweeteners, honey, lactose, maltose, various syrups, invert sugars, concentrated fruit juice) and reduced energy sugar alcohols (e.g., sorbitol, mannitol, xylitol, isomalt, and hydrogenated starch hydrolysates. Nonnutritive sweeteners (saccharin, aspartame, acesulfame-K, and sucralose) provide no energy; small amounts provide much sweetness.

If sucrose, or basic table sugar, is used as a standard of sweetness, other sweeteners can be compared with it as follows:

Sweeteners	Sweetness Compared with Sucrose
Sorbitol	50–70% as sweet
Mannitol	50–70% as sweet
Xylitol	As sweet
Erythritol	70% as sweet
Lactitol	30–40% as sweet
Isomalt	45–65% as sweet
Maltitol	90% as sweet
Saccharin	200–700% sweeter
Aspartame	160–220% sweeter
Acesulfame-K	200% sweeter
Sucralose	600% sweeter

Sweeteners differ in their behavioral properties in foods and beverages and in their response to heat. Information regarding their presence in specific foods is generally provided on the food label.

American Dietetic Association. 1998. Position of the American Dietetic Association: Use of nutritive and nonnutritive sweeteners. *J Am Diet Assoc* 98:580.

Adipose tissue
Fat storage sites composed of adipocytes (fat cells).

easily convert carbohydrates to fat and store it in various body **adipose tissues,** fat is an important form of body fuel for energy reserves. Food fats from both animal and plant sources yield the same amount of energy but have significantly different relationships to health. Excess dietary fat, especially fat from animal sources, and excess dietary cholesterol, which is synthesized only by animals and can be supplied in the diet only by animal

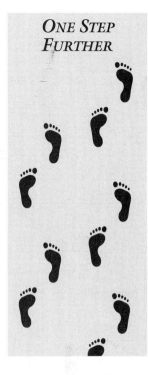

How Much Fat Are You Eating?

- Keep an accurate record of everything you eat or drink for one day. Be sure to estimate and add amounts of all fat or other nutrient seasonings used with your foods. (If you want a more representative picture and have a computer available with nutrient analysis programming, keep a one-week record and calculate an average of the seven days.)
- Calculate the total kilocalories (kcal) and grams of each of the energy nutrients (carbohydrates, fat, and protein) in everything you eat. Multiply the total grams of each energy nutrient by its respective fuel value:

fat _____ g × 9 = _____ kcal

protein _____ g × 4 = _____ kcal

carbohydrates _____ g × 4 = _____ kcal

- Calculate the percentage of each energy nutrient in your total diet:

$$\frac{\text{Fat kcal}}{\text{Total kcal}} \times 100 = \% \text{ fat kcal in diet}$$

- Compare with fat in American diet (40–45%) and with the U.S. dietary goals (25–30%).

From Williams, S.R. 1995. *Basic nutrition and diet therapy.* 10th ed. St. Louis: Mosby.

food sources, are health risk factors. The oils from fatty fish and from olives, on the other hand, appear to make positive contributions to overall health.

Protein: available energy if needed. As indicated, carbohydrates and fats are the primary fuel sources in the body's energy system. However, sometimes protein furnishes additional body energy, but it is a less efficient source. The fuel value of protein is the same as that of carbohydrates.

Measurement of nutrient energy value. The energy yielded by the macronutrients is measured in **kilocalories** (kcalories or kcal). Carbohydrates yield 4 kcal/g, fat 9 kcal/g, and protein 4 kcal/g. These values are called their respective fuel factors. The energy values of various foods, therefore, are based on their carbohydrate, fat, and protein composition. Any portion of these macronutrients not used for energy is restructured for body tissue storage as glycogen or fat for fuel use between meals, or for use in synthesizing other metabolic compounds needed in the body. Excess energy intake (kcalories) over energy use by the body to do its work results in weight gain. Insufficient energy intake to meet body needs results in weight loss. Any beverage alcohol is also metabolized by the body to yield 7 kcal/g. Excess alcohol intake, therefore, is harmful in terms of both weight gain (when it is converted to fat and stored) and its toxic effects.

The dietary guidelines for Americans recommend that we lower our daily dietary fat intake to less than 30% of total kcalories.[2] Do you know how much fat you are eating? Try calculating it by the directions given in the accompanying box.

Amino Acids and Protein Metabolism

Amino acids: basic building material. All protein, whether in our bodies or in the food we eat, is made up of its building units, the **amino acids.** These amino acids are joined by peptide linkages in a unique chain sequence to form specific proteins. When we eat protein foods, the protein (for example, casein in milk and cheese, albumin in egg white, and gluten in wheat products) is broken down into its constituent amino acids in the digestive process. According to need, from the body's overall metabolic "pool" of amino acids (fig. 1-1) specific ones are then reassembled in the body in the *specific* order to form *specific* tissue proteins (for example, collagen in connective tissue,

Kilocalorie (kcalorie, kcal)
Unit of measure of energy produced in the body by the energy-yielding macronutrients carbohydrates, fats, and protein.

Amino acids
Structural units of protein that supply essential nitrogen.

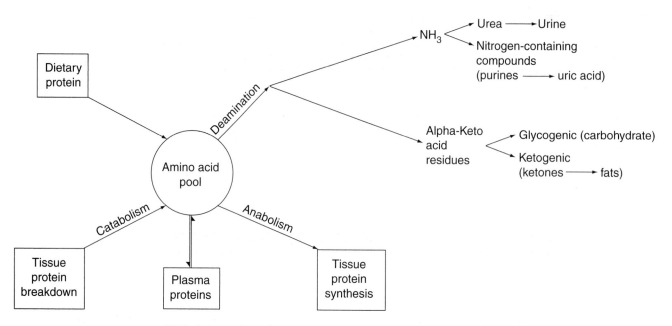

FIG. 1-1   Balance between protein compartments and amino acid pool.

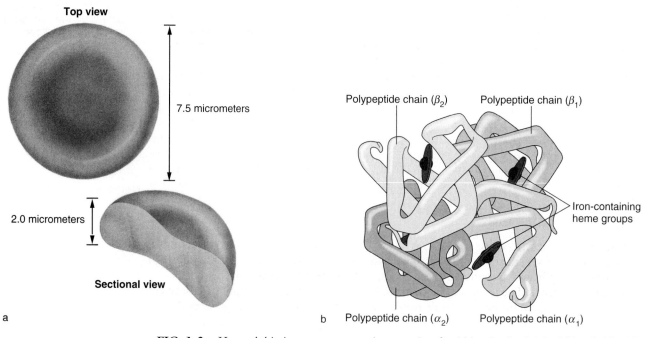

FIG. 1-2   Hemoglobin is an oxygen-carrying protein of red blood cells. (*a*) Red blood cells. (*b*) Hemoglobin molecule.

myosin in muscle tissue, hemoglobin in red blood cells (see fig. 1-2), cell enzymes, and insulin) that are required by the body.

Role as nitrogen supplier.   Amino acids are named for their chemical nature. The word *amino* refers to the monovalent chemical group—NH_2. Like carbohydrates and fats, proteins have a basic structure of carbon, hydrogen, and oxygen, but, unlike fats and carbohydrates, which contain no nitrogen, protein is about 16% nitrogen. In addition, some proteins contain small but valuable amounts of minerals, such as sulfur.

TABLE 1-5   *Amino Acids Required in Human Nutrition, Grouped According to Nutritional (Dietary) Essentiality*

Essential Amino Acids	Semiessential Amino Acids*	Nonessential Amino Acids
Histidine	Arginine	Alanine
Isoleucine	Cystine (cysteine)	Asparagine
Leucine	Tyrosine	Aspartic acid
Lysine		Glutamic acid
Methionine		Glutamine
Phenylalanine		Glycine
Threonine		Hydroxyproline
Tryptophan		Hydroxylysine
Valine		Proline
		Serine

*These are considered semiessential because the rate of synthesis in the body is inadequate to support growth; therefore, these are essential for children.

Essential amino acids. Nine amino acids are classed as **essential amino acids** because the body cannot manufacture them or cannot do so in sufficient amounts. Thus, the term *essential* means that they are necessary in the diet. In the strict physiologic sense, all amino acids are essential in overall body metabolism. Although the ninth amino acid added to the essential list, histidine, has previously been known as essential for infants, it has now been demonstrated to be required also by adults. The nine essential amino acids are histidine, isoleucine, leucine, lysine, methionine, phenylalanine, threonine, tryptophan, and valine (table 1-5). (See the box on p. 10.) Applying this concept of essentiality to our dietary food choices, we would need to obtain all of these nine essential amino acids in our diet to meet our protein needs for tissue growth and maintenance throughout the life cycle. A protein food that supplies all of these essential amino acids in sufficient quantities to meet human needs is called a **complete protein.** Since only foods of animal source—milk, cheese, egg, and meat—are complete proteins, a person following a vegetarian food pattern would need to plan carefully to obtain sufficient quantities of essential amino acids by using combinations of complementary plant proteins, as described in the box on p. 10. During the growth years, arginine is also essential to meet normal childhood growth demands. Although arginine is synthesized by the body, it may not be made in sufficient amounts to meet the rapid growth of infants, especially premature infants, and young children.

Nonessential amino acids. All amino acids have essential tissue-building and metabolic functions. However, the nonessential amino acids are twelve amino acids that the body can synthesize in sufficient amounts to meet needs, so they are not essential in the diet.

Protein balance. The term *balance* refers to the relative intake and output of substances in the body to maintain normal levels needed for health in various circumstances during the life cycle. We can apply this concept of balance to life-sustaining protein and the nitrogen it supplies. The body's tissue proteins are constantly being broken down, a process called **catabolism,** and then resynthesized into tissue protein as needed, a process called **anabolism.** To maintain nitrogen balance, the nitrogen-containing amino part of the amino acid may be removed by a process called **deamination,** the amino acid converted to ammonia (NH^3), and the nitrogen excreted as urea in the urine, as shown in fig 1-1. The remaining nonnitrogen residue can be used to make carbohydrates or fats, or it can be reattached to an amino group ($—NH^2$) to make another amino acid according to need. The rate of this protein and nitrogen turnover varies in different tissues, according to their degree of metabolic activity. This process involves a continuous reshaping and rebuilding, adjusting as needed to maintain overall protein balance within the body. Also, the body maintains an internal balance between tissue protein and plasma protein. In turn, these

Essential amino acid
An amino acid that the body cannot synthesize in sufficient amounts to meet body needs so it must be supplied by the diet—hence a *dietary* essential for nine such specific amino acids.

Catabolism
Metabolic process by which tissue is broken down.

Anabolism
Metabolic process by which tissue is built up.

Deamination
Process by which the nitrogen radical (NH_4) is split off from amino acids; important in maintaining nitrogen balance.

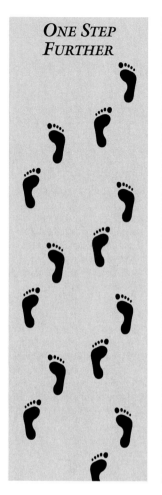

Essential Amino Acids (Nine or Eleven?) and Their Complementary Food Proteins

All of the nine essential amino acids must be supplied by the diet, but two of them, phenylalanine and methionine, have helpers as interactive backup. The body makes the amino acid tyrosine, which can spare some of the phenylalanine, and cystine, which can interact with methionine. Thus, although there are only nine essential amino acids the body cannot make, some may speak of eleven when they add the two helpers tyrosine and cystine.

The real-life concern in a vegetarian diet is to get a balanced amount of the essential amino acids to complement one another and to make complete food combinations. Only three of these nine essential amino acids are critical, however, because, if persons eat foods to supply enough of these three in a combined pattern, they will get sufficient amounts of the others too. These three amino acids are thus called the *limiting amino acids*—lysine, methionine, and tryptophan. Of these three, lysine is the most limiting.

The answer lies in mixing families of foods such as grains, legumes, and milk products to make complementary food combinations to balance these needed amino acids. For example, grains are low in lysine and high in methionine, while legumes are just the opposite—low in methionine and high in lysine. Basically, grains and legumes will always balance one another, and additions of milk products and eggs will enhance their adequacy. Following are a few sample food combination dishes to illustrate:

Rice + black-eyed peas: a southern United States dish called "Hopping John".

Whole wheat or bulgur + soybeans + sesame seeds: protein enhanced by the addition of yogurt.

Cornmeal + kidney beans: a combination in many Mexican dishes, protein enhanced by the addition of cheese.

Soybeans + peanuts + brown rice + bulgur wheat: an excellent sauce dish served over the rice and wheat.

Prepared with a variety of herbs, spices, onions, and garlic, to suit your taste, such dishes can supply needed nutrients and good eating.

---

two body protein stores are further balanced with dietary protein intake. With this finely balanced system, a metabolic "pool" of amino acids from both tissue protein and dietary protein is always available to meet construction needs.

Nitrogen balance. The body's **nitrogen balance** indicates how well its tissues are being maintained. The intake and use of dietary protein are measured by the amount of nitrogen intake in the food protein and the amount of nitrogen excreted in the urine. Total twenty-four-hour urinary urea nitrogen excretion measure is used with calculated dietary nitrogen intake over the same time period to determine a person's nitrogen balance:

Nitrogen balance

Metabolic balance between nitrogen intake in dietary protein and output in urinary nitrogen compounds such as urea and creatinine.

$$\text{Nitrogen balance} = \text{Protein intake} \div 6.25 - (\text{Urinary urea nitrogen} + 4)$$

The formula factor of 4 in the equation represents the additional nitrogen loss through feces and skin. Urinary urea nitrogen excretion reflects metabolism of dietary protein, as the nitrogen balance formula indicates, and is a measure of the adequacy of the protein nutriture. For example, 1 g of urinary nitrogen results from the digestion and metabolism of 6.25 g of protein. Therefore, if for every 6.25 g of protein consumed 1 g of nitrogen is excreted in the urine, the body is said to be in nitrogen balance. This is the normal pattern in adult health, but at different times during the life cycle, or in states of malnutrition or illness, this balance may be either positive or negative.

1. *Positive nitrogen balance.* A positive nitrogen balance exists when the body takes in more nitrogen than it excretes. This means that the body is storing nitrogen by building more tissue than it is breaking down. This situation occurs normally during periods of rapid growth, such as infancy, childhood, and adolescence, and dur-

ing pregnancy and lactation. It also occurs in persons who have been ill or malnourished and are being "built back up" with increased nourishment. In such cases, protein is being stored to meet increased needs for tissue building and associated metabolic activity.

2. *Negative nitrogen balance.* A negative nitrogen balance exists when the body takes in less nitrogen than it excretes. This means that the body has an inadequate protein intake and is losing nitrogen by breaking down more tissue than it is building up. This situation occurs in states of malnutrition and illness. For example, this nitrogen imbalance is seen not only in underdeveloped countries but also in America in cases where specific protein deficiency exists, even when kcalories from carbohydrates and fats may be adequate, causing the classic protein deficiency disease **kwashiorkor.** Failure to maintain nitrogen balance may not become apparent for some time, but it will eventually cause loss of muscle tissue, impairment of body organs and functions, and increased susceptibility to infection. In children, negative nitrogen balance will cause growth retardation.

Primary tissue building. Protein is the fundamental structural material of every living cell in the body. In fact, the largest portion of the body, excluding the water content, is made up of protein. Body protein, mainly the lean body mass of muscles, accounts for about three-fourths of the dry matter in most tissues other than bone and adipose fat. Protein not only makes up the bulk of the muscles, internal organs, brain, nerves, skin, hair, and nails but also is a vital part of regulatory substances, such as enzymes, hormones, and blood plasma. All of these tissues must be constantly repaired and replaced. The primary functions of protein are to repair worn-out, wasted, or damaged tissue and to build up new tissue. Thus, protein meets growth and developmental needs during early life and maintains tissue health during the adult years.

Micronutrients and Metabolic Control

As indicated, the body uses the macronutrients carbohydrates, fats, and protein to solve its major problems of energy production and tissue building and rebuilding to maintain life and health, processes that require thousands of interrelated physiologic and metabolic activities. However, meeting these two basic needs creates another major overall problem, that of metabolic regulation and control.[3] To maintain life and health, all of these multiple physiologic tasks must proceed in a highly organized and orderly fashion, without which metabolic chaos, illness, and death would occur. Such order requires specific control agents. In harmony with hormones and specific partnerships with key cell enzymes, the remaining nutrients, the micronutrients vitamins and minerals, operate mainly in a key role as **coenzyme factors,** as is the case with some vitamins, or essential enzyme components, as with some minerals, required in a specific enzyme system for a particular metabolic reaction to occur.

Vitamins

From 1900 to 1950, as the discoveries of the **vitamins** occurred, two characteristics marked a compound for assignment to the vitamin group: 1) it must be a vital organic dietary substance, which is neither carbohydrate, fat, or protein (hence, noncaloric), and it is necessary in only very small quantities to do special metabolic jobs or to prevent its deficiency disease and 2) it cannot be manufactured by the body and therefore must be supplied in food. With current knowledge, however, it has become evident that one of these organic substances—vitamin D—has been misassigned to the vitamin group. It is now known to behave as a hormone in its active form, now called vitamin D hormone, or *calcitriol,* but is still generally discussed with the vitamins in most source materials for the sake of convenience. Vitamins are usually grouped according to solubility in a medium. The fat-soluble vitamins—A, D, E, and K—are closely associated with lipids in their fate in the body. The water-soluble vitamins—B-complex and C—have fewer problems in absorption and transport throughout.

Fat-soluble vitamins. Vitamin A enters the body in two forms: 1) the preformed vitamin A from animal food sources, usually associated with lipids, and 2) the **precursor** beta-carotene pigment from plant food sources, which actually supplies about two-thirds of the vitamin A necessary in human nutrition. Its major physiologic roles relate to the eye's vision

Kwashiorkor
Classic protein deficiency disease, frequently encountered in children in developing countries but also seen in the United States in poverty areas and in metabolically stressed and debilitated hospitalized patients.

Coenzyme factors
Major metabolic role of the micronutrients vitamins and minerals as essential partners with cell enzymes in a variety of reactions in both energy and protein metabolism.

Vitamin
A nonenergy-yielding micronutrient, required in very small amounts for specific metabolic tasks, that cannot be synthesized by the body so must be supplied in the diet.

Precursor
Substance from which another substance is produced.

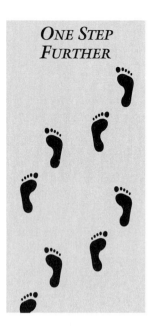

Iron Deficiency: Still a Problem in the United States

Iron deficiency and iron deficiency anemia are still relatively common in young children, adolescent girls, and women of childbearing age. A large national survey conducted between 1988 and 1994 showed that iron deficiency was found in 9% of the toddlers (aged one to two years) and 9–11% of the adolescent girls and women of childbearing age; iron deficiency anemia was found in 3% and 2–5% of the age groups, respectively. Iron deficiency occurred in no more than 7% of the older children and the adults aged over fifty years and in no more than 1% of the adolescent boys and young men. In the women of childbearing age, iron deficiency was positively related to minority ethnicity, low income, and possession of more than one offspring. Since iron deficiency (especially if manifested in anemia) is associated with increased risk of inferior pregnancy course and/or outcome and with impaired behavioral development in children, continued focus on assuring adequate iron nutrition in this population is justified.

Holst, M. 1998. Developmental and behavioral effects of iron deficiency anemia in infants. *Nutr Today* 33:27.
Looker, A.C., et al. 1997. Prevalence of iron deficiency in the United States. *J Am Med Assoc* 277:973.

Hemolytic anemia
(Gr *haima*, blood; *lysis*, dissolution) An anemia (reduced number of red blood cells) caused by breakdown of red blood cells and loss of their hemoglobin.

cycle—adaptation to light—and dark and to a more generalized role in the formation and maintenance of healthy-functioning epithelial tissue, the body's primary barrier to infections.

Vitamin D hormone is produced in the body, first by sunlight irradiation of a precursor cholesterol compound in the skin, intermediate product synthesis in the liver, and subsequent formation in the kidneys of the physiologically active form, *calcitriol*—1,25-dihydroxycholecalciferol [1,25 $(OH)_2D_3$]. Its major physiologic role is in regulation of bone and mineral metabolism. A more widespread tissue role relates to controlling basic cell processes associated with cellular proliferation and differentiation.

Vitamin E has a single vital physiologic role relating to its action in many tissues as an antioxidant, an agent that prevents tissue breakdown by oxygen—the process of oxidation. It acts as nature's most potent fat-soluble antioxidant, protecting the cell membrane fatty acids from damage. For example, vitamin E can protect fragile red blood cell membranes in premature infants from breaking down and causing *hemolytic anemia* (see the box on p. 13). It is interesting that vegetable oils, the richest sources of vitamin E, are also the richest sources of polyunsaturated fatty acids, which vitamin E protects.

Vitamin K has a basic physiologic role relating to the body's vital blood-clotting process through its essential presence in the formation of several proteins involved, including *prothrombin*. In this role, it can serve as an antidote for excess effects of anticoagulant drugs and is often used in the control and prevention of certain types of hemorrhages. A more recently discovered function of vitamin K relates to bone development. Specific proteins found in bone and bone matrix depend on vitamin K for their synthesis and are involved with calcium in bone development. Since intestinal bacteria usually synthesize adequate vitamin K, supporting food sources such as green leafy vegetables, a deficiency is unlikely except in clinical conditions related to blood clotting. For example, patients treated with antibiotics that kill intestinal bacteria and who are then placed on poor diets after surgery are susceptible to vitamin K deficiency with resulting blood loss and poor wound healing. A more detailed summary of the fat-soluble vitamins is given in table 1-6 for review.

Water-soluble vitamins. Nine vitamins, eight B-complex vitamins and vitamin C, constitute the water-soluble group. The letter name *B* remains loosely attached, from the initial name *water-soluble B* given to the food factor in rice polishings used by early investigators to cure beriberi. When an increasing number of water-soluble vitamins were discovered, however, their distinct and unique natures led to a new naming system, now in common use, based on individual chemical structure or function, and we now know that initial "water-soluble B" as *thiamin*, a name based on its ring-like chemical structure. These eight initial *B* vitamins are now recognized as unique individual compounds and are

TABLE 1-6 *A Summary of Fat-Soluble Vitamins*

Vitamins	Functions	Results of Deficiency	Food Sources
A (retinol); provitamin A (carotene)	Vision cycle—adaption to light and dark; tissue growth, especially skin and mucous membranes; toxic in large amounts	Night blindness, xerophthalmia, susceptibility to epithelial infection, changes in skin and membranes	Retinol (animal foods): liver, egg yolk, cream, butter or fortified margarine, fortified milk; carotene (plant foods): green and yellow vegetables, fruits
D (chole-calciferol)	Absorption of calcium and phosphorus, calcification of bones; toxic in large amounts	Rickets, faulty bone growth	Fortified or irradiated milk, fish oils
E (tocopherol)	Antioxidant—protection of materials that oxidize easily; normal growth	Breakdown of red blood cells, anemia	Vegetable oils, vegetable greens, milk, eggs, meat, cereals
K (phylloquinone)	Normal blood clotting	Bleeding tendencies, hemorrhagic disease	Green leafy vegetables, milk and dairy products, meat, eggs, cereals, fruits, vegetables

so named (although the previous letter name *B* is still commonly used for two of them): thiamin, niacin, riboflavin, pyridoxine (B_6), pantothenic acid, biotin, folate, cobalamin (B_{12}). Discovered later than the initial *B* vitamins, the remaining water-soluble vitamin, C, still carries its common letter name, although its true chemical name, *ascorbic acid*, based on its function in curing scurvy, is more precise.

Despite their remarkable diversity of chemical structure and physiologic roles, the water-soluble vitamins are alike in many ways. Aside from sharing enough likeness in chemical structure to have the common chemical characteristic of water-solubility, all these vitamins—with one exception in each case—share three additional characteristics significant in human nutrition:

1. *Food source.* All are synthesized by plants and are supplied in the diet by plant foods (as well as by animal foods)—except *cobalamin (vitamin B_{12})*.
2. *Storage.* All have no stable body "storage" form and must therefore be provided regularly in the diet—except *cobalamin (vitamin B_{12})*.
3. *Function.* All serve as coenzyme factors in cell enzyme reactions—except *ascorbic acid (vitamin C),* which serves mainly as a structural agent in building connective tissue.

Tables 1-7 and 1-8 provide water-soluble vitamin reviews for reference. Note that food sources of vitamin B_{12} are only animal foods. A nutrition concern centers on possible B_{12} deficiency states among vegans, strict vegetarians who use no animal foods (meat, milk, cheese, egg). A supplement of vitamin B_{12} may be needed when the demand is greater, especially in periods of rapid growth through the life cycle, such as pregnancy, infancy, childhood, and adolescence.

Minerals

The remaining micronutrients, the minerals, are single inorganic elements that are widely distributed in nature. During the eons in which the earth was forming, shifting oceans and mountains deposited a large number of minerals into earth materials. Over time, these minerals have moved from rocks to soil, then to plants, to animals, and to humans.

TABLE 1-7 *A Summary of B-Complex Vitamins*

Vitamins	Functions	Results of Deficiency	Food Sources
Thiamin	Normal growth; co-enzyme in carbohydrate metabolism; normal functions of heart, nerves, and muscle	Beriberi; GI: loss of appetite, gastric distress, indigestion, deficient hydrochloric acid; CNS: fatigue, nerve damage, paralysis; CV: heart failure, edema of legs especially	Pork, beef, liver, whole or enriched grains, legumes
Riboflavin	Normal growth and vigor; coenzyme in protein and energy metabolism	Ariboflavinosis; wound aggravation, cracks at corners of mouth, swollen red tongue, eye irritation, skin eruptions	Milk, meats, enriched cereals, green vegetables
Niacin (precursor: tryptophan)	Coenzyme in energy production; normal growth, health of skin; normal activity of stomach, intestines, and nervous system	Pellagra; weakness, lack of energy, and loss of appetite; skin: scaly dermatitis; CNS: neuritis, confusion	Meat, peanuts, legumes, enriched grains
Pyridoxine	Coenzyme in amino acid metabolism: protein synthesis, heme formation, brain activity; carrier for amino acid absorption	Anemia; CNS: hyperirritability, convulsions, neuritis	Grains, seeds, liver and kidney meats, milk, eggs, vegetables
Pantothenic acid	Coenzyme in formation of coenzyme A: fat, cholesterol, and heme formation and amino acid activation	Unlikely because of widespread occurrence	Meats, cereals, legumes, milk, vegetables, fruit
Biotin	Coenzyme A partner; synthesis of fatty acids, amino acids, purines	Natural deficiency unknown	Liver, egg yolk, soy flour, cereal (except bound form in wheat), tomatoes, yeast
Folic acid	Part of DNA, growth and development of red blood cells	Certain types of anemia: megaloblastic (large, immature red blood cells)	Liver, green leafy vegetables, legumes, yeast
Cobalamin	Coenzyme in synthesis of heme for hemoglobin, normal red blood cell formation	Pernicious anemia (B_{12} is necessary extrinsic factor that combines with intrinsic factor of gastric secretions for absorption)	Liver, kidney, lean meats, milk, eggs, cheese

GI: gastrointestinal; CNS: central nervous system; CV: cardiovascular
From Williams, S.R. 1995. *Basic nutrition and diet therapy*, 10th ed. St. Louis: Mosby.

TABLE 1-8 *A Summary of Vitamin C (Ascorbic Acid)*

Functions	Clinical Applications	Food Sources
Intercellular cement substance; firm capillary walls and collagen formation Helps prepare iron for absorption and release to tissues for red blood cell formation	Scurvy (deficiency disease) Sore gums Hemorrhages, especially around bones and joints Tendency to bruise easily Stress reactions Growth periods Fevers and infections Wound healing, tissue formation Anemia	Citrus fruits, tomatoes, cabbage, leafy vegetables, potatoes, strawberries, melons, chili peppers, broccoli, chard, turnip greens, green peppers, other green and yellow vegetables

From Williams, S.R. 1995. *Basic nutrition and diet therapy*, 10th ed. St. Louis: Mosby.

As a result, the mineral content of the human body is quite similar to that of the earth. Of the fifty-four known earth elements in the periodic table of elements, twenty-five have been shown to be essential to human life. In comparison with the vitamins, which are large, complex organic compounds, minerals—single inert elements—may seem very simple. However, in their activated form of **ions** (carrying a positive or negative charge), they perform a wide, fascinating variety of essential metabolic tasks. Minerals differ from vitamins in the variety of their physiologic roles and in the amounts, relatively large to exceedingly small, needed for these tasks.

Variety of physiologic roles. These seemingly simple, single elements, in comparison with the much larger organic structure of vitamins, perform an impressive variety of metabolic tasks. They build, activate, regulate, transmit, and control. For example, sodium and potassium control water balance. Calcium and phosphorus are building materials that structure body framework. Iron helps build the vital oxygen carrier hemoglobin in red blood cells (fig. 1-2). Cobalt is the central core of cobalamin (vitamin B_{12}). Iodine helps structure thyroid hormone, which in turn regulates the overall rate of all body metabolism. Thus, far from being static and inert, minerals are active essential participants, helping control many of the body's overall metabolic processes.

Variety in amount needed. As indicated, all vitamins are required in very small amounts for their specific metabolic tasks. On the contrary, minerals occur in varying amounts in the body. For example, calcium forms a relatively large amount of the body weight—about 2%. Most of this amount is in bone tissue. An adult who weighs 150 lb has about 3 lb of calcium in the body. On the other hand, iron occurs in very small amounts. This same adult has only about 3 g (about 1/10 oz) of iron in the body. In both cases, the amount of each mineral is essential for its specific task. This varying amount of individual minerals in the body provides the basis for classifying them into two main groups, major minerals and trace elements.

1. *Major minerals.* Certain elements are referred to as major minerals not because they are more important in metabolism but simply because they occur in larger amounts in the body; thus, their requirement is greater. On this basis, seven elements for which the requirement is greater than 100 mg/day are classed as **major minerals.** They contribute from 60% to 80% of the inorganic material in the human body. These seven major minerals are calcium, phosphorus, sodium, potassium, magnesium, chloride, and sulfur (table 1-9). A review of their physiologic roles is given in table 1-10. Our major food source of calcium for bone growth through the life cycle (see p. 30) is milk and other dairy products.
2. *Trace elements.* The remaining eighteen elements in table 1-9 make up the group of **trace elements.** These minerals are no less important, but they occur in very small

Ions
(Gr *ion*, wanderer) Activated form of certain minerals, such as sodium (NA^+), potassium (K^+), and chloride (Cl^-), that carry an electrical charge and perform a variety of essential metabolic tasks.

Major minerals
Minerals that occur in relatively large quantities in the body and hence have greater dietary requirements.

Trace elements
Minerals that occur in small amounts, or traces, in the body, and hence are required in very small amounts.

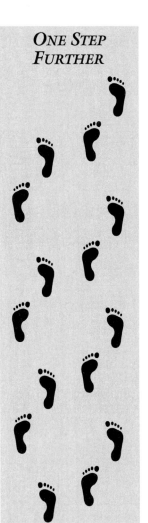

Fruits and Vegetables: Vitamin C Storehouses

Plenty of vitamin C can be had by emphasizing fruits and vegetables in the daily diet. Ingestion of these foods/beverages has been associated with reduced risk of cancer; this may be related to the vitamin contributions of these foods, but other nonnutrient components are now suspected of being beneficial. If one's daily goal is to consume 200 mg of vitamin C from food alone, the following sources are significant:

Food	Vitamin C (mg)
Orange juice (fresh-squeezed), 8 oz	124
Orange juice (from concentrate), 8 oz	97
Strawberries, fresh, 1 cup	84
Grapefruit juice (from concentrate), 8 oz	83
Orange, 1 medium	75
Kiwifruit, 1 medium	74
Cantaloupe, 1 cup pieces	68
Vegetable juice cocktail, 8 oz	60
Broccoli, cooked, 1/2 cup pieces	58
Sweet pepper, raw, 1/2 cup pieces	51
Brussels sprouts, cooked, 1/2 cup	48
Grapefruit, 1/2 medium	42
Potato, baked with skin, medium	31
Cauliflower, cooked, 1/2 cup pieces	27
Red cabbage, raw, 1/2 cup shredded	20
Green cabbage, cooked, 1/2 cup	15
Banana, medium	10

Anderson, J., and S.C. Garner. 1997. Phytoestrogens and human function. *Nutr Today* 32:232.
Bowes and Church's 1998. Food values of portions commonly used, 17th ed. Philadelphia. J.B. Lippincott Co.
Craig, W. 1997. Phytochemicals: Guardians of our health. *J Am Diet Assoc* 97 (suppl 2):S199.
Steinmetz, K., and J. Potter. 1996. Vegetables, fruit, and cancer prevention: A review. *J Am Diet Assoc* 96:1027.

traces in the body, contributing only 20–40% of all the inorganic material in the human body. For example, the human body contains only about 45 mg of iron per kilogram body weight. Nonetheless, each of these trace elements is necessary for its specific metabolic task. A review of the main physiologic roles of some of the trace elements is given in table 1-11.

The concept of essentiality. Note in table 1-9 that the trace elements are divided into two subgroups on the basis of essentiality in human nutrition. In the first subgroup, labeled "essential," ten trace elements have been deemed definitely essential on the basis of defined function and requirement determined from research. The remaining group of eight elements is probably essential also, but a more complete understanding of their status requires finer means of analysis and tests for function.

By the simplest definition, an essential element is one required for the existence of life; conversely, its absence brings death. However, for components that occur in very small amounts in the body, this determination of essentiality is not easy to make. Most living

TABLE 1-9   *Major Minerals and Trace Elements in Human Nutrition*

| Major Minerals (Required Intake over 100 mg/day) | Trace Elements | |
	Essential (Required Intake Under 100 mg/day)	Essentiality Unclear
Calcium (Ca)	Iron (Fe)	Silicon (Si)
Phosphorus (P)	Iodine (I)	Vanadium (V)
Sodium (Na)	Zinc (Zn)	Nickel (Ni)
Potassium (K)	Copper (Cu)	Tin (Sn)
Magnesium (Mg)	Manganese (Mn)	Cadmium (Cd)
Chlorine (Cl)	Chromium (Cr)	Arsenic (As)
Sulfur (S)	Cobalt (Co)	Aluminum (Al)
	Selenium (Se)	Boron (B)
	Molybdenum (Mo)	
	Fluorine (Fl)	

matter, as we know it, is made up of five fundamental elements, carbon (C), hydrogen (H), oxygen (O), nitrogen (N), and sulfur (S), which make up the macronutrients. We know these elements well because their concentrations are relatively large, hence more easily studied, and their requirements for human function can be expressed in multiples of grams per kilogram body weight. We have means for analysis of such quantities and can easily see that these are essential elements. Also, the major minerals occur in respectable quantities in the body, and their essentiality has been more easily studied and determined. However, the much larger number of trace elements occurs in biologic matter in very small amounts, and we know less about them. It is harder to determine essentiality of these trace elements because we require so little of them in the face of relatively large amounts found in our diet and environment. This makes it experimentally difficult to demonstrate essentiality, which requires removing it from the diet and the environment—an almost impossible task.

Nonetheless, despite the difficulties in determining essentiality of these small amounts of trace elements in our bodies, studies have indicated that essentiality can be determined on the basis of function and deficiency effect. Studies in trace element metabolism have indicated that in the simplest terms an element is essential when a deficiency causes an impairment of function and when supplementation with that substance, but not with others, prevents or cures this impairment. However, in relation to health care today, a leading researcher in trace elements also reminds us that major modern disease is often multifactorial, and a complex of nutritional interventions is often required. His studies of human metabolism have identified the function of trace elements in terms of catalytic and structural components of larger molecules.

1. *Catalytic components.* Small amounts of various trace elements may act as an enzyme component in a catalytic manner in essential cell metabolic reactions.
2. *Structural components.* Additional elements act as a structural molecule component in building materials used in cell and tissue formation.

These trace elements carry out their function in three ways 1) they may amplify the full function of the larger molecule of which they are a part, 2) they are specific to the particular function involved, and 3) they contribute to homeostatic regulation through their absorption-excretion balance and the degree of their carrier transport situation. Stages of research concerning trace element needs can be compared in terms of how far advanced our knowledge is: 1) longstanding knowledge, as is the case with iron and iodine; 2) recent history and questions, as for elements such as chromium, copper, zinc, and selenium; and 3) newer but incomplete knowledge, such as exists for silicon, vanadium, nickel, and arsenic. For example, metabolic studies of vanadium in laboratory-cultured cells and test animals have shown that, among other actions, this ultratrace element

Catalyst
(Gr *katalysis,* dissolution) A substance, such as enzymes and their component trace elements, that controls specific cell metabolism reactions but is not changed or consumed itself in the reaction, as are the specific substances on which it works.

TABLE 1-10 *A Summary of Major Minerals*

Minerals	Metabolism	Physiologic Functions	Clinical Applications	Requirements	Food Sources
Calcium (Ca)	Absorption according to body need, aided by vitamin D; hindered by binding agents (oxalates) or excessive fiber Parathyroid hormone controls absorption and mobilization	Bone and tooth formation Blood clotting Muscle contraction and relaxation Heart action Nerve transmission	Tetany—decrease in ionized serum calcium Rickets Osteoporosis	Adults: 1,200 mg Pregnancy and lactation: 1,200 mg Infants: 400–600 mg Children: 800–1,200 mg	Milk Cheese Whole grains Egg yolk Legumes, nuts Green leafy vegetables
Phosphorus (P)	Absorption with calcium aided by vitamin D; hindered by excess binding agents (aluminum)	Bone and tooth formation Overall metabolism Energy metabolism (enzymes) Acid-base balance	Bone loss Poor growth	Adults: 800–1,200 mg Pregnancy and lactation: 1,200 mg Infants: 300–500 mg Children: 800–1,200 mg	Milk Cheese Meat Egg yolk Whole grains Legumes, nuts
Sodium (Na)	Readily absorbed	Major extracellular fluid control Water balance Acid-base balance Muscle action; transmission of nerve impulse and resulting contraction	Fluid shifts and control Buffer system Losses in gastrointestinal disorders Dehydration	Limit to 2.4 g or less	Table salt (NaCl) Milk Meat Eggs Baking soda Baking powder Carrots, beets, spinach, celery
Potassium (K)	Secreted and reabsorbed in digestive juices	Major intracellular fluid control Acid-base balance Regulation of nerve impulse and muscle contraction Glycogen formation Protein synthesis Energy metabolism	Fluid shifts Heart action—low serum potassium (cardiac arrest) Insulin release Blood pressure factor	About 2,000–3,500 mg Diet adequate in protein, calcium, and iron contains adequate potassium	Fruits Vegetables Meats Whole grains Legumes

Mineral	Metabolism	Physiologic functions	Clinical application	Food sources
Magnesium (Mg)	Absorption increased by parathyroid hormone	Aids thyroid hormone secretion, normal BMR Activator and coenzyme in carbohydrate and protein metabolism Muscle, nerve action	Tremor, spasm; low serum level following gastrointestinal losses or renal losses from alcoholism; convulsions	Adults: 280–350 mg Pregnancy and lactation: 320–355 mg Deficiency in humans unlikely	Whole grains Legumes, nuts Green vegetables (chlorophyll)
Chlorine (Cl)	Absorbed readily	Acid-base balance—chloride shift Gastric hydrochloric acid—digestion	Hypochloremic alkalosis in prolonged vomiting, diarrhea, tube drainage	Parallel requirement of sodium	Table salt
Sulfur (S)	Absorbed as such and as constituent of sulfur-containing amino acid methionine	Essential constituent of cell protein Hair, skin, nails Vitamin structure Collagen structure High-energy sulfur bonds in energy metabolism	General protein malnutrition	Diet adequate in protein contains adequate sulfur	Meat Eggs Cheese Milk Legumes, nuts

From Williams, S.R. 1995. *Basic nutrition and diet therapy*, 10th ed. St. Louis: Mosby.

TABLE 1-11 *A Summary of Selected Trace Elements*

Elements	Metabolism	Physiologic Functions	Clinical Applications	Requirements	Food Sources
Iron (Fe)	Absorption according to body need; aided by vitamin C Heme and nonheme forms Excretion from tissue in minute quantities; body conserves then reuses	Hemoglobin formation Cellular oxidation of glucose Myoglobin in muscle Antibody production Drug detoxification Carotene conversion to vitamin A Collagen synthesis	Growth Pregnancy demands Deficiency—anemia	Men: 10 mg Women: 15 mg Pregnancy: 30 mg Lactation: 15 mg Children: 150 mg	Liver Meats Egg yolk Whole grains Enriched bread and cereal Dark green vegetables Legumes, nuts
Iodine (I)	Absorbed as iodides, taken up by thyroid gland under control of thyroid-simulating hormone (TSH) Excretion by kidney	Synthesis of thyroxine, the thyroid hormone, which regulates cell oxidation BMR regulation	Deficiency—endemic colloid goiter, cretinism Hypothyroidism Hyperthyroidism	Men: 150 µg Women: 150 µg Infants: 35–45 µg Children: 70–150 µg	Iodized salt Seafood
Zinc (Zn)	Transported with plasma proteins Excretion largely intestinal Stored in liver, muscle, bone, and organs	Essential enzyme constituent Combined with insulin for storage of the hormone Immune system leukocytes	Wound healing Taste and smell acuity Retarded sexual and physical development	Men: 15 mg Women: 12 mg Children: 10–15 mg Infants: 5 mg	Meat Seafood, especially oysters Eggs Milk Whole grains Legumes
Copper (Cu)	Stored in muscle, bone, liver, heart, kidney, and central nervous system Iron twin	Associated with iron in energy production, hemoglobin synthesis, and absorption and transport of iron	TPN deficiency Anemia	Adults: 1.5–3.0 mg Children: 1.0–2.5 mg (estimated)	Liver Seafood Whole grains Legumes, nuts

Mineral	Function	Clinical significance	Requirement	Food sources
Manganese (Mn)	Absorption limited / Excretion mainly by intestine / Activates reactions in urea formation, protein metabolism, glucose oxidation, and lipoprotein clearance and synthesis of fatty acids	Clinical deficiency in protein-energy malnutrition / Inhalation toxicity in miners	Adults: 2–5 mg (estimated) / Children: 1–5 mg	Cereals, whole grains / Soybeans / Legumes, nuts / Tea / Vegetables / Fruits
Chromium (Cr)	Improves faulty uptake of glucose by body tissues as part of glucose tolerance factor / Associated with glucose metabolism; raises abnormally low fasting blood sugar levels	Possible link with cardiovascular disorders and diabetes	Adults: 50–200 µg (estimated) / Children: 20–200 µg	Cereals, whole grains
Cobalt (Co)	Absorbed chiefly as constituent of vitamin B_{12} / Constituent of vitamin B_{12}; essential factor in red blood cell formation	Deficiency associated with deficiency of vitamin B_{12}—pernicious anemia	Unknown	Supplied by preformed vitamin B_{12}
Selenium (Se)	Active as cofactor in cell oxidation enzyme systems / Associated with vitamin E as antioxidant; protects lipid in cell membrane	Keshan disease, heart muscle failure / TPN deficiency	Men: 70 µg / Women: 55 µg / Children: 20 µg	Seafoods / Kidney / Liver / Meats / Whole grains
Molybdenum (Mo)	Minute traces in the body / Constituent of specific enzymes involved in purine conversion to uric acid / Aldehyde oxidation		Adults 75–250 µg (estimated)	Organ meats / Milk / Whole grains / Leafy vegetables / Legumes
Fluorine (Fl)	Deposited in bones and teeth / Associated with dental health	Small amount prevents dental caries / Excess causes endemic dental fluorosis	Adults 1.5–4.0 mg (estimated) / Children 0.5–2.5 mg	Fluoridated water (1 ppm Fl)

From Williams, S.R. 1995. *Basic nutrition and diet therapy*, 10th ed. St. Louis: Mosby.

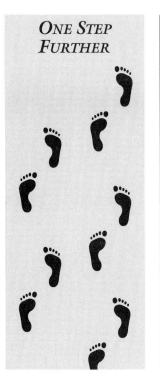

What Are the Differences Among Waters—
Purified, Spring, Distilled, Mineral . . .?

Not only does water come from the household tap, but it also comes from wells and is available in a variety of packaged forms in the marketplace. *Artesian well water* comes from a well that taps into an underground, water-bearing layer of rock or sand; the water level in this well is higher than the top layer of rock or sand from which it is drawn. *Mineral water* can be labeled as mineral water only if it contains at least 250 parts per million of total dissolved solids. *Purified water* is produced after water is treated through distillation, deionization, or reverse osmosis. *Sparkling bottled water* contains the same amount of carbon dioxide the water had when it left the source, and it maintains this level either naturally or after the bottler adds it during the bottling process. *Spring water* is collected either directly from a spring or through a borehole, which is a hole that has been bored into the ground and taps the underground source that supplies the spring. It also may be collected using an external force, as long as the product maintains the same chemical and physical properties as the spring water that flows naturally to the surface. *Seltzer water, soda water,* and *tonic water* are regulated differently than are the kinds of water previously mentioned and may contain sugar and calories and are considered to be soft drinks.

Kleiner, S.M. 1999. Water: An essential but overlooked nutrient. *J Am Diet Assoc* 99:200.
Levine, B. 1996. . . . About water. *Nutr Today* 31:209.

may affect glucose metabolism by altering or mimicking the action of insulin, possibly by altering membrane function for ion transport processes. These continuing studies, as well as knowledge of its food sources and nutritional requirement, suggest that vanadium may have an essential functional role in human beings, which in turn may yet indicate possible future clinical roles—for example, in diabetes management.

Water

The final basic nutrient, water, underlies all the functions of the other nutrients and, next to air, is the most essential substance to our survival. It creates the water-based environment necessary for the vast array of chemical actions and reactions that constitute body metabolism and sustain life. Also, it provides the means for maintaining a stable body temperature and helps give structure and form to our bodies through the turgor it provides for the tissues. We obtain this life-giving water in fluids we drink, including water and other beverages; in foods we eat; and the water of oxidation created within from the end products of cell metabolism. The average adult metabolizes from 2.5 to 3 L of water/day in a constant turnover balanced between intake and output. This water enters and leaves the body by various routes, controlled by basic mechanisms such as thirst and hormonal activity.

THE HUMAN LIFE CYCLE AND CHANGING NUTRIENT NEEDS ≈

Growth and Development

Physical growth. *Growth* may be defined as an increase in size, but it encompasses far more than that. Biologic growth of an organism occurs through cell multiplication. Development is the associated process in which growing tissues and organs take on an increased complexity of function. Both processes combine to form a unified whole in the many aspects of human growth and development throughout the life cycle. This dual concept indicates the magnitude and quality of maturational changes that establish early embryonic cells through cell multiplication and differentiation; that set the pattern for subsequent rapid fetal growth and development; that produce a fully formed, small dependent newborn; and that transform this newborn infant through successive childhood growth periods into a fully functioning, independent adult.

Physiologic and psychosocial development. Physiologic growth depends on a variety of nutrients in the food a child eats. It also depends on the vast number of biochemical processes of metabolism that supply the right materials in the right place at the right time for forming and maintaining unique body tissues. Human growth and development, however, involves far more than the physical process alone. It takes in social and psychologic influences and relationships—indeed, the entire environment and culture that promote individual growth potential. Food and feeding, especially during the early formative childhood years but also throughout the life cycle, do not and cannot exist apart from this broader, overall personal growth and development. Although we are concerned about necessary nutrients at any age, we do not eat nutrients; we eat food, with all the uniquely different social, cultural, and personal meanings it holds for each of us.

Changing nutrient needs. Through the successive age groups of the life cycle, changing nutrient needs reflect an increasing differentiation based on age and sex as the physical body grows and develops. There is a general, steady increase in nutrient and energy needs through early age groups to about age ten to twelve years, with individuals within any age group often having different needs according to individual growth patterns. With the onset of puberty and the differing sexual development of boys and girls, nutrient needs for the two sexes begin to vary. During this adolescent period, the final growth spurt of childhood occurs. Maturation during this period varies so widely that chronological age as a reference point for discussing growth ceases to be useful (if it ever was, for individual differences occur at all ages). **Physiologic age** becomes more important in dealing with individual adolescent girls and boys (see chapter 10). It accounts for wide fluctuations in metabolic rates, food requirements, scholastic capacity, and even illness. These capacities can be more realistically viewed in individual physiologic growth terms. The profound growth period of adolescents requires increases in energy, protein, minerals, and vitamins. Boys usually eat well enough to receive all necessary nutrients, whereas girls often do not.

Body Composition

Individual variation. Throughout the life cycle, the physical composition of the human body is changing. From conception and birth, throughout childhood growth and adult aging, to old age decline and death, the human body and its basic components change and adapt in a remarkable fashion to meet physiologic needs. Given the genetic imprint of its heritage and the physical and psychosocial nature of its environment, the human body, in the most literal sense, is the product of its nutrition throughout life. Through profound and fascinating transformations, food makes possible the living body and all its functions, as well as the varying mass of tissue it produces and maintains. There is no precise "ideal" or "standard" **body composition** except for purposes of study in the laboratory. In reality, this is a hazardous assumption, for, within the limits of genetic potential, individuals differ widely. There is great variability among healthy persons in both body composition and body response to internal and external environmental influences and to disease. However, a general knowledge of body composition components and their interrelatedness provides an important basis for measuring and determining the nutritional status of specific individuals of all ages, as well as the many influences that shape it.

Basic concepts of compartments and balance. With the two basic physiologic concepts of body compartments and balance for a foundation, we can identify and describe the gross components of body composition, especially in relation to body changes and nutritional needs through the life cycle. The concept of *balance* provides a dynamic view of the body, ever changing and adjusting to its internal and external environments. The biologic term **compartment** is used to describe the body's internal collection of a given vital substance. The concept of compartments gives a comprehensive view of the human

Physiologic age
Rate of biologic maturation in individual adolescents, which varies widely and accounts for more than does chronologic age for wide and changing differences in their metabolic rates, nutritional needs, and food requirements.

Body composition
The relative sizes of the four body compartments that make up the physical body—lean body mass, fat, water, and mineral mass.

Body compartment
The collective quantity of a particular vital substance in the body—for example, the mineral compartment, composed mainly of the skeletal bone mass.

body—not of static mechanical parts but of **homeostasis,** a state of dynamic equilibrium within an interdependent whole. The nutritional needs of individuals throughout growth and development can be understood through the application of these two basic concepts.

Body Composition Compartments Based on Metabolic Activity

Nutritional scientists, who are interested in nutritional status as a means of determining nutritional needs throughout life, usually use the criterion of metabolic activity to define the gross components of body composition. On this basis, many researchers commonly distinguish four main components in two divisions: 1) those parts that are most active in energy metabolism—*lean body mass*—and 2) those parts that are relatively inactive—*body fat, extracellular water,* and the *mineral mass of bones and smaller structural parts.*

Lean body mass compartment. The body's lean cell mass is the primary determinant of its energy requirements and thus its overall nutrient needs. Its relative size and metabolic activity, as well as its relation to weight changes, are important considerations.

1. *Compartment size and metabolic activity.* Lean body mass, as a collective compartment of the body's active fat-free mass of cells, accounts for 30–65% of the total body weight. However, it accounts for almost all the energy consumption. As a percentage of body weight, for example, the values for this lean cell mass range from low levels in very fat, sedentary persons to higher levels in very muscular persons.

2. *Relation to weight changes.* When individuals gain or lose weight because of dietary changes, it is a reflection of changes not merely in the body fat mass but also in the lean body mass. The density of the tissue added or lost is never that of pure fat. The density of the nonfat lean part also changes with nutritional status. Added exercise enhances its relative size.

Body fat compartment. The gross amount of the body fat compartment can vary widely and affect individual health status. In general, it reflects the number and size of fat cells—**adipocytes**—making up the adipose tissue. However, adipose tissue is not pure fat. It also contains parts of other compartments, such as blood vessels, connective tissue, cell membranes, and water.

Adipocytes
(L *adipis,* fat; Gr *kytos,* hollow vessel, cell) Fat cells.

1. *Compartment size.* In relation to a standard "reference body" and from body water measurements, the body fat compartment has been variously estimated in healthy persons to range in an adult man, for example, from about 14–28% of the total body weight. The woman's "reference body" would have a somewhat larger fat compartment, about 15–29% of total body weight. These percentages vary with factors such as age, climate, exercise, and fitness. About half of the total body fat is in the subcutaneous fat layers, which serve the important task of helping maintain body temperature.

2. *Relation to health.* Extremes in size of the body fat compartment can affect health status. For example, some athletes, especially compulsive runners, may strive for a very low level of body fat, even in some cases to an unhealthy deficit. Conversely, at the other extreme, massively obese sedentary persons carry increased health risks from an excessively large body fat mass. However, common beliefs that even moderate overweight brings poorer health and a shorter life span seem unfounded. Studies of various populations, such as the classic data from the long-standing Framingham study as well as later work, appear to indicate that it is the extremes of both underweight and obesity that increase health risks and contribute to higher mortality rates, concluding that moderate amounts of overweight, especially in older adults, may actually be a health protection.[4]

Body water compartment. The total body water content varies widely with relative body composition in terms of leanness and fatness, since lean muscle tissue contains more water than any other body tissue except blood. It also varies with age, being relatively higher in infants, and with hydration status, being lower in conditions causing dehydration and higher in conditions causing edema or ascites. In pregnancy the total maternal body water increases normally to support the increased metabolic work and sometimes abnormally in complications of pregnancy-induced hypertension.

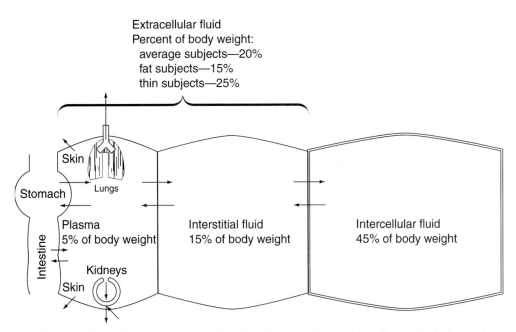

FIG. 1-3   Body fluid compartments. Note the relative total quantities of water in the intracellular compartment and in the extracellular compartment.

1. Total body water compartments. The total body water is divided into two subcompartments—the collective water inside the cells and the remaining collective water outside of cells. The water inside of cells is part of the active cell mass or lean body mass. Thus, it is the remaining collective water outside of cells, the **extracellular fluid (ECF)**, that makes up this designated water compartment of gross body composition.

2. ECF compartment. The size of the ECF compartment varies with individual fatness or leanness, being higher in thin persons and lower in fat persons. In average-weight adults, the collective water outside cells makes up about 20% of the total body weight; in fat persons, about 15%; in thin persons, about 25%. The ECF consists of four parts: 1) *blood plasma,* which accounts for about 25% of the ECF and 5% of body weight; 2) *interstitial fluid,* water surrounding the cells; 3) *secretory fluid,* circulating secretions in transit; and 4) *dense tissue fluid,* water in dense connective tissue, cartilage, and bone (fig. 1-3).

Body mineral compartment. The body's major mineral content by far is found in its large skeletal mass, with much smaller amounts in teeth, nails, and hair. Of all the minerals in the human body, calcium is present in far greater amounts than any other, comprising about 2% of the total body weight.

1. *Skeletal mass.* The human skeleton is a relatively large structure, comprising in the living body about one-sixth of the total body mass. Most of the body calcium—about 99%—is in the skeleton, accounting for most of the total body mineral compartment. Other minerals occur in varying lesser amounts.

2. *Mineral ash.* Only a small part of the skeletal mass, however, is comprised of mineral matter. The other components of bone—water, protein, and fat—are accounted for in their respective body composition compartments. In its dried, defatted state, the skeleton represents only about 6% of the gross body weight. Bone mineral mass as estimated from bone ash values is about 5% of total body weight.

DIET: INFLUENCES DURING THE LIFE CYCLE ≋

Although food likes and dislikes probably determine largely what people eat, food choices also reflect socioeconomic status and budget, cultural experiences, religious beliefs, time constraints, health-related concerns, susceptibility to advertising, and other such factors. As one expert stated, "Food symbolizes much of what we think about ourselves."

Extracellular fluid (ECF)
The total body water compartment composed of the collective water outside of cells.

Mineral compartment
Smallest part of the body composition, found mainly in the skeletal bone mass.

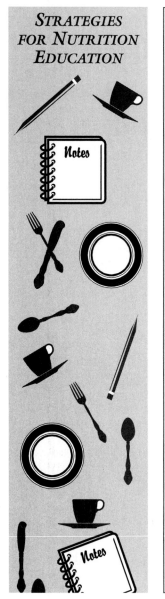

America's Changing Food Habits: Implications for Nutrition Education

The American public has been receiving increasing numbers of messages from public health agencies and private health organizations regarding the relationship between diet and health. Food companies are also directing their attention to health concerns in the development and marketing of new food products. Of the nearly 13,000 new food products introduced to the marketplace in 1993, about 2,500 made a health claim. Over two-thirds of the products making a health claim were low or reduced in fat, cholesterol, or kilocalories, and about one-third were low or reduced in sugar or sodium. Relatively few of the new products contained high levels or added amounts of fiber or calcium. Over the past thirty-five years, the typical American diet has undergone many changes that are consistent with the Dietary Guidelines for Americans issued by the U.S. Departments of Health and Human Services and Agriculture. Food consumption data indicate that since 1960 intakes per person of cholesterol, sugar, and eggs have declined by 18–36%, while intakes of fresh vegetables, fish, pasta, and chicken have increased by 45–70%. Use of low-fat milk has increased by 4,000%. Recent surveys suggest that over half of today's consumers are concerned about the level of fat in the foods they eat, and the demand for reduced and low-fat food products continues to grow. Increasing their intakes of fruits and vegetables is a major concern of consumers who are seeking more healthful diets. Other trends, however, are less encouraging. Americans are increasing their total energy intakes—up by 12% since 1980—despite their reduction in dietary fat, and all age groups are gradually gaining weight. Many new foods that are low or reduced in fat, or even fat free, are still high in kilocalories and can contribute to weight gain. Moreover, other important dietary goals are receiving little attention. Only 3% of consumers interviewed in 1994 were making an effort to lower their intake of cholesterol, and only 7–8% were attempting to increase their use of fish or high-fiber foods or to decrease their intake of salt, yet these patterns are also critical to the development of healthy food behavior. It would appear that nutrition education messages have emphasized the reduction of dietary fat at the expense of other food issues. A more effective approach might be to encourage:

- Eating a balanced diet to include a wide variety of foods.
- Using all foods in moderation.
- Limiting intakes of fat, cholesterol, added sugar, and added salt.
- Increasing intakes of complex carbohydrates, fiber, and calcium.
- Monitoring total energy intake and expenditure to maintain a healthy body weight.

American Institute for Cancer Research Newsletter, Issue 47, Spring 1995.
Stillings, B.R. 1994. Trends in foods. *Nutr Today* 29:6.
Stillings, B.R. 1997. . . . "What we eat in America" survey. *Nutr Today* 32:37.

Childhood Experiences

The food environment in which we are raised has a significant effect on our food choices later in life. Environment reflects social and cultural preferences, which in turn are influenced by monetary constraints, limitations in the food supply, parental decisions about introduction of new foods to children, and an array of other variables. Innate food preferences exist also, such as the universal enjoyment of sweet foods and the dislike of sour or bitter substances. It is possible, however, to modify these preferences through the process of conditioning, or learning. Some people learn, for example, to like very hot and spicy foods or foods that are very salty.

Social Situations

Special occasions are associated with the serving of specific foods. Foods often represent long-established traditions within a family or cultural group. Also, family schedules dictate the family mealtime group. The traditional family meal occurs less frequently now than in times past, and busy schedules often lead to eating outside the home. Some Americans have developed a pattern of **"grazing,"** as opposed to "meal eating." Negative nutritional effects may follow.

Financial Resources

Family income certainly determines the kinds of foods selected. More affluent people tend to purchase more fresh vegetables and fruits and more meat, poultry, and fish. Income also dictates in most families the pattern of eating away from home. However, since the cost of food in the United States is *relatively* inexpensive, differences in Americans' food choices are less than one might suspect.

Advertising

Billions of dollars are spent annually to entice the public to choose certain foods. Although the impact of such efforts was minimal at one time, the sophistication of modern advertising has markedly affected our pattern of product selection today. Whereas some of the advertising may promote important nutrition considerations, emphasis is often placed on sweets and other "goodies." Whatever the case, the force of advertising is now recognized to be substantial. This is true not only in the supermarket but also in the fast-food restaurant industry.

Daily Routine

Although we think of America as a society with much variation, a close look at any individual often discloses that the patterns of daily living include a rather limited food menu. People become locked into food choices that they enjoy, are readily available and affordable, and don't test their limited wishes to stray from "what is familiar." Children raised in an environment in which trying new foods is encouraged may accept the challenges of new food experiences better than do children exposed to limited options.

Health Concerns

A growing number of Americans are concerned enough about health that they select foods in part based on this factor. Some surveys indicate that half of the U.S. population considers health maintenance important when shopping for or ordering food. Attention to proper food choices for promotion of health was sparked in the late 1960s by the "back to nature" movement, along with the recommendations of the American Heart Association that fat and cholesterol may contribute to coronary heart disease. Recent years have seen the publication of evidence that some cancers may also be "preventable" with choice of a good diet. These findings have not gone unnoticed by the general public. The food industry recognizes this and is now providing an array of products that are specifically of low-calorie, low-fat composition. Also, government regulatory agencies are in the process of reforming food labeling to present sound nutrition information for the consumer. These directions are very likely to continue beyond the year 2000.

LIFE CYCLE NUTRITIONAL NEEDS ≋

From the moment of conception, the human organism depends on nutrition for growth, development, and long-term survival. Prior to birth, the fetus must draw from maternal nutrient supplies, and this process may continue after birth if the mother chooses to breast-feed her baby. Ultimately, an outside food supply provides the ongoing nutritional support for life. This nutritional support may come from both animal and plant food sources. An unlimited number of food combinations are known to satisfy nutrient needs. Consequently, people worldwide, consuming vastly different foods and food mixtures, demonstrate satisfactory growth and health.

Stages of the Life Cycle

Gestation. The **mammalian** fetus is completely dependent on nutritional support from the mother. The quantitative requirements are very small in the beginning but increase gradually until birth. During this time, it is absolutely essential that a correct equilibrium

Grazing
Informal descriptive label for food pattern of frequent small snacks throughout the day, rather than more formal, regular meals. Term taken from animal pattern of constant eating in a pastureland.

Milieu

(Fr *milieu,* surroundings) Environment, social or physical. An important concept in nutrition, referring to both external sociophysical setting and internal biochemical environments and the interacting balances between them.

Gestation

(L *gestare,* to bear) Intrauterine fetal growth period from conception to birth.

Neuromotor

(Gr *neuron,* nerve; L *motorium,* movement center) Movement involving nerve impulses to muscles.

be maintained among the various nutrients circulating in the maternal blood. This required biochemical **milieu** depends entirely on the mother's diet, her nutritional stores, and her metabolic idiosyncrasies. The adverse effects of nutritional-biochemical imbalance during **gestation** have been examined most frequently in animal models. Fortuitous observations of human experience, however, have contributed to our slowly growing knowledge base in this field. In general, the repercussions of abnormal nutrition depend on the stage at which a given nutrient factor acts, the nature of the nutrient considered, the intensity of the disequilibrium, and the species or strain of the animal studied. The types of repercussion are very different. They include death, tissue alterations, delayed growth, alterations of cellular differentiation, and malformations. Improvement in pregnancy outcome depends in part on motivating the pregnant woman to establish satisfactory diet and supplementation practices.[5]

Lactation. Establishment of **lactation** and continued production of sufficient high-quality milk also demands that the mother consume an adequate diet. While lactation is a high-priority physiologic process maintained even in the face of serious nutritional deprivation, without continuing nutritional support the quantity of milk production is generally hampered and milk quality eventually deteriorates. In either case, the nutritional well-being of the mother is compromised, as is eventually her health and preparedness for "mothering."[5]

Infancy. The first year after birth is a time in the life cycle when many changes occur in relation to food and nutrient intake. A number of factors influence these dramatic changes: 1) a rapid then gradually declining rate of physical growth, 2) maturation of oral structures and functions, 3) development of fine and gross motor skills, and 4) establishment of relationships with parents and family. As a result of these tremendous changes, infants prepared at birth to suck liquids from a nipple are at one year of age making attempts to feed themselves table foods with culturally defined utensils. The need for nutrients and energy depends on the infant's requirement for physical growth, maintenance, and energy expenditure. The foods offered to infants reflect culturally accepted practices. Infants' acceptance of food is influenced by **neuromotor** maturation and by their interactions with their parents. Well-nourished children at any month during infancy consume a variety of food combinations.[6]

Preschool. During the preschool years, the decreased rates of growth bring decreased appetites. Children learn to understand language and to talk and ask for food. Development of gross motor skills permits them to learn to feed themselves and to prepare simple foods, such as cereal and milk and sandwiches. They learn about food and the way it feels, tastes, and smells. Preschool children learn to eat a wider variety of textures and kinds of food, give up the bottle, and drink from a cup. They demand independence and refuse help in many tasks, such as self-feeding, in which they are not yet skillful. As they grow older, they become less interested in food and more interested in their environment. They test and learn the limits of acceptable behavior.[6]

School age. Between preschool and adolescence, children continue to grow slowly and demonstrate maturation of fine and gross motor skills. Individual personality develops and degree of independence increases. All of these changes influence the amounts of food consumed, the manner in which it is eaten, and the acceptability of specific foods. Food habits, likes, and dislikes are established, some of which are transient but many of which form the base for a lifetime of food experiences. Environmental influences and parental behaviors reinforce or extinguish food-related behaviors. Parents need to provide appropriate foods and supportive guidance, so that appropriate food patterns develop. The nutrition knowledge of the parents and other care providers positively influences children's requests for and acceptance of various foods. School feeding programs provide an opportunity for nutrition education.[6]

Adolescence. The adolescent period is a unique stage in the process of growth and development. It is characterized by a wide variability in norms of growth, increasingly independent behavior, and testing of adult roles. This critical period of human development occurs at physiologic, psychologic, and social levels. These tumultuous changes do not occur simultaneously but at varying rates. Although adolescence may be defined as

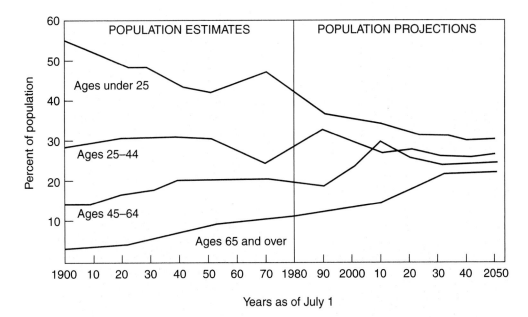

FIG. 1-4 Trend in age distribution of U.S. population (including Armed Forces overseas). From Insel, P.M., and W.T. Roth. 1988. *Core concepts in health,* 5th ed. Mountain View, CA: Mayfield.

the teenage years between twelve and twenty, physical maturation and changes in nutrient requirements actually begin at younger years and sometimes extend into the third decade.[7]

Teenagers assume greater responsibility for decision making in their own lives. In contrast to younger children, adolescents themselves most often determine their food intake. Their food choices reflect various factors, including family eating patterns, peer influence, the media, appetite, and food availability. Some of these factors can be positive for nutritional quality, but others may leave a lot to be desired. Body image plays a very important role in the eating behaviors of adolescents. Eating disorders account for a large number of nutritional concerns during adolescence.[7]

Adulthood. The adult years span a number of decades, during which nutritional needs change very little, but family circumstances and lifestyle often undergo substantial change. Marital status, living environment, job setting and responsibilities, income, and a variety of other factors significantly affect specific food choices and long-term dietary patterns. Ideally, a major focus during these years is health promotion and disease prevention. This goal entails, among other things, establishing nutritional practices that maximize health and minimize risk for developing preventable chronic diseases. Appropriate practices vary somewhat among individuals due in large part to differences in genetic bases. Of primary concern, however, is maintaining desirable body fatness by eating moderate amounts of a variety of wholesome foods.[4]

Aging. Persons who are sixty-five years of age or older comprise the fastest-growing segment of the population in most developed countries (fig. 1-4). Of these older individuals, 95% live within the community, many of them on incomes barely sufficient for survival. Financial limitations adversely affect food purchasing power. However, an assortment of other factors also contribute to the increased prevalence of malnutrition in this age group. Important contributors to the problem include loneliness, depression, oral discomfort, and chronic diseases, all of which lead to poor appetite. Physical and mental handicaps may limit the ability to shop for food or to prepare it. Use of an assortment of drugs, both prescription and over-the-counter, may further interfere with the maintenance of satisfactory nutritional status. The aging process itself may reduce nutrient absorption, increase urinary loss, and interfere with normal pathways of nutrient utilization.[8]

GUIDELINES FOR HEALTH MAINTENANCE AND DISEASE PREVENTION ≋

During the past twenty years, the understanding of the role of nutrition in health promotion and disease prevention has improved. Relationships between specific nutrient deficiencies and inferior health status have long been recognized, but, in recent years, diet has been associated with a number of chronic diseases, such as cardiovascular disease, cancer, and diabetes. The focus of concern about human nutrition has moved from the issues of nutritional deficiencies toward chronic disease prevention and health maintenance in all phases of the life cycle.

Dietary Guidelines

The Dietary Guidelines for Americans of the USDA define desirable basic goals for a daily diet (table 1-12).[9,10] However, putting these goals into practice requires choosing the right foods from the hundreds of items available. To aid in this undertaking, the United States Department of Agriculture (USDA) has developed a Food Guide Pyramid (fig. 1-5) that goes along with the Dietary Guidelines for Americans. The food groups are arranged in pyramid form to emphasize that it is wise to choose an abundance of foods from the category at the broad base (bread, cereal, rice, pasta) and to use sparingly foods from the peak (fats, oils, sweets). The other food groups appear in between these two, indicating the importance of vegetables and fruits and the need for some moderation when it comes to dairy products and meats. The pyramid suggests a reasonable number of servings to choose from each group daily; the range takes into account that need differs according to age and sex.[11]

It should be noted that other food pyramids have been developed based on the pattern proposed by the USDA, such as the following:

Mediterranean
Asian
Latin American
Puerto Rican
Vegetarian
Soul Food

These pyramids, used in conjunction with guidance offered by the USDA, can help the public choose foods that fit a specific ethnic or cultural pattern (fig. 1-6).[11]

Recommended Dietary Allowances (RDAs): Now Dietary Reference Intakes (DRIs)

While the USDA has been active in issuing nutrition guidelines, the National Academy of Sciences (NAS) has continued its practice of establishing and continually updating the more specific "nutrition standards" that define human nutrition needs. The Recommended Dietary Allowances (RDAs) (see inside front cover)[12] have been around since 1943, when the first efforts were made to describe what a normal person needs to eat each day to stay healthy. The stimulus for the creation of this list of requirements was the need

---

TABLE 1-12   *Dietary Guidelines for Americans*

Eat a variety of foods.
Balance the food you eat with physical activity; maintain or improve your weight.
Choose a diet with plenty of grain products, vegetables, and fruits.
Choose a diet low in fat, saturated fat, and cholesterol.
Choose a diet moderate in sugars.
Choose a diet moderate in salt and sodium.
If you drink alcoholic beverages, do so in moderation.

From U.S. Dept. of Agriculture. 1995. *Dietary guidelines for Americans,* 4th ed. Washington, DC: U.S. Government Printing Office, Home and Garden Bull. #232.

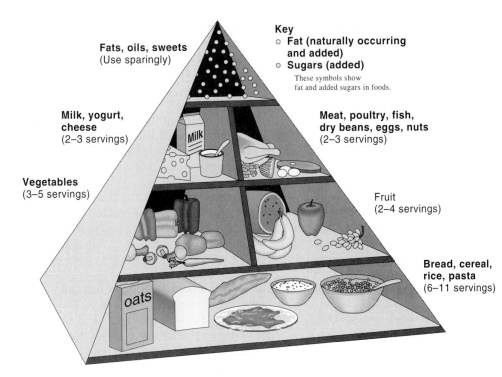

FIG. 1-5 USDA's Food Guide Pyramid—a Guide to Daily Food Choices. This guide lists the food groups and the number of servings of each to consume.

**The healthy traditional
Latin American diet pyramid**

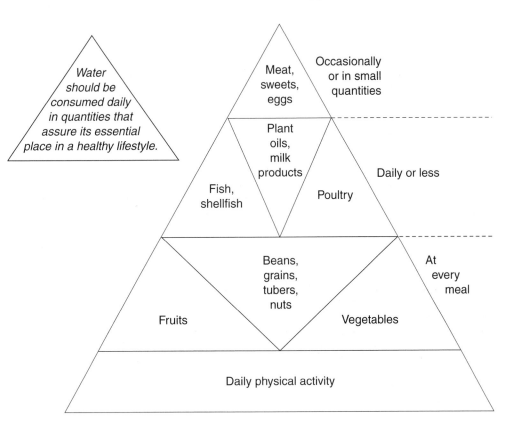

FIG. 1-6

to feed thousands of World War II soldiers in a variety of places around the world. Each of these sites had to be provided enough of the right kinds of foods to maintain the health of their men (and a few women). Since 1943, the RDAs have been updated periodically to reflect new knowledge of nutrient needs. The official definition of an RDA is the following: the amount of a nutrient that should decrease the risk of chronic disease for almost all healthy individuals of specified age and gender.

The terms used to define nutrient needs are calories, grams, milligrams, micrograms, and a few others, such as retinol equivalents. These terms have little meaning to many people, so information provided to the general public largely avoids these terms and often speaks of percentage of daily need found in a given product. For example, one medium orange provides 100% of an adult's daily vitamin C requirement.

In the late 1990s, the National Academy of Sciences decided that the original intent of the RDAs, to prevent nutrient deficiencies, was insufficient for optimizing the health of Americans.[13-15] This government agency set out to improve its recommendations. Other terms are now beginning to appear in published material:

Adequate Intake (AI)—Same as RDA, but lacking enough scientific evidence to set an RDA.

Estimated Average Requirement (EAR)—The amount that meets the optimal nutrient needs of half the individuals in a specified group.

Tolerable Upper Intake Level (UL)—Total intake from food, fortified food, and supplements should not exceed this amount, or adverse health effects may result.

Dietary Reference Intakes (DRIs)—An umbrella term for RDAs, AIs, EARs, and ULs.[16,17]

This array of terms is confusing. As each RDA is updated, these new terms will be used as deemed appropriate. No matter which tag is attached to a nutrient, it represents *the best available estimate of intake for optimal health*. For example, calcium now has an AI, not an RDA, because the NAS panel believes scientists do not yet know how much calcium is needed to prevent osteoporosis (aging bone loss) and the fractures that often occur from it in later life. That is because other factors, such as genetics and physical activity, are also influential. Calcium also now has an upper limit (UL)—2,500 mg/day. Above this, says the panel, excess calcium in the blood raises the risk of kidney stones and kidney failure. It can also interfere with the absorption of iron, zinc, and magnesium.

More recently, the Institute of Medicine issued its report on DRIs for the B vitamins. It recommends that all adult men and women consume 400 μg dietary folate per day—more than double the former RDA for this vitamin. Emphasizing that folate is particularly important for women of childbearing age, the report says that women capable of becoming pregnant should consume 400 μg folic acid daily from fortified foods and/or vitamin supplements, in addition to the naturally occurring food folate obtained from a varied diet, to reduce their risk of having a child with a neural tube defect. For choline, a B-complex vitamin with no previously established DRI, the report recommends intakes of 425 mg/day for women and 550 mg/day for men. Recommended intakes of other B vitamins have not been changed substantially from levels established in 1989.

National Nutrition Objectives (Healthy People 2000 and 2010)

In the late 1970s, efforts began at the national level in the United States toward health promotion and disease prevention. Healthy People 2000 is a national initiative to improve the health of Americans through prevention. Its goals are to increase the span of a healthy life for Americans, reduce health disparities, and achieve access to preventive services for all Americans. Nutrition is one of the twenty-two priority areas in which the objectives are organized. General goals related to nutrition include the reduction of:

Coronary heart disease deaths
Cancer deaths
Overweight

Desirable Nutrition Trends of the Future

A knowledgeable nutrition educator recently summarized the major challenges facing consumers who desire to establish diet and lifestyle patterns conducive to health. Self-care is deemed to be a sensible pattern of living. Prevention of disease, to the extent possible, should be a high priority. The following are defined as key nutrition trends for the future:

1. *Personal nutrition balance.* Individuals take charge of their health, making food and lifestyle choices that work for them.
2. *Food safety.* Concern about safe food takes priority as government, industry, and consumers push for action.
3. *Vitamins and minerals.* Evolving science shifts focus on micronutrients from alleviating deficiency to preventive health.
4. *Healthy eating.* Attention to ethnic cuisines attracts consumers to plant-based eating patterns.
5. *Functional foods.* Consumer interest gains momentum for foods and ingredients that may play a role in optimal health.
6. *Weight control.* "Magic bullets" come and go, whereas obesity continues to rise.
7. *Dietary fat versus carbohydrates.* Debate on fundamental dietary recommendations, fueled by beliefs, not science, inappropriately increases popularity of high-protein diets.
8. *Vitamin E.* Research demonstrates health benefits, shedding new light on the use of supplements.
9. *Women's nutrition and health.* Unique health needs of women are addressed through customized nutrition products and services.
10. *Childhood nutrition.* New approaches are in the works to motivate children to improve their nutrient intake and lifestyles.

McMahon, K. 1998. Consumers and key nutrition trends for 1998. *Nutr Today* 33:19.

ONE STEP FURTHER

Growth retardation in children
Stroke deaths
Colorectal cancer deaths
Diabetes incidence and prevalence

Goals to reduce the risk of these problems include:
Reduce (modify) fat intake
Improve vegetable, fruit, and grain intake
Increase weight loss practices
Increase intake of calcium-rich foods
Reduce salt and sodium intake
Prevent iron deficiency
Encourage breast-feeding
Prevent baby bottle tooth decay
Increase use of food labels
Reduce high blood cholesterol levels
Control blood pressure

Some progress has been made toward these goals, and evaluation of this progress has been ongoing.[10]

As the year 2000 approaches, efforts are underway to develop and implement year 2010 objectives. This project is being overseen by the U.S. Department of Health and Human Services. Use will be made of the Internet to acquire input from any American who chooses to become involved (http://odphp.osophs.dhhs.gov/pubs/hp2000). Healthy People 2010 objectives are scheduled for release in the year 2000.

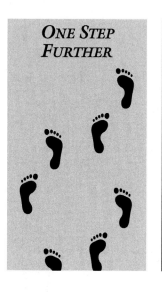

Food Fortification: An Effort to Prevent Micronutrient Deficiencies

During the past sixty years, as the processing of foods has increased, efforts have been made to prevent specific vitamin and mineral deficiencies through the addition of these nutrients to selected foods and beverages. This procedure is referred to as "fortification" or "enrichment." Iodine has been added to salt. Vitamin A has been added to margarine. Vitamin D has been added to milk. The vitamins thiamin, riboflavin, and niacin and the mineral iron have been added to flour. Recently, folic acid has been added to grain products. Overall, fortification has had a positive effect on the health of Americans. However, as time goes on, care must be taken to avoid "overfortification," since regular excessive intake of some nutrients is harmful. The responsibility for control rests with the scientists and regulatory agencies that oversee important decisions regarding food safety.

Mertz, W. 1997. Food fortification in the United States. *Nutr Rev* 55:44.

Nutrition Labeling

Many people obtain most of their nutrition information from labels on foods. Nutrition labeling is mandatory for most foods that contain more than one ingredient, the bulk of which are processed foods and dietary supplements. Labeling remains voluntary for raw meats and fresh fruits and vegetables; this is also the case for foods produced by small businesses and those sold in restaurants, food stands, and local bakeries (unless a health or nutrient content claim is made on the menu or package).

The nutrition information label is known as the Nutrition Facts Panel (Fig. 1-7). This panel highlights a product's content of fat, saturated fat, cholesterol, sodium, dietary fiber, two vitamins (A and C), and two minerals (calcium and iron). The food's content of these nutrients must be based on a standard serving size (defined by the Food and Drug Administration). Information about other nutrients *may* be put on the label if the producer wishes to do so. If any claim is made on the label, however, nutrient content *must* be listed. For example, if the label says "high in folic acid," then the folic acid content must be given.

The Nutrition Facts Panel contains a column headed "% Daily Value (DRV)." The percentages listed show the contribution of a serving of the food to the recommended diet of a person who consumes about 2,000 calories each day on average. The DRVs are "scientifically agreed upon daily levels of fat, saturated fat, cholesterol, carbohydrate, dietary fiber, and protein intake compatible with health." They are intended for use on nutrition labels only. For the vitamins and minerals listed on the label, the percentage is that of the nutrient's RDI.[18]

More and more people have begun to use nutrition labels in making food choices. For example, a daily diet containing 2,000 calories (with 30% of the calories from fat) contains about 56 g of fat. The label may indicate that a serving of macaroni and cheese contains 14 g of fat and the % Daily Value is 25%. This says to the consumer that a serving of macaroni and cheese provides about one-fourth of the suggested safe level of daily fat intake. If another brand of macaroni and cheese displays a % Daily Value of 10%, a nutrition-conscious person may opt to buy the latter.

Nutrition labels are an important tool for helping people make informed food purchasing decisions. However, labels do not now, or will they ever, provide all the information needed to make wise decisions about food. Only people who are well informed about nutrition can do that.

Since there is still much to learn about how nutrients and nonnutrients affect human health, speculators and outright "quacks" take opportunities to market food and supplement products with enticing health claims. Millions of dollars are spent each year

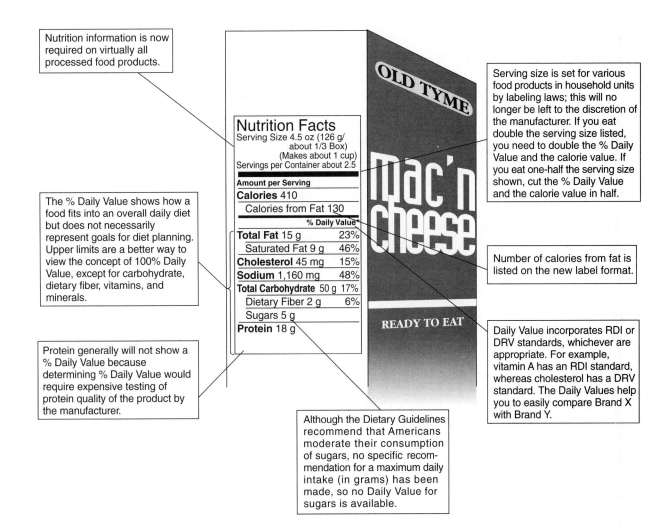

FIG. 1-7 The Nutrition Facts panel on a current food label.

Nutrition information is now required on virtually all processed food products.

The % Daily Value shows how a food fits into an overall daily diet but does not necessarily represent goals for diet planning. Upper limits are a better way to view the concept of 100% Daily Value, except for carbohydrate, dietary fiber, vitamins, and minerals.

Protein generally will not show a % Daily Value because determining % Daily Value would require expensive testing of protein quality of the product by the manufacturer.

Serving size is set for various food products in household units by labeling laws; this will no longer be left to the discretion of the manufacturer. If you eat double the serving size listed, you need to double the % Daily Value and the calorie value. If you eat one-half the serving size shown, cut the % Daily Value and the calorie value in half.

Number of calories from fat is listed on the new label format.

Daily Value incorporates RDI or DRV standards, whichever are appropriate. For example, vitamin A has an RDI standard, whereas cholesterol has a DRV standard. The Daily Values help you to easily compare Brand X with Brand Y.

Although the Dietary Guidelines recommend that Americans moderate their consumption of sugars, no specific recommendation for a maximum daily intake (in grams) has been made, so no Daily Value for sugars is available.

on such products, most of which have minimal health benefits at best. When it comes to nutrition, money is best spent on a variety of high-quality foods; however, under special circumstances, nutritional supplements may be justified.[19-21]

DIET THERAPY AS A COMPONENT OF DISEASE MANAGEMENT ≋

Although the maintenance of health and prevention of disease are primary goals throughout the life cycle, circumstances arise in every stage of life when dietary interventions are required to treat disease, trauma, or other undesirable situations. The basic principles governing diet therapy are simple: meet nutritional needs while modifying the diet to solve the health problem under treatment. Some changes in diet may be easily implemented, but others require special planning and in some cases major changes from established food habits. The degree to which an individual—with the help of family, friends, health care providers, and others—is able to follow short-term or permanent changes in diet varies in each case. The needed dietary changes may impact significantly on quality of life and in some cases even on chances of survival. While the focus of this book is health maintenance and disease prevention, some discussion must include selected problems that require diet and nutrition intervention.

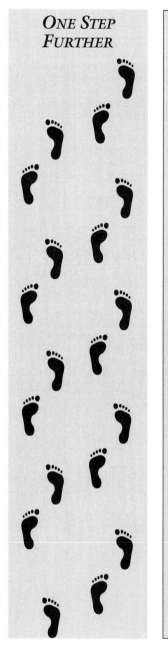

ONE STEP FURTHER

A New Resource for Nutrition Information: The Internet

The emergence of the computer era and the development of the Internet have allowed for the access of much nutrition data without opening a book. It can be a fascinating experience to "surf the web" and find sites that provide information that meets your needs. It is important to recognize, however, that there is no monitoring or evaluation of web site data to determine their accuracy. This is a valuable service built into the publication process of scientific journals and most textbooks. Admitting this shortfall, it is still possible to make good use of the Internet.

The references listed at the end of this box provide useful information about nutrition Internet resources, and the following web sites are worth noting:

American Dietetic Association
http://www.eatright.org
Arbor Nutrition Guide
http://arborcom.com
Dietary Guidelines for Americans
http://www.nal.usda.gov:80/fnic/dga/dguide95.html
Dietetics Online
http://www.dietetics.com
Food and Drug Administration
http://vm.cfsan.fda.gov/list.html
Food Guide Pyramid
http://www.nal.usda.gov:8001/pylpmap.htm
International Food Information Council
http://ificinfo.health.org
United States Department Agriculture (USDA)
http://www.usda.gov
USDA Center for Nutrition Policy and Promotion
http://www.usda.gov/fcs/cnpp.htm
USDA Food and Consumer Services
http://www.usda.gov/fcs/fcs.htm
USDA National Agriculture Library Food and Nutrition Information Center
http://www.nalusda.gov/fnic
USDA WIC Program
http://www.usda.gov/fcs/wic.htm

Capellano, K.L. 1998. Internet 101: A guide for food and nutrition professionals. *Nutr Today* 33:77.
————. 1998. More food and nutrition Internet resources. *Nutr Today* 33:94.
————. 1998. The wheat from the chaff: Sorting out nutrition information on the Internet. *J Am Diet Assoc* 98:1270.

Summary

Growth, development, reproduction, and the maintenance of health require that the human organism satisfy basic biologic needs. Nutrition is a basic need that can be met minimally to prevent death or optimally to help achieve maximum genetic potential. The goal of this book is to approach the issue of optimum nutrition from the developmental framework of specific stages of the life cycle. Attention to normal needs and feeding practices will predominate, but management strategies for selected special problems will be addressed. For more detailed coverage of special problems requiring diet therapy, the reader is referred to other available clinical texts.

Review Questions

1. Outline the key functions of the basic nutrients.
2. Describe the major influences on food choices of Americans.
3. Define the key nutritional concerns at each stage of the life cycle.
4. Describe the food pyramid concept.
5. Summarize the concept of Dietary Reference Intakes.
6. In your community, what factors do you think are of major importance in the development of dietary patterns?
7. The national nutrition objectives for the year 2000 are intended to reduce risk of what health problems in the United States?

THE ASSESSMENT
OF NUTRITIONAL NEEDS

Sue Rodwell Williams

≋ ≋ ≋ ≋ ≋ ≋ ≋ ≋ ≋

Basic Concepts

❑ *An integral component of health promotion for all persons throughout the life cycle is optimal personal and community nutrition.*

❑ *Through their specific and interdependent physiologic roles, certain nutrients in the food we eat are essential to life, health, and well-being.*

❑ *Changing nutrient needs throughout the life cycle relate to normal growth and development and resulting changes in body composition.*

❑ *The overall process of nutrition assessment reflects individual and community nutritional status and provides an important basis for personal health care plans and public nutrition intervention programs.*

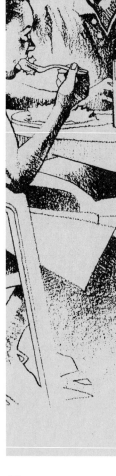

*W*e live in a rapidly changing world, one of changing environment, food supply, scientific knowledge, and population. Our numbers are increasing, not only in total population and age distribution but also in ethnic diversity. Then, within individual environments and communities, with physical growth and development through the life cycle come personality changes and changing personal needs and goals. These *constant changes* of life must be in *balance* to produce healthy living at any age.

Thus, to be realistic, within these life concepts of change and balance our study of life cycle nutrition focuses on health promotion through good food and its basic nutrients and an ongoing assessment of nutritional status and health needs. In this introductory chapter, we will focus on the process of assessing basic nutritional needs of both individuals and population groups. Because the background nutrition knowledge of students using this book varies widely, and to set the overall learning focus, we will look at a brief overview of nutritional assessment basics to provide a foundation for planning and providing sound nutritional care. This basic care must always assure the three fundamental physiologic components that must be present for the human body to survive and remain healthy: 1) energy to do its work, 2) building materials to maintain its form and functions, and 3) control agents, such as vitamins and minerals, to regulate these processes efficiently.

NUTRITIONAL STATUS OF PERSONS AND POPULATIONS ≈

Throughout the life cycle, in the health care of individuals and communities, **nutritional assessment** is the first step in developing nutritional care plans and programs. At both levels of care, individual clinical care plans and Public Health programs—although the scope of the work may vary from a simple conversation with a clinic patient or parent to a complex, nationwide survey including all ages—the basic goal of the assessment process remains the same—to identify nutritional status and needs on which to base care plans and programs designed to meet these identified needs.

Nutritional assessment
Process of determining individual or group nutritional status as a basis for identifying needs and goals and planning personal health care or community programs to meet these identified goals.

PERSON-CENTERED CLINICAL CARE ≈

Levels of Care

Nutrition is essential to individual health on two levels:
1. *Tissue level.* Nutrients and energy from the food we eat build and maintain body tissues. It is on the integrity of these tissues that the physiologic functioning and health of the body depend.
2. *Personal level.* Food has many meanings that help fulfill personal needs. It is on the integrity of these personal psychosocial and cultural values that health as a human being depend.

Needs and Goals

In personal health care or clinical nutrition, assessment of individuals helps health care providers, together with the patient or client, determine nutritional and health status on both physiologic tissue level and psychosocial personal level and plan nutritional care according to personal needs and goals. The overall goals are health promotion and disease prevention, or treatment of disease. If an underlying chronic disorder, such as diabetes mellitus, is present or if risk factors for potential health problems, such as heart disease, have begun to develop, the goal is healthy control of the disorder or prevention of the health problem by reduction of risk factors. All of these nutritional and health goals involve personal health and nutrition education and skills in self-care, as well as collaboration of a skilled and sensitive team of health care professionals, including a clinical nutritionist.

Phases of the Clinical Care Process

Five distinct yet interactive phases are essential in the **clinical care process:**
1. *Assessment.* A broad base of information about the person's body composition, nutrition and health status, food habits, and personal living situation provides necessary knowledge for assessing initial nutritional status and needs. Useful background information comes from various sources, primarily the individual and family, as well as health care records and other health care team members.
2. *Analysis.* The data collected must be analyzed carefully to determine specific needs. Some are evident immediately. Others develop as the situation unfolds. On the basis of this analysis, a list of problems forms.
3. *Care planning.* As problems are identified, valid care can be planned with the individual and family to solve them. This plan must be based on personal needs and goals, as well as any health problem involved.
4. *Implementation of the plan.* Realistic and appropriate actions planned are carried out. In nutritional care and education, this involves decisions and actions about the diet, mode of feeding as needed, and training of the person, staff, and family to carry out the plan.
5. *Evaluation and recording of the results.* As the plan is carried out, the results are monitored carefully to see if the needs are being met or if revisions in the plan must be made. Records of data, plans, procedures, and progress guide actions and instructions for continuing self-care.

Clinical care process
Interactive process of planning personal health care through five phases of assessment and data collection, analysis of findings, planning of care according to a written individual care plan, implementation of the plan, and evaluation and recording of the results.

COMMUNITY-CENTERED PUBLIC HEALTH ≈

Changing Population Patterns and Health Goals

As the 1990 census reported, the U.S. population continues to increase, reflecting rapid change, not only in total numbers but also in greater ethnic diversity, especially in border states such as California and Texas, and increasing age. In community nutrition, the assessment of population groups helps Public Health officials determine health goals and allocation of resources according to priority of need. Often the focus of this nutrition and health assessment is on groups of people bearing higher health risks: pregnant women, infants and children, adolescents, and elderly adults, especially those under the added stress of poverty, malnutrition, and illness.

Phases of the Community Care Process

Community care process
Program planning to meet defined community health needs through assessment procedures, objectives, program plan, and evaluation.

At whatever level of community nutrition work—national, state, or local—nutrition is an integral component of health and health care. The program-planning process to identify and meet health care needs involves four basic areas of activity:

1. *Assessment.* The two-fold process of assessment includes 1) data collection about the population of concern and 2) an analysis of the information to identify nutrition needs and problems.
2. *Objectives.* In relation to the identified needs or problems, both general goals and specific contributory objectives are determined to meet these needs. These goals involve staff and agency decisions about what actions are to be taken and a projected timeline for doing the work.
3. *Program plan.* To reach the established objectives, a specific plan of action is developed and carried out as projected. The program plan must consider such items as staff, tools, and documents required; sources of funding; and budget for cost control.
4. *Evaluation.* Assessment of program activities and results continues throughout the nutrition project for health promotion or disease prevention. On the basis of this monitoring information, revisions may be made for study purposes or for conversion to a regular, ongoing program status.

Community Groups with Special Life Cycle Needs

Several higher-risk groups in the general population require special nutritional attention, especially if their normal growth and development needs are compounded by such basic problems as poverty:

1. *Pregnant women.* During a woman's pregnancy, she must meet increased nutrient and energy needs to support this period of rapid fetal growth and to bring the pregnancy to a successful outcome. At best, this period is one of physiologic stress. In poor circumstances, this normal stress is compounded by inadequate nutrition, bringing increased stress to both mother and baby. Ongoing nutritional assessment can identify specific needs, help prevent problems and complications, and promote a healthy pregnancy for both mother and baby.
2. *Infants and children.* The highest nutrient requirements per kilogram of body weight during the entire life cycle occur during infancy, when rates of growth and metabolism are at their highest point. Because of this direct relation between growth and nutritional status, careful nutritional assessment is required to monitor progress. Over the following period of young childhood, the growth pattern slows and becomes erratic, with alternating small growth spurts and plateaus. Continued assessment of progress is essential to promote health.
3. *Adolescents.* With puberty comes the second large growth spurt for the child. In both sexes, intensive growth and hormonal changes profoundly affect nutritional needs. The continued monitoring of growth, changing body composition, and nutritional status helps ensure the foundations of a healthy adulthood.

4. *Adults and the elderly.* With our increasing life span, the gradual aging process through adulthood requires a sound nutritional base to maintain health and prevent or control chronic diseases, which account for 75% of all deaths in the United States. Nutritional risk factors are associated with most of these chronic diseases of aging.

METHODS OF ASSESSMENT: CLINICAL AND POPULATION ≋

Whether the assessment is being done in a clinical or community setting, four basic methods are used—anthropometric, biochemical, clinical, and dietary. Community assessment centers mainly on dietary intake surveys and nutrient analyses, but comparative data from biochemical tests, body measurements, and various clinical observations are also used to evaluate individual nutritional status, as well as to provide practical information about response to nutrition intervention programs. Clinical assessment may include a broader focus on related disease processes, with more extensive biochemical and clinical assessment. Whatever the situation, all four methods together provide essential information to identify needs and to plan health care. The American Dietetic Association has developed comprehensive guidelines and components for appropriate nutrition screening and assessment and determination of nutritional risk.[1] To review assessment basics, a few of the commonly used measures in each method category are briefly outlined in the following sections.

Anthropometry

Anthropometry is the process of measuring various dimensions of the human body. Several of these body measures provide valid estimates of the muscle and fat components of body composition. They have the advantage of being inexpensive and simple to obtain. Skill gained through careful practice will minimize the margin of error. The selection and maintenance of proper procedures and equipment, as well as attention to careful technique, will help secure accurate data.

> **Anthropometry**
> (Gr *anthropos*, man, human; *metron*, measure) The process of measuring various dimensions of the human body to help determine basic body composition and needs.

1. *Weight.* For accuracy, use regular clinic beam balance scales with nondetachable weights, with an additional weight attachment for use with very obese persons. Metric scales with readings to the nearest 20 g provide specific data, but the standard clinic scale is satisfactory. Read and record the person's weight; then obtain information about usual body weight and check standard height-weight tables for comparison. However, approach these tables with caution in applying them to individuals as specific ideals, remembering that wide *normal* variations occur in healthy bodies. Keeping this in mind, interpret present weight in terms of percentage of the person's usual body weight, with general reference to standard tables. Check for any significant weight loss.

2. *Height.* Use a true vertical bar, such as a flat wall-attached measuring stick or the movable measuring rod on the platform clinic scales. Have the person put his or her back to the measuring rod and stand as straight as possible, without shoes or hat, heels together, looking straight ahead. The heels, buttocks, shoulders, and head should be touching the vertical measuring surface. Read and record the measure. Compare it with previous recordings to detect possible errors and to note the growth of children or diminishing height of older adults.

3. *Body mass index (BMI).* The weight and height measures can be used to calculate the person's body mass index (BMI), a value often used in clinical assessment:

> **Body mass index (BMI)**
> A calculated assessment of body mass based on weight and height: BMI = weight (kg) ÷ height (m)^2.

$$BMI = \text{weight (kg)} \div \text{height (m)}^2$$

The metric conversion factors involved are 1 kg equals 2.2 lb and 1 m equals 39.37 in. This weight/height ratio is commonly used in evaluating obesity states in relation to risk factors. The desired health maintenance BMI range for adults is 20 to 25 kg/m^2. Health risks associated with obesity begin in the range of 25 to 30 kg/m^2. Values above 40 kg/m^2 indicate severe obesity.

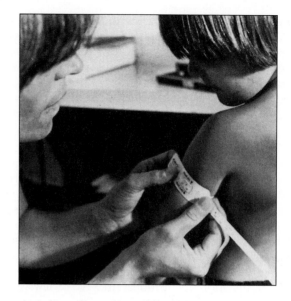

FIG. 2-1 Mid-upper-arm circumference is measured with paper tape that touches skin but does not compress tissue.

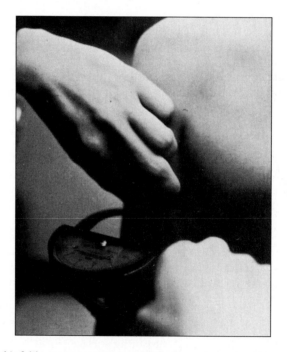

FIG. 2-2 Triceps skinfold measurements are taken midway between the acromion and olecranon processes.

4. *Mid-upper-arm circumference (MAC)*. On the nondominant arm, unless it is affected by edema, use a nonstretchable centimeter tape to locate the midpoint of the upper arm (Fig. 2-1). Measure the circumference at this midpoint. Read this measure accurately to the nearest tenth of a centimeter and record. Compare this result with previous measurements to note possible changes and with standard reference tables.
5. *Triceps skinfold thickness (TSF)*. With thumb and forefinger, grasp a vertical pinch of the skin and subcutaneous fat at this previously marked upper-arm midpoint and gently pull away from the underlying muscle (Fig. 2-2). Using a standard millime-

ter skinfold caliper and avoiding excessive pressure, measure the skinfold thickness quickly, within 2 or 3 seconds, to the nearest full or fraction of a millimeter. For increased accuracy, take three measures and use the mean for calculations. Record the results and compare them with standard reference tables. This measure provides a good estimate of the subcutaneous fat reserves.[2]

6. *Mid-upper-arm muscle circumference (MAMC)*. Using the two previous measures, calculate this value to provide a good indirect measure of the body's skeletal muscle mass:

$$MAMC(cm) = MAC(cm) - [\pi \times TSF(cm)]$$

If desired, the TSF can be left in millimeters as measured and the value of the mathematical factor *pi* in the formula changed accordingly to 0.314. The formula then is

$$MAMC(cm) = MAC(cm) - [0.314 \times TSF(mm)]$$

Standard reference tables for all of these body measures are given in appendix F.

Biochemical Tests

Numerous biochemical tests are available for assessing nutritional status. The following are most commonly used. Further description, formulas, and reference standards are given in appendix H.

1. *Plasma protein*. Basic measures of plasma protein include serum albumin, hematocrit, and hemoglobin. Also, for persons with diabetes the standard monitoring tool, especially during an intensive insulin therapy program, is the **glycosylated hemoglobin A_{1c}**. Additional general tests may include serum transferrin or total iron-binding capacity (TIBC) and ferritin.

2. *Protein metabolism*. Basic twenty-four-hour urine tests are used to measure urinary creatinine and urea nitrogen levels. These materials are products of protein metabolism. The twenty-four-hour excretion of creatinine is interpreted in terms of ideal creatinine excretion for height, the creatinine-height index (CHI). The twenty-four-hour urea nitrogen excretion is used with the calculated dietary nitrogen intake (6.25 g protein = 1 g nitrogen) over the same twenty-four hour-period to calculate nitrogen balance:

$$Nitrogen\ balance = (Protein\ intake \div 6.25) - (Urinary\ urea\ nitrogen + 4)$$

3. *Immune system integrity*. Any diminished capacity of the immune system *(anergy)* is reflected in basic measures such as lymphocyte count and by additional skin testing, observing for any delayed sensitivity to common recall antigens such as mumps or purified protein derivative of tuberculin (PPD).

Clinical Observations

Careful observations of physical signs of nutritional status provide an important added dimension to the overall assessment of individuals. Using a general examination guide for such physical signs, as given in table 2-1, check for any possible evidence of malnutrition. Also, other physical data may include such vital signs as pulse rate, respiration, temperature, and blood pressure. A study of the common procedures of a normal physical examination will provide useful background orientation.

Dietary Evaluation

Information about the food intake of different groups of people or individuals is usually obtained by the use of several basic tools. Choices among these procedures are guided by the purposes of the assessment, as well as by the available staff and funds. More than one tool may be used for cross-checking or expanding the data received. For example, an initial nutritional history to learn basic food patterns may be followed with specific food records to provide some examples of actual food choices and quantities, as well as a meal/snack schedule. A brief review of commonly used diet evaluation methods follows.

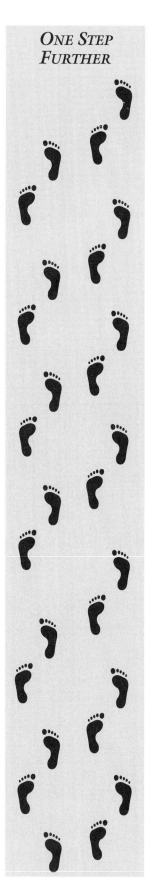

How Tall Is the Child in the Wheelchair?

A variety of conditions affecting children make it difficult to assess growth. Children who cannot stand are among those who may be evaluated using either tibial length (Fig. 2-3) or measurements of armspan (Fig. 2-4). Tibial length is defined as the distance between the medial tibial epicondyle to the medial malleolus. To measure tibial length, subjects are seated with their feet resting as flat on the floor as possible. The appropriate points are located and marked. An anthropometer is used to measure the distance between the two points. Height is estimated from the equation

$$\text{Height (cm)} = 3.54 \times \text{Tibial length} + 32.23$$

Armspan is defined as the greatest distance between the outstretched fingers of the left and right hands with the arms and forearms extended horizontally sideways and the back pressed against a flat surface. Researchers have found a correlation of armspan to linear height (normal armspan/height ratio = 1). While both of these measurements provide only estimates, they have been useful in some clinical settings.

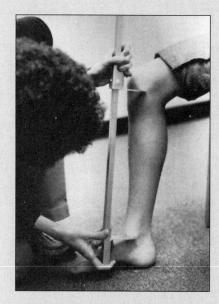

FIG. 2-3   Tibia length measurement.

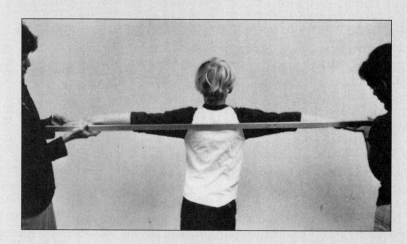

FIG. 2-4   Arm span is measured from the tip of one middle finger to the other.

TABLE 2-1   *Clinical Signs of Nutritional Status*

	Good	Poor
General appearance	Alert, responsive	Listless, apathetic; cachexia
Hair	Shiny, lustrous; healthy scalp	Stringy, dull, brittle, dry, depigmented
Neck glands	No enlargement	Thyroid enlarged
Skin, face and neck	Smooth, slightly moist; good color, reddish pink mucous membranes	Greasy, discolored, scaly
Eyes	Bright, clear; no fatigue circles	Dry, signs of infection, increased vascularity, glassiness, thickened conjunctiva
Lips	Good color, moist	Dry, scaly, swollen; angular lesions (stomatitis)
Tongue	Good pink color, surface papillae present, no lesions	Papillary atrophy, smooth appearance; swollen, red, beefy (glossitis)
Gums	Good pink color; no swelling or bleeding; firm	Marginal redness or swelling; receding, spongy
Teeth	Straight, no crowding; well-shaped jaw; clean; no discoloration	Unfilled cavities, absent teeth, worn surfaces, mottled, malpositioned
Skin, general	Smooth, slightly moist; good color	Rough, dry, scaly, pale, pigmented, irritated; petechiae, bruises
Abdomen	Flat	Swollen
Legs, feet	No tenderness, weakness, or swelling; good color	Edema, tender calf; tingling, weakness
Skeleton	No malformations	Bowlegs, knock-knees, chest deformity at diaphragm, beaded ribs, prominent scapulae
Weight	Normal for height, age, body build	Overweight or underweight
Posture	Erect, arms and legs straight, abdomen in, chest out	Sagging shoulders, sunken chest, humpback
Muscles	Well developed, firm	Flaccid, poor tone; undeveloped, tender
Nervous control	Good attention span for age; does not cry easily; not irritable or restless	Inattentive, irritable
Gastrointestinal function	Good appetite and digestion; normal, regular elimination	Anorexia, indigestion, constipation, diarrhea
General vitality	Good endurance; energetic, vigorous; sleeps well at night	Easily fatigued, no energy, falls asleep in school, looks tired, apathetic

1. *Diet history.* Depending on the assessment needs, information about food habits may be obtained by a comprehensive nutrition interview or a tested questionnaire filled out by the individual or parent and followed up by a brief personal review by the nutritionist as needed. Whatever its form, a careful nutritional history—including related living situation and other personal, psychosocial, and economic problems, as well as any drugs being used—is a fundamental base of nutritional assessment.

2. *Twenty-four-hour recall.* Individuals are asked to recall the specific food items they ate during the previous day, describing the nature and amount of each. Sometimes this method is used because it is simpler and less costly than a longer diet history, but it has disadvantages in some groups, such as elderly persons whose memory may be limited. Also, there are measurement problems in determining portion sizes.

3. *Food records.* At times a full dietary analysis of all nutrient and energy values is needed and a three- to seven-day food record supplies the detailed information. Individuals are asked to record their food intake for a brief period, or on certain days periodically. Each person is taught how to describe food items used singly and in combination and how to measure amounts eaten. Studies indicate that a three-day record is usually sufficient and the best choice to provide accurate information for nutritional analysis.[3] Currently, computer analysis of these daily food records is common, using a computer program with a large database of food values for analysis of the person's intake of kcalories (energy) and nutrients as compared with the Recommended Dietary Allowances. A simple food analysis may be made by comparison with the five food groups of the Food Guide Pyramid.[4]

4. *Food frequency questionnaire.* This assessment tool provides information about an individual's food intake over an extended period of time, useful data when studying a group's disease risk and incidence.[5] It has two basic parts: 1) a list of foods and 2) a scale for checking frequency of use over a given period of time.

ASSESSMENT EVALUATION CRITERIA ≋

Well-Nourished Persons

Throughout the life cycle, nutritional status monitoring, guided by reference growth standards for each age group and general signs of good or poor nutrition as were outlined in table 2-1, helps assure sound nutrition and healthy development. The rapid growth and development of the early years of life and the stress of aging in later adult years carry risks and require special attention.

1. *Pregnancy.* During a woman's pregnancy, she must meet increased nutrient and energy needs to support this period of rapid fetal growth and bring the pregnancy to a successful conclusion. Sufficient weight gain to meet maternal-fetal-placental demands during the pregnancy must be assured. Recent criteria for this weight gain, which reflects a positive nutritional status, have been established by the National Academy of Sciences' Institute of Medicine and can serve as a general guide.[6] Optimal nutrient and energy intake to meet both pregnancy and lactation needs can be monitored in general terms by the Recommended Dietary Allowances (see inside book covers) and guidelines discussed in chapters 3 through 5. As previously mentioned, at best, pregnancy is a period of physiologic stress; in poor circumstances, this normal stress is compounded by inadequate nutrition, bringing increased stress to both mother and baby. Ongoing nutrition assessment can identify specific needs, help prevent problems and complications, and promote a healthy pregnancy for both mother and baby.

2. *Early growth and childhood.* As previously discussed, the highest nutrient requirements per kg body weight during the entire life cycle occur during infancy, when rates of growth and metabolism are at their highest point. Because of this direct relation between growth and nutritional status, close nutrition assessment is required to monitor progress. Over the following period of young childhood, the growth pattern slows and becomes erratic as the child grows in spurts and plateaus. Con-

tinued assessment of progress is essential to promote health. Commonly used monitoring tools are the age-specific growth charts from birth through adolescence, such as the National Center for Health Statistics percentile charts (included in appendix A). Age-specific RDA nutrient and energy levels can serve as general criteria (see chapters 8, 9, and 10 for interpretations and guidance).

3. *Adolescence.* As mentioned, with puberty comes the second large growth spurt for the child. In both sexes, intensive growth, under control of hormonal changes, profoundly affects nutritional needs. The continued monitoring of growth, changing body composition, and nutritional status helps ensure foundations for a healthy adulthood. In addition to the growth charts through age eighteen, extensive height-weight tables for the adolescent years are included in appendix B. The RDA reference standard provides general evaluation criteria for monitoring nutrient and energy needs. Refer to chapters 10, 11, and 12 for specific monitoring guidelines.

4. *Aging and the aged.* As previously stated, with our increasing life span, the gradual aging process through adulthood requires a sound nutritional base to maintain health and prevent or control chronic diseases, which account for 75% of all deaths in the United States. Nutritional risk factors are associated with most all of these chronic diseases of aging. The age-adjusted height-weight table (see appendix C) provides better evaluation criteria for older adults than does the regular standard tables. Also, alternate measures of height and weight for stooped or nonambulatory older adults are included in the appendix C. The RDA provide general nutrient-energy standards, although more specific individual analysis of needs may be required for elderly persons. These needs are discussed in detail in chapter 14.

Malnourished Persons

Poorly nourished persons can be found at both extremes of the nutrient- energy intake range. On one hand, gross deficits are obvious in children suffering from protein-energy malnutrition; on the other, extreme nutrient deficits may be masked by obesity from excess caloric intake.

1. *Protein-energy malnutrition.* The high risk of malnutrition in low-income families caught in a cycle of poverty, as well as among the "new poor," is well known and documented. There is also a growing awareness of the extent of various degrees of malnutrition among persons in hospitals, rehabilitation centers, and other long-term care facilities, especially among elderly patients or residents. Assessment procedures in Public Health Services and medical/nursing facilities are designed to identify persons at risk for malnutrition. This assessment can provide the base for planning community intervention programs or individual care plans for needed nutritional support and family food assistance programs, especially for pregnant women, infants, and young children to meet crucial growth needs.

2. *Obesity.* Obesity, especially extreme forms, is a dangerous form of malnutrition, because it carries an increased risk of chronic disease, such as hypertension, heart disease, and diabetes. Weight assessment and early monitoring, especially of children in families at high risk for obesity and chronic disease, are important health promotion and disease prevention practices.

IMPORTANCE OF NUTRITIONAL ASSESSMENT TO HEALTH CARE AND PUBLIC POLICY ≋

Nutritional Care Management

In both preventive health care and clinical care of disease, nutritional assessment is the essential first step in identifying individual nutritional needs and in planning valid care to meet these needs. Careful assessment in health care can detect underlying risk factors early, so that programs for reducing these risks and helping prevent related disease can be initiated. In clinical care, assessment of nutritional needs can identify and help change lifestyle

CASE STUDY

*The Patient with Insulin-Dependent Diabetes Mellitus**

Anne Davis is a forty-five-year-old woman diagnosed two years ago with insulin-dependent diabetes mellitus (IDDM)–Type 1. She has three children whose birth weights were in the range of 4.5 to 5.0 kg (10 to 11 lb). The children, now teenagers, show no signs of diabetes and their weights are reported to be within normal limits, despite their mother's fondness for cooking. Her husband, an underpaid construction worker, is slightly overweight.

Six months ago, Mrs. Davis was seen with a complaint of a series of infections during the past two months that lasted longer than usual. At that time, she was measured as 165 cm (5 ft 5 in) and 93 kg (205 lb). Her glucose tolerance test was positive. She was seen for follow-up twice during the following month, each time showing hyperglycemia and glycosuria. At the second follow-up, an oral hypoglycemic agent was prescribed, and she was referred to the clinic dietitian for weight management counseling.

Mrs. Davis did not keep this appointment or her subsequent medical appointment. She was not seen again until a month ago, when she was admitted with ketoacidosis. She responded well to treatment and was placed on a weight reduction diet and a mixture of intermediate- and rapid-acting insulin given in two injections a day. On discharge, she was again referred to the clinic dietitian for individual counseling and diabetes education classes.

Questions for analysis
1. What factors do you think contributed to the ketoacidosis? Why? What relation do these factors have to diabetes control?
2. What additional information about Mrs. Davis is necessary to understand her major nutritional problems? Why? How could this information be obtained?
3. Based on the information provided, what nutritional problems can be identified? What is the scientific basis for each problem?
4. Outline an appropriate day's food plan for Mrs. Davis using meals and interval snacks to guide her weight reduction and diabetes control. Also outline a schedule of self-monitoring of blood glucose for Mrs. Davis. Assume that she administers the insulin before breakfast and before the evening meal, and that she is using the Food Exchange System for meal and snack planning with the clinical dietitian's guidance.
5. Identify any personal factors that may affect Mrs. Davis' follow-through with her treatment plan. Do you anticipate any problems? If so, how would you attempt to help her solve them? Outline a diabetes education plan for Mrs. Davis.

*Used with permission from *Essentials of Nutrition and Diet Therapy*, 7th edition, S. Rodwell Williams, Mosby.

factors and food habits that contribute to the disease process and, thus, control its progress. A number of these health promotion and disease prevention or management approaches are discussed in chapter 13.

Public Nutrition Intervention Programs

In a similar manner, Public Health intervention programs must include careful assessment of community need and resources, identifying persons with problems that hinder care as well as the higher cost in the long run of unmet needs. For example, the community cost, (in taxes), of simple supportive prenatal care for poor pregnant women is far less than the high long-term cost of neonatal medical technology for salvaging tiny, **low birth weight** babies, premature and with multiple medical problems, who then die in infancy or require continuous disability care. Similar situations exist in the care of young children and older adults.

low birth weight
Birth weight less than 2,500 g (5.4 lb). Very low birth weight: birth weight less than 1,500 g (3.3 lb).

Poor childhood nutrition, especially during important early growth and development years, contributes to learning disabilities and educational problems. Unmet older adult nutritional needs contribute to progressive chronic disease and long-term costly care.

Summary

Nutrition is an integral component of both health and health care. Thus, nutritional assessment, both community and clinical, is basic to meeting nutritional needs. This assessment process includes a variety of methods, including anthropometric, biochemical, clinical, and dietary procedures, and is important to both health care and public policy.

Review Questions

1. What basic role does assessment play in meeting nutritional needs? Compare this role in both clinical and community nutrition.
2. Identify the four basic methods of nutrition assessment and give examples of each.
3. Describe the importance of this basic assessment to nutritional health care and public policy.
4. Describe a process of estimating height in a wheelchair-bound person.

MATERNAL NUTRITION: THE BEGINNING OF LIFE AND THE PHYSIOLOGY OF PREGNANCY

Bonnie S. Worthington-Roberts

≋ ≋ ≋ ≋ ≋ ≋ ≋ ≋ ≋ ≋

Basic Concepts

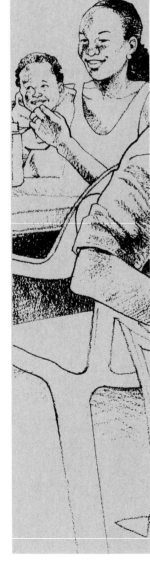

❏ *Human fetal growth is an amazing phenomenon.*

❏ *Maternal nutrition influences fetal growth.*

❏ *Physiologic changes during pregnancy impact the maternal diet and nutritional needs.*

*F*ood is essential to life and growth. Without an adequate supply of food, and the nutrients it contains, an organism cannot grow and develop normally. Eventually it dies.

In spite of these simple and well-established facts, the role that nutrition plays in the course and outcome of pregnancy has not always been recognized. In the controlled conditions of the laboratory, researchers have been able to demonstrate harmful effects of deficient diets on pregnant animals and their offspring in a number of species. However, when studies are made on free-living human populations, direct relationships between what a mother eats during the nine months of gestation and the course and outcome of her pregnancy are not always evident. Consequently, the emphasis that nutrition has received in prenatal care has varied over the years.

Part of the problem is that the changes occurring during pregnancy, their influence on nutritional needs, and the effects of long-term nutritional status on reproductive performance are not fully understood. The application of nutrition principles to pregnancy has had to depend on progress in scientific knowledge about reproduction itself, and, as in any science, one of the most important advances is simply learning to ask the right questions. The emphasis of research has changed as more has become known about nutrition, reproduction, and human growth. It is therefore easy to understand why different dietary recommendations for pregnant women have been made.

Before launching into consideration of the nutrition issues associated with fetal development and maternal needs during pregnancy, this chapter will outline the amazing events in utero and their impact on maternal physiology.

STAGES OF HUMAN FETAL GROWTH [1] ≋

After the ovum is released from the mature follicle in the ovary, it enters the fallopian tube (fig. 3-1). It moves slowly through the tube toward the uterus, encountering potentially fertilizing sperm along the way. The stages of human embryonic-fetal growth are illustrated in fig. 3-2. Fertilization usually occurs in the fallopian tube within forty-eight

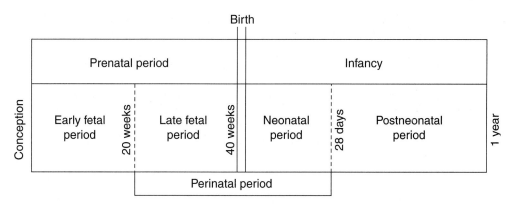

FIG. 3-1 Periods of prenatal and infant life.

hours, after which cell division rapidly proceeds. The resulting solid ball of cells, the **morula,** enters the uterus, where it undergoes reorganization into a hollow ball, the **blastocyst.** The blastocyst ultimately buries itself in the endometrial lining of the uterus (five to seven days postovulation). There the precursor cells of the placenta begin to arrange themselves into a functioning placental unit. Nutritional support for the embryo at this time comes from the endometrial lining of the uterus. After its initial development, the placenta grows rapidly throughout gestation. By thirty-four to thirty-six weeks, the fetus has completed cell division. From that time until term, growth continues only by increases in the size of the existing cells.

Embryologic studies indicate three stages of fetal growth:

1. *Blastogenesis stage.* The fertilized egg divides into cells that fold in on one another. An inner cell mass evolves, giving rise to the embryo and an outer coat, the *trophoblast,* which becomes the placenta. This process is complete about two weeks after fertilization.
2. *Embryonic stage.* This is the critical time when cells differentiate into three germinal layers. The **ectoderm,** outer layer, gives rise to the brain, nervous system, hair, and skin. The **mesoderm,** middle layer, produces all of the voluntary muscles, bones, and components of the cardiovascular and excretory systems. The **endoderm,** inner layer, forms the digestive and respiratory systems and glandular organs. By sixty days' gestation, all of the major features of the human infant have been achieved.
3. *Fetal stage.* This is the period of most rapid growth. From the third month until term, fetal weight increases nearly 500-fold from 6 g (0.2 oz) to 3,000–3,500 g (6.5 to 7.5 lb) at birth. The average weight curve from ten weeks to term is shown in fig. 3-3.

Measurements of DNA and protein in embryonic and fetal tissues show that embryonic growth occurs only by increase in number of cells, **hyperplasia.** Fetal growth continues in cell number but now also involves increase in cell size **hypertrophy.** The stages of cell growth involving hyperplasia and hypertrophy are illustrated in fig. 3-4.

Growth-Retarded Infants

From the sequence described, it is possible to estimate the effects of malnutrition on growth at different stages of gestation. In the early months of pregnancy, a severe limit on supply or transport of nutrients would have to occur to cause retarded growth, because the quantitative requirements of the embryo are extremely small. Nevertheless, a restriction of materials and energy needed for cell synthesis and cell differentiation could produce malformations or cause the embryo to die. Malnutrition after the third month of gestation would not have teratogenic effects, but it could interfere with fetal growth. Nutrient requirements are greatest in the last trimester of pregnancy, when cells are increasing rapidly in both number and size. Even a relatively mild restriction could have serious effects at this time.

Morula
(L *morus,* mulberry) Solid mass of cells resembling a mulberry, formed by cleavage of a fertilized ovum.

Blastocyst
(Gr *blastos,* germ; *kystic,* sac, bladder) A stage in the development of the embryo in which the cells are arranged in a single layer to form a hollow sphere.

Ectoderm
(Gr *ektos,* outside; *derma,* skin) Outermost of the three primitive cell layers of the embryo.

Mesoderm
(Gr *mesos,* middle; *derma,* skin) Intermediate layer of embryonic cells developing between the ectoderm and endoderm.

Endoderm
(Gr *endon,* within; *derma,* skin) Innermost of the three primitive embryonic cell layers.

Hyperplasia
(Gr *hyper,* above; *plasis,* formation) Enlargement of tissue due to a process of rapidly increasing cell number.

Hypertrophy
(Gr *hyper,* above; *trophe,* nutrition) Enlargement of an organ or a part due to the process of increasing cell size.

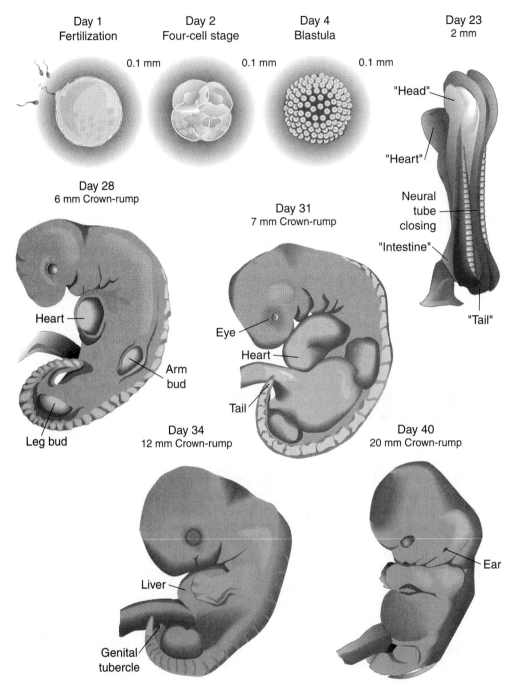

FIG. 3-2   Stages of fetal development.

Characteristics of SGA Infants

Gestational age
Stage of fetal growth and development at birth, varying from a premature delivery to full term.

The effects of fetal malnutrition are reflected in the characteristics of small-for-**gestational-age** (SGA) infants, who, although full term, are poorly developed. Their conditions are variable, suggesting the multiple causes and importance of timing shown in animal studies. Among the SGA infants who do not have birth anomalies, there are two patterns of growth retardation. One type affects weight more than length; the other affects weight and length equally:

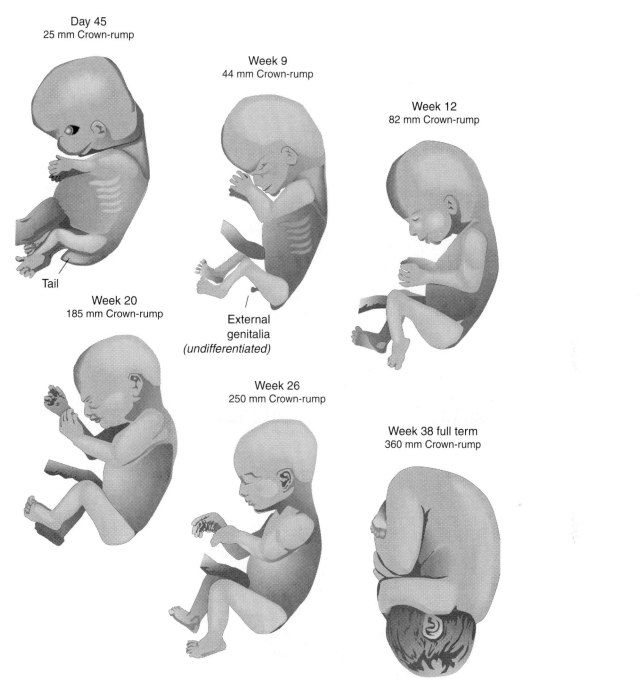

Day 45
25 mm Crown-rump

Tail

Week 9
44 mm Crown-rump

External
genitalia
(undifferentiated)

Week 12
82 mm Crown-rump

Week 20
185 mm Crown-rump

Week 26
250 mm Crown-rump

Week 38 full term
360 mm Crown-rump

FIG. 3-2   cont'd.

1. *Type I: growth retardation primarily affecting weight.* Head size (circumference) and skeletal growth are about normal, but the infants have poorly developed muscles and almost no subcutaneous fat. The resemblance of these infants to the large head and small body features of animals malnourished during the last weeks of gestation, either by maternal dietary restrictions or uterine ligation, is remarkable.

2. *Type II: growth reduction in both weight and height.* Size of all parts of the body, including head circumference and skeleton, is reduced proportionally. The physical

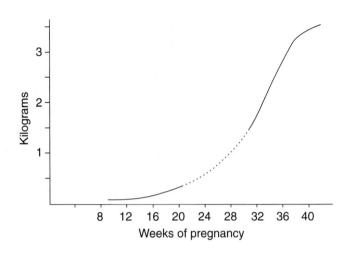

FIG. 3-3   Average curve of fetal growth.

From Hytten, E.E., and I. Leitch. 1971. *The physiology of human pregnancy,* 2d ed. Oxford: Blackwell Scientific Publications; reprinted from Thompson, A.M., et al. 1965. *J Obstet Gynaec Brit Commonw* 75:903.

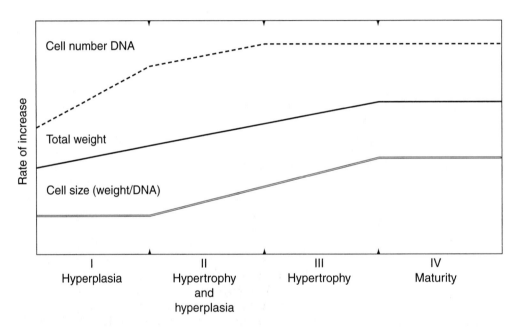

FIG. 3-4   Stages of cell growth.

Modified from Winick, M. 1968. *Nutr Rev* 26:195.

characteristics of these infants are similar to those of rat pups whose mothers had deficient diets throughout all of gestation.

NUTRITIONAL INFLUENCES ON FETAL GROWTH ≋

It is not possible, for obvious reasons, to examine maternal-fetal relationships directly at the cellular and molecular levels in humans. Consequently, work toward understanding how maternal nutrition influences growth and development in utero must be done on animals. The technique has usually been to manipulate the diets of pregnant animals and study the effects on cellular morphology and physiology in the offspring at various stages of gestation. Over the past 50 years, much information has accumulated from studies of this type.[2]

Experiments in Animals

Energy and nutrient restriction. Two types of dietary restrictions have been imposed on laboratory animals to study the effects of maternal nutrition on fetal growth and development. One restriction is simply not giving the animals enough food, so that the diet is low in kilocalories. The other restriction holds kilocalories at an adequate level but reduces or completely eliminates one or more essential nutrients. The effects of deficiencies of almost all of the known nutrients have been studied this way, but restrictions of protein and kilocalories have more relevance to humans than restrictions of vitamins or minerals. All animals need energy and use protein in essentially the same way, but the need for vitamins and minerals and their specific functions differ from species to species.

A number of investigators have demonstrated what can happen to fetuses when pregnant animals are fed kilocalorie- or protein-restricted diets. Maternal malnutrition can interfere with the mother's ability to conceive, it can produce death and resorption or abortion of the fetuses, and it can produce malformations or retarded growth. Of course, the more severe the dietary restrictions are, the more serious the effects will be. A reduction of as little as 25% of the total kilocalories without an imbalance in the quality of the maternal diet in rats can reduce both the number of pups born and their ability to survive.

Biochemical studies show why this occurs. One effect of protein-kilocalorie malnutrition is an impairment of cell energy metabolism through interference with the enzymes involved in glycolysis and the citric acid cycle. Without adequate supplies of amino acids and energy, cell functions break down, and the normal processes of growth cannot occur. The effects are most damaging when cells are normally undergoing rapid division. This implies that the timing of the dietary deficiency, as well as its severity, is important.

Types of growth failure. It is now clear that a number of things can produce growth failure in utero. The cause can be either "intrinsic" or "extrinsic." In differential diagnosis, the condition of the placentas of animals born small for gestational age is considered. In *intrinsic intrauterine growth failure,* placentas are usually of normal size. This implies that fetal growth retardation was not caused by inadequate maternal-fetal transport but was the result of other factors. Some examples include chromosomal abnormalities and maternal infections. *Extrinsic intrauterine growth failure* is usually manifested by placentas that are reduced in size. This indicates that they were incapable of supplying the fetus with adequate nutrition.

The principle feature of intrinsic growth failure is the presence of multiple malformations in the fetuses. These are absent in growth failure produced experimentally by ligation of the blood vessels supplying the placenta. They are variable in maternal malnutrition, depending on the timing of the restriction. In both vascular and nutritional failure, placentas are reduced in proportion to fetal weight. In the ligated animals and in late maternal malnutrition, the reduction is caused by a decrease in the average size of the cells. Maternal protein restriction maintained throughout most of the gestation, however, decreases both the number and size of placental cells.

The fetuses themselves also show different patterns of growth retardation. Those subjected to vascular insufficiency show an asymmetric retardation. The fetuses have relatively normal brain size and head circumference, but their livers are greatly reduced, by as much as 50%, and glycogen reserves are completely absent. Proportionally, these animals have bigger brains and heads compared with the rest of their bodies. They are extremely hypoglycemic at birth.

When maternal protein restriction is limited to the last few days of gestation, the fetuses show a pattern of growth retardation similar to that produced by vascular insufficiency—proportionally big heads and small bodies. However, when the restriction is imposed throughout most of the gestation period, the pattern of fetal growth retardation becomes more symmetric. There is a 15–20% decrease in cell number in all organs, including the brain. Head circumference is also reduced. The reduced cell number is greatest in the regions of the brain that are undergoing the most rapid rates of cell division.

Consequences of growth failure. These findings make it obvious that fetuses are *not* perfect parasites that can survive intrauterine insults without adverse effects. Data suggest

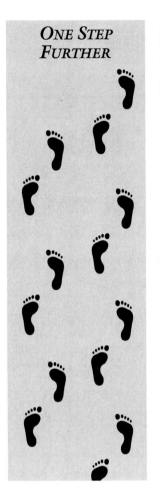

Does Prenatal Nutrition Influence Risk of Adult Disease?

Recent research suggests that human fetuses have to adapt to a limited or excessive supply of nutrients; in so doing, their physiology and metabolism are permanently changed. These changes can be said to be "programmed" and may be the origins of a number of diseases in later life. One disease suspected to be related to this fetal environment is coronary heart disease and the related disorders of stroke, diabetes, and hypertension. Another adult condition suggested to be influenced by the in utero environment is obesity.

The mechanisms by which a fetus may be permanently "programmed" are now the focus of considerable research. It is believed that there are critical periods for the development of specific organs and functions and that nutritional factors affect first the proliferation of cells at specific periods of life and then the developmental changes during a second phase of growth. In addition, nutrition (of specific nutrients) are known to affect early embryonic development; it can also affect metabolic regulation and cellular function through variations in gene expression and other molecular mechanisms.

The importance of this new field of investigation is substantial, since most attention to the development of these adult problems has focused on the adult lifestyle and dietary factors that contribute to disease onset and progression. If risk reduction can begin in the prenatal period, aggressive efforts can be made at this time that can change the course of a human life.

1996. Early nutrition and lifelong health. *Nutr Rev* 54:S1–S76.
Barker, D.J.P. 1996. The fetal origins of adult disease. *Nutr Today* 31:108.
Barker, D.J.P., C.N. Martyn, C. Osmond, and C.N. Hales. 1993. Growth in utero and serum concentrations in adult life. *BMJ* 307:1524.
Langley-Evans, S., and A. Jackson. 1996. Intrauterine programming of hypertension: Nutrient-hormone interactions. *Nutr Rev* 54:163.
Ravelli, A.C.J. et al. 1998. Glucose tolerance in adults after prenatal exposure to famine. *Lancet* 351:173.
Whitaker, R.C., and W.H. Dietz. 1998. Role of the prenatal environment in the development of obesity. *J Pediatr* 132:768.

that inadequate maternal nutrition can affect the fetus in ways that coincide with the stages of cell growth and that the body reserves of the mother cannot always insulate the fetus from dietary deficiencies. What happens to animals whose mothers were nutritionally deprived during pregnancy depends to a great extent on how they are fed after birth.

Perhaps the finding of most concern is the effect of continued deprivation on the growth of brain cells. If prenatally malnourished pups are restricted after birth by feeding them in litters of eighteen pups per dam, they demonstrate a 60% reduction in brain cell number by the time they are weaned. This contrasts with the 20–25% reduction associated with prenatal or postnatal malnutrition alone. Thus, it seems that continued malnutrition throughout the time the brain cells are dividing produces greater deficits than would be expected if the separate effects were simply added together. Experiments have shown that nutritional rehabilitation does not enable these animals to recover their normal size once the period of cell proliferation has passed. They continue to be small no matter how well fed they are after weaning. Other data suggest that maternal malnutrition may even have an intergenerational effect; brain cell numbers were reduced in rats whose mothers were prenatally malnourished, even though these mothers had adequate diets during gestation and after weaning.

These studies would not be so disturbing if size were not related to function. The fact is, however, that alterations in normal biochemical and developmental processes accompany fetal and neonatal malnutrition in several species of animals. Changes in the usual constituents of cells, as well as the delayed appearance of specific enzyme systems, are observed. Depending on the timing of the dietary deficiency, degeneration of the cerebral cortex, the medulla, and the spinal cord occurs. Muscular development is also impaired because of a reduced number of muscle cells and fibers.

What has been learned from animal research. Much can still be learned from experiments with animals about the processes of fetal growth and development and the consequences of maternal malnutrition. However, the work to date has produced important results:

1. *Growth failure.* Although a number of prenatal influences affect fetal growth, maternal malnutrition can be one cause of growth failure that results in low birth weight.
2. *Nature of tissue effects.* Animals malnourished from restrictions of their mothers' diets throughout most of gestation are characterized by 1) reduced number and size of cells in the placenta, 2) reduced brain cell number and head size, 3) proportional reductions in the size of other organs, and 4) alterations in normal cell constituents and biochemical processes.
3. *Influencing factors.* The fetal consequences of malnutrition depend on the timing, severity, and duration of the maternal dietary restriction. These consequences may be reversible if the restriction primarily affects growth in cell size, but a reduction in the number of cells may be permanent if the restriction is maintained throughout the entire period of hyperplastic growth.

Human Experience in Fetal Growth

Low birth weight. In view of the risks of early death or permanent disability associated with low birth weight, it is apparent that the animal research on intrauterine failure may have great implications for human problems. Of the annual incidence of low birth weight infants, it is estimated that 10–20% are a result of intrauterine growth failure. This means that 80,000 to 120,000 infants who have experienced malnutrition in utero are born each year in the United States. An important thing to understand when interpreting these statistics is that there is no one cause—a number of factors can retard fetal growth. When the term *fetal malnutrition* is applied to human infants, it simply means that there was a reduction in the maternal supply or placental transport of nutrients so that fetal growth was retarded significantly below genetic potential. It does not necessarily mean that the mother's nutrition was at fault. At present there is no way to judge how many growth-retarded infants are the result of maternal malnutrition.

Relation to animal studies. Although the animal experiments are highly suggestive, caution should be taken in making direct applications to humans. A primary reason for doing animal research is to find out what can possibly happen when certain conditions are imposed. The findings do not guarantee that these things actually happen in the course of human events. There are a number of reasons that the dramatic results of maternal malnutrition demonstrated in animals may not occur as readily in human beings. In effect, the consequences of maternal malnutrition on fetal growth and development are all magnified in the animal studies. This is because 1) the relative rates of growth and development are much slower in humans than in laboratory animals, 2) the timing of maximum growth also differs, 3) the number and size of fetuses a mother must nourish in utero compared with her own body size and nutritional reserves are much smaller in humans than in laboratory animals, and 4) the magnitude of dietary deprivation used for experimentation is rarely encountered in human populations under ordinary circumstances.

PHYSIOLOGY OF PREGNANCY ≋

Normal pregnancy is accompanied by anatomic and physiologic changes that affect almost every function in the body. Many of these changes are apparent in the very early weeks. This indicates that they are not merely a response to the physiologic stress imposed by the fetus but are also an integral part of the maternal-fetal system, which creates the most favorable environment possible for the developing child. The changes are necessary to regulate maternal metabolism, promote fetal growth, and prepare the mother for labor, birth, and lactation.[3]

The changes that occur in pregnancy are too complex to be given full treatment here, but a look at some changes that have effects on general metabolism will lay the foundation for interpreting nutritional requirements and dietary allowances (see the box on page 58).

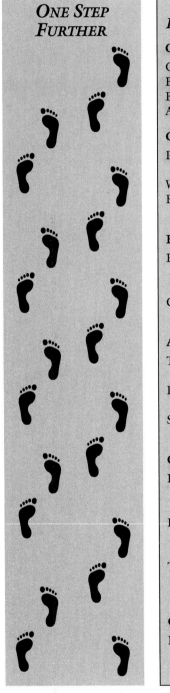

Key Physiologic Changes During Pregnancy and Nutritional Implications

Cardiovascular Changes

Cardiac output increases—a function of increased stroke volume and heart rate.
Blood volume increases.
Blood flow changes.
Arterial pressure decreases (first and second trimesters).

Changes in Blood Volume

Progressive plasma volume expansion occurs from weeks ten to twelve through weeks thirty-three to thirty-five.
Weekly increments are maximal during midgestation.
Expansion in red cell mass is proportionally smaller than that in plasma, resulting in the so-called physiologic anemia of pregnancy.

Blood Pressure During Pregnancy

Blood pressure tone decreases, and peripheral vascular resistance falls. Arterial pressure falls during the first trimester; it is used as the baseline to evaluate pregnancy-induced hypertension in the third trimester.
Changes occur in regional blood flow. For example, uterine blood flow increases from 15 to 20 ml/min in nonpregnant to 500 to 600 ml/min near term.

Adjustments in Respiratory System

The enlarging uterus results in increased intraabdominal pressure and elevation of the diaphragm by as much as 4 cm. As a result, thoracic breathing replaces intraabdominal breathing.
Resting ventilation increases by about 48%; this exceeds increments in either oxygen consumption (21%) or metabolic rate (14%) and expanded title volume.
Since respiratory rate remains constant throughout gestation, there is more efficient exchange of lung gases in the alveoli. The oxygen-carrying capacity of the blood is increased accordingly.

Changes in Renal Functions

In normal pregnancy, changes include ureteral dilation, slowed velocity of urine, increased susceptibility to urinary tract infections, and uterine compression of the ureters as they go over the pelvic brim.
Renal function is altered considerably. Renal blood flow and glomerular filtration rates are increased to facilitate the clearance of waste products resulting from fetal and maternal metabolism.
The increase in glomerular filtration rate presents the tubules with greater quantities of nutrients than they can reabsorb, sometimes resulting in proteinuria and glycosuria in healthy women.

Changes in Gastrointestinal Function

Due to the influence of hormonal changes during pregnancy, it is normal to observe adaptations such as taste changes, heartburn, nausea and vomiting, and constipation.

Blood Volume and Composition

Plasma is the fluid component of blood; serum is the part of plasma that remains after its coagulation factors have been removed. Total plasma volume in a nonpregnant woman averages 2,600 ml. Near the end of the first trimester of pregnancy, plasma volume begins to increase, and by thirty-four weeks it is about 50% greater than it was at conception.

There is considerable variation from these averages. Women who have small volumes to begin with usually have a greater increase, as do **multigravidae** and mothers with multiple births.

Multigravidae
(L *multus*, many; *gravida*, pregnant) Women who have had two or more pregnancies

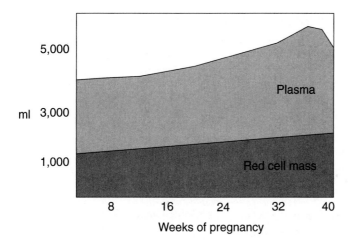

FIG. 3-5   Increase in plasma volume and red cell mass during the course of human pregnancy.
From Worthington-Roberts, B.S., and S.R. Williams. 1993. *Nutrition in pregnancy and lactation,* 5th ed. St. Louis: Mosby.

Researchers have shown that the increase in plasma volume is correlated with obstetric performance. They found that women who have a small increase when compared with the average are more likely to have stillbirths, abortions, and *low birth weight* babies. Clearly, the restriction of a normal expansion of plasma volume is undesirable in pregnancy.

If the availability of nutrients or the synthesis of normal blood constituents does not keep pace with the expansion of plasma volume, concentrations per 100 ml of blood will decrease, even though the total amount may rise. This is apparently what happens with red blood cells, serum proteins, minerals, and water-soluble vitamins.

Red cell production is stimulated during pregnancy, so that their numbers gradually rise, but the increase is not as large as the expansion of plasma volume (fig. 3-5). The **hematocrit (HCT),** which is normally around 35% in women, may be as low as 29–31% during pregnancy. The amount of hemoglobin in each red blood cell does not change, but, because there are fewer red blood cells per 100 ml of blood, hemodilution occurs. Nonpregnant **hemoglobin** values of 13 to 14 g per 100 ml can drop as low as 10 or 11 g/ 100 ml in the early months. In a nonpregnant woman, this level of hemoglobin would indicate anemia, but in pregnancy the red blood cells are **normochromic** and **normocytic.**

Serum levels of the major nutrients typical for pregnant and nonpregnant women are compared in table 3-1. The values for pregnant women must be interpreted with caution. Investigators have obtained different values depending on the laboratory methods used. Moreover, levels of certain nutrients can be influenced by a number of maternal factors, such as age, parity, smoking, and the use of various medications before or during pregnancy. Even the sex of the fetus can influence the mother's blood levels of some nutrients. The levels also fluctuate at different times during **gestation.**

The Cardiovascular System

Extensive anatomic and physiologic changes occur in the cardiovascular system during the course of pregnancy. These adaptations protect the woman's normal physiologic functioning to meet the metabolic demands pregnancy imposes on her body and provide for fetal development and growth needs.

The slight cardiac *hypertrophy* is probably secondary to the increased blood volume and cardiac output. As the diaphragm is displaced upward, the heart is elevated upward and to the left. The degree of shift depends on the duration of pregnancy and the size and position of the uterus.

Hematocrit (HCT)
(Gr *haima,* blood; *krinein,* to separate) The volume percentage of red blood cells (RBCs) in whole blood, normally about 35% in women. Shows the ratio of RBC volume to total blood volume.

Hemoglobin
(Gr *haima,* blood; L *globus,* a ball) Oxygen-carrying pigment in red blood cells; a conjugated protein containing four heme groups combined with iron and four long globin polypeptide chains; formed by the developing RBC in bone marrow.

Normochromic
Normal red blood cell color.

Normocytic
Normal red blood cell size.

Gestation
(L *gestare,* to bear) Intrauterine fetal growth period (forty weeks) from conception to birth.

TABLE 3-1   *Serum Nutrient Levels in Pregnant and Nonpregnant Women*

Nutrients	Normal Nonpregnancy Range	Values in Pregnancy
Total protein	6.5–8.5 g/100 ml	6.0–8.0
Albumin	3.5–5.0 g/100 ml	3.0–4.5
Glucose	<110 mg/100 ml	<120
Cholesterol	120–190 mg/100 ml	200–325
Vitamin A	20–60 μg/100 ml	20–60
Carotene	50–300 μg/100 ml	80–325
Ascorbic acid	0.2–2.0 mg/100 ml	0.2–1.5
Folic acid	5–21 ng/100 ml	3.15
Calcium	4.6–5.5 mEq/L	4.2–5.2
Iron/iron-binding capacity	>50/250–400 μg/100 ml	>40/300–450

Modified from Aubry, R.H., A. Roberts, and V. Cuenca. 1975. *Clin Perinatol* 2:207.

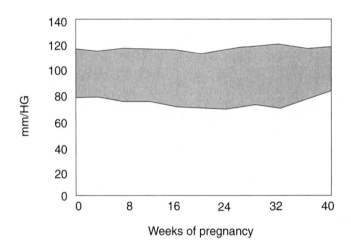

FIG. 3-6   Change in blood pressure during the course of human pregnancy.

From Worthington-Roberts, B.S., and S.R. Williams. 1993. *Nutrition in pregnancy and lactation,* 5th ed. St. Louis: Mosby.

Vasodilation
(L *vas*, vessel; *dilatare*, to spread out) Expansion or stretching of a blood vessel.

During the first half of pregnancy, there is a decrease in both systolic and diastolic pressure of 5 to 10 mm Hg. The decrease in blood pressure is probably the result of peripheral **vasodilation** from the hormonal changes during pregnancy. During the third trimester, maternal blood pressure should return to the values obtained during the first trimester (fig. 3-6).

Cardiac output increases from 30% to 50% by week thirty-two of pregnancy; it declines to about a 20% increase at week forty. The elevated cardiac output is largely a result of increased stroke volume and is in response to increased demands for oxygen (normal value is 5 to 5.5 L/min). The cardiac output decreases with the woman in the supine position and increases with any exertion, such as labor and delivery. The circulation time decreases slightly by week thirty-two. It returns to near normal near term.

Respiration

Respiration adaptations occur during pregnancy to provide for both maternal and fetal needs. Maternal oxygen requirements increase in response to the acceleration in metabolic rate and the need to add to the tissue mass in the uterus and breasts. The fetus requires oxygen and a way to eliminate carbon dioxide.

CASE STUDY

Drugs in Early Pregnancy

A woman visits her health care provider because she is concerned about missing three menstrual periods. She is found to be pregnant. The pregnancy was not planned. She admits to having taken an assortment of over-the-counter drugs and vitamin/mineral supplements. She also has been taking several prescription drugs. She is concerned about the well-being of the fetus, as is the clinician. What questions should be asked of the woman, and what advice can be provided by the clinician?

As previously mentioned, the level of the diaphragm is displaced by as much as 4 cm during pregnancy. With advancing pregnancy, thoracic breathing replaces abdominal breathing, and descent of the diaphragm with respiration becomes less possible.

The pregnant woman breathes deeper (greater **tidal volume,** the amount of gases exchanged with each breath) but increases her respiratory rate only slightly (about two breaths per minute). There is a more efficient exchange of lung gases in the **alveoli;** the oxygen-carrying capacity of the blood is increased accordingly.

Tidal volume
> The amount of gases passing into and out of the lungs in each respiratory cycle.

Alveoli
> (L *alveus,* hollow) Small sac-like formations; thin-walled chambers in the lungs surrounded by networks of capillaries through whose walls exchange of carbon dioxide and oxygen takes place.

Renal Function

In normal pregnancy, renal function is altered considerably. The woman's kidneys must manage the increased metabolic and circulatory demands of the maternal body, as well as the excretion of fetal waste products. Changes in renal function are caused by pregnancy hormones, an increase in blood volume, the woman's posture, and nutritional intake.

To facilitate the clearance of creatinine, urea, and other waste products of fetal and maternal metabolism, blood flow through the kidneys and the glomerular filtration rate are increased during pregnancy. The change in glomerular filtration rate is partially caused by the lower osmotic pressure, which results from the fall in serum albumin. This is one adaptation that appears to be purely mechanical, since no effects of hormones on this aspect of kidney function have been shown. However, there are consequences for nutrition.

Normally, most of the glucose, amino acids, and water-soluble vitamins that are filtered by the nephrons are reabsorbed in the tubules to preserve the body's balance. However, in pregnancy substantial quantities of these nutrients appear in the urine. The most satisfactory explanation is that the higher glomerular filtration rate offers the tubules greater quantities of nutrients than they can feasibly reabsorb. Because the change in filtration rate is largely mechanical, there may not be an accompanying mechanism by which the tubules can readjust.

Gastrointestinal Function

The functioning of the gastrointestinal system undergoes a number of interesting changes during the course of pregnancy. The appetite increases, nausea and vomiting may occur, motility is diminished, intestinal secretion is reduced, sense of taste is altered, and absorption of nutrients is enhanced.

Increased progesterone production causes decreased tone and motility of the smooth muscles of the gastrointestinal tract. This leads to esophageal regurgitation, decreased emptying of the stomach, and reverse **peristalsis.** As a result, the pregnant woman may experience heartburn. The decreased smooth muscle tone also results in an increase in water absorption from the colon, and constipation may result. In addition, constipation is secondary to hypoperistalsis, unusual food choices, lack of fluids, abdominal pressure by the pregnant uterus, and displacement of intestines with some compression. **Hemorrhoids** may be everted or may bleed during straining at stool.

Peristalsis
> (Gr *peri,* around; *stalsis,* contraction) A wave-like progression of alternate contraction and relaxation of the muscle fibers of the gastrointestinal tract.

Hemorrhoids
> (Gr *haima,* blood; *rhoia,* to flow) Enlarged veins in the mucous membranes inside or outside of the rectum; causes pain, itching, discomfort, and bleeding.

Flatulence

(L *flatus,* a blowing) Excessive formation and expulsion of gases in the gastrointestinal tract.

Decreased emptying time of the gallbladder is typical. This feature, together with slight hypercholesterolemia from increased progesterone levels, may account for the frequent development of gallstones during pregnancy.

Intraabdominal alterations that can cause discomfort include pelvic heaviness or pressure, **flatulence,** distention and bowel cramping, and uterine contractions. In addition to displacement of intestines, pressure from the expanding uterus increases venous pressure in the pelvic organs. Although most abdominal discomfort is a consequence of normal maternal alterations, occasional bowel obstruction or an inflammatory process may be present.

Insofar as taste is concerned, one study[4] examined the ability of the pregnant woman to discriminate among different concentrations of salt and sucrose solutions. Results of tests with salt solutions showed that the pregnant women were significantly less able to identify concentration differences correctly and preferred significantly stronger salt solutions than did the nonpregnant women. The researchers suggest that these observations may reflect a physiologic mechanism for increasing salt intake during pregnancy.

Hormones

The pregnant woman secretes more than thirty different hormones throughout gestation. Some, like those just mentioned, are present only in pregnancy, whereas others that are normally present have altered rates of secretion that are modified by the pregnant state.

Most hormones are proteins or steroids that are synthesized from precursors such as amino acids and cholesterol in endocrine glands throughout the body. Their production is influenced by the mother's general health and nutritional status. Under normal circumstances, they are controlling factors in a complex feedback system that maintains homeostasis between cellular and extracellular constituents and metabolism. During pregnancy, many of these homeostatic mechanisms are "reset," so that changes occur in the retention, utilization, and excretion of nutrients. Some of the hormones that exert important effects on nutrient metabolism are summarized in table 3-2, where only those that have more general implications for nutritional management are singled out for discussion.

Progesterone and estrogen are two hormones that have major effects on maternal physiology during pregnancy. The chief action of progesterone is to cause a relaxation of the smooth muscles of the uterus, so that it can expand as the fetus grows, but it also has a relaxing effect on other smooth muscles in the body. Relaxation of the muscles of the gastrointestinal tract reduces motility in the gut, allowing more time for the nutrients to be absorbed. The slower movement is also a cause of the constipation commonly experienced by pregnant women. The general metabolic effects of progesterone are to induce maternal fat deposition, to reduce alveolar and arterial Pco_2 (partial pressure or tension of carbon dioxide, facilitating exchange of lung gases in respiration and ensuring buffer capacity), and to increase renal sodium excretion.

Hydroscopic

(Gr *hydro,* water; *skopein,* to measure or examine) Possessing the tendency to take up and hold water readily.

Edema

(Gr *oidema,* swelling) Accumulation of fluid in the intercellular tissue spaces of the body.

Preeclampsia

(L *prae,* before; *eklampein,* to shine forth) Condition in late pregnancy in which hypertension and edema occur, with or without proteinuria.

The secretion of estrogen is lower than that of progesterone during the early months of pregnancy, but it rises sharply near term. Its role is to promote the growth and control the function of the uterus, but it also has generalized effects on nutrition. One effect that has caused some difficulties for clinicians is the alteration of the structure of mucopolysaccharides in connective tissue. This alteration is beneficial because it makes the tissue more flexible and therefore assists in dilating the uterus at birth, but it also increases the affinity of connective tissue to water. This **hydroscopic** effect of estrogen and the sodium-losing effect of progesterone produce a confusing clinical picture of the pregnant woman's fluid and electrolyte balance. Because of estrogen, many pregnant women complain of excess fluid retention in the skin. Their faces and fingers become puffy, and there are other indications of generalized **edema.** In addition, changes in cardiovascular dynamics cause extracellular fluid to accumulate in the feet and legs.

Since excess fluid retention is one of the hallmarks of **preeclampsia,** some clinicians view these changes with alarm and may initiate rather rigorous treatment with diuretics and a sodium-restricted diet to promote water loss. The evidence, however, weighs strongly against this practice. It is now apparent that, while the incidence of generalized

TABLE 3-2   *Hormonal Effects on Nutrient Metabolism in Pregnancy*

Hormones	Primary Sources of Secretion	Principal Effects
Progesterone	Placenta	Reduces gastric motility; favors maternal fat deposition; increases sodium excretion; reduces alveolar and arterial P_{CO_2}; interferes with folic acid metabolism.
Estrogen	Placenta	Reduces serum proteins; increases hydroscopic properties of connective tissue; affects thyroid function; interferes with folic acid metabolism.
Human placental lactogen (HPL)	Placenta	Elevates blood glucose from breakdown of glycogen.
Human chorionic thyrotropin (HCT)	Placenta	Stimulates production of thyroid hormones.
Human growth hormone (HGH)	Anterior pituitary	Elevates blood glucose; stimulates growth of long bones; promotes nitrogen retention.
Thyroid-stimulating hormone (TSH)	Anterior pituitary	Stimulates secretion of thyroxine; increases uptake of iodine by thyroid gland.
Thyroxine	Thyroid	Regulates rate of cellular oxidation (basal metabolism).
Parathyroid hormone (PTH)	Parathyroid	Promotes calcium resorption from bone; increases calcium absorption; promotes urinary excretion of phosphate.
Calcitonin (CT)	Thyroid	Inhibits calcium resorption from bone.
Insulin	Beta cells of pancreas	Reduces blood glucose levels to promote energy production and synthesis of fat.
Glucagon	Alpha cells of pancreas	Elevates blood glucose levels from glycogen breakdown.
Aldosterone	Adrenal cortex	Promotes sodium retention and potassium excretion.
Cortisone	Adrenal cortex	Elevates blood glucose from protein breakdown.
Renin-angiotensin	Kidneys	Stimulates aldosterone secretion; promotes sodium and water retention; increases thirst.

[handwritten margin note: relaxes smooth muscle ⇒ overbreathing]

From Worthington-Roberts, B.S., and S.R. Williams. 1997. *Nutrition in pregnancy and lactation,* 6th ed. Dubuque, IA.:WCB/McGraw-Hill.

and peripheral ankle edema is high, it is not associated with an increase in perinatal mortality when the two other symptoms of preeclampsia—hypertension and proteinuria—are absent. In fact, women with mild edema have slightly larger babies and a lower rate of premature births.

The propensity of women to lose sodium from the action of progesterone is compensated for by an increased secretion of aldosterone from the adrenal glands and renin from the **juxtaglomerular apparatus** of the kidneys. If sodium restriction is imposed, this renin-aldosterone system must work harder to maintain normal sodium concentrations in the body. Pushed beyond the stress naturally induced by pregnancy, the system could become exhausted, so that in the long run less aldosterone and renin are produced. The sodium and water depletion that would result is more dangerous than the mild degree of edema that the treatment is supposed to prevent. This effect has been demonstrated in pregnant rats that are placed on sodium-restricted diets that would be equivalent to 1 g/day of sodium or a "no added salt" diet in humans.

Juxtaglomerular apparatus
(L *juxta,* near; *glomus,* ball) Complex of cells located near or adjoining a nephron at the head of a glomerulus of the kidney, responsible for sensing the level of sodium in the blood.

Although more research is needed on hormonal effects on fluid and electrolyte balance, the mechanisms that are understood to date suggest that a mild degree of edema is physiologic in pregnancy and that the measures commonly used to prevent it impose an unnecessary risk.

Metabolic Adjustments

The basal metabolic rate (BMR) usually rises by the fourth month of gestation, although small increments may occur before that time. It is normally increased by 15–20% by term. The BMR returns to nonpregnant levels by five or six days postpartum. The elevation in BMR reflects increased oxygen demands of the uterine-placental fetal unit as well as oxygen consumption from increased maternal cardiac work. Peripheral vasodilation assists in the release of the excess heat production, though some women may continue to experience heat intolerance. Lassitude and fatigability after only slight exertion are described by many women in early pregnancy. These feelings may persist along with a greater need for sleep.

A complex series of adjustments in carbohydrate, protein, and fat metabolism occur during gestation to ensure that the fetus receives a continuous supply of fuel when the needs are maximal in late pregnancy. These adjustments are induced by changes in the endocrine milieu and by development of new endocrine tissue, the placenta.

Approximately 50–70% of the kilocalories required daily by the fetus in the third trimester (43 kcal/kg/day) is derived from glucose; about 20% of the kilocalories are derived from amino acids, and the remainder from fat. When maternal blood glucose levels fall, the rate of glucose transfer to the fetus declines, and fatty acids may become a more dominant fuel source. The net effect of maternal fuel adaptations is to increase the use of fat as a fuel source by the mother to conserve glucose for the fetus. During the second trimester, the mother prepares for the anticipated fetal glucose demand by storing fat. Then, in the third trimester, when the fetal glucose demand causes maternal plasma glucose levels to fall, **lipolysis** increases in the maternal compartment.

Lipolysis
(Gr *lipus,* fat; *lysis,* dissolution) The breakdown of fat.

During a brief fast, such as overnight, maternal plasma glucose concentrations fall significantly below that of nonpregnant women because of continual placental uptake of glucose and impaired hepatic gluconeogenesis. The reduced capacity for gluconeogenesis is related in part to the reduced availability of alanine; the latter is the result of increased placental alanine uptake and restrained maternal muscle breakdown. Lipolysis is enhanced and mild ketosis may occur. In the postprandial period, maternal glucose uptake is lower than in nonpregnant women, despite increased plasma insulin concentrations. More of the glucose removed by the liver is converted to triglycerides; these are stored in maternal adipose tissue to be available for later fasting periods.

Overall, the major adjustment in energy during pregnancy is a shift in the fuel sources. Fat becomes the major maternal fuel, whereas glucose is the major fetal fuel. Since the size of the maternal tissue is considerably greater than the size of the fetal mass, lipolysis dominates, causing the respiratory quotient to fall in fasting women. Pregnant women gain weight readily without appreciable changes in energy intake, because water normally comprises about 65% of the weight gain, not because energy is used more efficiently. However, there is still some question about the efficiency of energy use, especially in a pregnant woman exposed to severe food deprivation.

Role of the Placenta

The **placenta** is not a passive barrier between the mother and the fetus. Rather, it plays an active role in reproduction. The placenta is the principal site of production for several important hormones that regulate maternal growth and development. For the fetus, it is the only way that nutrients, oxygen, and waste products can be exchanged.

Structure and development. Evolving from a tiny mass of cells in the first weeks of pregnancy, the placenta becomes a complex network of tissue and blood vessels weighing about 1.4 lb (650 g) at term. The vital role it plays as a link between mother and child is represented by the two principal parts of the placenta—one uterine and the other fetal.

Placenta
(L *placentas,* a flat cake) Characteristic organ of mammals during pregnancy joining mother and offspring, providing supportive nourishment and endocrine secretions for embryonic-fetal development and growth.

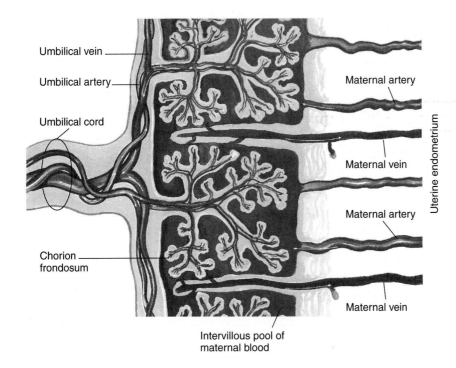

Umbilical vein

Umbilical artery

Umbilical cord

Chorion
frondosum

Maternal artery

Maternal vein

Uterine endometrium

Maternal artery

Maternal vein

Intervillous pool of
maternal blood

FIG. 3-7   Diagrammatic representation of a section through a mature placenta showing the relationship of the fetal placenta (villous chorion) to the maternal placenta (decidua basalis), fetal placental circulation, and maternal placental circulation. Maternal blood is forced into the intervillous space, and exchanges occur with the fetal blood as the maternal blood flows around the villi. Incoming arterial blood pushes venous blood into the endometrial veins, which are scattered over the surface of the maternal placenta. Umbilical arteries carry deoxygenated fetal blood to the placenta, and the umbilical vein carries oxygenated blood to the fetus.

On the maternal side, the placenta is part of the uterine mucosa. When the tiny blastocyst implants itself in the uterus six to seven days after fertilization of the **ovum,** the uterine tissue and blood vessels break down to form small spaces called **lacunae,** which fill with maternal blood. These spaces are eventually bounded on the maternal side by the decidua, or basal plate. Blood begins to circulate in the spaces at about twelve days' gestation.

Meanwhile, the **trophoblast** grows and sends out root-like villi into the pools of maternal blood. The villi contain capillaries, which exchange nutrients and metabolic waste products between the mother and the fetus. In the early weeks of pregnancy, the villi are thick columns of cells, but as they subdivide throughout gestation the villi become thinner and produce numerous branches. Some branches become anchored in the maternal tissue, and others remain free or floating in the intravillous spaces. The multiple villus branches provide a large surface membrane area for the efficient exchange of nutrients and metabolic waste products between mother and fetus (fig. 3-7). Even though uterine and embryonic tissues are intermingled, the blood of the mother and the embryo never mix, because they are always separated by the placental membrane (fig. 3-8).

Mechanisms of nutrient transfer.   The efficiency of placental nutrient transfer is a determinant of fetal well-being. Reduced surface area of the villi, insufficient vascularization, or changes in the hydrostatic pressure in the intervillous space can limit the supply of nutrients available to the fetus and inhibit normal growth.

Nutrient transfer in the placenta is a complex process. It employs all the mechanisms used for the absorption of nutrients from the gastrointestinal tract: simple diffusion, facilitated diffusion, active transport, and **pinocytosis** (table 3-3). The difference, however, is that in the placenta two completely separate blood supplies are maintained. The

Ovum
(L *ovum,* egg) The female reproductive cell (egg), which develops into a new organism.

Lacunae
(L *lacuna,* small pit or hollow cavity) Blood spaces of the placenta in which the fetal villi are found.

Trophoblast
(Gr *trophe,* nutrition; *blastos,* germ) Extraembryonic ectodermal tissue on the surface of the cleaving, fertilized ovum, which is responsible for contact with maternal circulation and the supply of nutrients to the embryo.

Pinocytosis
(Gr *pinein,* to drink; *kytos,* cell) Uptake of fluid nutrient material by a living cell by means of incupping and invagination of the cell membrane, which closes off, forming free cell vacuoles.

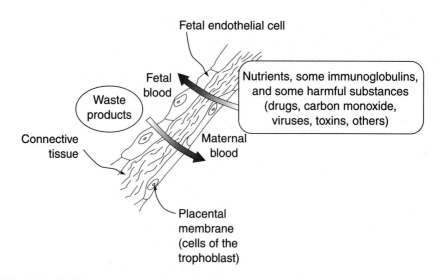

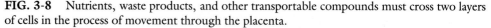

FIG. 3-8 Nutrients, waste products, and other transportable compounds must cross two layers of cells in the process of movement through the placenta.

maternal circulation remains in the intervillous space. The fetal capillaries are separated from the maternal blood by two layers of cells. Their thickness is approximately 5.5 μm (fig. 3-8).

Although the same nutrient may be simultaneously transferred by more than one mechanism, the major means of transport can be estimated by comparing nutrient concentrations in maternal and cord blood. If the concentrations are equal, the transfer has most likely occurred by simple or facilitated diffusion. Simple diffusion is a passive process in which nutrients move from high concentrations in the maternal blood to lower concentrations in fetal capillaries until equilibrium is reached. Facilitated diffusion differs from simple diffusion in that the rate of transfer is faster than would be expected. The mechanism of facilitated diffusion is not established, but it is thought that a carrier in the membrane is used. Active transport requires both a carrier protein and metabolic energy to move a nutrient against an electrochemical gradient.

Most proteins do not cross the placenta, since their molecular size is too big to allow penetration through the cells of the villi. This protects the fetus from acquiring harmful agents of high molecular weight, but it also means that the fetus must synthesize its own proteins from its supply of amino acids. An exception is the maternal immunoglobulin IgG. It is not known why this particular protein crosses the placenta, but it appears that the selectivity is related to the structure and not to the size of the molecule. IgG is probably transported by pinocytosis. The benefit to the fetus is that it has the same resistance to infectious diseases as the mother.

Respiratory and excretory exchange. Besides serving as a lifeline for nutrients, the placenta functions in the exchange of respiratory gases and waste products between the mother and fetus.

The delivery of oxygen to the fetus is just as important to proper metabolism as an adequate supply of nutrients. The mother makes adjustments in her breathing to meet fetal oxygen needs, but the amount ultimately depends on the blood flow through the uterus to the placental villi. Near term, the rate of flow through the intervillous space is 375 to 560 ml/min. Exchange is made between maternal red cells, which characteristically have a lower affinity for oxygen during pregnancy, and fetal red cells, which have a high affinity.

Maternal nutrition can influence oxygen exchange through the production of hemoglobin. Each gram of hemoglobin carries 1.34 ml of oxygen. In normal concentrations, it

TABLE 3-3   *Placental Transport Mechanisms and Materials Transported by Each Mechanism*

Transport Mechanisms	Substances Transported
Passive diffusion	Oxygen
	Carbon dioxide
	Fatty acids
	Steroids
	Nucleosides
	Electrolytes
	Fat-soluble vitamins
Facilitated diffusion	Most monosaccharides
Active transport	Amino acids
	Some cations (calcium, iron)
	Iodine
	Phosphate
	Water-soluble vitamins*
Solvent drag[†]	Electrolytes

*At very high concentrations, vitamin C has been shown to cross the placenta via diffusion.
[†]Movement of ions with water as it flows back and forth across the membrane

can deliver up to 16 ml of oxygen per 100 ml of blood to the placenta. If maternal hemoglobin levels are depressed from iron deficiency, the supply of oxygen per 100 ml of blood is reduced. Since the fetus can tolerate little variation in the rate at which oxygen is supplied, the mother must compensate by increasing her cardiac output.

Another function of the placenta is to rid the fetus of metabolic wastes. The placenta is freely permeable to carbon dioxide, water, urea, creatinine, and uric acid. **Hyperventilation** by the mother reduces her PCO_2, so that carbon dioxide exchange from the fetus is accomplished by simple diffusion. Urea, creatinine, and uric acid, which are the wastes of fetal amino acid metabolism, move through the placenta by diffusion and active transport.

Placental hormones. The production of hormones to regulate the activities of pregnancy is one of the most interesting special functions of the placenta. From the earliest days of pregnancy, the cells of the trophoblast and their successors in the placenta manufacture a large variety of hormones. The first to be manufactured in appreciable amounts is the protein hormone *human chorionic gonadotropin (HCG)*. Early in the differentiation of the trophoblast, this hormone is found coating the trophoblast's outer cell surfaces, where it is believed to act as an immunologically protective layer, preventing the rejection of the blastocyst and thereby facilitating implantation. HCG also stimulates the synthesis of *estrogen* in the placenta. Synthesis of estrogen actually begins in the free-floating blastocyst, where it facilitates implantation. The fact that the cells of the small, primitive blastocyst are already equipped to conduct complex steroid manipulation is a measure of the importance of these hormones at this early stage.

As pregnancy proceeds, large amounts of progesterone are synthesized in the placenta, principally from maternal cholesterol. In addition to sustaining pregnancy, this hormone serves as a raw material for the production of estrogens, mainly estrone, estradiol, and estriol, which in turn act on many organs and tissues of both the mother and fetus. Interestingly, the human placenta lacks the enzymes needed for converting the large amounts of progesterone it makes into certain essential estrogens and other steroids. Consequently, these synthetic events are carried out in the *fetal zone* cells, which are clusters of transient cells found in the developing adrenal glands of the fetus. These cells lack the enzymes necessary to manufacture progesterone but possess the requisite ones for its conversion. In

Hyperventilation
(Gr *hyper,* over; L *ventilatio,* ventilation) Increased respiration with larger consequent air intake and oxygen–carbon dioxide exchange in the lungs above the normal amount.

this way, the fetal and placental tissues complement each other. When the fetus's endocrine glands become sufficiently mature to take over the manufacture of steroid hormones, the fetal zone cells gradually diminish and eventually disappear. Presumably, this sophisticated collaboration is organized and timed by precise genetic instructions and is regulated by equally precise releasing hormones.

Because a great variety of regulatory hormones are synthesized in the placenta, including HCG, human placental lactogen (HPL), chorionic somatomammotropin, and human chorionic thyrotropin (HCT), the placental control during pregnancy must be as comprehensive as that maintained by the pituitary gland throughout life. By means of these hormones, the placenta not only carries out the functions of the fetus's pituitary until the organ is ready to perform on its own but also conducts the entire "endocrine orchestra of pregnancy," which performs largely in the placenta itself.

Immunologic protection.   During pregnancy, it is absolutely vital that the embryo be protected from immunologic rejection by maternal tissue. One of the mechanisms that seems to play a part in this task is the nonspecific suppression of lymphocytes, the cells that normally mediate the rejection of a graft. Experiments have shown that lymphocytes can be suppressed by HCG, HPL, prolactin, cortisone, progesterone, the estrogens, and a variety of proteins and glycoproteins.

It is also likely that the embryo is protected by the large, tightly packed cells that enclose it soon after the implantation of the blastocyst. This protective barrier prevents the drainage of lymphocytes to maternal tissues. In addition, the maternal blood vessels do not invade the trophoblast of the placenta, so this potential means of graft rejection is blocked. In the early days of the development of the trophoblast, further protection is provided by the absence of the expression of antigens. Thus, even though the embryonic tissue is "foreign," it manages to conceal the fact, at least for a while.

Maternal malnutrition.   Maternal malnutrition has also been found to interfere with normal placental growth and function (fig. 3-9). This is reflected by lower placental weight, smaller placental size, and reduced deoxyribonucleic acid (DNA) content. Affected placentas also have a reduced peripheral villous mass and villous surface.

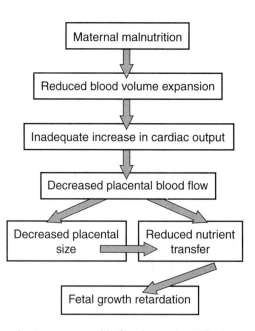

FIG. 3-9   Postulated mechanisms responsible for placental and fetal growth retardation as seen with maternal malnutrition in animal models and in human subjects.

Modified from Rosso, P. 1980. *Fed Proc* 39:250.

Summary

During the nine months of fetal development, the minute embryo matures into a human being capable of surviving in the outside world. For this process to unfold without flaws, the fluid environment in which thousands of chemical reactions take place must provide all of the nutrients necessary to support these important events. The mother adapts to the physiologic changes associated with pregnancy. The mother and her fetus(s) share available nutrition, which, under ideal conditions, is sufficient to meet the needs of both without compromise.

Review Questions

1. Describe the three stages of human gestation.
2. List the major changes in maternal physiology during pregnancy.
3. Trace the course of a nutrient from the maternal bloodstream to the fetal bloodstream.
4. Describe the changes in hemoglobin and hematocrit levels during a normal pregnancy.
5. Women with established renal or cardiac disease are considered to be at high risk during pregnancy. Why?
6. Why can a urine test during early pregnancy determine the pregnant state?

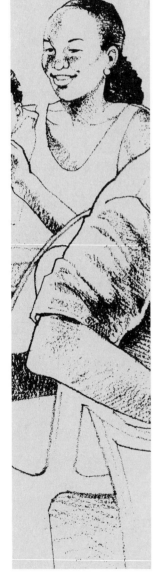

CHAPTER
4

MATERNAL NUTRITION: OVERALL NUTRITION AND THE ROLES OF SPECIFIC NUTRIENTS

Bonnie S. Worthington-Roberts

≋ ≋ ≋ ≋ ≋ ≋ ≋ ≋ ≋

Basic Concepts

❐ *Progress has been slow in understanding maternal nutritional needs during pregnancy.*

❐ *Preconception care (including nutrition counseling) has been a recent thrust.*

❐ *Obvious effects of maternal malnutrition during pregnancy have been documented.*

❐ *Weight gain during pregnancy has served as a useful gross measure of pregnancy progress.*

❐ *Nutrition supplementation studies have shown the value of nutrition intervention when serious dietary deficits are present.*

❐ *Specific nutritional deficiencies and excesses affect maternal health and fetal development.*

Some information is now available about the roles of energy, protein, and micronutrients in the course and outcome of pregnancy. However, data have been slow to accumulate. This is not to say that recommendations about diet for a healthful pregnancy have been absent. Efforts to encourage and mandate adequate maternal nutrition have been made for years.

HISTORICAL DEVELOPMENT ≋

Early Beliefs and Practices[1]

During the nineteenth century, much of what was known and recommended about diet during pregnancy was based on casual observation rather than controlled studies. Little information was available on the nutrient composition of foods or their biologic values. Dietary advice was influenced by belief in imitative magic: belief that the mother or child would acquire the attributes of the foods in the mother's diet. For example, pregnant women were sometimes forbidden to eat salty, acidic, or sour foods for fear the infant would be born with a "sour" disposition. The beliefs were often colored by the emotional and mystical aura surrounding the pregnant state. The consumption of eggs was sometimes restricted because of their association with the reproductive function. On the other hand, certain foods were encouraged for their presumed beneficial effects. Pregnant women were often advised to eat broths, warm milk, and ripe fruits to soothe the fetus and ease the birth process.

Problems in nineteenth-century obstetric practice also influenced dietary recommendation. During the Industrial Revolution, children in Europe had poor diets and worked long hours in dark factories. Rickets, which impairs normal bone formation during the growth years, was a common disorder. A contracted pelvis resulting from rickets was a major obstetric risk. Physicians did not have the modern means of delivering infants from these mothers. Death of both mother and child during childbirth was common.

Experience with his own patients in the 1880s led a German physician, Prochownick, to advocate a fluid-restricted, high-protein, low-carbohydrate diet for women with contracted pelvises to be followed for six weeks before birth. Women following this diet produced smaller infants and had easier deliveries. The diet may have had some justification in the 1880s, but it later gained in popularity and became a standard recommendation throughout pregnancy, even when the original rationale no longer applied. Remnants of the Prochownick diet, restricting fluid and carbohydrate, persist today.

There is very little specific information available about diet and pregnancy before the 1930s, other than reports on effects of food shortages during and after World War I. After the war, there was much effort to relate food shortages to the size of the baby, but most of the evidence presented was inconclusive and even contradictory.

Reevaluation and Redirection

It was not until the mid-1960s that renewed interest in infant mortality and morbidity rates led to a reappraisal of the influence of diet on pregnancy. Once attention was redirected toward this problem, a number of significant steps were taken. The resulting progress has been rapid. First, two important events occurred in rapid succession.

The White House conference. The White House Conference on Food, Nutrition, and Health was held in Washington in December 1969. The immediate stimulus was the nationwide shock at the disclosures of widespread hunger and malnutrition in the United States. The determination to do something about it produced the conference as the first organizational step. Many experts there, involved in the Panel on Pregnancy and Very Young Infants, were also involved with the soon-to-be-published National Research Council (NRC) report on maternal nutrition and the course of pregnancy. They saw the conference as a priceless opportunity to address the applied issues of diet and pregnancy within the context of their needed health services.

Benchmark NRC report. The NRC report, *Maternal Nutrition and the Course of Pregnancy*,[2] was issued in 1970. It remains the major source of research information on the role of nutrition in human reproduction. One of the principal findings of that report was the limited and fragmentary nature of studies on diet and pregnancy. The report singled out the need for long-term longitudinal studies on women and their families, a need that still remains.

Follow-Up Guidelines and Programs ≈

Initial Guidelines for Practice

In 1973, two sets of guidelines appeared as a direct outgrowth of the stimulus given to nutrition services at the White House Conference: 1) the American Public Health Association[3] guidelines and standards issued primarily for public health workers as an aid to assessments and program planning and 2) the NRC[4] guidelines for uses and limitations of supplementary food provided during pregnancy. Technical issues, practical problems, and political realities were explored, along with the inherent difficulties involved in multidisciplinary and multifactorial studies.

WIC Program

In 1978, the now well-known WIC program—Special Supplemental Food Program for Women, Infants, and Children[5]—was initiated under court order. The purpose of the WIC program was to provide food as an adjunct to health care during critical times of growth

TABLE 4-1   *The Special Supplemental Food Program for Women, Infants, and Children (WIC)*

1. Sponsored by the Food and Nutrition Service of the U.S. Department of Agriculture.
2. Originally authorized in 1972.
3. Target population: pregnant and postpartum women up to six months after delivery if not breast-feeding and up to twelve months if breast-feeding; infants; children up to five years of age.
4. Eligibility criteria: nutritionally at risk and members of low-income families.
5. Program administered by state health departments.
6. Regulations require that WIC agencies offer nutrition education and that appropriate health services be available directly or by referral.

and development. Table 4-1 summarizes the main features of this important program. The WIC program has grown from a pilot program costing $40 million in 1973 to one costing over $1 billion today. Many of the same problems addressed in the 1969 White House Conference are still being encountered in the WIC program, leading to questions of what the program is accomplishing.

ACOG-ADA Guidelines

In 1981, the American College of Obstetricians and Gynecologists (ACOG) and the American Dietetic Association (ADA) issued a joint publication, *Guidelines for Assessment of Maternal Nutrition.*[6] This was indeed a milestone. The report produced the first national consensus on the relevant risk factors before and during pregnancy. This original listing has been updated by the more recent material in the NRC perinatal guide.

NRC Perinatal Guide

In 1981, the NRC produced the highly useful guide *Nutrition Services in Perinatal Care.*[7] This report was particularly timely because it was designed for use with the rapidly growing regional networks for maternal and perinatal services. It is very helpful because it addresses the nutritional issues of infant feeding and the increasingly important concerns about substance abuse—cigarettes, drugs, and alcohol.

The Most Recent Landmark Document

The increasing visibility of maternal services in the United States motivated the National Academy of Sciences to appoint an expert committee with a mandate to evaluate data related to prenatal weight gain and nutrient supplements. The committee's final report entitled *Nutrition During Pregnancy: Weight Gain and Nutrient Supplements,* was issued in July 1990.[8] Recommendations made in this report are cited throughout this chapter.

More About WIC

WIC has strong support from Congress and the public. About 4.9 million participants receive monthly WIC benefits. This is about 60% of those eligible. The goal of those who favor the program is to make it available to *all* who are eligible.[9,10]

WIC has been more thoroughly evaluated than any publicly funded program in history. Early management studies compared using vouchers (such as bank checks) at local grocers with warehousing and direct distribution of food. More recently, new ideas have been evaluated, such as the use of vouchers at farmer's markets and a computerized "credit card" in place of food vouchers. Individual states make constant efforts to control food costs in order to serve more people.

Studies of the nutrition and health benefits of WIC have found that participation in WIC has positive effects on iron nutriture and growth and development of infants and children. WIC participation during pregnancy has been found to decrease the risk of delivering a low birth weight or very low birth weight infant by 25% and 44%, respectively.

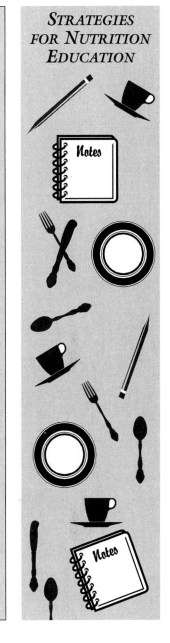

STRATEGIES FOR NUTRITION EDUCATION

WIC: Providing Supplemental Food with Nutrition Education

The Special Supplemental Food Program for Women, Infants, and Children (WIC) was established in 1972. Its goal is to improve the diets of pregnant and lactating mothers and infants and children up to the age of five who, because of low income or inadequate health care, are at high risk. Although all WIC programs must provide foods from each major food group, there is some flexibility at the state and local level. Foods commonly included are:

- Milk: skim, lowfat, whole or buttermilk; infant formula; cheese
- Protein: eggs, peanut butter, dried peas, beans, or lentils; tuna fish
- Fruit/vegetable: orange, grapefruit, pineapple, tomato, or apple (with added vitamin C) juices; carrots
- Cereal: iron-fortified infant cereal; others for children and mothers (a program may exclude sugar-coated cereals)

The amounts of food provided are intended to include $3\frac{1}{2}$ servings from the milk group, 1 serving from the protein group, 2 servings of fruit or vegetable, and 1 to 2 servings of cereal per participant per day.

A major component of the WIC program is the distribution of foods representing all the major food groups; however, an equally important mission is providing food and nutrition education to participating mothers. WIC participants in Ohio considered the nutritionists and dietitians at the WIC clinic to be their major source of nutrition information and over half were interested in additional classes. Surprisingly, the employed mothers were more likely to attend WIC nutrition classes than the unemployed mothers. This points to the need for classes scheduled at other than usual office hours. Teenage mothers and homeless mothers may have a special need for food and nutrition classes. The following are possible topics for WIC educators:

Food buying: making a shopping list and planning purchases; appropriate use of store specials; unit pricing; using the nutrition label in food selection.

Food preparation: easy-to-prepare recipes using supplemental foods; healthy cooking methods; safe food-handling practices.

Infant/child feeding: appropriate meal patterns (quantity and selection of food to be provided); nutritious snacks, nutrient-dense food choices; mealtime behavior; parenting issues (food as a reward, forcing food intake); prevention of baby bottle tooth decay; prevention of inappropriate weight gain.

Concerns of homeless mothers: food storage if no refrigeration is available; meal preparation with limited (a hotplate, electric frying pan) or no cooking equipment.

Hamilton, C.V., M.R. Schiller, and L. Boyne. 1994. Nutrition attitudes, practices, and views of selected Ohio WIC participants. *J Am Diet Assoc* 94:899.
Siegler, M.B., G.K. Franklin, and M.A. Lynch. 1993. Lesson plans for WIC homeless. *J Nutr Educ* 25:294A.

A comprehensive, national evaluation of WIC was completed in 1985. Major findings include the following:

1. Pregnant WIC participants were more likely to register for prenatal care in the first trimester and were less likely to have inadequate prenatal care, compared with nonparticipants.
2. WIC children were more likely to have a regular source of medical care and were better immunized, compared with nonparticipating children.
3. Women's dietary intake improved for protein, iron, calcium, and vitamin C, as well as for energy, magnesium, phosphorus, thiamin, riboflavin, niacin, vitamin B_6 and vitamin B_{12}.
4. Women participants had a longer length of gestation by 1.4 days than nonparticipants.
5. The rate of preterm deliveries was significantly reduced among less educated white and black mothers.
6. Infants of participating mothers had bigger head circumferences.

WIC has also been the subject of cost-benefit analyses.[11–15] These studies have focused on cost savings resulting from heavier infants with longer periods of gestation and fewer infants requiring neonatal intensive care. The most comprehensive study involved five states and found benefit-to-cost ratios ranging from $1.77 to $3.13 for WIC services provided to children. The government's General Accounting Office estimated that each dollar invested in WIC saves $2.89 in Medicaid, SSI, and special education and other health care within the first year after birth, and it saves $3.50 over eighteen years.

It is believed that the most positive effects of WIC are related directly to the nutrition education that all participants get as part of WIC benefits. Every participant receives assessment and counseling geared to his or her individual needs and problems. Monthly contacts allow for reinforcement of education and recommendations.

Because of the success of WIC in reaching out to large numbers of low-income women and children, several special activities have been piggybacked on the WIC staff; these include immunization outreach, drug and alcohol screening, cholesterol screening, and food stamp and Medicaid eligibility determination. These activities support the principle of one-stop social services. Hopefully, this diffusion of effort will not adversely affect the proven merits of the original WIC program.

WIC provides selected foods, nutrition education, counseling, and support and referral to or coordination with health care. In so doing, it has become an extremely important program for fostering food security and increasing access to health services for the youngest and most vulnerable members of our society.

Continued Needs

There is increasing realization of the seamless web of variables that influences the outcome of pregnancy. Within the constellation of income, health, education, family, and fertility, food and nutrition are just one part, but an important and modifiable one. As one observer stated, "Special efforts to improve prenatal, child, and maternal health showed clear evidence that the services did make a difference. . . . No one has yet teased out the relative effects of different variables." This is the clearest statement of the nature of the problems that need to be addressed in the years ahead.

A New Thrust—Preconception Care ≋

A major movement is underway to motivate potential new parents to participate in advanced planning of their pregnancies.[16] This effort, now referred to as "preconception care," allows for preparation of the best possible prenatal environment for the conceptus. The components of preconception care include risk assessment, health promotion, and interventions to reduce risk. Risks identifiable prior to conception may involve medical, social, psychologic, or lifestyle conditions. Risk assessment provides an opportunity to identify social factors related to poor obstetric outcome, including inadequate housing, low income, less than a high school education, and problems related to being a single parent. Once risks are known, some women may benefit from counseling and referral to social, mental health, and substance abuse treatment programs or vocational training.

Preconception assessment of nutritional status should identify individuals who are underweight or overweight; conditions such as bulimia, anorexia, pica, or hypervitaminosis; and special dietary habits such as vegetarianism. Nutrition counseling may prove useful; this may include information about dietary control of chronic diseases such as diabetes mellitus. The same applies to phenylketonuria; strict control of maternal serum phenylalanine levels is essential to optimizing chances for normal development of the offspring.

It is hoped that eventually preconception care will be shown to yield such positive results that insurance coverage will routinely be provided and clinicians will urge their clients of reproductive age to prepare for conception in every possible way. This preparation should include a formal preconception evaluation to determine 1) if reproduction is associated with high risk that is not modifiable and, thus, suggestive that serious consideration

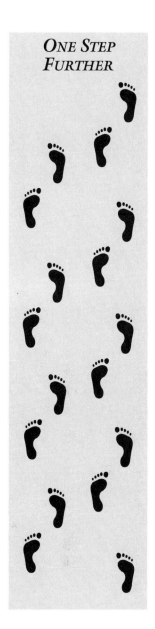

ONE STEP FURTHER

Components of Preconception Care as Part of Primary Care Services

Risk Assessment

Individual and social conditions (age, diet, education, housing, and economic status).

Adverse health behaviors (tobacco, alcohol, and illicit drug abuse).

Medical conditions (immune status; medications; genetic illness; illnesses, including infection; and prior obstetric history).

Psychologic conditions (personal and family readiness for pregnancy, stress, anxiety, and depression).

Environmental conditions (workplace hazards, toxic chemicals, and radiation contamination).

Barriers to family planning, prenatal care, and primary health care.

Health Promotion

Promotion of behaviors (proper nutrition; avoidance of smoking, alcohol, teratogens; and practice of "safe sex").

Counseling about the availability of social, financial, and vocational assistance programs.

Advice of family planning, pregnancy spacing, and contraception.

Counseling about the importance of early registration and compliance with prenatal care, including high-risk programs if warranted.

Identification of barriers to care and assistance in overcoming them.

Arrangements for ongoing care.

Interventions

Treatment of medical conditions, including changes in medications, if appropriate, and referral to high-risk pregnancy programs.

Referral for treatment of adverse health behaviors (tobacco, alcohol, and illicit drug abuse).

Rubella and hepatitis immunization.

Reduction of psychosocial risks that may involve counseling or referral to home health agencies, community mental health centers, safe shelters, enrollment in medical assistance, and assistance with housing.

Nutrition counseling, supplementation or referral to improve adequacy of diet.

Home visit to further assess and intervene in the home environment.

Provision of family planning services.

Jack, B. and L. Culpepper. 1990. Preconception care: Risk reduction and health promotion. *JAMA* 264:1147.

should be given to avoiding pregnancy and 2) if modifiable risks exist, if they are identified and addressed, can it be expected that there will be a marked increase in the likelihood of good pregnancy outcome.

EFFECTS OF MALNUTRITION DURING PREGNANCY ≈

The observations previously discussed provide fertile grounds for speculation, but what is the evidence in human populations that maternal malnutrition causes fetal malnutrition? Of necessity, much of the information is incidental. Nonetheless, there have been three kinds of studies that have addressed this question with highly significant results: 1) natural experiments in which birth statistics before, during, and after periods of acute famine are studied and compared; 2) measurements of organ size and cell numbers in stillbirths and neonatal deaths in which all causes not related to maternal malnutrition have been ruled out; and 3) epidemiologic studies of the nutritional correlates of birth weights.

CASE STUDY

Preconceptional Counseling

A professional woman thirty-five years of age visits her health care provider for advice. She and her husband are planning a pregnancy, and she wishes to approach this project systematically. An interview and physical examination reveals that she:
- Has been using oral contraceptives for ten years
- Smokes
- Is 10 pounds underweight
- Enjoys wine with her meals
- Has a family history of diabetes
- Has a sixty-hour work week
- Intends to continue her career during and after pregnancy

Questions for analysis
1. Outline appropriate recommendations for the preconception period.
2. Define the issues that require discussion about the pregnancy period itself.
3. Summarize appropriate anticipatory guidance for the postpartum period.

Natural Experiments[1]

The hardships of war afford researchers an opportunity to study the effects of severe dietary restrictions during pregnancy under conditions that are seldom duplicated. Throughout most of Europe at various times during World War II, food shortages were common. Reports were made on the effects of these shortages during the 1940s, but they are being considered with renewed interest today in light of the findings from animal research. Experiences in Russia and Holland provide examples of these effects.

1. *Russia*. During the siege of Leningrad in 1942 and its immediate aftermath, there was an eighteen-month period of severe starvation. Comparison of statistics for infants born before, during, and after the siege revealed an expected toll in the course and outcome of pregnancy under such desperate conditions. During the famine period, there was a twofold increase in fetal mortality, as well as an increase in the number of infants weighing less than 2,500 g (5.4 lb) at birth.

2. *Holland*. Similar findings were reported from Holland. Here the results are more insightful because the famine began suddenly and was limited to about six months during the winter of 1944 to 1945. It was not accompanied by other deprivations as severe as those experienced during the siege of Leningrad, and the women of Holland had fairly good diets before the food shortage. During the famine period, dietary intake dropped to less than 1,000 kcal per day, and protein was limited to 30 to 40 g. Since the famine lasted only six months, babies conceived before and during that period were exposed for varying lengths of time, but none was exposed for the entire course of gestation. On the average, birth weights of infants exposed to the famine were reduced by 200 g (7 oz). Weights were lowest for babies exposed to the famine during the entire last half of pregnancy. Added exposure before that time did not reduce birth weights further. In fact, babies exposed to the famine during the first twenty-seven weeks of gestation, but finishing their terms after the famine ended, had higher average birth weights than those who were exposed only during the last three weeks of gestation. The data for stillbirths and congenital malformations followed a different pattern. The rates were lowest for infants conceived before the famine and highest for those conceived during it.

   The findings are in line with what is anticipated from knowledge of the stages of human growth. Poor nutrition in the last part of pregnancy affects fetal growth, whereas poor nutrition in the early months affects development of the embryo and its capacity to survive.

3. *Great Britain*. It is interesting to note that, in contrast with the experiences in Russia and Holland, the prenatal mortality rate in Great Britain, which had been fairly constant before the war, actually declined between 1940 and 1945, despite the poor environmental conditions and no discernible improvements in prenatal care. One possible explanation is that pregnant and lactating women were given priority status for food in Britain as a matter of national policy.

Organ Studies

Studies that attempt to relate the size of organs in human infants to maternal nutrition must control for other conditions known to affect fetal growth. One group of researchers looked at the organs of 252 American stillborn infants and infants who died in the first forty-eight hours of life, excluding all multiple births, maternal complications, and congenital defects. The infants were grouped as coming from poor or nonpoor families according to income. Comparisons of organs between the two groups showed that the mass of adipose tissue and the size of individual fat cells were smaller in the poor infants. These infants also had smaller livers, adrenal glands, thymuses, and spleens. Heart, kidney, and skeleton were also reduced, but the differences were not as great. The ranking in organ size is consistent with reductions noted in animals that have been prenatally malnourished and in humans who have experienced uterine or placental disorders. Since the last two conditions were ruled out of the study, the investigators concluded that undernutrition could be responsible for prenatal growth retardation in infants from low-income families.

The organs in infants who survive intrauterine malnutrition cannot be studied to see if cells are reduced in number or size, but one organ is available. This is the placenta. One scientist reported that the size of placentas and the number of placental cells are 15% and 20% below normal when infants experience growth failure.[17] By comparing placentas from different sources, he has shown that those from indigent populations in developing countries have reductions in cell numbers similar to the reductions noted in placentas from American infants with intrauterine growth failure. In one interesting case in the United States, a mother who was severely undernourished from anorexia nervosa during pregnancy gave birth to an infant weighing less than 2,500 g (5.4 lb). When the placenta was examined, it was found to have only 50% of the normal number of cells.

Nutritional Correlates of Birth Weight

Studies of the relationship between maternal nutrition and the birth weight of the infant have tended to focus directly on the nutrient composition of the diet during pregnancy. Because of variations in the nutritional requirements of individuals, these studies have produced conflicting results. However, there are two indicators of long-term and immediate nutritional status that have shown consistent associations with birth weight: 1) *maternal body size*, height and prepregnancy weight of the mother, and 2) *maternal weight gain*, the amount of weight gained by the mother during the pregnancy itself.

Maternal body size. It should not be surprising that big mothers have big babies. What is less often appreciated is that the size of the infant at birth largely depends on the size of the mother and is not influenced to a great degree by the size of the father. This was shown years ago in a classic experiment in which Shire stallions were bred with Shetland mares and Shetland stallions with Shire mares. The newborn foals were always an appropriate size to the mothers' breeds. No intermediate sizes were ever produced. The same effects have been demonstrated in a number of animals, and there is indirect evidence for the same phenomenon in humans.

It has been further demonstrated in humans that height and prepregnancy weight of the mother have independent and additive effects on the birth weight of a child. In an analysis of 4,095 mothers in Aberdeen, Scotland,[18] it was found that, on average, the

Neonatal mortality
Number of newborn deaths during the neonatal period (birth to one month postpartum) per 1,000 live births.

tallest and heaviest mothers had babies who weighed 500 g (1 lb) more at birth than babies of the shortest and lightest mothers. It is postulated that maternal size is a conditioning factor on the ultimate size of the placenta and thus controls the blood supply of nutrients available to the fetus.

This idea has support in findings from the Collaborative Perinatal Project of the National Institutes of Health. In this project, Naeye[19] analyzed data from nearly 60,000 pregnancies to discover causes of fetal and **neonatal mortality** among different racial groups. He found that Puerto Ricans experience a higher rate of placental growth retardation than whites. However, this difference disappears when women with prepregnancy weights of 45 kg (101 lb) or less are excluded from the analysis. Naeye concludes that the high rate of placental growth retardation in Puerto Ricans is a result of the greater proportion of women who enter pregnancy with low body weights. Further data from Naeye's study show that, regardless of race or ethnic origin, mothers with low prepregnancy weights have much lighter placentas than do heavier mothers.

Maternal underweight. Infants of underweight women show several kinds of morbidity. Edwards and colleagues[20] compared outcomes for women who entered pregnancy at 10% or more below standard weight for height with outcomes for women who entered pregnancy at normal weight (table 4-2). The women were matched for age, race, parity, and socioeconomic status. The incidence of both low birth weight and prematurity were significantly higher among the underweight mothers. Infants of underweight women also scored lower on the Apgar scale. This scale measures the general condition of the neonate as evidenced by heart rate, respiration, muscle tone, reflex irritability, and color at delivery. Differences in **Apgar scores** were even greater when only the infants of women who were excessive cigarette smokers were compared. Underweight women who smoked more than one pack of cigarettes a day during pregnancy had three times the number of infants with low Apgar scores, compared with their normal weight controls.

Apgar score
Number defining an infant's condition at one minute after birth by scoring the heart rate, respiratory effort, muscle tone, reflex irritability, and color; named for its developer, American anesthesiologist Virginia Apgar (1909–1974).

Underweight women were also subject to different rates of pregnancy complications.[20,21] Anemia occurred more frequently in the underweight group, and those who were both underweight and anemic had an incidence of low birth weight of 17.4%, compared with 3.6% among women who were anemic but of normal weight. The investigators point out that both underweight status and iron deficiency anemia reflect long-term suboptimum nutritional intake. They suggest this as a possible explanation for the apparent influence of anemic underweight mothers on the incidence of low birth weight.

The condition of underweight is potentially modifiable, since it is often related to abusive dieting practices and/or exercise programs. A woman motivated toward improvement of her body weight-for-height status may successfully and healthfully achieve her goal within a relatively short period of time (three to six months).

Maternal Weight Gain

The weight gained in a normal pregnancy is the result of physiologic processes designed to foster fetal and maternal growth. Much of the weight gain can be accounted for by the products of gestation.

The total number of pounds gained in pregnancy varies among women. Young mothers and **primigravidae** usually gain more than older mothers and multigravidae. A normal

Primigravida
(L *prima*, first; *gravida*, pregnant) Woman pregnant for the first time.

TABLE 4-2   Infant Morbidity in Underweight Women and Normal Weight Controls

Infant Morbidity	Low Pregnancy Weight (% of Births)	Normal Weight Controls (% of Births)
Low birth weight	15.3	7.6
Prematurity	23.0	14.0
Low Apgar score	19.0	12.0

From Edwards, L.E. et al. 1979. Pregnancy in the underweight woman: Course, outcome and growth patterns of the infants. *Am J Obstet Gynecol* 135:297.

gain for most healthy women is about 11 to 15 kg (25 to 35 lb), but current guidelines from the National Academy of Sciences specify appropriate ranges for weight gain related to maternal prepregnancy weight-for-height, height, age, and race (table 4-3). A chart incorporating these recommendations for underweight, normal weight, and overweight women is provided in fig. 4-1.

TABLE 4-3 *Recommended Total Weight Gain Ranges for Pregnant Women,* by Prepregnancy Body Mass Index (Weight/Height^2)†*

Weight-for-Height Categories	Recommended Total Gain	
	kg	lb
Low (BMI <19.8)	12.5–18.0	28–40
Normal (BMI of 19.8–26.0)	11.5–16.0	25–35
High‡ (BMI >26.0–29.0)	7.0–11.5	15–25

*Young adolescents and black women should strive for gains at the upper end of the recommended range. Short women (<157 cm or 62 in) should strive for gains at the lower end of the range.
†Body mass index (BMI) is calculated using metric units.
‡The recommended target weight gain for obese women (BMI >29.0) is at least 7.0 kg (15 lb).
From Institute of Medicine. 1990. *Nutrition during pregnancy: Weight gain and nutrient supplements.* Washington, DC: National Academy Press.

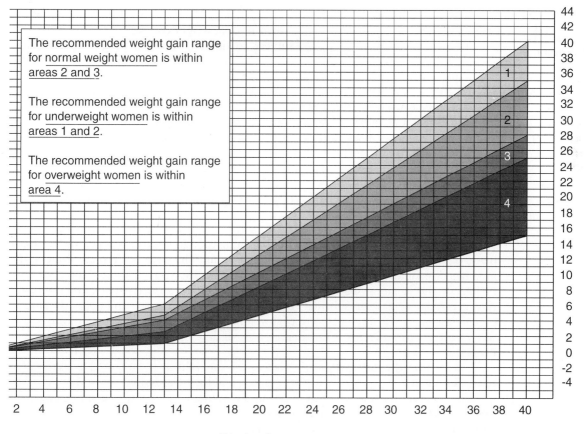

FIG. 4-1 A "modern" weight gain chart for pregnant women.
Modified from the National Academy of Science. 1990. *Nutrition during Pregnancy.*

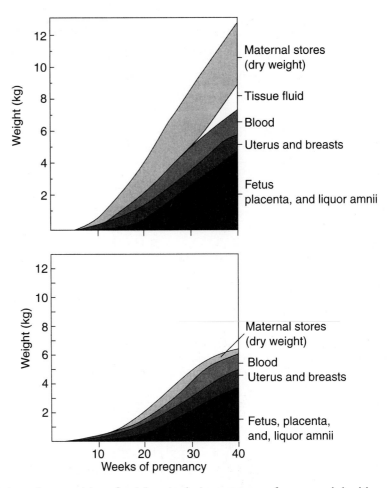

FIG. 4-2   Estimated composition of weight gain during pregnancy for a normal, healthy, Northern European woman *(top)* and a poor, underfed woman from India *(bottom)*.

Modified from Hurley, L.S. 1980. *Developmental nutrition.* Englewood Cliffs, NJ: Prentice-Hall.

The normal pattern of weight gain is illustrated in fig. 4-2. Less than half the total weight gain resides in the fetus, placenta, and amniotic fluid. The remainder is found in maternal reproductive tissues, fluid, blood, and "stores." The weight component labeled "maternal stores" is largely composed of body fat, although some increase in the lean body mass, other than reproductive tissue, may also occur. The action of progesterone in the pregnant woman dictates that a fat pad be produced to serve as a caloric reserve for both pregnancy and lactation. Fatfold measurements from ten to thirty weeks' gestation have shown gradual increases in subcutaneous fat at the abdomen, back, and upper thigh. The pregnant woman who attempts to restrict weight gain to avoid development of the fat pad will simultaneously affect to some degree normal development of the other products of pregnancy (fig. 4-2).

A sudden weight gain that greatly exceeds this rate is likely to be caused by excess fluid retention. As stated repeatedly in this chapter, mild generalized edema and some accumulation of fluid in the lower limbs is not unphysiologic. Women with edema can gain as much as 9 liters of fluid and still have clinically normal pregnancies. However, it should be emphasized that this accumulation is gradual. A large shift in water balance reflected by a sudden increase in weight is usually an indication of preeclampsia, particularly if it occurs after the twentieth week.

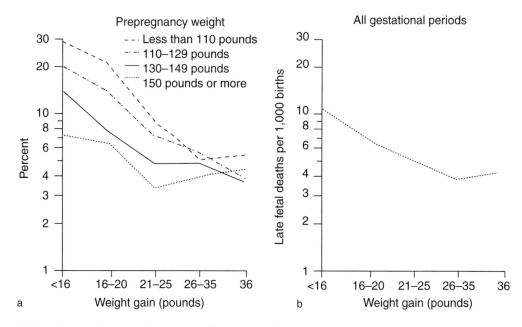

FIG. 4-3 *(a)* Percent of live-born infants of low birth weight by maternal weight gain during pregnancy, according to mother's prepregnancy weight: United States, 1980, *National Natality Survey. (b)* Fetal death ratio by weight gain during pregnancy: United States, 1980, *National Natality and Fetal Mortality Surveys.*

The more liberal attitude about weight gain during pregnancy that prevails today should not detract from the logic of avoidance of excessive weight gain. While large weight gain may have little or no adverse impact on the developing fetus, it may be detrimental to the mother during pregnancy and afterward.[22,23] Women who gain excessively large amounts of weight during pregnancy are at greater risk for the development of hypertension and are more likely to require cesarean delivery. Figure 4-3 illustrates the correlation between maternal weight and infant weight. Evidence also suggests, not surprisingly, that excessive weight gain during pregnancy may increase risk of long-term problems in controlling weight gain later in life. Tips for the health professional when evaluating maternal weight loss and weight gain can be found in the box on p. 82.

Women exceeding their desirable body weight by more than 35% are at greater risk than normal weight women for unsatisfactory pregnancy course and outcome. Numerous studies have shown that obese women are at higher risk for antenatal complications, especially pregnancy-induced hypertension, gestational diabetes, urinary tract infections and pyelonephritis; they also are more likely to demonstrate prolonged labor followed by difficult vaginal delivery and thus are more frequently delivered by cesarean section. Perinatal mortality is likewise higher. Surviving babies of obese mothers may present more challenges in management during the neonatal period, since they often demonstrate difficulty in regulating blood glucose. Suffice to say, reducing the degree of maternal obesity prior to conception theoretically should improve pregnancy progress and outcome. Attempts along this line are worth making if time allows and the woman appears to be properly motivated. Unfortunately, such motivation may not exist or, if it does, ability to follow a prescribed program may be limited. In any case, attempts should be made throughout the reproductive period (if not before) to prevent the development of excessive adiposity.

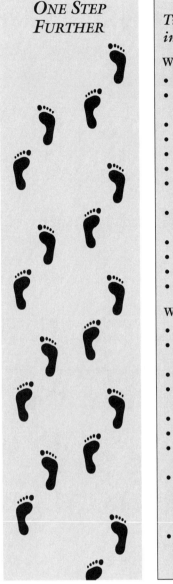

Tips for the Health Professional: Managing Weight Gain and Loss in Pregnancy

What to Look for If Weight Gain Is Slow or If Weight Loss Occurs

- Is there a measurement or recording error?
- Is the overall pattern acceptable? Was a lack of gain preceded by a higher than expected gain?
- Was there evidence of edema at the last visit and is it resolved?
- Is nausea, vomiting, or diarrhea a problem?
- Is there a problem with access to food?
- Have psychosocial problems led to poor appetite?
- Does the woman resist weight gain? Is she restricting her energy intake? Does she have an eating disorder?
- If the slow weight gain appears to be a result of self-imposed restriction, does she understand the relationship between her weight gain and her infant's growth and health?
- Is she smoking? How much?
- Is she using alcohol or drugs (especially cocaine or amphetamines)?
- Does her energy expenditure exceed her energy intake?
- Does she have an infection or illness that requires treatment?

What to Look for If Weight Gain is Very Rapid

- Is there a measurement or recording error?
- Is the overall pattern acceptable? Was the gain preceded by weight loss or a lower than expected gain?
- Is there evidence of edema?
- Has the woman stopped smoking recently? The advantages of smoking cessation offset any disadvantages associated by gaining some extra weight.
- Are twins a possibility? (A large increase in fundal height may be the earliest sign.)
- Are there signs of gestational diabetes?
- Has there been a dramatic decrease in physical activity without an accompanying decrease in food intake?
- Has the woman greatly increased her food intake? Obtain a diet recall, making special note of high-fat foods. However, rapid weight gain is often accompanied by normal eating patterns, which should be continued. If intake of high-fat or high-sugar foods is excessive, encourage substitutions.
- If serious overeating is occurring, explore why. Does stress, depression, an eating disorder, or boredom play a factor? Is there need for special support or a referral?

Supplementation/Intervention Trials

It is now well recognized that the provision of extra food, with or without education, improves pregnancy outcome in groups of high-risk, low-income pregnant women. The value of supplemental food varies from woman to woman, but obviously the severity of the original deficit is predictive of the value of the added food resources. A series of supplementation studies in developing countries has proved the positive impact on birth weight that such interventions can have. Even in developed countries, however, the benefits of nutrition intervention programs for high-risk women have been demonstrated.

The experiences at the Montreal Diet Dispensary in Canada show that the benefits of extra kilocalories and special dietary management during pregnancy are not confined to chronically malnourished women in developing countries.[24,25] They can also improve the pregnancy performance of high-risk mothers in more affluent nations. Knowing the risk of reproductive problems associated with low income, Higgins and colleagues selected

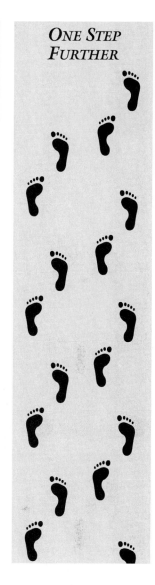

Are Current Weight Gain Recommendations Satisfactory?

Efforts have been made to evaluate the most recent weight gain recommendations for pregnant women, which were developed in the early 1990s by the Institute of Medicine of the National Academy of Sciences. Evaluations of these recommendations have sought to determine if the recommended weight gains are associated with the least perinatal mortality and morbidity. To date, the follow-up studies indicate that relatively new standards are appropriate for the general population of U.S. women.

In evaluating the adequacy of current weight gain recommendations, attention has been drawn to the consequences of maternal weight gain on postpartum weight retention. Since weight gain recommendations exceed those used in the past, concern has been expressed about the potential of these new guidelines to contribute to the growing level of obesity in the United States. Since obesity increases risks of problems developing during later pregnancies as well as in the postreproductive period, any factor seen to be contributing to adiposity is of concern.

Results to date suggest that the Institute of Medicine's pregnancy weight gain ranges recommended for underweight and normal weight women appear reasonable, but the recommendations for overweight and obese women require further evaluation. Also, the recommendation that black women strive for gains toward the upper ends of the ranges is not supported by available data.

Brown, J.E., S.A. Kaye, and A.R. Folsom. 1992. Parity-related weight changes in women. *Intern J Obesity* 16:627–31.

Hickey, C.A., S.F. McNeal, L. Menefee, and S. Ivey. 1997. Prenatal weight gain within upper and lower recommended ranges: Effect on birth weight of black and white infants. *Obstet Gynecol* 90:489.

Parker, J.D., and B. Abrams. 1993. Differences in postpartum weight retention between black and white mothers. *Obstet Gynecol* 81:768–74.

———. 1992. Prenatal weight gain advice: An examination of recent weight gain recommendations of the Institute of Medicine. *Obstet Gynecol* 79:664–69.

Schieve, L.A., M.E. Cogswell, and K.S. Scanlon. 1998. An empiric evaluation of the Institute of Medicine's pregnancy weight gain guidelines by race. *Obstet Gynecol* 91:878.

Siega-Riz, A.M., L.S. Adair, and C.J. Hobel. 1994. Institute of Medicine maternal weight gain recommendations and pregnancy outcome in a predominantly Hispanic population. *Obstet Gynecol* 84:565–73.

Smith, D.E. et al. 1994. Longitudinal changes in adiposity associated with pregnancy. The Cardia Study. *JAMA* 271:1747–51.

the hospital handling the highest percentage of poor patients in Montreal. All patients from two of the hospital's public maternity clinics were enrolled, a total of 1,544 women, between 1963 and 1970. A unique feature was that dietary needs for kilocalories and protein were individually calculated for each woman based on her body weight for height, with adjustments for protein deficiency, underweight, and other stress conditions. Women whose family incomes fell below specified levels (70% of all women in the study) were given supplies of milk, eggs, and oranges every two weeks. All of the women received counseling on food selection to meet their individual needs every time they visited the clinic, and nutritionists visited them at home at least once during their pregnancies.

Such intensive nutritional care enabled the women to average 93% of their total kilocalorie needs and 96% of their total protein requirements throughout gestation. Since the majority started out with large average daily deficits, they all showed significant improvements in the quality of their diets. Birth statistics indicate how the mothers and their infants benefited from these measures. The incidence of low birth weight in this high-risk study group decreased to the point that it equaled the all-Canada rate and was lower than

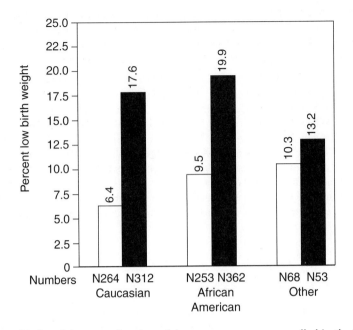

FIG. 4-4 Low birth weight rates of underweight pregnant women enrolled in the Virginia Nutrition Intervention Project, 1984 to 1988, who were ≤90% of expected weight at the initial visit and either >90% *(open bars)* or ≤90% *(solid bars)* of expected weight at the last visit.

From Clements, D.F. 1988. The Nutrition Intervention Project for underweight women. *Clin Nutr* 7:205. Reprinted with permission from Churchill Livingston Medical Journals.

Perinatal mortality

(Gr *peri,* around; L *natus,* born) Infant deaths in the perinatal period (before and after birth, from approximately week twenty through twenty-eight of gestation to one to four weeks postpartum) per 1,000 live births.

the rate for Quebec province. Stillbirths, neonatal mortality, and **perinatal mortality** were also lower than the rates prevailing in Canada and Quebec.

It is impossible to know how much of the improvements in pregnancy performance and outcome demonstrated in this study can be attributed to the diets of the women, the food supplements, or the special attention they received. What is important about the study is that it shows how high-risk mothers, against all odds, can experience successful pregnancies when superior nutritional guidance is a part of their prenatal care.

Other clinicians have made aggressive efforts to improve pregnancy outcome through nutrition intervention for underweight pregnant women and women demonstrating poor weight gain during pregnancy. Between 1984 and 1988, approximately 2,000 women receiving prenatal services in Virginia Health Department clinics were provided individualized nutrition interventions based on techniques developed at the Montreal Diet Dispensary.[26] Those responding to the food intake and weight gain guidelines showed a marked reduction in low birth weight deliveries (fig. 4-4).

Similarly, in a large urban clinic, a group of fifty-two underweight pregnant women who received no counseling was compared with a similar group of fifty-seven underweight and failure-to-gain pregnant women who received extensive nutrition counseling during the course of pregnancy. Women in the counseled group gained significantly more weight during their pregnancies than did the controls. They also delivered babies that averaged 300 g heavier than those born to women in the control group, a difference not related to ethnic background, income status, age, or smoking habit. The percentage of women having low birth weight babies was 8% in the counseled group, compared with 17% among controls.[27]

Orstead and colleagues took the process one step further by estimating the cost-effectiveness of individualized nutrition counseling for a group of high-risk women in Chicago. The nutrition services for the counseled group cost about $44,500 more than the usual program, but the cost of caring for the extra low birth weight babies in the control group was approximately $230,700. The benefit-to-cost ratio was therefore close to five to one.[28]

Finally, numerous efforts have been made over the years to evaluate the massive Special Supplemental Food Program for Women, Infants, and Children (WIC). In 1986, the U.S. Department of Agriculture published a five-volume report based on a nationally representative low-income population.[29] The researchers concluded after five years of study that WIC had a significant beneficial effect on the duration of pregnancy, birth weight, head growth, fetal mortality, and neonatal mortality. The program's effects were most clearly seen in high-risk pregnant women.

Not all nutrition intervention programs provided to high-risk pregnant women have demonstrated the degree of positive impact that was shown in the previously cited studies. This varied response should be expected, given the different populations served, the different supplements used, the various methods of supplement administration, and a variety of other differing variables. Overall, however, the findings appear to suggest that *the poorer the nutritional condition of the mother entering pregnancy, the more valuable the prenatal diet and nutritional supplement is in improving her pregnancy course and outcome.*

RECOMMENDED DIETARY ALLOWANCES/ DIETARY REFERENCE INTAKES ≈

As mentioned previously, the Recommended Dietary Allowances[30] are in the process of reevaluation such that the new Dietary Reference Intakes will provide guidance toward achieving optimum health. In the meantime, the current 1989 edition of the RDAs for pregnant and nonpregnant women are summarized in table 4-4. Developing DRIs may differ from the 1989 directives; special note should be taken of current folic acid recommendations for all women capable of becoming pregnant. In addition, guidelines like the RDAs and the DRIs may not be adequate for women who enter pregnancy in very poor

TABLE 4-4 *Recommended Dietary Allowances for Women of Reproductive Age*

	Age				
Nutrients	11–14	15–18	19–24	25–50	Pregnancy
Energy (kcal)	2,200	2,200	2,200	2,200	+300*
Protein (g)	46	48	46	50	60
Vitamin A (μg RE)	800	800	800	800	800
Vitamin D (μg)	10	10	10	5	10
Vitamin E (mg α-TE)	8	8	8	8	10
Vitamin C (mg)	50	60	60	60	70
Folate (μg)	150	180	180	180	400
Niacin (mg NE)	15	15	15	15	17
Riboflavin (mg)	1.3	1.3	1.3	1.3	1.6
Thiamin (mg)	1.1	1.1	1.1	1.1	1.5
Vitamin B_6 (mg)	1.4	1.5	1.6	1.6	2.2
Vitamin B_{12} (μg)	2.0	2.0	2.0	2.0	2.2
Calcium (mg)	1,200	1,200	1,200	800	1,200
Phosphorus (mg)	1,200	1,200	1,200	800	1,200
Iodine (μg)	150	150	150	150	175
Iron (mg)	15	15	15	15	30
Magnesium (mg)	280	300	280	280	320
Zinc (mg)	12	12	12	12	15
Selenium (μg)	45	50	55	55	65

*Second and third trimesters

From Food and Nutrition Board, National Council, National Academy of Sciences. 1989. *Recommended Dietary Allowances,* 10th ed. Washington, DC: National Academy Press.

nutritional status or who suffer from chronic disease or other complicating conditions. They may not be appropriate for the young pregnant adolescent or the woman who is very overweight.

NUTRIENT FUNCTIONS AND NEEDS ≋

Energy

During pregnancy, two factors determine energy requirements: 1) changes in the mother's usual physical activity and 2) increase in her basal metabolism to support the work required for growth of the fetus and the accessory tissues. The cumulative energy cost of pregnancy has been estimated at 40,000 to 70,000 kilocalories.[31] This amount is derived from the kilocalorie equivalents of protein and fat stored in the products of conception and from increased oxygen consumption of the mother. The total 40,000 to 70,000 kilocalories break down to an addition of only 200 to 300 extra kilocalories during the second and third trimesters of pregnancy to the daily allowance of the nonpregnant reference woman. A portion of the energy increment may be offset by the tendency of pregnant women to reduce their physical activity in the last trimester.

Protein

Pregnancy requirements. Requirements for protein during pregnancy are based on the needs of the nonpregnant reference woman plus the extra amounts needed for growth. The easiest way to determine how much extra protein is needed daily to support the synthesis of new tissue is to divide the amounts contained in the products of conception and maternal body by the average length of gestation. About 925 g of protein are deposited in a normal weight fetus and in the maternal accessory tissues.[32] When this is divided by the 280 days of pregnancy, the average is 3.3 g of protein that must be added to normal daily requirements. The rate at which new tissue is synthesized, however, is not constant throughout gestation. Maternal and fetal growth does not accelerate until the second month, and the rate progressively increases until just before term. The need for protein follows this growth rate. Only about an extra 0.6 g of protein is used each day for new tissue synthesis in the first month of pregnancy, but by thirty weeks' gestation protein is being used at the rate of 6.1 g per day. If this is added to the normal maintenance needs of the reference woman, 18.6 to 24 g of protein per day are required.

Protein utilization. These calculations of protein need would equal dietary allowances if 100% of the protein eaten could be used in the body. Actually, however, the efficiency of protein utilization depends on its digestibility and amino acid composition. Proteins that do not contain all of the essential amino acids in amounts proportional to human requirements are utilized less efficiently. Even a high-quality protein, such as that in eggs, is utilized much less than 100%. Protein utilization from a mixed diet is about 70% and, from a totally vegetarian diet, it is even less efficient. Protein utilization also depends on kilocalorie intake. It has been shown that an extra 100 kcal during pregnancy has the same effect on nitrogen retention as an additional 0.28 g of nitrogen itself. This means that kilocalories from nonprotein sources—that is, carbohydrates and fats—have a protein-sparing effect. If these kilocalories are inadequate, protein requirements increase. Finally, the trials that measure nitrogen loss are conducted on a limited number of subjects. There is a great deal of variation from the averages obtained. Since a dietary allowance must cover the needs of all healthy women, room for individual differences must be built in.

RDA standard. Because of these considerations, RDAs for protein are set much higher than calculated requirements of 18.6 to 24 g per day. The National Research Council allows 50 g of protein a day for the nonpregnant reference woman, with an extra 10 g per day starting in the second month of pregnancy. If individual allowances are calculated on the basis of body weight, daily need is about 1.3 g/kg of pregnant body weight, or about 0.6 g/lb. The RDA standard is based on a mixed diet in which at least one-third of the protein comes from high-quality animal foods. Thus, vegetarian diets that exclude all an-

TABLE 4-5   *Current Supplementation Recommendations: National Academy of Sciences (1990)*

Nutrients	Candidates for Supplementation	Levels of Nutrient Supplementation
Iron	All pregnant women (second and third trimesters)	30 mg ferrous iron daily
Vitamin D	Complete vegetarians and others with low intake of vitamin D–fortified milk	10 μg/day
Calcium	Women under age twenty-five whose daily dietary calcium intake is less than 600 mg	600 mg/day
Vitamin B_{12}	Complete vegetarians	2 μg/day
Zinc/copper	Women under treatment with iron for iron deficiency anemia	15 mg Zn/day 2 mg Cu/day
Multivitamin-mineral supplements	Pregnant women with poor diets and those who are considered high risk: multiple gestation, heavy smokers, alcohol/drug abusers, other	Preparation containing iron—30 mg zinc—15 mg copper—2 mg calcium—250 mg vitamin B_6—2 mg folate—300 μg vitamin C—50 mg vitamin D—5 μg

From Institute of Medicine. 1990. *Nutrition during pregnancy: Weight gain and nutrient supplements.* Washington, DC: National Academy Press.

imal products can be made adequate only when more total protein is consumed, or when foods are selected so that those low in a particular amino acid are complemented by foods in which that amino acid is high.

Protein deficiency. Adverse consequences of protein deficiency during pregnancy are difficult to separate from the effects of kilocalorie deficiency in real-life situations. Most cases of limited protein intake are accompanied by limitation in availability of kilocalories. Under such circumstances, decreased birth weight has been reported. As indicated in a Guatemalan study,[33] provision of supplemental kilocalories alone to pregnant women with deficient levels of protein intake was just as effective as provision of both protein and kilocalories in influencing birth weight of babies.

Protein excess. Adverse effects of excessive protein during pregnancy are poorly understood at the present time.

Micronutrients: General

Food is the optimal vehicle for delivering nutrients. Supplementation requires justification. As will be discussed in the next section, folic acid supplementation of the diet is recommended for all women of reproductive age who are capable of becoming pregnant. The National Academy of Sciences has also identified individual circumstances in which other nutrient supplements are justified (table 4-5).[34]

Folate

The B-complex vitamin folate is required for cell division to proceed. If this vitamin is lacking, detrimental effects are especially great in body tissues that have high turnover rates. One of the first signs of folate deficiency is megaloblastic anemia, caused by the production of abnormal red blood cells. These cells are arrested in their development, so bone marrow contains a large number of immature megaloblasts and hemoglobin levels are

TABLE 4-6   *Current Definition of Anemia*

Trimesters	Hemoglobin (g/dl)
First	<11.0
Second	<10.5
Third	<11.0

Data from National Academy of Sciences. 1990. *Nutrition during pregnancy: Weight gain and nutrient supplements.* Washington, DC: National Academy Press.

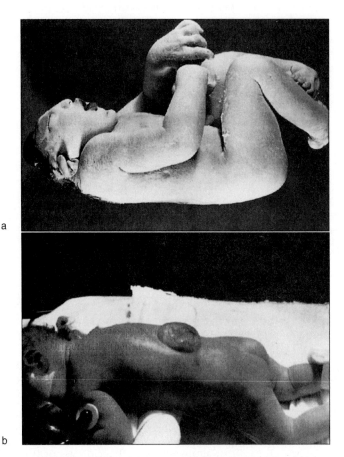

FIG. 4-5   Examples of neural tube defects. *(a)* Anencephaly. *(b)* Spina bifida.

reduced. Hemoglobin levels below 11 g/dl during the first and third trimesters or below 10.5 g/dl during the second trimester are criteria for diagnosis of anemia (table 4-6). Anemia is associated with increased risk of adverse pregnancy course and outcome.

Maternal folic acid deficiency in experimental animals has long been associated with increased incidence of congenital malformations in the offspring. Malformations have also been described in the offspring of women who used drugs that are folate antagonists. Limited evidence in humans also suggests that deficiency of this vitamin may be associated with spontaneous abortion. Recently, the importance of folic acid in the prevention of neural tube defects (NTDs) in human infants has been well established, but this has come only after many years of observation and experimentation.[1]

Neural tube defects (NTDs) are among the most serious congenital malformations; they are usually seen as anencephaly and spina bifida (fig. 4-5). Babies with anencephaly die before or shortly after birth, whereas most babies born with spina bifida grow to adulthood with paralysis of the lower limbs and varying degrees of bowel and bladder incontinence. This NTD may occur between postconceptional days fifteen and twenty-eight in humans. Thus, NTDs occur so early that most women are unaware of their pregnancy.

In the 1980s, the introduction and efficacy of maternal alpha-fetoprotein and ultrasound screening, in addition to amniotic alpha-fetoprotein and other examinations, have had a substantial effect. Nevertheless, selective abortion of a seriously malformed fetus should be considered a last resort rather than an optimal solution. Informed parents have to choose between two evils: to terminate their pregnancy or to have a malformed baby, with its long-term medical and social consequences. Many parents choose the lesser evil and prevent the birth of the affected fetus. This scenario may be called secondary prevention, but virtually everyone agrees that primary prevention is preferable. This is where folic acid comes in.

What is known to date is that neural tube defects appear to have some genetic base. That is, while they occur in about 0.1% of all pregnancies, the risk of occurrence is 0.3–1% if there is a close relative with NTD, and recurrence risk is 3–4%. Chromosomal aberrations, gene mutations, and teratogenic factors (i.e., valproic acid) appear to account for a small fraction of the cases. The other 92% of cases may have multifactorial origins, such as polygenic liability triggered by environmental factors.[35]

Among the triggering environmental factors, undernutrition has been found to be a factor in the well-known association between NTDs and poverty, seasonality, and rapid secular changes in the prevalence of NTDs. Clinicians in Northern Europe suggested in the 1960s that folic acid might prevent neural tube defects. Limited evidence was available at that time and little attention was paid to the idea. However, scientists examined the impact of vitamin supplementation (or, specifically, folic acid) on the recurrence of NTDs among women who had previously given birth to such offspring. Their findings yielded favorable outcomes, with supplementation positively associated with reduction in risk of recurrence. However, these researchers were criticized for methodological errors in study design and execution. Only after the British Medical Research Council issued its impressive study did the world take notice. This randomized prevention trial began in July 1983 and was halted in April 1991. It involved thirty-three centers, seventeen in the United Kingdom and sixteen in six other countries. Study participants were women who had a previous pregnancy that resulted in an infant with a neural tube defect and who were planning a subsequent pregnancy. Each participant was randomly assigned to one of four supplementation groups (Groups A, B, C, and D). Group A received 4 mg of folic acid daily; Group B, a multivitamin preparation plus 4 mg folic acid; Group C, neither the multivitamin nor folic acid; and Group D, the multivitamin preparation without folic acid. All capsules contained two mineral supplements.[36]

During the study period, complete information was available on 1,195 pregnancy outcomes. Folic acid supplementation was associated with a 71% reduction in the recurrence of neural tube defects. Use of the multivitamins without folic acid was not associated with a protective effect. Because of the substantial protective effect, the study data monitoring group recommended halting the study early, so that all women at risk could receive the potential benefits of supplementation. The Centers for Disease Control and Prevention in the United States then recommended the use of folic acid supplementation (4 mg/day) for women who previously had an infant or a fetus with spina bifida, anencephaly, or encephalocele.

Concurrent with and following this folic acid research activity, effort was underway to test the value of folic acid supplementation periconceptionally on the *occurrence* of NTDs. Czeizel and colleagues in Hungary[37] recruited women who were planning a pregnancy and assigned them randomly to receive (before and during early pregnancy) a 0.4 mg folic acid supplement or a placebo containing trace elements. None of the women had previously delivered an abnormal offspring. The results of the study were very impressive—a markedly reduced incidence of NTDs in the folic acid supplemented group.

This landmark study was accompanied by a series of observational studies, many of which were conducted in various parts of the United States. Groups of women were interviewed about their vitamin supplementation patterns around the time of conception. Patterns of vitamin use among women who had delivered babies with NTDs were compared with patterns of women who had delivered normal infants. Of nine studies conducted, only one was negative. That is, eight of the studies showed that taking vitamins around the time of conception was associated with a significantly reduced risk of delivering an infant with NTDs.

With this abundance of data in hand, the Centers for Disease Control and Prevention and the U.S. Public Health Service recommended that "all women of childbearing age who are capable of becoming pregnant should consume 0.4 mg of folic acid per day for the purpose of reducing their risk of having a pregnancy affected with spina bifida or other neural tube defects." This recommendation was followed by several other countries.

The underlying mechanisms of periconceptional multivitamin or folic acid supplementation in the prevention of NTDs are still not understood. In general, women who have NTD-affected pregnancies have not been found to have lower serum or red blood cell folate values during pregnancy. However, several researchers found a difference in red blood cell folate levels between women who had NTD pregnancies and controls. While the risk of NTDs is not dramatically altered by raising the red blood cell folate status from very low to a more normal value, the risk is significantly reduced by attaining a red blood cell folate status of > 300 or 400 ug/L. Thus, a small change in folate status may profoundly reduce risk.

Recent epidemiologic and biochemical evidence has suggested that the problem is not primarily a lack of sufficient folate in the diet. Instead, the problem appears to be rooted in changes in metabolism of folate in both maternal and fetal cells. (Absorption of folate has been found to be normal in women with NTD pregnancies, and all pregnant women experience accelerated breakdown of folate during pregnancy.) It is proposed that there is an interaction between a vitamin *dependency* (i.e., an inborn error of folate metabolism) and nutrition (e.g., a dietary vitamin deficiency) that may have a causal role in the origin of folic acid–related NTDs. The effect on the embryo may be a localized folate deficiency. The supply of folate may be limited even in women with normal folate nutrition, resulting in impaired embryonic cell division at the crucial time of neural tube closure. Folate supplementation may cause an increase in folate concentrations in tissue fluids, and it may overcome this failure of local folate supply.

While the pathogenesis of NTDs is still unproven, three studies shed some light on the subject.[35] One found a possible role of methionine deficiency in the origin of NTDs, based on cultures of whole rat embryos. Methionine is an essential amino acid, which is converted to S-adenosylmethionine; it is the ultimate methyl donor in humans.

$$\text{methionine} \xrightarrow{\quad} \overset{\displaystyle \text{CH-3}}{\text{S-adenosylmethionine}}$$
$$\text{homocysteine} \longleftarrow$$

Methionine deficiency may cause NTDs at the period when the folds of the neural tube first become elevated and have started to appose opposite ridges. Other researchers reported that 31% of infants with NTDs had methionine intolerance (with abnormally high serum homocysteine concentrations after an oral methionine load), whereas only 1% of people in the general population had such intolerance. This finding may indicate a metabolic block of demethylation of homocysteine to methionine. Bunduki et al.[38] reported a study of fourteen NTD mothers and fourteen controls. Mothers of NTD offspring had a significantly lower folate methylation rate than did mothers of normal infants. A study by Kirke et al. showed that plasma vitamin B_{12} level is an independent risk factor for NTD offspring. *Only one function in humans is independently influenced by both plasma folate and plasma vitamin B_{12}, and that is the action of the enzyme methionine synthase.*[35]

Finally, Mills and colleagues[39] obtained blood during the pregnancies of 81 women who produced infants with NTDs and 323 women who produced normal infants. Mothers of children with NTDs had significantly higher homocysteine values than did matched controls. The difference was significant in the 50% of women with the lowest plasma B_{12} concentrations. These researchers propose that an abnormality in homocysteine metabolism, apparently related to methionine synthase, is present in many women who give birth to children with neural tube defects (fig. 4-6). They also suggest that the most effective periconceptional prophylaxis to prevent NTDs may require B_{12} as well as folic acid.

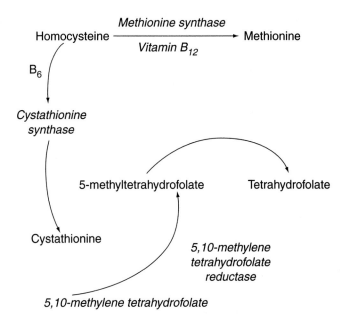

FIG. 4-6 Pathways of homocysteine metabolism.

From Worthington-Roberts, B., and S.R. Williams. 1994. Nutrition in pregnancy and lactation, 6th ed. Dubuque, IA: WCB/McGraw-Hill.

The mechanism of NTD prevention is receiving much research attention. An example of this is a recent report by Irish and American investigators who studied 550 pregnant and nonpregnant women.[40] They found that a substantial number of the women carried a gene mutation for an enzyme defect that leads to folate deficiency. They suggest that people who carry two copies of the abnormal gene may need additional folate to reduce their risk of abnormal fetal development.

Folic acid is available over-the-counter in dosages up to 0.8 mg and is available by prescription in 1 mg tablets. Prenatal vitamins contain 0.8 or 1.0 mg of folic acid. Folic acid is water-soluble, with no known toxicity; however, at high doses (more than 1.0 mg/day) the anemia of vitamin B_{12} deficiency (pernicious anemia) can be obscured, with progression of neurologic sequelae. Because pernicious anemia is rare before the age of fifty, this is likely to be an uncommon occurrence among women receiving folic acid during the reproductive years. Studies that definitively address the question of maternal and fetal safety of folic acid are not available. However, folic acid has been used extensively during later pregnancy without adverse effects.

Based on the evidence available to date, the Public Health Service (PHS) has recommended that *all women of childbearing age who are capable of becoming pregnant should take 0.4 mg of folic acid daily.* Implementation of this recommendation is believed to have the potential of reducing the rate of NTD pregnancies by 50%. Regular and continuous ingestion of folic acid is necessary, so that offspring of unplanned pregnancies benefit from this intervention. The PHS also points out that this recommendation should be followed by women who have previously had an affected pregnancy, even though they are not planning a pregnancy; by couples with a close relative with an NTD; by women with insulin-dependent diabetes mellitus; and by women with seizure disorders being treated with valproic acid or carbamazepine. Currently, the most direct way to achieve this goal is to ingest a 0.4 mg tablet of folic acid.

It might be asked, "Can current recommendations for folate be met by diet alone?" It might also be asked, "Is it practical to expect that women will be able to select foods to allow them to ingest 400 ug of folate daily?" If the diet is meticulously designed according to the U.S. Food Guide Pyramid or Canada's Food Guide to Healthy Eating, it is possible to provide the level of folate currently recommended to reduce the risk of an NTD-affected pregnancy. However, women in the United States and Canada consistently select diets with less than 400 ug/day of folate. Nutrition education may help. The U.S. Food and Drug Administration recently authorized a health claim on food labels relating diets adequate in folate to reduction in risk of NTD pregnancies.

The U.S. Food and Drug Administration (FDA) approved folate fortification of enriched flour, breads, corn meals, rice, noodles, macaroni, and other grain products early in 1996. This action was effective January 1, 1998. The FDA concluded that it is unlikely that vitamin B_{12} deficiency will be masked in the older population when daily intakes of folate are below 1 mg/day.

Before leaving the topic of folic acid, another important and unexpected finding of the Hungarian NTD occurrence trial was a lower prevalence at birth of major congenital abnormalities *other than* neural tube defects diagnosed during pregnancy and at birth after periconceptional multivitamin supplementation (9.0 per 1,000 vs. 16.6 in the trace element or placebo group).[37] Some congenital abnormality groups, such as congenital cardiovascular malformations, defects of the urinary tract, and congenital limb deficiencies, occurred less frequently in the multivitamin group than in the trace element group, and Shaw et al.[41] reported in 1995 a reduced risk of orofacial clefts if a mother used multivitamins containing folic acid periconceptionally (overall risk reduction of 25–50%). Also in 1995, Li et al.[42] reported a case-control study using the Washington State Birth Defect Registry; their results indicated that early prenatal multivitamin use was associated with a reduced risk of congenital urinary tract defects. The bottom line is that folic acid (or another vitamin) may play a role in the prevention of birth defects other than those related to neural tube closure.

Czeizel points out in his recent discussion of this issue that the hour may have come for a more effective and primary prevention of birth defects.[43] The recognition of this challenge led some experts to establish the World Alliance of Organizations for the Prevention of Birth Defects. Its manifesto declares, "We believe that children have the right to be free of preventable birth defects and that prevention must be accessible to all segments of the population."

Just what do women know about folic acid and birth defects? A Gallup poll was taken in 1997 with the sponsorship of the March of Dimes Birth Defects Foundation. This telephone survey (random-digit dialing) of 2,001 women aged eighteen to forty-five asked questions about vitamins and birth defects. The response rate was 50%. Overall, 30% of nonpregnant women reported taking daily and multivitamin supplements containing folic acid; 19% of nonpregnant women under twenty-five reported taking vitamin supplements daily, compared with 33% of nonpregnant women aged greater than or equal to twenty-five. Among the women who had had a pregnancy during the two years preceding the 1997 survey, 23% reported taking a daily vitamin containing folic acid before pregnancy.

A total of 66% of the respondents said yes to the question "Have you ever read or heard anything about folic acid?; 22% said they had heard of the PHS recommendation about folic acid. Of women who were familiar with folic acid, 16% reported knowing that folic acid helps prevent birth defects and 9% that folic acid should be taken before pregnancy. Few women knew which foods were good sources of folic acid. While this survey was small and the response rate was low, it is clear that strategies need to be improved to increase awareness of the benefits of this vitamin.[44]

Vitamin B_{12}

Vitamin B_{12}, or cobalamine, like folate, is also an important contributor to the process of cell division. Deficiency of this vitamin can therefore lead to the development of megaloblastic anemia with consequences described in the previous section. Fortunately, deficiency of vitamin B_{12} is rare; high-risk women include those who choose a strict vegetarian diet. Such women need vitamin B_{12} supplements of 2 μg per day.

Vitamin B_6

Vitamin B_6, or pyridoxine, is concerned with amino acid metabolism and protein synthesis. In its active form of pyridoxal phosphate, the vitamin is a cofactor in reactions involving a group of enzymes known as transaminases. Vitamin B_6 requirements increase in pregnancy not only because of the greater need for nonessential amino acids in growth but also because the body is making more niacin from tryptophan.

Fetal needs. Urinary excretion of vitamin B_6 metabolites during pregnancy is ten to fifteen times higher than in nonpregnant women, but blood values are typically reduced. Investigators are not sure of the clinical significance of this. There is evidence that the placenta concentrates vitamin B_6 and that levels in cord blood are much higher than in the maternal circulation. This could mean that the reduced maternal blood levels are simply the result of physiologic adjustments. On the other hand, there is also evidence that the fetus takes up more vitamin B_6 and that maternal levels increase when oral supplements are used. Limited animal data suggest adverse pregnancy outcome in the presence of vitamin B_6 deficiency. In addition, European researchers observed that the depth of pregnancy depression correlated negatively with serum vitamin B_6 concentration. Others observed significantly lower Apgar scores in newborns of mothers with evidence of vitamin B_6 deficiency when compared with offspring of controls. The meaning of these observations remains to be determined.[1]

Maternal nausea and vomiting. While the precise etiology of nausea and vomiting during pregnancy remains unknown, interest continues in the possibility that vitamin B_6 status may be important. Vitamin B_6 is known to catalyze a number of reactions involving neurotransmitter production and, in that capacity, could conceivably affect an assortment of physiologic states. However, a clear connection between vitamin B_6 and pregnancy nausea remains to be observed.

Most recently, Thai investigators conducted a large, well-controlled trial in which women in early pregnancy received either 30 mg B_6/day or a placebo for five consecutive days. Patients graded the severity of their nausea by a visual analog scale and recorded the number of vomiting episodes over the previous twenty-four hours. Pyridoxine proved quite effective in decreasing both the severity of nausea and the number of vomiting episodes.[45]

Vitamin C

Vitamin C deficiency has not been shown to affect the course or outcome of pregnancy in humans, but questions have arisen about the possible association of vitamin C with several specific conditions made known through isolated clinical observations. For example, low plasma levels of vitamin C have been reported in association with premature rupture of the membranes and preeclampsia. An extra 10 mg of vitamin C a day is recommended for the pregnant woman. This total recommendation of 70 mg a day is easily met by the U.S. diet. Large intakes of vitamin C supplements may adversely influence fetal metabolism. Metabolic dependency on high doses may develop in the fetus, causing possible scurvy in the neonatal period.

Thiamin, Riboflavin, and Niacin

Since thiamin, riboflavin, and niacin are all part of the reactions that produce energy in the body, requirements are related to caloric intake. Since kilocalorie allowances increase during pregnancy, the allowances for thiamin, riboflavin, and niacin automatically increase also. In addition, evidence from urinary excretion studies indicates that pregnant women have higher requirements for thiamin and riboflavin than do nonpregnant women. The RDA for these two nutrients, therefore, include additional adjustments.

In animals, severe deficiencies of thiamin, riboflavin, or niacin during pregnancy have resulted in fetal death, reduced growth, and congenital malformation. The skeleton and organs that arise from the ectoderm appear to be especially susceptible to riboflavin deficiency. Lack of riboflavin in the mother's diet was once thought to be a cause of prematurity in humans, but recent studies have failed to find a correlation.

Researchers have evaluated the thiamin status of pregnant women at various stages of gestation and have found that 25–30% have values that would be considered deficient by nonpregnant standards. Although there have been some reported cases of congenital beriberi from maternal thiamin deficiency, there is no evidence of impairment at the levels consumed by women in developed countries. The niacin status of pregnant women has been inadequately investigated. However, there are no cases indicating that niacin deficiency in humans produces the malformations noted in experimental animals.

Vitamin D

Vitamin D has long been appreciated for its positive effects on calcium balance during pregnancy. Evidence suggests that vitamin D may be involved in neonatal calcium homeostasis. Observations in Great Britain indicate that the peak season for neonatal hypocalcemia coincides with the time of least sunlight. In addition, serum vitamin D levels are often low in such infants, suggesting that some cases of neonatal hypocalcemia and enamel hypoplasia may relate to maternal vitamin D deficiency and subsequent limitation in placental transport of vitamin D to the fetus. A study of pregnant Asian women showed that vitamin D supplementation during the third trimester was associated with an improved rate of maternal weight gain, higher maternal and newborn serum 25 (OH)D levels at term, a reduced incidence of symptomatic hypocalcemia in newborns, and a lower percentage of small-for-gestational-age infants. However excessive amounts of vitamin D may be harmful during gestation. Severe infantile hypercalcemia and associated problems have been reported in newborn animals and in human infants.[1]

Vitamin A

Vitamin A is an essential nutrient for all animal species because of its critical role in reproduction, the immune system, and vision, as well as in the maintenance of cellular differentiation. Both vitamin A and carotene cross the placenta. Most of our information regarding requirements for vitamin A during pregnancy are extrapolations from animal studies, studies of nonpregnant adult women, or observational studies of women who report night blindness while consuming diets of a certain vitamin A content. Although the need in pregnancy is increased above the nonpregnant state, this additional amount is relatively small and confined mostly to the last trimester. Maternal reserves are generally adequate (at least in developed countries) to meet the need. Therefore, the RDA during pregnancy is not different from that of the nonpregnant state. A chronically inadequate intake below the basal requirement must take place to critically deplete maternal body stores before detrimental effects occur in the mother.[1]

Excessive consumption of vitamin A is believed to be teratogenic in humans, but most of the scientific evidence describes developmental anomalies in animals. Over the past forty years, isolated reports have appeared in the literature which imply that abnormal babies have been born to human mothers who took very large amounts of vitamin A during pregnancy (greater than ten times the RDA).[1] Since 1990, several epidemiologic studies have tended to confirm the findings from earlier case studies. One such study[46] conducted at Boston University involved more than 22,000 pregnant women who were asked many questions about their diets and behaviors during early pregnancy. Information about pregnancy outcomes was obtained largely from their obstetricians. Among other things, results indicated that, the higher the vitamin A intake during the first trimester, the greater the risk of specific birth defects. This increased risk began to show up with intakes greater than 10,000 IU/day. However, Mills and colleagues[47] reported in 1997 that daily intake of vitamin A in excess of 10,000 IU was not associated with the specific birth defects reported by the Boston group. They concluded that, if vitamin A is teratogenic, doses well above 10,000 IU/day taken during early pregnancy would be required to disturb embryonic development.

Vitamin A analog. The adverse effects of excessive vitamin A intake in early pregnancy have also been illustrated by the introduction of isotretinoin (Accutane) into the marketplace. This drug, used to treat cystic acne, is an analog of vitamin A. Since its first appearance on pharmacy shelves in the early 1980s, cases of birth defects and spontaneous abortion have been associated with its use. This toxicity syndrome has been called the *isotretinoin teratogen syndrome.* Major features include prominent **frontal bossing, hydrocephalus, microphthalmia,** and small, malformed, low-set, undifferentiated ears (fig. 4-7). More cautionary labeling has now been provided with the product, and physicians are warned about the possible dangers of prenatal exposure.

Frontal bossing
(ME *boce,* lump, growth) A rounded protuberance of the forehead. In general, a boss is a knob-like rounded protuberance on the body or a body organ.

Hydrocephalus
(Gr *hydro,* water; *kephale,* head) Condition characterized by enlargement of the cranium caused by abnormal accumulation of fluid.

Microphthalmia
(Gr *mikros,* small; *ophthalmos,* eye) Abnormal smallness of one or both eyes.

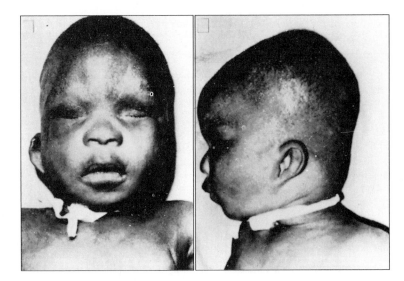

FIG. 4-7   Front and lateral views of a child affected prenatally by isotretinoin.
From Benke, P.J. 1984. *JAMA* 251:3267.

Topical vitamin A. Parenthetically, topical application of retinoids does not appear to pose a problem. Researchers in Seattle used information from the Group Health Cooperative of Puget Sound, Washington, to evaluate the risk of birth defects in mothers exposed to topical tretinoin—a retinoid preparation used to treat acne—in the first trimester of pregnancy.[48] Two hundred fifteen women were identified who had delivered live or stillborn infants at Group Health Cooperative hospitals and who were exposed to topical tretinoin early in pregnancy; 430 age-matched nonexposed women who had delivered live or stillborn babies at the same hospitals served as controls. The prevalence of major anomalies among infants born to the exposed women was 1.9%, and among babies born to the nonexposed women was 2.6%. It was concluded that topical tretinoin is not associated with an increased risk of major congenital disorders.

Vitamin E

Requirements for vitamin E are believed to increase somewhat during pregnancy, but deficiency in humans rarely occurs and has not been linked with either reproductive causality or reduced fertility. Since vitamin E deficiency in experimental animals has long been associated with spontaneous abortion, interest in the use of vitamin E for prevention of abortion has been a popular idea. In general, however, studies in humans have not supported this preventive measure. Several studies have shown, however, that the fetal vitamin E level is one-third to one-fourth the maternal concentration in both premature and term infants. Maternal levels of vitamin E rise during pregnancy such that by the third trimester these levels become 60% greater than in the nonpregnant controls. It has been found, however, that the maternal level must be from 150% to 500% of the value of the nonpregnant controls if the cord blood values are to reach the low normal adult vitamin E concentrations.

Although the vitamin E level in the infant at birth is significantly less than in the mother, the infant's level has been shown to correlate directly with the maternal concentration. Attempts to raise the fetal level by supplementing the mother with vitamin E during the last trimester confirmed the direct correlation of fetal and maternal vitamin E concentrations. It has been concluded, however, that parenteral vitamin E administration to the mother before delivery is not enough to prevent an infant from having the hemolytic anemia of vitamin E deficiency. Since this problem develops within six weeks after birth, it can best be prevented by oral supplementation of the infant during the postnatal interval.

TABLE 4-7 *Estimated Safe and Adequate Daily Dietary Intakes of Additional Selected Vitamins and Minerals for Adolescents and Adults*

	Age Group	
	Adolescents	Adults
Age	11+	
Vitamins		
Biotin (µg)	30–100	30–100
Pantothenic acid (mg)	4–7	4–7
Trace elements (mg)		
Copper	1.5–2.5	1.5–3.0
Manganese	2.0–5.0	2.0–5.0
Fluoride	1.5–2.5	1.5–4.0
Chromium	0.05–0.2	0.05–0.2
Molybdenum	0.075–0.250	0.075–0.250

Modified from Food and Nutrition Board, National Research Council, National Academy of Sciences. 1989. *Recommended dietary allowances.* Washington, DC: U.S. Government Printing Office.

Vitamin K

Data are insufficient for the RDA committee of experts to establish a standard for vitamin K during pregnancy. Additional increments to usual intakes are not recommended, because consumption of this vitamin by adult women usually exceeds the RDA. Efforts to determine if vitamin K supplementation of pregnant women can improve the vitamin K status of their preterm offspring have yielded conflicting results.

Other Vitamins

Little is known about the dietary requirements for biotin and pantothenic acid. Safe and adequate dietary intakes for these vitamins were suggested in the 1989 edition of the RDA (table 4-7).

Iron

During pregnancy, iron is needed for the manufacture of hemoglobin in both maternal and fetal red blood cells. The fetus accumulates most of its iron during the last trimester. At term, a normal weight infant has about 246 mg of iron in blood and body stores. An additional 134 mg are stored in the placenta. About 290 mg are used to expand the volume of the mother's blood.

Erythropoiesis
(Gr *erythros*, red; *poiesis*, making) Production of erythrocytes, red blood cells.

Maintenance of **erythropoiesis** is one of the few instances during pregnancy when the fetus acts as a true parasite. It assures its own production of hemoglobin by drawing iron from the mother. Maternal iron deficiency, therefore, does not usually result in an infant who is anemic at birth. The most common cause of iron deficiency anemia in the infant is prematurity. The infant who has a short gestation simply does not have time to accumulate sufficient iron during the last trimester.

Iron deficiency in the mother may have adverse effects on her obstetric performance. A reduction in hemoglobin concentration means that the mother must increase her cardiac output to maintain adequate oxygen use by placental and fetal cells. This extra work fatigues the mother and makes her more susceptible to other sources of physiologic stress. A very low maternal hemoglobin places the mother at risk of cardiac arrest and leads to a poor prognosis for survival should she hemorrhage on delivery.

Setting requirements for iron during pregnancy is complicated by changes in the erythropoiesis system. Even when women have adequate iron status at conception, the plasma volume increases faster than the number of red blood cells, so that hemodilution occurs. However, erythropoiesis is stimulated in the last half of pregnancy, and the rate of red blood cell production goes up. If sufficient iron is available, hemoglobin levels should rise to at least 11 mg/100 ml by term.

Generally, the initial drop in hemoglobin is a normal physiologic phenomenon, but there is concern that the usual iron intakes of pregnant women may not support increased erythropoiesis and fetal demands in the last half of pregnancy. Iron absorption increases during pregnancy (to as much as 30%), compared with the usual 10% absorption from the diet. Also working in the mother's favor is the 120 mg or so that she saves over the course of gestation because she is not menstruating. However, even when these adjustments are taken into account, the pregnant woman still may need to consume about 30 mg of iron each day to maintain iron reserves. This amount could be supplied if large servings of iron-rich foods were eaten, but, unfortunately, such foods are limited to organ meats, oysters, clams, and prune juice. These are not foods that people typically consume. From an average mixed diet, about 6 mg of iron are obtained from each 1,000 kcal of food. At this rate, a pregnant woman would have to eat 3,000 to 5,000 kcal of food per day to meet her iron needs. Furthermore, studies have shown that most women enter pregnancy with low iron stores, so they have little to draw on to maintain normal hemoglobin.

For this reason, the expert panel from the National Academy of Sciences[49] concluded, "Iron is a nutrient for which requirements cannot be met reasonably by diet alone. To meet the increased need for iron during the second and third trimesters of pregnancy, the average woman needs to absorb approximately 3 mg of iron per day in addition to the amount of iron usually absorbed from food. Evidence from iron supplementation studies indicates that low-dose supplements (e.g., 30 mg of ferrous iron daily during the second and third trimesters) can provide this amount of extra iron." The committee went on to say that, since low doses of iron pose no known dangers to the mother or fetus, the potential benefits of iron supplementation outweigh the risks.

Calcium

The fetus acquires most of its calcium in the last trimester, when skeletal growth is maximum and teeth are being formed. The fetus draws about 13 mg per hour of calcium from the maternal blood supply, or 250 to 300 mg per day. At birth, the infant has accumulated approximately 25 g. Additional calcium is stored in the maternal skeleton as a reserve for lactation.

The reproductive process promotes extensive adjustments in calcium homeostasis. Hormonal factors play a significant role. Over the years, many efforts have been made to clarify the role of the intestines, kidneys, and bones in maintaining calcium balance during pregnancy and lactation and after the resumption of menstruation. Since it has been estimated that the physiologic demands for calcium during pregnancy and lactation are elevated by about 200–300 mg/day, the mother must consume more, absorb more, or lose less to avoid permanent damage to her bones.

Research to date indicates that the maternal organism adjusts to the demands of reproduction.[50] During pregnancy, calcium intake generally increases, as does calcium absorption; this occurs in the face of increased urinary calcium losses. Fetal bone mineralization proceeds normally without substantial net loss of maternal bone. The current recommendation for daily calcium intake during pregnancy is 1,200 mg; this level of intake should satisfy the needs of both fetus and mother.

In 1980, an inverse relationship was reported between calcium intake and hypertensive disorders of pregnancy. It was proposed that satisfactory calcium intake may be protective against elevation in blood pressure during pregnancy. The hypothesis was based on the observation that Mayan Indians in Guatemala, who traditionally soak their corn in lime before cooking, had a high calcium intake and a low incidence of preeclampsia and eclampsia. Reports from other parts of the world have confirmed an inverse relationship between calcium intake and blood pressure during pregnancy. If calcium intake via food or supplements can significantly lower the risk of preeclampsia, strategies to achieve this goal are attractive interventions.

In recent reports,[51,52] available randomized trials in which the intervention included calcium supplementation during pregnancy were evaluated and summarized. These trials suggest that calcium supplementation during pregnancy is associated with a substantial

CASE STUDY

Calcium Needs During Pregnancy

Marcia Nahikian-Nelms Ph.D., R.D., Southwest Missouri State University

Mrs. Romano is a thirty-three-year-old woman who is pregnant with her third child. At twelve weeks' gestation, she is referred to you for general nutrition counseling at her routine prenatal appointment. Mrs. Romano's previous pregnancies were complicated by both eclampsia and preterm labor. These pregnancies were eventual successful outcomes, but both infants were born at about thirty-five weeks' gestation with birth weights of 5 lbs 5 oz and 5 lbs 20 oz, respectively. In addition, both pregnancies required that Mrs. Romano spend much of the last trimester at bedrest, because she experienced preterm labor.

Mrs. Romano gives you the following food frequency:
- (A.M.) toast or bagel, fresh fruit, coffee, and juice
  (midday) sandwich, soup and/or salad; fresh fruit; fruit juice or iced tea
- (P.M.) beef, chicken, or fish; pasta, rice, or potato; one or two fresh or frozen vegetables, including broccoli, romaine lettuce, asparagus; fruit juice or iced tea
  (snacks) popcorn, fruit, frozen yogurt

When you ask her about her intake of milk and dairy products, she tells you that she has never really liked milk and that her parents and other family members tend to avoid dairy products. She occasionally eats cheese but states that it is too high in fat. The only other dairy product she consumes occasionally is frozen yogurt. She says, "I do take my prenatal vitamin everyday, and I know that it has calcium in it. I also eat lots of dark green vegetables, and I know there is lots of calcium there too. And I use an antacid for heartburn that is advertised as containing calcium."

Questions for analysis
1. Compare Mrs. Romano's diet history with her recommended needs during pregnancy.
2. What is the physiologic role of calcium in the body?
3. Mrs. Romano appears to eat a variety of foods, but can she meet her calcium requirements without the consumption of dairy products? Using a food composition table in the appendix, calculate the amount of calcium from her typical diet. Compare this with the requirements during pregnancy.
4. How may calcium intake be related to preeclampsia and the incidence of preterm labor?
5. How could you use this information to convince Mrs. Romano to increase her intake of dairy products? What strategies might you use to increase her calcium intake? At what point would you recommend calcium supplementation?
6. You also notice during your assessment that Mrs. Romano has multiple dental caries. Is this probably a result of low calcium intake during her previous pregnancy?

reduction in the risk of hypertension during pregnancy and of preeclampsia. There was also evidence of a moderate but promising reduction in preterm labor. The authors concluded that calcium supplementation during pregnancy appears to reduce the risk of preeclampsia, and there is promising evidence of a reduction in the risk of preterm delivery. If these benefits were to lead to a reduction in the number of perinatal deaths or disabled survivors, this would be a substantial advance in the care of women during pregnancy. However, the newly published multicenter Calcium for Prevention of Preeclampsia trial conducted in the United States found no measurable benefit of 2000 mg/day calcium supplementation for blood pressure control or prevention of preeclampsia. Since the women participating in this study were already consuming approximately 1100 mg/day of calcium, relative calcium deficiency was unlikely.

In the spring of 1997, a spokesperson for the obstetrics and gynecology community made the following statement: "Because of the efficacy and safety of calcium supplementation, current evidence supports administering 1.5–2.0 g/day of elemental calcium for pregnant women who are at high risk for developing preeclampsia, e.g., women with multiple pregnancies, chronic hypertension, diabetes mellitus, or prior preeclampsia. Studies indicate that many pregnant women consume only about half the Recommended Dietary Allowance of 1.2 g/day. Thus, a case can be made on a nutritional basis alone for supplementing calcium in all pregnant women."[53]

Phosphorus

The RDA standard for phosphorus is the same as that for calcium, 800 mg with an extra 400 mg during pregnancy. It is so widely available in foods that a dietary deficiency is rare. In fact, many problems may be caused by too much phosphorus rather than too little. Most adults can tolerate relatively wide variation in dietary calcium-phosphorus ratios when vitamin D is adequate.

Calcium-phosphorus balance relates to the maintenance of normal neuromuscular action. Twenty years ago, it was suggested that sudden clonic or tonic contractions of the *gastrocnemius muscle* (posterior "calf" muscle that flexes knee and ankle joints), occurring often at night, was caused by a decline in serum calcium. Prevention or relief was proclaimed to come from reduction of milk intake, a high phosphorus and calcium beverage. Supplementation with nonphosphate calcium salts was also recommended, along with regular use of aluminum hydroxide to form insoluble aluminum phosphate salts in the gut. While anecdotal reports have suggested some benefit of these measures, controlled and double blind studies have failed to show any correlation between leg cramps and either the intake of dairy products or the type of calcium supplement used.

Magnesium

Magnesium is much like calcium and phosphorus in that most of it is stored in the bones. The amounts that are biochemically active are concentrated in nerve and muscle cells. Deficiencies of magnesium produce neuromuscular dysfunction characterized by tremors and convulsions. Magnesium-deficient pregnant rats show impaired abdominal contractions during parturition. Not a great deal is known about the need for magnesium during pregnancy. The RDA standard is based on estimates of the amounts accumulated by the mother and the fetus.

Studies of leg cramps have included both magnesium and calcium. Magnesium therapy as treatment for nightly leg cramps has been studied in several populations, including elderly men and women and people with Type I diabetes; good results have apparently been found. Leg cramps have been reported in 5–30% of all pregnant women, most often during the latter months of pregnancy and without relationship to other complications or to unfavorable fetal outcome. Low serum magnesium levels have been reported in pregnant women with leg cramps.

Recently, Dahle et al.[54] sought to determine whether low levels of serum magnesium occur in women with pregnancy-related leg cramps and whether the symptoms can be alleviated by oral magnesium substitution. Seventy-three pregnant women with leg cramps participated in this controlled, prospective, randomized, double-blind trial. Interviews and laboratory tests were performed before and after the three-week intervention. The serum magnesium levels of these patients were at or below the lower reference limit, which is common for pregnant women. Oral magnesium substitution decreased leg cramp distress significantly but did not increase serum magnesium levels; excess magnesium was excreted as measured by an increase in urinary magnesium levels. The authors concluded that magnesium supplementation seems to be a valuable tool in the treatment of pregnancy-related leg cramps.

Zinc

Zinc has an active role in metabolism for several reasons: 1) it is a component of insulin, 2) it is part of the carbonic anhydrase enzyme system that helps maintain acid-base balance in the tissues, and 3) it acts in the synthesis of DNA and RNA, which gives it a very important role in reproduction.

Much recent interest has centered on the significance of zinc deficiency in adversely affecting pregnancy course and outcome. Zinc is a known constituent of a number of important metalloenzymes and a necessary cofactor for other enzymes. Zinc deficiency in rats leads to development of congenital malformations. Nonhuman primates also are affected. Abnormal brain development and behavior have been described in offspring of zinc-deficient monkeys. Evidence from human populations suggests that the malformation rate and other poor pregnancy outcomes may be higher in populations where zinc deficiency has been recognized. However, since conflicting reports also appear in the literature and questions remain about satisfactory measures of zinc status, the true role of zinc deficiency in adverse course and outcome of human pregnancy remains unknown. The potential hazard of prenatal zinc supplements has not been determined in human populations. Haphazard use of such supplements, however, has no role in wise prenatal care.[1]

Iodine

Iodine deficiency is by far the most common preventable cause of mental deficits in the world.[1] The most severe form of endemic cretinism is characterized by a combination of mental deficiency, deafmutism, and motor rigidity, and sometimes hypothyroidism occurs in parts of the world where iodine deficiency is sufficiently severe to cause goiter in 30% of the population. It is found in southern and Eastern Europe and is common in Asia, Africa, and Latin America. Iodine injections in the form of iodized oil before but not during pregnancy prevent cretinism. Studies in China showed that 2% of infants of mothers who had had injections in the second trimester of pregnancy compared with 9% of those whose mothers had had injections in the second trimester had moderate or severe neurodevelopmental abnormalities. The importance of maternal thyroid hormone is supported by research results showing that maternal thyroxine is transported across the placenta to the fetus and that iodine-replete but hypothyroid women have an increased frequency of stillbirths as well as cretinism and less severe neurological defects of motor and cognitive performance in live-born infants.

In 1990, the World Health Organization estimated that 20 million people in the world had preventable brain damage due to the effects of iodine deficiency on fetal brain development. It also set at 1 billion people the number at risk for iodine deficiency caused by low levels of iodine in the soil. Twenty percent of these had goiter. Prevalence of neonatal hypothyroidism varied from 1% to 10% in these areas.[55]

Other dietary compounds may affect iodine bioavailability. This is suspected to be the case in the Republic of Guinea, where the overall prevalence of goiter is 70% among adults. Thyroid swelling is sometimes present at birth and affects 55% of schoolchildren. In this region, iodine deficiency is the primary causative factor, but the diet also contains substantial amounts of thiocyanate anions, which are likely to further depress iodine bioavailability. Other dietary components, notably flavonoids, are suspected to contribute.[56]

Fluoride

The role of fluoride in prenatal development is poorly understood. Some questions have existed over the past fifty years about the degree of fluoride transport across the placenta. Should it cross the placenta, questions still remain about its value in the development of caries-resistant permanent teeth.

Development of the primary dentition begins at ten to twelve weeks of pregnancy. From the sixth to ninth months of pregnancy, the first four permanent molars and eight of the permanent incisors begin to form. Thus, thirty-two of the ultimate teeth are forming and developing during human pregnancy. Since there is no indication that color of the teeth is adversely affected and some evidence that caries resistance and morphologic characteristics are improved, prenatal fluoride supplementation may be justified. *It should be recognized, however, that this issue is highly controversial and to date formal support for routine prenatal fluoride supplementation has not been voiced by any established medical or dental organization.*

Sodium

The metabolism of sodium is altered during pregnancy under the stimulus of a modified hormonal milieu. Glomerular filtration increases markedly over time to "clean up" the increased maternal blood volume. An additional filtered sodium load of 5,000 to 10,000 mEq daily is typically seen during pregnancy. Compensatory mechanisms come into play to maintain fluid and electrolyte balance.

Dietary sodium restriction has been used in various countries for the prevention of preeclampsia. This is still the case in The Netherlands, but recent research has shown that it does not work.[57] It may, however, alter the diet in some negative respects. Dutch scientists studied the effects of long-term sodium restriction on the intake of other nutrients and the outcome of pregnancy.[58] Sixty-eight healthy pregnant women were randomly assigned to either a low-sodium diet or an unrestricted diet; the diet was consumed between week fourteen of gestation and delivery. Rigid dietary sodium restriction was associated with reduced intake of fat, protein, and calcium; it tended to reduce energy intake, limit weight gain, and reduce maternal fat stores. It had no major effect on birth weight. However, the undesirable impact that sodium restriction had on dietary pattern may be of concern for women who have poor nutritional status before pregnancy.

Other Minerals

One of the more recent advances in nutrition research is the discovery that many other trace elements are necessary for human growth, general health, and reproduction. Chromium, manganese, copper, selenium, molybdenum, vanadium, tin, nickel, and silicon have all been shown to be needed by the body. Like iodine, calcium, and phosphorus, these elements (and likely others as well) participate in reactions that control body processes. Studies in animals have revealed that deficiencies produce widespread and serious metabolic defects. Limited knowledge of requirements in humans makes it impossible to establish RDA standards for most of these minerals. The current RDA does, however, list estimated safe and adequate daily dietary intakes for copper, manganese, fluoride, chromium, and molybdenum (review table 4-7). No figures are available for pregnant women. Since toxic levels for many of the trace elements may be much higher than usual intakes, pregnant women should not take supplements that would greatly exceed the upper limits recommended.

GENERAL COMMENTS ABOUT NUTRIENT SUPPLEMENTATION ≋

Commonsense supplementation of pregnant women with vitamin and/or minerals is justifiable. The decision to supplement is best based on evidence that the woman is in need of such. Time taken to pursue information about dietary patterns is indicated for high-risk women; the use of a registered dietitian may be cost-effective. Whether or not nutrient supplementation can be clearly justified or is simply suspected to be advantageous, care should be taken to provide recommendations for safe levels of daily intake.

Summary

While much remains to be learned about the roles that nutrients play in assuring satisfactory pregnancy course and outcome, much has been learned during the past fifty years. Nutrition guidelines for pregnant women (and those planning a pregnancy) are based on current available information. Good overall nutrition optimizes birth weight; prevention of specific vitamin/mineral deficiencies and excesses reduces risk of congenital malformations. Under the best of circumstances, after delivery of her infant, the mother remains, with satisfactory nutritional stores to recover rapidly, lactate successfully, and take on the responsibilities of caring for an infant.

Review Questions

1. Describe the WIC program.
2. Define total weight gain recommendations for normal pregnant women.
3. Cite the current recommended daily folic acid intake for women of reproductive age.
4. Identify these nutrients for which excessive intake during pregnancy is believed to be harmful.
5. Discuss how pregnancy does or does not modify a woman's need for iron and calcium.
6. List ten foods that contribute significant folic acid to the diet.

5

MATERNAL NUTRITION: ISSUES BEYOND THE NUTRIENTS

Bonnie S. Worthington-Roberts

≈≈ ≈≈ ≈≈ ≈≈ ≈≈ ≈≈ ≈≈ ≈≈ ≈≈

Basic Concepts

☐ *Unusual eating behaviors that occur during pregnancy require evaluation.*

☐ *Some nonnutrient components of foods may harm the fetus.*

☐ *Commonsense attention to physical activity during pregnancy is justified.*

☐ *Common discomforts of pregnancy may be minimized by attention to maternal diet.*

☐ *High-risk pregnancies often require specific dietary manipulations.*

Discussion of maternal nutrition during pregnancy would be incomplete without mention of a variety of diet and lifestyle issues that may impact the mother and/or the fetus. These include food cravings, early-pregnancy nausea, potentially harmful nonnutrient food components, substance abuse, exercise, and certain chronic diseases, which themselves are treated with dietary manipulation. In this chapter, a brief discussion of each of these topics is provided.

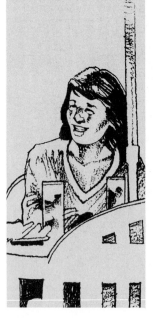

FOOD BELIEFS, CRAVINGS, AVOIDANCES, AND AVERSIONS ≈≈

Most women change their diets during the course of pregnancy. Some changes are based on medical advice, others on folk medical beliefs, and others on changes in preference and appetite that may be idiosyncratic or culturally patterned. Since those changes that are culturally sanctioned affect a woman's willingness to follow prescribed dietary regimens, the health care provider should be sensitized to their existence.

Food Beliefs and Food Behaviors

Many beliefs have been recorded about prenatal diet, such as the idea that the mother can mark her child before birth by eating specific foods.[1] Overuse of a craved food during pregnancy is thought to explain physical or behavioral peculiarities of the infant. More often, unsatiated cravings are thought to explain birthmarks that mimic the shape of the desired food (such as strawberry- or drumstick-shaped marks). Behavioral markings have also been thought to derive from the prenatal diet; that is, the mother's consumption of many foods has been said to cause the child to like such foods after birth.

Another important group of beliefs concerns dietary means by which the mother can ensure an easier delivery. Most important, from the biomedical viewpoint, are beliefs that lead a woman to avoid animal protein foods or to avoid "excessive" weight gain. Most laypeople know very well that a smaller weight gain during pregnancy produces a smaller

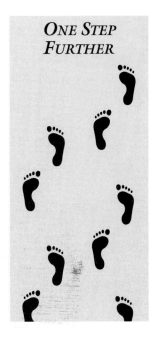

ONE STEP FURTHER

Should Supplements Be Recommended for All Women with Childbearing Potential?

Potential Supplement Benefits

1. Improved nutritional status.
2. Reduced risk of some developmental defects.
3. Improved antioxidant and immune status.
4. Lower incidence and slower progression of some diseases.
5. Harmonization of government and health professionals' dietary recommendations for optimal health.

Questions

1. Will the supplement reduce the women's motivation to maintain and/or improve dietary quality?
2. Will the supplement result in excessive nutrient intakes and adverse nutrient/nutrient interactions?
3. Will supplement use encourage the perception that all women are, by definition, well nourished?

---

infant. Thus, since a smaller baby may be "easier to deliver," low weight gain has been proposed as desirable, especially since it is commonly believed that the baby can "catch up" after birth.

Food avoidances are behaviors away from foods the mother consciously chooses not to consume during her pregnancy, usually for a reason she can articulate and that seems reasonable to her. The four most commonly avoided foods are sources of animal protein: milk, lean meats, pork, and liver. Cravings and aversions are powerful urges toward or away from foods, including foods about which women experience no unusual attitudes outside of pregnancy. The most commonly reported craved foods are sweets and dairy products. The most common aversions are reported to be to alcohol, caffeinated drinks, and meats. However, cravings and aversions are not limited to any particular food or food groups.

The nutritional significance of these food-related behaviors is difficult to evaluate. Available information has often been collected in an anecdotal or one-sided manner. Thus, there is limited detailed information on dietary alterations that appear to be detrimental and little knowledge of total subcultural prenatal dietary intakes. As a result, it is difficult to quantify the nutritional effect of restrictive beliefs, avoidances, cravings, or aversions. The nutritional importance of such practices cannot be assessed without reference to the rest of the woman's diet. Overall, however, most cravings result in increased intakes of calcium and energy, whereas aversions often result in decreased intake of animal protein. Such cravings and aversions are not necessarily deleterious.

Pica

One type of compulsive food behavior or craving during pregnancy, however, does carry potential danger.[2–4] This practice is termed *pica* (from the Latin word for magpie, with reference to the bird's **omnivorous** appetite). Human pica is the compulsion for persistent ingestion of unsuitable substances having little or no nutritional value. Pica of pregnancy most often involves consumption of dirt or clay (geophagia) or starch (amylophagia). However, compulsive ingestion of a variety of nonfood substances, such as ice, burnt matches, hair, stone or gravel, charcoal, soot, cigarette ashes, mothballs, antacid tablets, milk of magnesia, baking soda, coffee grounds, and tire inner tubes, has been noted. The practice of pica is not new, nor is it limited to any one geographic area, race, creed, culture, sex, or status within a culture.

The medical implications of pica are not well understood, although several speculations have been made. The displacement effect of pica substances could result in reduced intake

Omnivorous
(L *omnis,* all; *vorare,* to eat)
Eating all kinds of foods, both animal and plant.

of nutritious foods, leading to inadequate dietary intakes of essential nutrients. Alternatively, substances that provide kilocalories, such as starch, could lead to obesity if ingested in large amounts above the usual dietary intakes. Some pica substances may contain toxic compounds or quantities of nutrients not tolerated in disease states. Some pica substances interfere with the absorption of certain mineral elements, such as iron.[5] Other less commonly reported complications of pica include:

1. *Lead poisoning.* Congenital lead poisoning secondary to maternal pica for wall plaster.
2. *Irritable uterus.* Tender, irritable uterus with dystocia associated with fecal impaction from clay ingestion.
3. *Anemia.* Fetal hemolytic anemia caused by maternal ingestion of mothballs and toilet air fresheners.
4. *Obstruction.* Parotid enlargement and gastric and small bowel obstruction from ingestion of excessive laundry starch.
5. *Infection.* Parasitic infection from ingestion of contaminated soil or clay.

The etiology of pica is poorly understood, although several proposals have been made. One theory suggests that the ingestion of nonfood substances relieves nausea and vomiting. Another theory suggests that the deficiency of an essential nutrient, such as calcium or iron, results in the eating of nonfood substances that contain these nutrients. When pregnant women were questioned about the practice of pica, they gave a variety of answers:

- A taste for clay existed.
- Clay kept the baby from being marked at birth.
- Nervous tension was relieved.
- Starch made the newborn lighter in color.
- Starch helped the baby "slide out" more easily during delivery.
- Clay quieted hunger pains.

 ## CASE STUDY

Pica Cases

Case 1

In England a twenty-one-year-old woman was hospitalized at thirty-eight weeks' gestation because of severe anemia. She was generally tired, was occasionally dizzy, and had edema of the ankles and mild anorexia. After three weeks of concentrated treatment with iron and folic acid, she showed no improvement. Through further questioning, it was found that throughout her pregnancy she had been eating toilet air freshener blocks at the rate of one to two per week. Cessation of this practice led to immediate improvement.

Case 2

A thirty-one-year-old black woman was admitted to a rural emergency room with extreme weakness, severe nausea and vomiting, and fever. The patient reported no bowel movements during the preceding two weeks. On examination, she was lethargic and appeared critically ill. Within ten minutes of arrival, she experienced a grand mal seizure followed by cardiorespiratory arrest. Efforts at resuscitation were unsuccessful and the woman died. Autopsy findings included 3 L of pus within the peritoneal cavity and a 4 cm perforation of the sigmoid colon. Free within the cavity were stones measuring 2.5 cm in diameter and a clay ball measuring 5 cm in diameter. Near the site of perforation, the colon was impacted with hardened clay-like material. Subsequent inquiry of the family revealed that clay ingestion in the rural area was commonplace, and the husband noted that three of the patient's four children occasionally ate clay from the same bank their mother had used.

- Clay and starch were pleasant to chew.
- Pica carries social approval.

Many of these reasons are based on superstition, customs, and traditions or on practices passed from mother to daughter over generations. Two examples of pica, one of which caused maternal death, are described in the case study.

EFFECTS OF POTENTIALLY HARMFUL FOOD COMPONENTS ≋

A number of food components have shown harmful effects on the course and outcome of pregnancy. Several of these agents and their effects are alcohol, caffeine, food additives, and food contaminants.

Alcohol

Fetal alcohol syndrome (FAS). During the past twenty-five years, health researchers have become aware of the adverse effect of excessive consumption of alcohol on fetal development. In 1973, pediatricians in Seattle, Washington, described a unique set of characteristics of infants born to women who were chronic alcoholics. These infants exhibited specific anomalies of the eyes, nose, heart, and central nervous system that were accompanied by growth retardation, small head circumference, and mental retardation (fig. 5-1). The investigators named the condition *fetal alcohol syndrome* (FAS) (tables 5-1 and 5-2). The condition does not necessarily lead to death but is associated with permanent disabilities (fig. 5-2).

There is a high rate of prenatal mortality among infants with FAS. Infants who survive are generally irritable and hyperactive after birth. These symptoms are attributed

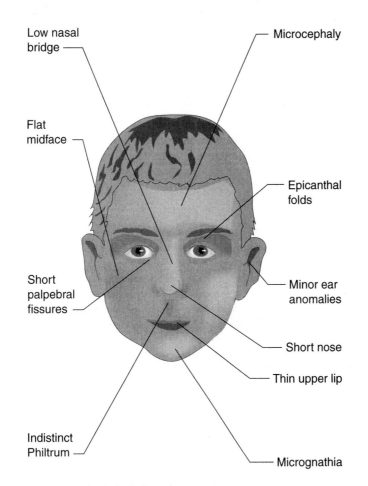

FIG. 5-1   Facial characteristics in fetal alcohol syndrome.

TABLE 5-1 *Facial Characteristics in Fetal Alcohol Syndrome*

	Features Necessary to Characteristic Face	Associated Features
Eyes	Short palpebral fissures	
Nose	Short and upturned in early childhood, hypoplastic philtrum	Flat nasal bridge; epicanthal folds
Maxilla	Flattened	
Mouth	Thinned upper vermilion	Prominent lateral palatine ridges, cleft lip with or without cleft palate; small teeth
Mandible		Retrognathia in infancy; micrognathia or relative prognathia in adolescents
Ears		Posterior rotation, abnormal concha

From Clarren, S., and D. Smith. 1978. *N Engl J Med* 298:1063–67. Reprinted with permission from *The New England Journal of Medicine.*

TABLE 5-2 *More Subtle Features of Fetal Alcohol Syndrome*

Characteristics	Indicators of Central Nervous System Dysfunction
Growth deficiency for height and weight	Microcephaly (small head circumference)
Distinct pattern of facial features and other physical abnormalities	Poor coordination
Central nervous system dysfunction	Lower average IQ
	Hyperactivity
	Attention problems
	Learning difficulties
	Developmental delays
	Motor problems

to alcohol withdrawal. Physical and mental development is impaired. FAS infants exhibit poor rates of weight gain and failure to thrive, despite concerted efforts at nutritional rehabilitation. The box on p. 107 illustrates the occurrence of FAS due to maternal ingestion of alcohol—in this instance, in the unusual form of large amounts of cough syrup.

Fetal alcohol effects. The impact of more moderate levels of alcohol consumption on fetal development has been the focus of much research during the past twenty years. It is now recognized that moderate drinkers may produce offspring with fetal alcohol effects (FAE); this term refers to the more subtle features of FAS.

Diagnosis of FAE is by no means an easy task. For this reason, the term *possible fetal alcohol effects (PFAE)* has been coined to describe individuals who have been prenatally exposed to alcohol and present with cognitive and behavioral problems but do not have all of the facial characteristics of FAS. Simply put, PFAE is "FAS without a face." In the absence of the characteristic facial features, the cognitive/behavioral dysfunction in an individual cannot be directly and exclusively linked to the prenatal alcohol exposure. Therefore, FAE is not a medical diagnosis at this time, and it is more accurate to use the term *PFAE*. PFAE is also not a mild form of FAS. In fact, individuals with PFAE can be just as severely affected cognitively and behaviorally as those with FAS. The needs of individuals with PFAE and their families may be just as acute as those with full FAS. However, it is often difficult for affected individuals to access services because they do not have a medical diagnosis.[6]

General actions of alcohol. At present, the mechanisms by which alcohol produces such widespread effects on the fetus are not completely understood.[7,8] Scientists have used experimental animals and in vitro methods—whole embryos or cells grown in a test tube or petri dish—to help them determine the molecular and cellular events affected by expo-

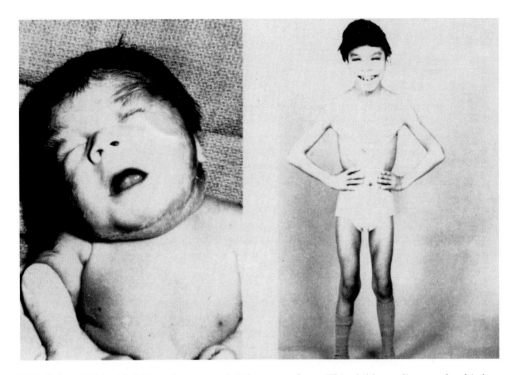

FIG. 5-2 Child with FAS at day one and eight years of age. This child was diagnosed at birth and has spent all his life in a foster home where the quality of care has been excellent. His IQ has remained stable at 40 to 45. Although he is more seriously retarded than most children with FAS, he demonstrates the resistance of the disability to environmental intervention.

Courtesy of Dr. Ann P. Streissguth, University of Washington, Seattle.

 ## CASE STUDY

Fetal Alcohol Syndrome

An infant with typical features of FAS, including a head circumference below the tenth percentile on the National Center for Health Statistics growth chart, was born at term to a twenty-four-year-old mother who reported consumption of 480 to 840 ml per day of a nonprescription cough syrup. The alcohol content of the syrup was 9.5%, or 36.5 to 63.8 g per day, equivalent to the alcohol content of 1 to 2 L of 4% beer or 0.5 to 1.0 L of wine.

Intensive prenatal care had been instituted with entry into an addiction treatment program at an undefined point in pregnancy. No evidence of distortion of truth was found with urinary test for substance abuse. Whether pregnancy outcome was related to alcohol, to other drugs, or to their interactive effects is not clear. The case emphasizes the need for awareness of the full content of over-the-counter drugs used in pregnancy.

Questions for Analysis
1. What other over-the-counter medications contain alcohol?
2. What items on shelves in the kitchen contain significant amounts of alcohol?

Answers
1. A variety of sleep inducers and cold remedies contain alcohol.
2. Besides wine, flavorings are an example of alcohol-containing products.

CASE STUDY

Lifestyle Issues

Beth appears for prenatal care at 12 weeks gestation. She is concerned about the baby's well-being and seems to know much about what she should and should not do during pregnancy. She cries and tells you that she celebrated her anniversary about eight weeks ago with a bottle of champagne; she did not know that she was pregnant and now she is afraid of what damage might have been done to the fetus.

Questions for Analysis
1. This is not an uncommon scenario. What do you tell this woman?
2. It is very important that the rest of this pregnancy goes well. Outline your approach to counseling this woman the duration of this prenatal period.

sure of embryonic tissues to alcohol. Since alcohol can cross the placenta, the current hypothesis is that high levels build up in the fetus and produce direct toxic effects that are most adverse in the early phases of pregnancy. Another theory is that some of the effects of alcohol may be caused by maternal malnutrition. Women who derive a substantial portion of their daily caloric needs from alcohol may not have an appetite for more nutritious foods. Micronutrient deficiencies are frequently seen in alcoholics.

Besides the possible role of nutritional deficiencies in the manifestation of FAS, other theories have been introduced. Adverse changes have been proposed to occur in the following:
- Hormonal factors
- Local growth factors
- Level and variety of prostaglandins
- Diminished oxygen delivery to fetal tissues
- Impaired cell migration and adhesion

Many crucial biochemical and cellular events are affected by exposure of the fetus to alcohol during gestation. It is too early to speculate whether any one of alcohol's effects on molecular or cellular function is more significant than others.

Prevention of FAS and FAE. In the developed world, fetal alcohol syndrome is the major cause of significant lifetime disabilities. Unlike many other birth defects, however, it is preventable. Prevention of FAS is a national health priority included in the *Healthy People 2000* objectives for health promotion and disease prevention. The specific health objective is *to reduce the rate of FAS to no more than 1.2 cases per 10,000 live births by the year 2000.* Surveillance programs allow for the tracking of the prevalence of a condition over time. Tracking the prevalence of FAS poses particular problems, however, since there is no "gold standard" of diagnosis. At the present time, the reported incidence rate of FAS is high.[9,10]

It is imperative to identify alcohol and other drug use in pregnant women as early as possible during the course of prenatal care so that interventions may be applied. However, many health professionals do not feel comfortable asking pregnant women about alcohol and other drug use. In addition, the time constraints of many busy prenatal clinics and private practices encourage health professionals to avoid adding time-consuming assessments to their already busy schedules. However, there are a number of quick screening tests for unsafe alcohol use. One is called T-ACE, which asks four questions about *tolerance* to alcohol *(T)*, being *annoyed* about other comments about drinking *(A)*, attempts to *cut down* (C) and having a drink first thing in the morning (E—*eye-opener*). A recent study showed its sensitivity for detecting lifetime alcohol diagnoses, risk drinking, and current alcohol consumption.[11]

A recent survey examined alcohol use among pregnant women in the United States. An attempt was made to characterize pregnant women who use alcohol with an emphasis on frequent use (at least five drinks per occasion or at least seven drinks per week). Overall, about 15% consumed alcohol and about 2% consumed alcohol frequently. Pregnant women who were at high risk for alcohol use were college-educated, were unmarried, were unemployed (or students), had annual household incomes of more than $50,000, or were smokers. Pregnant women who were at high risk for frequent alcohol use were more likely to be unmarried or smokers.[12]

Paternal alcohol exposure. The possibility exists that paternal alcohol consumption affects fetal development through a direct effect on the father's sperm or gonads. There are three possible mechanisms for the effect of paternal alcohol consumption on the offspring. First, alcohol may directly affect the characteristics and properties of sperm, perhaps by causing mutations in the sperm's genetic material. Second, sperm may be "selected," such that only a specific population is functionally intact following prolonged exposure to alcohol. Third, alcohol consumption might alter the chemical composition of semen so as to influence the activity of ejaculated sperm. Animal studies suggest that any of these possibilities holds true. Much more investigation of human males is required before useful light can be shed on this issue.[13]

Caffeine

In 1980, the Food and Drug Administration warned pregnant women to restrict or even eliminate consumption of coffee based on studies showing teratogenic effects in rodents. While this advisory remains in effect, the implications of caffeine consumption during pregnancy remain controversial.

The results of studies in rodents indicate that caffeine, when administered in large single doses, has teratogenic effects.[14] In addition to fetal resorptions, the most frequently seen malformations are those of the limbs and digits, as well as cleft lips and palates. Such malformations are observed, however, only in relatively high doses. Teratogenic effects usually appear only at doses high enough to cause toxicity in the mother and far higher than those consumed by humans, even those who drink large amounts of coffee. For example, a woman weighing 60 kg would have to drink about ten to fourteen cups of coffee in one sitting in order to achieve plasma caffeine concentrations comparable to those associated with teratogenic effects in rats. Animal studies in which more moderate doses were administered over the course of a day (to mimic the typical pattern of human caffeine intake) have not shown teratogenic effects.

The available human evidence indicates that there is at most a very slight relationship between moderate caffeine consumption and the incidence of common congenital abnormalities.[15,16] Most epidemiological surveys have not shown an association between caffeine intake and the frequency of malformations. However, very little is known about the potential teratogenic effect of very large amounts of coffee (more than eight cups per day).[17,18]

Just how caffeine may interfere with the normal reproductive process is open for debate. Of interest, however, is a recent report by Norwegian researchers interested in the now popular topic of plasma homocysteine and risk of cardiovascular disease.[19] In a population of more than 15,000 men and women, daily use of coffee was reported by 89.1% of the participants, of whom 94.9% used caffeinated filtered coffee. There was a marked positive dose-response relation between coffee consumption and plasma homocysteine. The combination of cigarette smoking and high caffeine intake was associated with particularly high homocysteine concentrations. Since elevated levels of plasma homocysteine has been mentioned as a distinct risk factor for adverse pregnancy outcome, this observation is particularly provocative.

In light of the inconclusive data regarding caffeine and pregnancy outcome, several experts have concluded the following: "In the absence of more precise data and to avoid any fetotoxic risk, women should be advised to moderate their consumption of coffee during pregnancy and above all, to avoid tobacco and alcohol as well as other vasoconstricting medications such as anti-migraine drugs the innocuity of which has not yet been proven."[15]

CASE STUDY

Fetal Arrhythmia Caused by Excessive Intake of Caffeine by Pregnant Women

Case 1

A twenty-six-year-old woman experienced preterm labor from thirty-four to thirty-six weeks' gestation. Ten days later, she gave birth to a boy who weighed ~3100 g; his Apgar score at five minutes was 8. Management of this infant was "touch and go" from the beginning, but the ultimate result was that this baby seemed fine when released from the hospital. The only remarkable finding was that the woman had drunk ten cups of coffee during the last hours before delivery. The baby's urine contained caffeine.

Case 2

A twenty-three-year-old woman was admitted to a hospital at forty weeks' gestation to deliver her first baby. The fetal heart rate was very irregular, but laboratory tests of cardiac performance were fine. During and after delivery, the fetal heart rate remained irregular. The point of interest is that the woman reported that she had drunk 1.5 L of cola each day during the past two weeks because of the hot weather. Although the baby was small, she did well, even though her cardiac performance was abnormal. However, caffeine could have taken its toll.

Case 3

A twenty-two-year-old woman was admitted to the hospital at twenty-three weeks' gestation because of fetal arrhythmia. The fetal heart seemed fine, but the heart rate was totally irregular. Laboratory tests were normal. The woman reported that she had drunk more than 1.5 L of cola, two cups of coffee, and one cup of cocoa daily. She was told not to drink anything that contained caffeine; one week later, the arrhythmias stopped and the pregnancy continued without problems.

From Oei, S., R.P.L. Vosters, and N.L.J. van der Hagen. 1989. Fetal arrhythmia caused by excessive intake of caffeine by pregnant women. *BMJ* 298:568.

Food Additives

The teratogenicity of common food additives is largely unknown in human situations.[1] Metabolism of cyclamate and red dye no. 2 reportedly damages developing rat embryos, but both of these additives have now been banned for use in the U.S. food supply. Saccharin, mannitol, xylitol, aspartame, and other artificial sugar substitutes have come under careful scrutiny in the past several decades. Kline and co-workers have reported, however, that incidence of spontaneous abortion in a human population is not associated with ingestion of any sugar substitute.

Saccharin. Because saccharin has been shown to be weakly carcinogenic in rats, moderation in its use seems appropriate. This is especially true for women of reproductive age, since studies in rats indicate that saccharin can most effectively initiate bladder cancer when the mother is exposed to high doses before pregnancy and the offspring are exposed in utero and throughout their lives. Saccharin can also markedly promote or enhance the potential of other carcinogens in rats, providing another reason for moderation in use.

Aspartame. The increasing use of aspartame in the American food supply has been associated with outcries from a minority of scientists who propose that one or more of the breakdown products of aspartame may interfere with normal fetal development. Chemically, aspartame is L-aspartyl-L-phenylalanine methyl ester. The dipeptide ester is metabolized into three moieties in the small intestine, so that studies of the safety of aspartame are essentially studies of aspartic acid, phenylalanine, and methanol.

Human studies with pregnant women. Human subjects have been fed up to six times the 99th percentile of the projected daily intake (6 × 34 = 200 mg/kg). No evidence of risk to the fetus has been observed. Aspartate does not readily cross the placenta. Small elevations of blood methanol following the above-abuse doses of aspartame have not led to measurable increases in blood formic acid, which is the product responsible for the acidosis and ocular toxicity of methanol poisoning. Phenylalanine is concentrated on the fetal side of the placenta.

Phenylalanine and PKU. The phenylalanine component of aspartame has raised the most concern due to the unknown damaging impact of phenylalanine on brain tissue of children with phenylketonuria (PKU). Individuals with this genetic disease lack the liver enzyme that converts phenylalanine to tyrosine. Thus, blood levels of phenylalanine rise to high levels, and mental retardation is the ultimate result. Aspartame in abuse doses up to 200 mg/kg in normal subjects, or to 100 mg/kg in PKU **heterozygotes** (carriers of the gene for PKU), have not been found to raise blood phenylalanine levels to the range generally accepted to be associated with mental retardation in offspring.

Conclusions. One might conclude that, under foreseeable conditions of use, aspartame poses no risk for use in pregnancy. However, since limited data are available to date on pregnancy course and outcome in heavy aspartame users, it may be wise to recommend moderation in aspartame use during pregnancy, especially in women known to be PKU heterozygotes.

> **Heterozygotes**
> (Gr *hetero,* other; *zygotos,* yoked together) Individuals possessing different *alleles* (gene forms occupying corresponding chromosome sites) in regard to a given trait.

Food Contaminants[1]

General toxicity. A number of "contaminants" are found in food. Some of these may adversely affect pregnancy course and outcome if consumed in sufficient amounts. Most heavy metals are embryotoxic, but only mercury, lead, cadmium, and possibly nickel and selenium have been implicated in this regard. Lead toxicity has long been known to be associated with abortion and menstrual disorders. Evidence as to whether lead is teratogenic is conflicting. Some authors report a correlation between atmospheric lead levels and congenital malformations, whereas others deny these associations. In sheep, prenatal lead exposure has also been shown to affect the offspring's learning ability. Cadmium (which is derived accidentally from tobacco smoke, the electroplating industry, and deterioration of rubber tires) is a known cause of developmental malformations in rodents. Low doses of nickel cause embryotoxicity and eye malformations in the progeny of rats. Selenium is also a suspect teratogen.

Mercury. Probably the earliest instance of massive, unplanned exposure of a local population to an environmental toxicant occurred in 1953 in and around Minamata, a town located on a bay in southern Japan. Unusual neurologic problems (For example, mental confusion, convulsions, and coma) began afflicting villagers. Over one-third of the affected individuals died, and many infants and children suffered permanent brain damage from prenatal and neonatal exposure. Mercury was transported across the placenta and appeared in breast milk of mothers consuming contaminated fish. Eventually, the source of the mercury was traced to the effluent discharged from a local plastics factory into Minamata Bay. A similar incident occurred in Niigata, Japan, in 1964.

A massive methylmercury disaster occurred in Iraq during the winter of 1971 to 1972. In this case, barley and wheat grain treated with methylmercury as a fungicide had been purchased from Mexico. The grain sacks carried a written warning—but only in Spanish. Thirty-one pregnant women who ate the grain were hospitalized with methylmercury poisoning. Almost half of them died. Infants born to surviving mothers showed evidence of cerebral palsy, blindness, and severe brain damage. Similar outbreaks have occurred in Russia, Sweden, and elsewhere.

Lower exposures to methylmercury during early development has been suspected of effecting permanent damage to the nervous system. A recent effort to evaluate this idea was reported in 1998. Mother-infant pairs were identified in the Republic of Seychelles, a Westernized archipelago in the middle of the Indian Ocean, where 85% of the population consumes marine fish daily. Neurodevelopmental tests were administered to the children at sixty-six months of age. Mercury exposure was confirmed by analysis of maternal and child hair samples, and no adverse outcomes were associated with either prenatal or post-natal methylmercury exposure.[20]

Pesticides. A number of pesticides have been a major concern among public health professionals for quite some time. The Environmental Protection Agency reports that about one-third of the 1,500 active ingredients in registered pesticides are toxic, and one-fourth are mutagenic and carcinogenic. Although the agency has established limits on the amounts of pesticide residues that are allowed in foods, it has restricted the use of only five: heptaclor, chlordane, DDT, Mirex, and DBCP. Once deposited in the food chain, they are almost impossible to eliminate. The effects of exposure to low concentrations of these toxins is not only unknown but also difficult to investigate because of the problem of finding pesticide-free control populations.

PCBs. Polychlorinated biphenyls (PCBs), used as plasticizers and heat exchange fluids, constitute another group of chemicals that endanger health. In Kyushu, Japan, in 1968, a number of pregnant and lactating women ingested cooking oil contaminated with PCBs. As a result, they had small-for-gestational-age infants with dark skin, eye defects, and other abnormalities. Although prenatal exposure was probably significant, evidence indicated that transfer of PCBs through breast milk was the most significant route of exposure. Polybromated biphenyl (PBB), produced commercially as a fire retardant, also provoked attention after its accidental entry into cattle feed in Michigan in 1973 to 1974. More than 30,000 cattle and many sheep, swine, and poultry died or were slaughtered. Contaminated meat, milk, and eggs were identified in local food supplies, and stillbirths among affected cattle increased. Adverse effects in human pregnancy have not been reported, but considerable concern still exists.

EFFECTS OF RIGOROUS PHYSICAL ACTIVITY ≈

For many years, questions have been raised about the effect of heavy maternal physical activity during pregnancy on fetal growth. Some insight may be gained from studies related to heavy physical labor, modern fitness programs, and athletic training.

Heavy Physical Labor

In a study conducted in Ethiopia, trained nutritionists visited pregnant women in their homes for three consecutive days. During this time, dietary surveys were conducted. Two groups of women who had similar energy and protein intakes during pregnancy were then compared. One group of mothers was forced by circumstances beyond their control to engage in hard physical work throughout pregnancy. The second group of mothers had servants to do such physical labor. Mothers in both groups ate on the mean about 1,550 kcal a day.

When the two groups of Ethiopian women were compared, the women who engaged in hard physical labor had significantly lower pregnancy weight gains and smaller babies than did mothers who did not have to engage in such work. Kilocalorie deficiency was likely involved in the etiology of the fetal growth retardation that was seen. In addition, however, the oxygen debt incurred by moderate exercise is increased in human pregnancies, and this may lead to fetal hypoxia. This response is also evident in animal studies, where uterine blood flow decreases during maternal exercise.

Fitness Programs

The circumstances of mandatory physical labor described in the previous section, further imposed on an underlying state of moderate undernutrition, may seem far removed from today's modern fitness-conscious woman who opts to engage in a rigorous exercise program during pregnancy. However, some useful comparisons can be made.

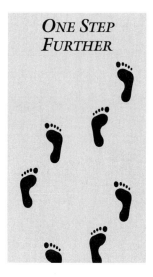

ONE STEP FURTHER

What Is the Real Caloric Cost of Pregnancy If the Mother Is Sedentary?

The basal metabolic rate, activity pattern, and energy costs of some daily activities were measured in twenty-five Dutch women throughout pregnancy and in the first year postpartum. Typical women in this population demonstrated very low basal metabolic needs and very low levels of physical activity. The end result was that daily kcalorie needs were modest at best. Basal metabolic requirements at one year postpartum were 1,440 kcal per day; the costs of physical activity were modest. The conclusions of the researchers in this study were as follows:

For women with sedentary lifestyles, the energy saved during pregnancy and lactation because of decreased physical activity and decreased costs of activities will be limited.

van Raaji, J.M.A. et al. 1990. Energy cost of physical activity throughout pregnancy and the first year postpartum in Dutch women with sedentary lifestyles. *Am J Clin Nutr* 52:234.

The fitness-conscious pregnant woman often gets conflicting advice from her physician and other health professionals. The obstetric textbooks rarely offer more than a single paragraph concerning physical activities during pregnancy. Obstetricians tend to form their own philosophies about various physical activities or athletic participation during pregnancy, and their recommendations often are based on their own (or their wives') experiences. Traditional advice to women from the obstetric community has been to decrease activity and increase periods of rest during pregnancy, particularly in the third trimester.

Over the past fifteen years, a number of studies have been conducted to examine the true relationship between physical activity programs and pregnancy course and outcome. A variety of fitness and training regimens have been evaluated. Most studies have reported no difference in pregnancy outcome related to physical activity. However, most pregnant women followed by these investigators decreased frequency, duration, or intensity of exercise in the latter part of pregnancy.

Of interest is a series of reports from researchers at the University of Vermont[21–26]. These scientists were able to compare the pregnancy course and outcome of two groups of women: those who were modestly active during pregnancy and those who maintained frequent vigorous exercise routines. The results included the following:

1. The women who continued regular exercise during pregnancy gained less weight and less body fat than did the women who were minimally active during this time. However, weight gain for all was within normal limits and all the babies were healthy.
2. The babies of the very active women were not more likely to abort spontaneously.
3. The very active women had fewer difficulties in the labor and delivery process.
4. The babies of the very active women were smaller than those of the minimally active women. However, at five years of age, the developmental progress of the children was similar in the two groups.

Some high-risk women, such as those with diabetes, heart disease, or history of spontaneous abortion, may be well advised to be particularly cautious about their selection of exercise programs. The American College of Obstetricians and Gynecologists provides exercise guidelines for all pregnant women that go well beyond discouraging endurance training in the third trimester (table 5-3). While these guidelines may be overly restrictive for many pregnant women, they provide a commonsense base from which to start.

TABLE 5-3 *American College of Obstetricians and Gynecologists' Guidelines for Exercise during Pregnancy and Postpartum*

1. Regular exercise (at least three times per week) is preferable to intermittent activity. Competitive activities should be discouraged.
2. Vigorous exercise should not be performed in hot, humid weather or during a period of febrile illness.
3. Ballistic movements (jerky, bouncy motions) should be avoided. Exercise should be done on a wooden floor or a tightly carpeted surface to reduce shock and provide a sure footing.
4. Deep flexion or extension of joints should be avoided because of connective tissue laxity. Activities that require jumping, jarring motions, or rapid changes in direction should be avoided because of joint instability.
5. Vigorous exercise should be preceded by a five-minute period of muscle warm-up. This can be accomplished by slow walking or stationary cycling with low resistance.
6. Vigorous exercise should be followed by a period of gradually declining activity that includes gentle stationary stretching. Because connective tissue laxity increases the risk of joint injury, stretches should not be taken to the point of maximum resistance.
7. Heart rate should be measured at times of peak activity. Target heart rates and limits established in consultation with the physician should not be exceeded.
8. Care should be taken to gradually rise from the floor to avoid orthostatic hypotension. Some form of activity involving the legs should be continued for a brief period.
9. Liquids should be taken liberally before and after exercise to prevent dehydration. If necessary, activity should be interrupted to replenish fluids.
10. Women who have led sedentary lifestyles should begin with physical activity of very low intensity and advance activity levels very gradually.
11. Activity should be stopped and the physician consulted if any unusual symptoms appear.

Pregnancy Only

1. Maternal heart rate should not exceed 140 beats/minute.
2. Strenuous activities should not exceed fifteen minutes in duration.
3. No exercise should be performed in the supine position after the fourth month of gestation is completed.
4. Exercises that use the Valsalva maneuver should be avoided.
5. Caloric intake should be adequate to meet not only the extra energy needs for pregnancy but also of the exercise performed.
6. Maternal core temperature should not exceed 38° C.

Reprinted with permission from the American College of Obstetricians and Gynecologists: Exercise during pregnancy and the postnatal period (ACOG Home Exercise Programs), Washington, DC, 1985, American College of Obstetricians and Gynecologists.

EFFECTS OF CIGARETTE SMOKING ≋

Fetal growth retardation is often seen in offspring of cigarette smokers, as shown in fig. 5-3. It has been postulated that this condition is due to the reduced food intake of the mother. Observations have shown that this is not true. Women who smoke often consume more kilocalories per day than women who do not smoke.

The growth-retarding impact of smoking relates to the effects of carbon monoxide, nicotine, and possibly other compounds on placental perfusion and oxygen transport to the fetus. It is also likely that efficiency of kilocalorie utilization is reduced in women who smoke.

In 1992, 16.9% of all U.S. mothers reported to have smoked during pregnancy. Smoking was more common in white mothers than in blacks. In both groups, there has been a small reduction in the level of smoking since 1989. Smoking rates for Asian American women are generally very low; this is also true of Hispanic mothers. In both cases, the level of smoking is observed to be less in foreign-born than in U.S.-born mothers.[27]

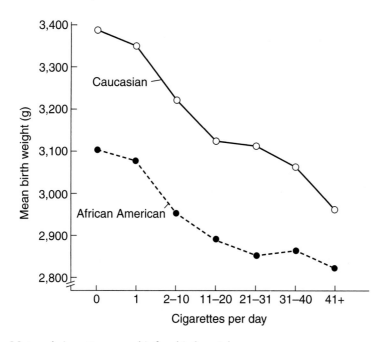

FIG. 5-3 Maternal cigarette use and infant birth weight.

Modified from Niswander, K.R., and M. Gordon. 1972. *The women and their pregnancies.* Philadelphia: W.B. Saunders. In Martin, J. 1982. *Neurobehav Toxicol Teratol* 4:421.

With regard to pregnancy outcome, in 1992, babies born to smokers were at nearly twice the risk of low birth weight as babies born to nonsmokers. The effect of smoking on infant birth weight becomes more severe with advancing maternal age. The percentage of low birth weight for infants of women who smoked even less than six cigarettes per day at the time of the study was still 41% higher than for infants of nonsmokers.[27]

COMMON COMPLAINTS WITH DIETARY IMPLICATIONS ≈

General nutritional guidance may also be needed during pregnancy for common functional gastrointestinal difficulties encountered. These complaints are highly individual in form and extent. They will therefore require individual counseling and assurances for control. Usually these difficulties are relatively minor, but, if they persist or become extreme, they will need medical care. In most cases, general investigation of food practices will reveal some areas where diet counseling may help relieve gastrointestinal problems. Some of the more common difficulties include nausea, constipation, hemorrhoids, and heartburn.

Nausea and Vomiting

Difficulty with nausea and vomiting is usually mild and limited to early pregnancy. It is commonly called "morning sickness," because it tends to occur early in the day, but it can come at any time of day. Usually it lasts only a brief period at the beginning of the pregnancy, but in some women it may persist longer.

A number of factors contribute to the usual mild condition. Some are physiologic, based on normal hormonal changes that occur early in pregnancy. Other factors are psychologic, such as various tensions and anxieties concerning the pregnancy itself. Simple treatment generally improves food toleration. Small, frequent meals—fairly dry and consisting chiefly of easily digested energy foods such as carbohydrates—are more readily tolerated. Cooking odors should be avoided as much as possible.

Other odors, such as stale cigarette smoke, also intensify discomfort. *There is no generally effective remedy for nausea in early pregnancy.* Finding foods that produce minimal sickness and avoiding particularly disgusting odors is the most potentially useful advice that can be given.

If the condition persists and develops into hyperemesis—severe, prolonged, persistent vomiting—medical attention is required to prevent complications and dehydration. However, such an increase in symptoms is rare. Most conditions pass early in the pregnancy and respond to the simple dietary remedies. Women should be reassured that mild short-term nausea is common in early pregnancy and will not harm the fetus.

Constipation

The condition of constipation is seldom more than minor. Hormonal changes in pregnancy tend to increase relaxation of the gastrointestinal muscles. Also, the pressure of the enlarging uterus on the lower portion of the intestine, especially during the latter part of the pregnancy, may make elimination somewhat difficult at times. Increased fluid intake, use of naturally laxative foods and fiber—such as whole grains with added bran, fibrous fruits and vegetables, dried fruits (especially prunes and figs), and other fruits and juices—generally induce regularity. Laxatives should be avoided. They should be used only in special situations under medical supervision.

Hemorrhoids

A fairly common complaint during the latter part of pregnancy is that of hemorrhoids. These are enlarged veins in the anus, often protruding through the anal sphincter. This vein enlargement is usually caused by the increased weight of the fetus and the downward pressure it produces. The hemorrhoids may cause considerable discomfort, burning, and itching. Occasionally, they rupture and bleed under the pressure of a bowel movement, causing more anxiety. The difficulty is usually remedied by the previously mentioned dietary suggestions to control constipation. Also, observing general hygiene recommendations concerning sufficient rest during the latter part of the day may help relieve the pressure of the uterus on the lower intestine.

Heartburn and Full Feeling

The related complaints of "heartburn" and "full feeling" are sometimes voiced by pregnant women. These discomforts may occur especially after meals and are usually caused by the pressure of the enlarging uterus crowding the adjacent digestive organ, the stomach, thereby causing some difficulty after eating. Food mixtures may sometimes be pushed back into the lower part of the esophagus, causing a "burning" sensation from the gastric acid mixed with the food mass. This burning sensation is commonly called heartburn simply because of the proximity of the lower esophagus to the heart. Obviously, however, it has nothing to do with the heart and its action. A full feeling comes from general gastric pressure, caused by a lack of normal space in the area, and is accentuated by a large meal

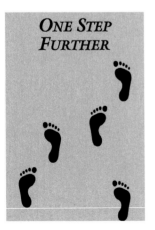

ONE STEP FURTHER

What About Alternative Therapies for the Nausea and Vomiting of Pregnancy?

A recent review (1996–1997) of thirteen large national and international databases sought to examine the value of various alternative treatments for nausea, vomiting, and hyperemesis. There was a dearth of research to support or refute the efficacy of a number of common remedies. The best studied alternative remedy was found to be acupuncture, which reportedly afforded relief to many women; ginger and vitamin B_6 were also judged to be potentially beneficial.

Murphy, P.A. 1998. Alternative therapies for nausea and vomiting of pregnancy. *Obstet Gynecol* 91:149.

or gas formation. These complaints are generally remedied by dividing the day's food intake into a number of small meals during the day. Attention may also be given to relaxation, adequate chewing, slower eating, and avoidance of tensions during meals. Comfort is also improved by wearing loose-fitting clothing.

SELECTED EXAMPLES OF HIGH-RISK PREGNANCY[1] ≋

A number of risk factors may contribute to a poor pregnancy outcome. In a joint report, the American College of Obstetricians and Gynecologists and the American Dietetic Association have issued a set of risk factors to identify women with special nutritional and health care needs during pregnancy. These factors, summarized in table 5-4, relate to nutritional status, habits, needs, and problems. The nutritional factors identified in this report are based on clinical evidence of inadequate nutrition. A better approach provides useful criteria for predicting nutritional risk, instead of waiting for clinical signs of poor nutrition to appear. Three types of dietary patterns do not support optimal maternal and fetal nutrition: 1) insufficient food intake, 2) poor food selection, and 3) poor food distribution through the day. These patterns, added to the list of risk factors in table 5-4, would be much more sensitive for nutritional risk. On this basis, practitioners can plan personal care and provide for special counseling needs.

Pregnancy-Induced Hypertension (PIH)

Formerly labeled *toxemia*, pregnancy-induced hypertension (PIH) is a risk factor related to nutrition and treated according to its symptoms:

1. *Clinical symptoms.* PIH is generally defined according to its manifestations, which usually occur in the third trimester toward term. Among these symptoms are hypertension; abnormal and excessive edema; albumuria; and, in severe cases, convulsions or coma—*eclampsia.*

2. *Treatment.* Specific treatment varies according to the patient's symptoms and needs. In any case, optimal nutrition is a fundamental aspect of therapy. Adequate dietary protein is essential. Correction of plasma protein deficits stimulates normal operation of the capillary fluid shift mechanism and restores circulation of tissue fluid, inducing subsequent correction of the **hypovolemia.** In addition, adequate salt and sources of vitamins and minerals are needed for correction and maintenance of metabolic balances.

Hypovolemia
(Gr *hypo*, under; ME *volu(me)*, volume; Gr *haima*, blood) Low blood volume.

TABLE 5-4 *Nutritional Risk Factors in Pregnancy*

Risk Factors Present at the Onset of Pregnancy	Risk Factors Occurring During Pregnancy

Age
  Fifteen years or younger
  Thirty-five years or older
	Low hemoglobin or hematocrit
	  Hemoglobin less than 12.0 g
	  Hematocrit less than 35.0 me/dl

Frequent pregnancies: three or more during a two-year period	Inadequate weight gain
Poor obstetric history or poor fetal performance	Any weight loss
Poverty	Weight gain of less than 2 lb per month after the first trimester
Bizarre of faddist food habits	Excessive weight gain: greater than 1 kg (2.2 lb) per week after the first trimester
Abuse of nicotine, alcohol, or drugs	
Therapeutic diet required for a chronic disorder	

Inadequate weight
  Less than 85% of standard weight
  More that 120% of standard weight	

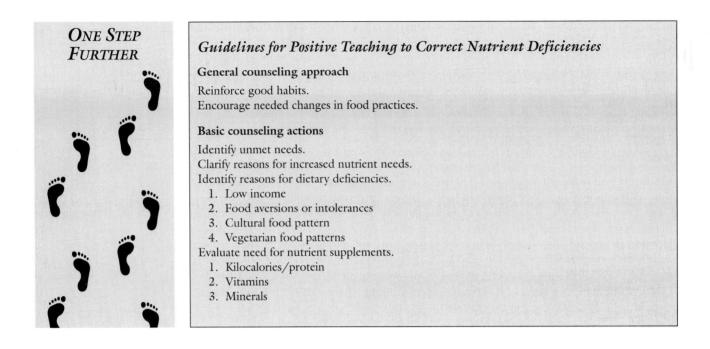

ONE STEP
FURTHER

Guidelines for Positive Teaching to Correct Nutrient Deficiencies

General counseling approach

Reinforce good habits.

Encourage needed changes in food practices.

Basic counseling actions

Identify unmet needs.

Clarify reasons for increased nutrient needs.

Identify reasons for dietary deficiencies.

1. Low income
2. Food aversions or intolerances
3. Cultural food pattern
4. Vegetarian food patterns

Evaluate need for nutrient supplements.

1. Kilocalories/protein
2. Vitamins
3. Minerals

Preexisting Disease

Preexisting clinical conditions complicate pregnancy and increase risks. They are managed according to the general principles of care related to pregnancy and to the particular disease involved. Examples of these preexisting conditions include hypertension, diabetes mellitus, and phenylketonuria (PKU).

Hypertension. Preventive screening and monitoring of blood pressure are essential. The hypertensive disease process begins long before any signs and symptoms appear, and later symptoms are inconsistent. Risk factors for hypertension before and during pregnancy are given in table 5-5. Nutritional care centers on prevention of weight extremes, either underweight or obesity, and correction of any dietary deficiencies by maintaining optimal nutrition. Sodium intake can be moderate but should never be unduly restricted because of its relation to fluid and electrolyte balances during pregnancies.

Diabetes mellitus. The management of diabetes in pregnancy presents special problems. Routine screening is therefore necessary to detect gestational diabetes, and team management is required to control preexisting insulin-dependent diabetes mellitus (IDDM) table 5-6.

Screening. Most prenatal clinics do routine screening for diabetes and provide careful follow-up for every patient who shows glycosuria. Risk factors detected in initial history include 1) family history of diabetes, 2) previous unexplained stillbirths, 3) large babies weighing 4 kg (9 lb) or more, 4) recurrent miscarriage, 5) births of babies with multiple congenital anomalies, and 6) excessive obesity.

Gestational diabetes. During pregnancy, glycosuria is not uncommon because of the increased circulating blood volume and its load of metabolites. However, only 20–30% of women showing glycosuria or somewhat abnormal glucose tolerance subsequently develop diabetes. Nonetheless, identification of women with this condition and close follow-up observation are important because of the higher risk of fetal damage during this period. Most of these women revert to normal glucose tolerance after delivery.

Preexisting IDDM. Because of the course of diabetes during pregnancy, as well as the altered course of pregnancy in the presence of diabetes, a team of specialists is necessary for sound management and prevention of problems to reduce risk of fetal death and increase the probability of a successful outcome. Close personalized nutritional care by the

TABLE 5-5 *Risk Factors in Pregnancy-Induced Hypertension*

Before Pregnancy	During Pregnancy
Nulligravida	Primigravida
Diabetes mellitus	Large fetus
Preexisting condition (Hypertension, renal or vascular disease)	Glomerulonephritis
Family history of hypertension or vascular disease	Fetal hydrops
Diagnosis of pregnancy-induced hypertension in a previous pregnancy	Hydramnios
Dietary deficiencies	Multiple gestation
Age extremes	Hydatidiform mole
Twenty years or younger	
Thirty-five years or older	

TABLE 5-6 *Classification of Diabetes Mellitus During Pregnancy**

New Classifications	Former Names	Clinical Characteristics
Type I insulin-dependent diabetes mellitus (IDDM)	Juvenile diabetes Juvenile-onset diabetes Brittle diabetes Ketosis-prone diabetes	Ketosis prone: insulin deficient because of loss of islet cells; often associated with human leukocyte antigen types, with predisposition to viral insulitis or autoimmune (islet-cell antibody) phenomena; can occur at any age, but more common in youth

Type II non-insulin-dependent diabetes-mellitus (NIDDM)
  Nonobese
  Obese
	Adult diabetes
	Adult-onset diabetes
	Maturity-onset diabetes
	Stable diabetes
	Ketosis-resistant diabetes
	Maturity-onset diabetes of youth
		Ketosis resistant; occurs at any age but more frequent in adults; majority are overweight; may be seen in families as an autosomal dominant genetic trait; may require insulin in times of stress; usually requires insulin during pregnancy

Gestational diabetes	Gestational diabetes	Classification retained for women whose diabetes begins (or is recognized) during pregnancy; carries increased risk of perinatal complications; transitory glucose intolerance, which frequently recurs; diagnosis: at least two abnormal values on a three-hour oral glucose tolerance test (100 g glucose) Fasting plasma glucose 105 mg/100 ml One hour 190 mg/100 ml Two hour 160 mg/100 ml Three hour 145 mb/100 ml

*This classification replaces the White classification for pregnancy, which was based on age at onset, duration of the disease, and complications.

team nutritionist is mandatory throughout. The insulin requirement increases during pregnancy and drops dramatically on delivery. The woman with IDDM must control blood glucose levels through careful food selection and scheduled meal timing in concert with the administration of insulin.

Maternal phenylketonuria (MPKU). Mandatory screening of all newborns for the genetic disease PKU and low phenylalanine diet have supported normal growth in PKU

≋ ≋

GUIDELINES FOR NUTRITIONAL MANAGEMENT FOR THE PREGNANT WOMAN WITH PHENYLKETONURIA

The goals of nutritional management are to:
1. Maintain serum phenylalanine levels as low as possible. The U.S. Maternal Collaborative Study recommends concentrations between 2 and 6 mg/dl, or 120 and 360 μmol/L.
2. Maintain adequate and consistent weight gain.
3. Maintain serum tyrosine in the normal range.
4. Meet nutrient requirements for protein, energy, vitamins, and minerals using the 1989 RDA as a guide.

The tasks of nutritional management are to:
1. Stress the special nutritional needs during pregnancy.
2. Stress the importance of strictly following the phenylalanine prescription to achieve the necessary rigid control of blood phenylalanine levels.
3. Calculate a food pattern to provide adequate energy, protein, phenylalanine, vitamins, and minerals.
4. Provide a food pattern for the individual that is based on a phenylalanine-free protein source (one of the medical foods).
5. Provide a meal guide and serving lists that indicate protein, energy, and phenylalanine content of foods.
6. Provide education on food selection, food purchasing, food preparation using low-phenylalanine recipes, and recording food intake as needed.
7. Review and calculate diet records for accuracy.
8. Compare recorded and calculated food intake with blood phenylalanine levels and weight gain.
9. Adjust the food pattern and meal guide as necessary to meet the individual's needs.

children. Now a generation of young women with childhood PKU are having children of their own. Maternal PKU presents potential fetal hazards associated with increased abortions and stillbirths, congenital anomalies often causing death, and intrauterine and postnatal growth and development retardation in surviving infants. A planned pregnancy, with careful management of the mother's diet *before* conception, and close follow-up care *throughout* the pregnancy can improve the outcome of these high-risk pregnancies (see the box on p. 120). A strict diet low in phenylalanine and a special formula of other amino acids are required.

It makes sense, therefore, that efforts should be made preconceptionally to motivate women with controllable diseases to prepare themselves for conception by initiating the dietary and other necessary lifestyle changes that will allow each of them to offer to her conceptus the optimum maternal metabolic milieu. This can certainly be said for women with IDDM and PKU, but it also applies to women with other chronic diseases. Not only will such efforts reduce morbidity and mortality of offspring, but they may also improve the health and well-being of the mother during the prenatal period.

Adolescent Pregnancy

Developmental issues. Teenage pregnancy must be studied in the light of the highly dynamic nature of adolescence. Both the psychologic and the physical status of the adolescent have implications for the course of any pregnancy. The many interactions of factors in adolescent development and in reproduction have great clinical significance for all aspects of the pregnancy, including the nutritional aspect. Indeed, adolescents are changing so profoundly that pregnancy for the younger, less mature teenager is different from that of the older, more mature adolescent.

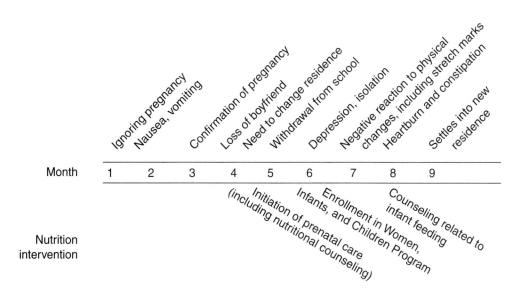

FIG. 5-4 Typical events in teenage pregnancy that could affect intake or utilization of nutrients.

Less mature teenagers are more dependent on others and less able to act and make decisions on their own. They are more **narcissistic** and less able to comprehend the needs of others. These young women are less realistic, engage in more fantasy and wishful thinking, and have less insight into their own behaviors and motives (see the box on p. 123). In general, younger teenagers have fewer intellectual and physical skills to cope with any situation, especially a complex reproductive experience. Many of the difficulties related to pregnancy in adolescence stem from this immaturity. As development advances, a person is able to carry out reproduction and childrearing in a more normal, less problem-fraught way. As seen in fig. 5-4, the timeline of events in teenage pregnancy has great potential for affecting the nutritional well-being of the adolescent.

Reproduction during adolescence. The pregnant adolescent's nutritional needs are influenced by many factors. Primary influences are her growth and nutrient stores, her **gynecologic age,** and her preconception nutritional status.

The assumption that pregnant adolescents need a supply of nutrients to support their own growth along with that of the growing fetus has been questioned. Because hormone levels are high in pregnancy, even the slower adolescent growth that usually follows menarche may not occur. According to recent studies, growth does continue to some degree during adolescent pregnancy. Whether or not actual growth continues for an adolescent who becomes pregnant, she will have experienced rapid growth more recently than her adult counterparts. There will have been less opportunity for storage of nutrients. Thus, there may be greater physiologic risk to young women who conceive in menarche.

The number of years between the onset of menses and conception is calculated to derive the gynecologic age. Adolescents who are more sexually mature—that is, of greater gynecologic age—share a vulnerability to physiologic stresses but appear to have no more physically based complications than adult women. It is the young women of lower gynecologic age who carry more risk and need more nutritional support. The number of adolescents who become pregnant in the first two years following menarche is relatively small, because most of them are not ovulating during that time, even though they are menstruating. Those who do become pregnant, however, are of great concern to clinicians and researchers in this area.

Pregnant adolescents who are of young gynecologic age and malnourished at the time of conception are at double risk. They appear to have the greatest need for nutrients to support a pregnancy and maintain optimal health themselves.

Hazards to the mother. Given the complexity of pregnancy in the adolescent period, it is logical to question how these young women fare during pregnancy. They have more

Narcissism
Self-love; drawn from Narcissus, a character in Greek mythology who saw his image mirrored in a pool of water and fell in love with his own reflection.

Gynecologic age
(Gr *gynaikos,* women) Length of time from onset of menses to present time of conception.

~~~~ ~~~~

RISKS ASSOCIATED WITH ADOLESCENT PREGNANCY

Maternal risks

Pregnancy-induced hypertension
Premature labor
Intrauterine growth retardation
Anemia
Maternal mortality
Increased incidence of cephalopelvic
disproportion

Neonatal risks

Increased perinatal mortality
Increased neonatal mortality

Prematurity
Lack of access to pediatric health care services
Poor parenting skills

Psychosocial risks for mother and baby

Failure to complete education
Unemployment
Poverty
Dependence on public assistance
Poor job satisfaction
Marital instability
Greater number of children per mother

---

complications, a higher risk of maternal mortality, and more problems in personal psychologic development and education that carry implications for economic well-being (see the box on p. 122).

The variety of complications often described for the teenage mother during gestation include:

- First and third trimester bleeding
- Anemia
- Difficult labor and delivery
- **Cephalopelvic disproportion**
- Pregnancy-induced hypertensive disorders, including **preeclampsia** and eclampsia
- Infections

Of these complications, the most common physical problem is infection, while the most common serious complication is preeclampsia. Preeclampsia usually occurs in the third trimester and is manifested in increased weight gain, fluid retention, high blood pressure, and proteinuria; it does not appear to run a different course in pregnant teenagers than in older women. Some researchers point out that it is a disease of first pregnancies. By and large, data support this observation. In addition, the harmful effects of preeclampsia, or the more serious state of eclampsia, may be greater in teenagers. Damage to the cardiovascular and renal systems initiated with a first pregnancy early in life and intensified by insults such as other pregnancies can increase the risk of developing renal and cardiovascular problems with increasing age.

The serious burden of maternal mortality is also a problem. The rate is $2\frac{1}{2}$ times greater for mothers under fifteen years of age than for those twenty to twenty-four years of age.

Apart from the physical sequelae, pregnancy often affects teenagers' psychologic development, education, and ability to gain economic independence. Clearly, these developmental steps are difficult to achieve in any case, and for many adolescents pregnancy is not a cause of failure but a coinciding event. The situations responsible for early pregnancy often remain unresolved, and many teenage mothers have additional pregnancies before the adolescent years are over.

Hazards to the infant. Infants born to teenage mothers suffer a higher incidence of morbidity and mortality in the perinatal period than do infants of older mothers. Problems seen more frequently include:

- Prematurity
- Stillbirth

Cephalopelvic disproportion
(Gr *kephale*, head; *pyelos*, an oblong trough, pelvis) Relationship of fetal head to size of the maternal pelvis.

Preeclampsia
(Gr *pre-*, before; *eklampein*, to shine forth) Abnormal condition of late pregnancy marked by rather sudden hypertension and increased edema, usually accompanied by proteinuria; may progress to more severe stage of preeclampsia with convulsions and coma.

Expectations vs. Reality

Pregnant adolescents often find their expectations are quite different from the reality of motherhood.

Expectation	Reality
Life with baby	
Life with baby will be wonderful.	Life with baby isn't wonderful.
Baby will meet their emotional needs.	Baby doesn't meet emotional needs. Baby may even interfere with their own need meeting.
They won't be lonely anymore.	They may be even more lonely with the demands and limitations of a baby.
Parenting	
Parenting is easy (based on baby-sitting experience). They will manage.	Parenting is not easy. The twenty-four hour responsibility is overwhelming.
Others (e.g., partner, family) will help them.	Many are parenting alone. There are limited resources for teen parents. Many are not ready to accept help, education, role modeling, etc.
Self-esteem	
Self-esteem will increase with pregnancy and parenthood. They now have a role.	They are self-conscious about body changes. Society disapproves. Self-esteem decreases. Baby takes attention away from them.
Relationships	
Their parents will be upset but supportive.	Many have family support, but some parents reject or do not support on their terms.
The parents will care for the teen mom and her baby.	
Relationship with partner will improve or he'll come back.	Some live common-law or are married. Relationship with partner is often strained and he frequently leaves.
Friendships will continue as they are.	Life is different from peers. They become isolated from friends.
Finances	
Somebody will provide welfare.	Welfare is not sufficient, and mothers are unable to manage. Many do not know how to budget.
Some plan to be self-sufficient (finish school, get a job).	Self-sufficiency takes a long time. Often, they don't have energy and/or the organizational skills to continue or reenter school/work.
Housing	
They want to find affordable, safe, clean housing to live on their own.	Landlords can be biased against single moms, children, and tenants on welfare. Rent may be too expensive to afford.
Goals	
Motherhood will make life meaningful.	Life may prove to be no longer meaningful.
They tend not to have long-term goals.	They find it difficult to follow through, even on short-term goals.

Modified from Browne, C., and M. Urback. June 1989. Pregnant adolescents: Expectations vs. reality. *Can J Public Health.*

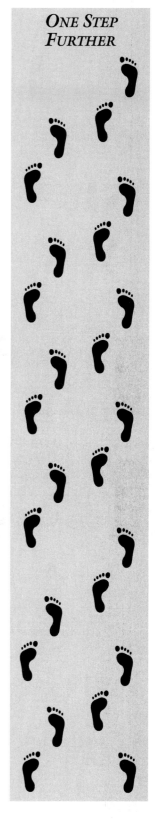

ONE STEP FURTHER

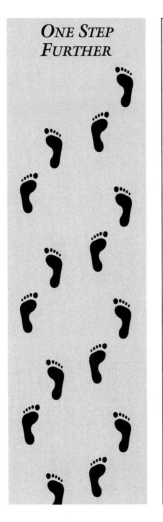

ONE STEP FURTHER

Is Biological Immaturity or "Environmental" Stress More Contributory to Pregnancy Outcome?

It has long been assumed that immature women probably have more low birth weight and preterm outcomes than older women because of their immature anatomy and physiology. However, a number of studies over the past fifteen years have refuted this concept. When researchers have controlled for sociodemographic factors, minimal differences in pregnancy outcomes have been reported between teens and women in their twenties. These observations have suggested that factors *associated with* young age, such as poverty, poor education, unmarried status, and inadequate prenatal care, are more powerful influences on outcomes than is maternal age. There is no question about the relevance of these sociodemographic factors.

A recent report, however, has reopened this controversy about biology versus environment. Vital statistics from the state of Utah were used, providing data on 134,088 white mothers thirteen to twenty-four years old. These mothers had delivered singleton, first-born children between 1970 and 1990. Age of mother and sociodemographic variables were examined. Among the white married mothers who had educational levels appropriate for their ages and who received adequate prenatal care, the teenage mothers (thirteen to seventeen years of age) had a significantly higher risk than did the mothers aged twenty to twenty-four years of delivering an infant who was low birth weight, premature, or small for gestational age. The older teenage mothers (eighteen and nineteen years of age) also had a significant increase in these risks. The researchers concluded that, in white, middle-class women, a younger age confers an increased risk of adverse pregnancy outcomes, which is independent of important sociodemographic factors. They speculate that two features of biologic immaturity could play a role in this relationship: a young gynecologic age (defined as conception within two years after menarche) and the effect of an adolescent becoming pregnant before her own growth has ceased.

Fraser, A.M., J.E. Brockert, and R.H. Ward. 1995. Association of young maternal age with adverse reproductive outcomes. *N Engl J Med* 332:1113.

- Low birth weight (the major hazard in adolescent pregnancy)
- Perinatal and infant deaths
- Physical deformities

It is difficult to compare the likelihood of these problems occurring in infants born to teenage versus older mothers, or to younger versus older teenage mothers, but it is generally agreed that the problems do occur in a considerable number of teenage pregnancies. For example, the incidence of low birth weight is far greater when the mothers are adolescent.

Growth of young mothers and the competition for nutrients. Growth patterns and the timing of menarche vary considerably from one young woman to another. The general sequence of events is similar but is not directly related to chronological age. Most young women begin their adolescent growth spurt between the ages of ten and fourteen. Peak height velocity is achieved within the following few years, and menarche occurs after that time. Therefore, by the time a young woman is capable of reproduction, her rate of growth has slowed considerably. It is to be emphasized, however, that the timing and levels of growth that occur in individual women vary significantly.

Do pregnant teens continue to grow? It has been tempting to conclude that if so, not much. Accurately assessing growth in stature during pregnancy is not an easy chore. Usual measures may underestimate it because of the tendency for compression of the spine and postural changes during pregnancy to cause apparent "shrinkage." A well-designed study by Scholl et al.,[28] however, has provided useful information. These researchers used a knee-height measuring device to track lower-leg length during pregnancy in a group of teenagers in New Jersey. In this study, maternal growth during adolescent pregnancy was present in approximately 50% of the young women (both primiparas and multiparas). After controlling for a number of variables, such as length of gestation, black ethnicity, smoking, prepregnant body mass index and weight gain, the infants born to the young mothers who were growing weighed 156 g less than the infants of the teens who were not growing; this was despite a significantly greater weight gain and less smoking.

Scholl et al. also examined the mothers themselves.[29] Body composition differences associated with maternal growth did not arise until after twenty-eight weeks of gestation, when the growing teenagers continued to accrue fat, had larger gestational weight gains, and retained more of this weight postpartum. Still, these mothers had smaller babies. The researchers concluded that "despite an apparently sufficient weight gain and the accumulation of nutritional stores during pregnancy, young growing women appeared not to mobilize stores after 28 weeks' gestation, reserving them instead for their own continued development."

This brings up the issue of competition for nutrients between mothers and fetuses. It has been proposed that fetal growth may be retarded in young mothers who are still growing, since both are seeking a potentially limited source of nutrients; diminished placental transfer may account for this phenomenon.[30] However, it was suggested more than fifteen years ago that fetuses grow more slowly in ten- to sixteen-year-olds than in older women; the same thing was observed in a population of 400 Peruvian adolescents. Because a recent study in black adolescents has provided data to counter the notion of maternal/fetal competition for nutrients,[31] this area remains controversial. Biologically, however, it makes sense that available nutrients will only go so far. A fetus may suffer (in an immature mother) when the mother's needs are substantial.

Thus, there is evidence that gestational weight gain in young, still-growing adolescents may have a greater impact on infant size than in older adolescents or mature women. This makes sense from the standpoint that both mother and fetus are growing and, if both are provided for, adequate growth of both can and may occur. The pattern of gestational weight gain also appears to significantly affect fetal growth. In nearly 800 adolescents, early inadequate weight gain increased the risk of having small-for-gestational-age infants, despite adequate total gains. Also, inadequate gains after twenty-four weeks of gestation increased the risk of preterm delivery in the same population.[29]

Until more formal guidelines are available on the amount and pattern of gestational weight gain in young adolescents, use of the Institute of Medicine guidelines of 1990 seems appropriate.[32] However, some question the legitimacy of one of the recommendations: "young adolescents should strive for weight gains at the upper end of the newly recommended ranges during pregnancy." The basis of this recommendation seems to be that there is a higher risk of young adolescents' having smaller infants. The fact is that younger adolescents have smaller infants for a number of reasons, including low income, lack of education, small prepregnancy size, cigarette smoking, cervical infections, and psychosocial stress. Increased weight gain during pregnancy may compensate for their smaller prepregnancy size but may do little to ameliorate the adverse effects of cigarette smoking, cervical infections, and psychosocial stress on their infants.

In 1983, one expert said the following:"Although it is true that larger weight gains during pregnancy do lead to increased birthweights and a lower incidence of prematurity, we do not urge a large weight gain for teenagers because this will lead to an elevated weight and an excess in body fat." Since the incidence of obesity has gradually increased in adolescents over time, this point may be well taken. This is especially true of high weight gains in young teens, a circumstance associated with more macrosomic infants, more cesarean sections, and more situations of birth asphyxia.[33]

CASE STUDY

Two Teenage Pregnancies

Two adolescent females in the same grade become pregnant. One is 16.5 years of age: her menses began at age 14, and her weight for height is below the 5th percentile. The other pregnant adolescent is 15 years of age: her menses began at age 9, and her weight for height is at the 50th percentile.

Questions for analysis
1. Describe the theoretical difference in nutritional needs of the two adolescents.
2. Which one should be given clinical priority? Why?
3. If neither young woman seeks prenatal care, what might you expect as the outcome for the respective infants? Why?

Caring for the mother-infant dyad. The importance of nurturing the "mother-infant dyad" was nicely summarized by McAnarney and Lawrence.[34] They point out that young adolescent mothers may successfully finish school, obtain jobs, and achieve financial independence during their children's formative years. At the same time, these children have more short-term and long-term cognitive and behavioral problems than do children of adult mothers. They also stress that if, for some young mothers to succeed, their children receive inadequate nurturing, minimal care, and little or no supervision, resulting in adverse developmental outcome, then the price of these mothers' success is unacceptably high for their children, for them, and for society. It obviously makes sense to provide these mother-child pairs with an environment in which both can flourish. Day care programs for young mothers and their children provide an appropriate setting, if they are located close to mothers' high schools and jobs.

There are now sufficient data to provide targeted interventions for teenagers and their children and to build on adolescents' assets. First, adolescent mothers often lack knowledge of child development, even though they may have previous experience baby-sitting other people's children. Young mothers should be given basic information about child development, focused on the specific age and stage of their children. Second, young mothers must learn to delay their own needs and place their children's needs above their own. Third, young mothers need to accept, without frustration, that their children may not respond immediately to their well-meaning overtures. Fourth, skilled older women might teach young mothers how to verbalize with their infants and children. Fifth, young people should be taught about nonverbal communication. They need to learn how to read their children's nonverbal signals and how to respond to them. Children's responses to their mothers' nonverbal communication can be positively reinforcing if the mothers learn to read their infants' signals and responses accordingly.[34]

The best time to intervene with young mothers and their children is early in the children's lives. Thus, ideally, young mothers and their infants should start a day care program together. Every effort should be made to keep young mothers and their children together in supervised settings. We have the opportunity to mold the young mother's behavior while she is still young and flexible by involving both her and her child in the program.[34]

Protocol for Assessment and Management of Normal Teenage Pregnancy

Initial evaluation (if possible)

Review intake material, social and lifestyle history.

Review clinical data.
  Height and weight
  Gynecologic age
  Physical signs of health
  Expected delivery date

Review laboratory data.
  Hematocrit or hemoglobin
  Urinalysis

Begin to build relationship with the client (and partner if available).

Assess client's perspective of nutrition issues.

Assess attitude about, and acceptance of, prepregnancy weight and feelings about weight gain during pregnancy.

Assess intake patterns using dietary methodology best suited to client and professional.

Make preliminary assessment of food resources and refer to supportive agencies if necessary.

Check for nausea and vomiting and suggest possible remedy.

Discuss supplemental vitamins and minerals.

Make initial plan that sets priorities for issues.

Come to agreement with patient about any initial changes and steps to take; have client state plan as she perceives it.

Determine client understanding of relation between nutrition and health.

Do initial anthropometrics, calculate reasonable weight gain.

Second visit

Check on referrals to other agencies.

Discuss results of initial evaluation and suggest any changes necessary in dietary patterns (use printed materials as appropriate).

Do any further investigations when necessary.

Laboratory studies.
  For specific diagnosis of anemia:
    Protoporphyrin heme or serum ferritin
    Serum or red cell folate
    Serum vitamin B_{12}

Further probe into dietary habits if necessary.

Monitor weight gain; discuss projected weight gain for following visit and total for gestation.

Assess and address issues affecting nutritional status in order of priority for the individual.
  Activity level
  Appetite changes
  Pica, food cravings, and aversions
  Allergies/food intolerances
  Supplementation practices (prescribed and self-selected)

Subsequent visits

Monitor and support appropriate weight gain; include discussion of fitness and encourage habitual safe exercise.

Support upgrade in nutritional pattern in support of the woman and the developing infant; augment knowledge of principles of nutrition; continue to address issues affecting nutritional status.

Check for heartburn, small food-intake capacity, and elimination problems; suggest dietary interventions.

Begin preliminary discussion and comparison of advantages/disadvantages of breast-feeding and formula feeding.

Final prenatal visit(s)

Discuss infant feeding if client will keep infant.

If breast-feeding is chosen, provide preliminary guidance about breast-feeding practices.

If formula feeding is chosen, discuss product selection and preparation; define important details about feeding techniques.

Postpartum visits

Help client understand safe methods of managing weight following delivery.

Review infant feeding practices and infant growth; provide assistance when problems are identified.

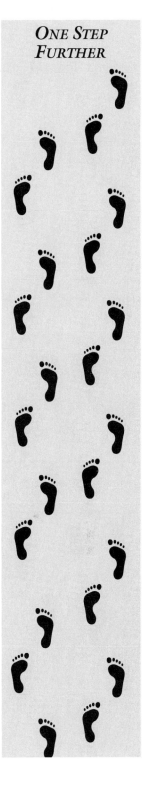

ONE STEP FURTHER

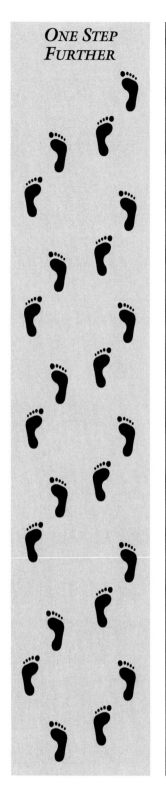

Issues in Adolescent Pregnancy That Influence Nutritional Well-Being

Acceptance of the pregnancy

Desire to carry out successful pregnancy.
Acceptance of responsibility (even if child is to be relinquished).
Clarification of identity as mother separate from her own mother.
Realistic acceptance versus fantasy and idealization.

Food resource

Family meals (timing, quantity, quality, responsibility).
Self-reliance.
School lunch.
Fast-food outlets.
Socially related eating.
Food assistance (WIC program and others).
Mobilization of all resources.

Body image

Degree of acceptance of an adult body.
Maturity in facing body changes throughout pregnancy.

Living situation

Acceptance by living partners and extended family.
Role expectations of living partners.
Financial support.
Facilities and resources.
Ethnic group (religious, cultural, and social patterns).
Emancipation versus dependency.
Support system versus isolation.

Relationship with the child's father

Presence or absence of father.
Quality of relationship.
Influence on decision making.
Contribution to resources.
Influence on mother's nutritional habits and general lifestyle.
Understanding of physiologic processes.
Tolerance of physical changes in pregnancy and physical needs of mother and child.
Influence on child feeding.

Peer relationships

Support from friends.
Influence on nutritional knowledge and attitudes.
Influence on general lifestyle.

Nutritional state

Weight-for-height proportion.
Maturational state.
Tissue stores of nutrients.
Reproductive and contraceptive history.
Physical health.
History of dietary patterns and nutritional status, including weight-losing schemes.
Present eating habits.
Complications of pregnancy (nausea and vomiting).
Substance use.
Activity patterns.
Need for intensive remediation.

Prenatal care

Initiation of and compliance with prenatal care.
Dependability of supporting resources.
Identification of risk factors.

Nutritional attitude and knowledge

Prior attitude toward nutrition.
Understanding of role of nutrition in pregnancy.
Knowledge of foods as sources of nutrients and of nutrients needed by the body.
Desire to obtain adequate nutrition.
Ability to obtain adequate nutrition and to control food supply.

Preparation for child feeding

Knowledge of child-feeding practices.
Attitude and decisions about child feeding.
Responsibility for feeding.
Understanding the importance of the bonding process.
Support from family and friends.

Summary

Besides the issues of nutrient intake and weight gain during pregnancy, other aspects of diet and lifestyle influence the course and outcome of pregnancy. Pregnant women experience altered "appetites" and frequently suffer from early pregnancy nausea and later pregnancy constipation and heartburn. An array of nonnutrient dietary components raise concerns about safety; some of these concerns are justified and others are not. A minority of women face additional challenges because of their high-risk conditions. In some of these cases, special dietary manipulation is recommended to optimize pregnancy outcome. In the face of all of these circumstances, it is amazing that the vast majority of pregnancies result in healthy offspring and equally healthy new mothers.

Review Questions

1. Define *pica* and discuss its relevance to the course of pregnancy.
2. Summarize the known effects of maternal alcohol ingestion during pregnancy.
3. How safe is caffeine intake during pregnancy?
4. Describe the differences, if any, between the nutrient needs of pregnant adolescents and those of pregnant adults.
5. What would you recommend to a pregnant woman who trains intensively for marathons?
6. Outline your nutritional advice to a seemingly healthy seventeen-year-old pregnant girl who started menstruating at age eleven.

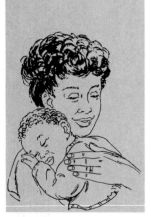

CHAPTER 6

LACTATION: THE MOTHER AND HER MILK

Bonnie S. Worthington-Roberts

≈ ≈ ≈ ≈ ≈ ≈ ≈ ≈ ≈ ≈ ≈

Basic Concepts

❏ *Female anatomy and physiology provide the required structures and functions for normal postpartum lactation.*

❏ *Human milk is designed to meet human infant needs.*

❏ *Successful lactation requires nutritional support.*

---

*L*actation is a physiologic process accomplished by females since the origin of mammals. Today, as in times past, the process of breast-feeding is successfully initiated by at least 99% of women who try. All that is required of the lactating mother is an intact mammary gland (or preferably two) and the presence and operation of appropriate physiologic mechanisms that allow for adequate milk production and release.

From this basic physiologic view, the establishment and maintenance of human lactation are determined by at least three factors:

1. The anatomic structure of the mammary tissue and the development of milk-producing cells (alveoli), ducts, and nipples to produce and then deliver the milk.
2. The initiation and maintenance of milk secretion.
3. The ejection or propulsion of milk from the alveoli to the nipple.

However, the most significant term is *human*. This brings an added personal dimension to the physiologic process. Breast-feeding is a very personal process for a mother.

In this chapter, we will look at lactation, human milk, and breast-feeding in physiologic terms. Clear knowledge of the physiologic factors, which include nutritional needs, is essential for effective lactation management.

BREAST ANATOMY AND DEVELOPMENT ≈≈

Anatomy of the Mammary Gland

Basic structure. The **mammary gland** of the human female consists of milk-producing cells (glandular epithelium) and a duct system embedded in connective tissue and fat (fig. 6-1). The size of the breast is variable, but in most instances it extends from the second through the sixth rib and from the central breast bone (sternum) to the arm pit. The mammary tissue lies directly over the large chest muscle (pectoralis major muscle) and is separated from this muscle by a layer of fat, which is continuous with the fatty tissue of the gland itself.[1]

Areola. The center of the fully developed breast in the adult woman is marked by the **areola,** a circular pigmented skin area from 1.5 to 2.5 cm in diameter. The surface of the areola appears rough because of the presence of large, somewhat modified fluid-producing glands, which are located directly beneath the skin in the thin subcutaneous tissue layer. The fatty secretion of these glands is believed to lubricate the nipple. Bundles of smooth muscle fibers in the areolar tissue stiffen the nipple for a better grasp by the sucking infant.[1]

Nipple and duct system. The nipple is elevated above the breast and contains fifteen to twenty **lactiferous ducts** surrounded by modified muscle cell tissues and covered by wrinkled skin. Partly within this compartment of the nipple and partly below its base, these ducts expand to form the short lactiferous sinuses in which milk may be stored. The sinuses are the continuations of the mammary ducts, which extend outward from the nipple toward the chest wall with numerous secondary branches. The duct system ends in masses of milk-producing cells, which form subsections, or **lobules,** of the breast (fig. 6-1).

Adolescent-adult development. During adolescence, the female breasts enlarge to their adult size. Frequently, one breast is slightly larger than the other, but this difference is usually unnoticeable. In a nonpregnant woman, the mature breast weighs approximately 200 g, the left being somewhat larger than the right. During pregnancy there is some increase in size and weight such that by term the breast may weigh between 400 and 600 g. During lactation, this weight increases to between 600 and 800 g.[1]

Mammary gland
(Gr *mamme,* mother's breast) Milk-producing gland in the females of all mammal species, humans and animals, distinguished from all other animal life by bearing live young and producing milk to nourish them.

Areola
(L *areola,* area, space) Pigmented area surrounding the nipple of the human breast.

Lactiferous ducts
(L *lac,* milk; *ferre,* to bear; *ducere,* to lead or draw) Vessels producing or conveying milk from producing cells to storage and release areas of the breast; tube or passage for secretions.

Lobules
(L *lobus,* lobe, a well-defined area) Smaller branching vessels that make up a lobe of the mammary gland.

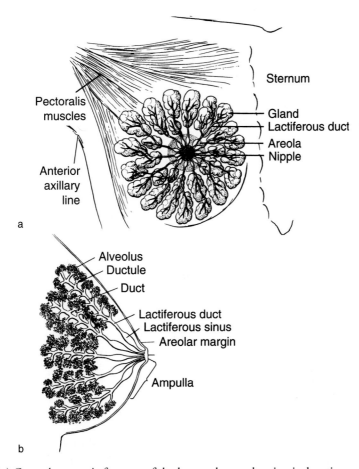

FIG. 6-1 (*a*) General anatomic features of the human breast showing its location on the chest—more specifically, the anterior region of the thorax between the sternum and the anterior axillary line. (*b*) Detailed structural features of the human mammary gland showing the terminal glandular (alveolar) tissue of each lobule leading into the duct system, which eventually enlarges into the lactiferous duct and lactiferous sinus. The lactiferous sinuses rest beneath the areola and converge at the nipple pore.

Lactation
(L *lactare,* to suckle) Process of milk production and secretion in the mammary glands.

Neonatal
(Gr *neos,* new; L *natus,* born) Relating to the period surrounding birth, especially the first four weeks after birth when the newborn is called a neonate.

Variation after childbirth. Wide variation in the structural composition of the human breasts has been observed in women after childbirth. Some breasts contain little secretory tissue; some large breasts contain less glandular tissue than much smaller organs. It is well known, however, that neither size nor structural composition of the breast significantly influences **lactation** success in the average woman. Almost all women who want to breast-feed find that they can.[1]

Breast Development

Infancy and childhood. In the human female newborn, the mammary glands are developed sufficiently to appear as distinct, round elevations, which feel like movable soft masses. Through the microscope, future milk ducts and glandular lobules can be recognized easily. These early glandular structures can produce a milk-like secretion ("witch's milk") two or three days after birth. All of these **neonatal** phenomena related to the mammary glands probably result from the intensive developmental processes that occur in the last stages of intrauterine life. Usually they subside in the first few weeks after birth. Some shrinkage, or involution, in the breast takes place by the time the infant is several weeks old, and this is followed by the "quiescent" period of mammary growth and activity during infancy and childhood.[1]

Adolescence. With the onset of puberty and during adolescence, an increased output of estrogenic hormone accomplishes ovarian maturation and follicular stimulation. As a result of this response, the mammary ducts elongate, and their lining cells reduplicate and proliferate. The growth of the ductal cells is accompanied by the growth of fibrous and fatty tissue, which is largely responsible for the increasing size and firmness of the adolescent gland. During this period, the areola and nipple also grow and become pigmented.[1]

Breast Maturation

Hormonal effects. As the developing woman matures and ovulation patterns become established, the regular development of progesterone-producing corpora lutea in the ovaries promotes the second stage of mammary development. Lobules gradually appear, giving the mammary glands the characteristic lobular structure found during the childbearing period. This differentiation into a lobular gland is completed about twelve to eighteen months after the first menstrual period, but further development continues in proportion to the intensity of the hormonal stimuli during each menstrual cycle and especially during pregnancies.[1]

Functional mammary tissue. Some young women enter reproductive life with insufficient functional mammary tissue to produce enough milk for their baby's total nourishment. In some cases, this relates to underdevelopment of the mammary ductwork associated with periodic cessation of menstruation (amenorrhea) or very late menarche. In addition, there are women who have had surgery to remove cysts, tumors, or other growths; others have undergone surgery for breast reduction or reconstruction. For whatever reason, circumstances exist in which functional mammary tissue is insufficient to fully support a nursing infant. Fortunately, these situations are rare.[1]

Preparation during pregnancy. The mammary gland of a nonpregnant woman is inadequately prepared for secretory activity. Only during pregnancy do changes occur that make satisfactory milk production possible. In the first trimester of pregnancy, the small ducts sprouting from the mammary ducts proliferate to create a maximum number of surface cells for future alveolar cell formation. In the midtrimester, the reduplicated small ductules group together to form large lobules. Their central cavities begin to dilate. In the last trimester, the existent clumps of milk-producing cells progressively dilate in the final preparation for the lactation process.[1]

Role of the placenta. The placenta plays an important role in mammary growth in pregnancy. It secretes ovarian-like hormones in large quantities. A number of these hormones have been identified as contributing to mammary gland growth.[1]

Antepartum preparation. Although mammary growth and development occur rapidly throughout pregnancy, additional proliferation of lining cells takes place in the **antepartum** period shortly before delivery of the baby or at **parturition.** The proliferation of these cells that begins just before parturition in response to increasing levels of the hormone **prolactin** results in new cells with a new complement of enzymes.[1]

The Physiology of Lactation ≋

General Activity

Initial postpartum secretions. Full lactation does not begin as soon as the baby is born. During the first two or three days **postpartum,** a small amount of **colostrum** is secreted. In subsequent days, a rapid increase in milk secretion occurs, and in usual cases lactation is reasonably well established by the end of the first week. In first-time mothers (primiparas), however, the establishment of lactation may be delayed until the third week or even later. Generally, therefore, the first two or three weeks are a period of lactation initiation, and this is followed by the longer period of maintenance of lactation.

Milk production stages. Initiation and maintenance of lactation constitute a complex process involving both nerves and hormones. Lactation involves the sensory nerves in the nipples, the spinal cord, the hypothalamus, and the pituitary gland with its various hormones. The process of milk production occurs in two distinct stages: 1) secretion of milk and 2) propulsion or ejection whereby the milk passes along the duct system. The two events are closely related and often occur simultaneously in the nursing mother.

The secretion of milk involves both the synthesis of the milk components and the passage of the formed product into the ducts (fig. 6-2). These events may be under independent control, since the accumulation of both fat and protein reaches a high level during the latter part of pregnancy. Shortly before delivery, the accumulated secretory products begin to pass into the duct system. The secretory process is activated again by the sucking stimulus of the infant.

In general, each milk-producing **alveolar** cell proceeds through a secretory process that is preceded and followed by a resting stage (fig. 6-3). Milk synthesis is most active during the suckling period but occurs at lower levels at other times. The secretory cells are square but change to a cylindric shape just before milk secretion while cellular water uptake is increased. As secretion commences, the enlarged cell with its thickened surface becomes club-like in shape. The tip pinches off, leaving the cell intact. The milk constituents are then free in the secreted solution, and the cell retains a cap of membrane. Between periods of active milk secretion, alveolar cells return to their characteristic resting state.

Fat Synthesis and Release

Initial synthesis. Fat synthesis takes place in the **endoplasmic reticulum** from compounds synthesized intracellularly or imported from the maternal circulation. Alveolar cells are able to synthesize short-chain fatty acids, which are derived predominantly from available acetate. Long-chain fatty acids and triglycerides are derived from maternal plasma; these fatty acids are predominantly used for the synthesis of milk fat. Synthesis of triglyceride from intracellular carbohydrate also plays a predominant role in fat production for human milk.

Final preparation and release. The process of esterification of fatty acids takes place in the endoplasmic reticulum. The resultant triglycerides accumulate as small fat droplets in the endoplasmic reticulum but eventually coalesce in the basal region of the cell to form large droplets that migrate toward the top of the cell. Ultimately, these droplets bulge into the lumen for eventual discharge. Apocrine secretion involves the protrusion of the cell surface into the lumen, with eventual pinching off of the protruded unit. This discharged material usually contains fat globules, protein, and a small amount of **cytoplasm,** all of which appear in human milk.

Antepartum
(L *ante,* before; *partum,* parting, a separate part) Period of gestation before onset of labor and the birth of the infant.

Parturition
(L *parturitio,* to give birth) Act or process of childbirth; labor and delivery.

Prolactin
(Gr *pro-,* before; L *lac,* milk) Hormone of the anterior pituitary gland that stimulates and maintains lactation in postpartum mammals.

Postpartum
The first 30 days after delivery.

Colostrum
(L *colostrum,* bee sting swelling and secretions) Thin, yellowish, milky liquid, mother's initial breast secretion before and immediately after birth of her baby; rich in immune factors and nutrition, especially protein and minerals; foremilk.

Alveoli
(L *alveolus,* hollow) Small sac-like, out-pouching areas in the mammary gland, secretory units that produce and secrete milk.

Endoplasmic reticulum
(Gr *endon,* within; *plassein,* to form; L *rete,* net) A protoplasmic network of flattened double-membrane sheets in cells; important metabolic cell organelles, some with rough surfaces bearing ribosomes for protein synthesis and other smooth surfaces synthesizing fatty acids.

Cytoplasm
(Gr *kytos,* hollow vessel; *plasma,* anything formed or molded) Protoplasm of the cell outside the nucleus, a continuous, gel-like aqueous solution in which the cell organelles are suspended; site of major cell metabolism.

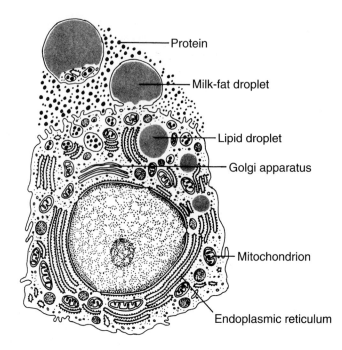

FIG. 6-2   Diagrammatic representation of a mammary gland cell showing the basic square shape with typical wavy surface border and nucleus. Cytoplasmic organization is characteristic of cells undergoing active protein synthesis and secretion. The synthetic apparatus consists of many free ribosomes and an extensive system of rough endoplasmic reticulum. A large Golgi body is located above the nucleus, and associated with it are some vacuoles containing particulate material that condenses into a central core or granule. Toward the top, the granules become progressively larger and contain more dense protein granules. The vacuoles fuse with the surface membrane and liberate their contents intact into the lumen. Fat droplets are found throughout the cell but are largest near the top. They protrude into the lumen and appear to pinch off from the cell proper along with a small bit of cytoplasm. Other cytoplasmic structures include large mitochondria lysosomes, and a small number of smooth membranous tubules and vesicles.

Modified from Lentz, T.L. 1971. *Cell fine structure: An atlas of drawings of whole cell-structure.* Philadelphia: W.B. Saunders.

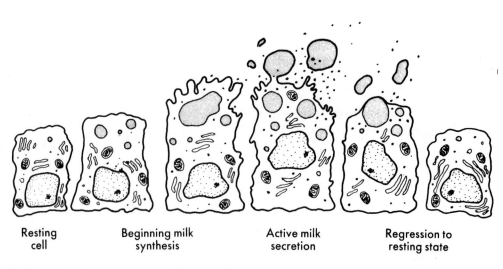

FIG. 6-3   Diagrammatic representation of the cycle of changes that occur in secretory cells of the alveoli from resting stage through milk production and secretion with eventual return to the resting stage.

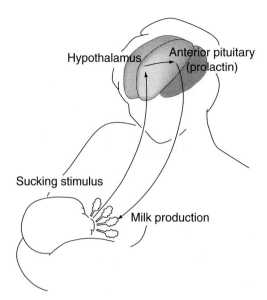

FIG. 6-4   Diagrammatic representation of the basic physiologic features of milk production. The sucking stimulus provided by the baby sends a message to the hypothalamus. The hypothalamus stimulates the anterior pituitary to release prolactin, the hormone that promotes milk production by alveolar cells of the mammary glands.

Protein Synthesis and Discharge

Initial synthesis.   The vast majority of proteins present in normal milk are specific to mammary secretions and are not identified in any quantity elsewhere in nature. The formation of milk protein including mammary enzymes is induced by prolactin and further stimulated by other hormones. Studies using sophisticated microscopic techniques have clearly shown that the abundant rough endothelial reticulum is the site of protein synthesis in the secretory cell.

Final preparation and release.   Protein granules accumulate within the Golgi complexes before transport through the cell and release into the lumen by apocrine secretion or reverse pinocytosis. The proteins in milk are derived from two sources: 1) some are synthesized **de novo** in the mammary gland, and 2) others are derived as such from plasma. Inclusion of plasma-derived proteins in the milk secretion occurs primarily in the early secretory product, colostrum. Thereafter, the three main proteins in milk—casein, alpha-lactalbumin, and beta-lactalbumin—are synthesized within the gland from amino acid precursors. All of the essential and some of the nonessential amino acids are taken up directly from the plasma, but some of the nonessential amino acids are synthesized by the milk-producing cells of the gland.

Carbohydrate Synthesis and Release

Lactose synthesis.   The predominant carbohydrate in milk is lactose. Its synthesis occurs within the **Golgi apparatus** of the alveolar cell. The synthesis of lactose combines glucose and galactose. Most of the intracellular glucose is derived continually from circulating blood glucose; galactose is synthesized from glucose.

Final preparation and release.   Once synthesized within the Golgi complex, lactose is attached to protein and carried to the cell surface in a **vesicle.** It is then released from the surface of the cell by reverse pinocytosis, as occurs with several other milk components.

The Role of Hormones

Milk secretion.   The stimulus for milk secretion derives largely from the hormone prolactin (fig. 6-4). This hormone acts on alveolar cells and promotes continual milk production and release. Maintenance of milk secretion, however, requires other hormonal

de novo
(L *anew,* from the beginning) To make a fresh from primary components; "from scratch," as in cooking.

Golgi apparatus
A complex, cup-like structure of membranes with associated vesicles first described by Italian Nobel Prize-winning histologist Camillo Golgi (1843–1926); synthesis site of numerous carbohydrate metabolic products such as lactose, glycoproteins, and mucopolysaccharides.

Vesicle
(L *vesica,* bladder) A small bladder or sac containing liquid; secretory transport sacs that move out into the cell cytoplasm to aid metabolism.

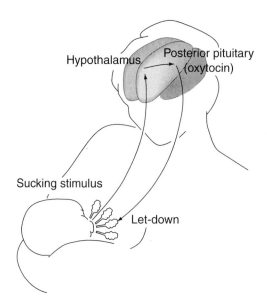

FIG. 6-5   Diagrammatic representation of the basic features of the "let-down reflex." The sucking stimulus arrives at the hypothalamus, which promotes the release of oxytocin from the posterior pituitary. Oxytocin stimulates the contraction of the muscle-like (myoepithelial) cells around the alveoli in the mammary glands. Contraction of these muscle-like cells causes the milk to be propelled through the duct system and into the lactiferous sinuses, where it becomes available to the nursing infant.

Estrogen
A steroidal hormone elaborated by the ovaries and, during pregnancy, by the placenta.

factors from the anterior pituitary. If sucking is discontinued during the lactation period, pituitary release of these necessary hormones ceases and milk secretion usually stops in the following few days, with accompanying deterioration and sloughing of alveolar cells.

Relation of oral contraceptive agents. **Estrogen** inhibits milk production, especially in the early stage of lactation. However, studies of the use of combined estrogen-progestin oral contraceptive agents (OCAs) indicate that lactation is not inhibited in women who wish to nurse their infants, as long as the pill is not used in the immediate postpartum period. Some dose-related suppression of the quantity of milk produced and the duration of lactation is found with extended use. Even though several reports suggest that measurable composition changes occur in the milk produced by women taking OCAs, the results are inconsistent and largely viewed as insignificant.

The Let-Down Reflex

Primary stimulus.   Once milk production and secretion have been accomplished, the baby may then obtain this milk by promoting its ejection from the ducts. The milk ejection, or "let-down," reflex is a mechanism involving both nerves and hormones that is regulated in part by central nervous system factors (fig. 6-5). The primary stimulus is sucking on the nipple, which triggers the discharge of the hormone **oxytocin** from the posterior pituitary. Oxytocin is carried in the bloodstream to the muscle-like **(myoepithelial) cells** around the alveoli and along the duct system, where it is easily available to the nursing baby.

Oxytocin
(Gr *oxys*, sharp, sour; *tokos*, birth) Pituitary hormone causing uterine contraction and milk ejection.

Myoepithelial cells
(Gr *mys*, muscle; *epi*, on; *thele*, nipple) Tissue composed of contractile epithelial cells surrounding the alveoli and duct system of the lactating breasts.

Psychologic influences.   The milk ejection reflex appears to be sensitive to small differences in circulating oxytocin level. Thus, even minor emotional and psychologic disturbances can influence the degree to which breast milk is released to the baby. The significance of psychologic influences on the milk ejection reflex in humans has been demonstrated by numerous case histories. These experiences illustrate the fact that milk ejection can be inhibited by embarrassment or stress, or it can be set off by the mere thought of the baby or the sound of the baby's cry. This observation has been confirmed by experimental stimulation (or inhibition) of the milk ejection reflex. Signs of successful let-down of milk are easily recognized by the nursing mother. Common and significant occurrences include 1) milk dripping from the breasts before the baby starts nursing, 2) milk dripping from the breast opposite the one being nursed, 3) contractions of the uterus during breast-feeding, often causing slight pain or discomfort, and 4) a tingling sensation in the breast.

Sucking stimulus. Sucking stimulation is widely accepted as the most effective means of maintaining adequate lactation. There is considerable evidence in human subjects that the restriction of sucking significantly inhibits lactation. Artificial sucking stimulation in the form of manual expression or a breast pump has repeatedly been recommended as a means of increasing milk yield or maintaining yield in the absence of the baby. Evidence suggests that feeding on demand optimally stimulates the lactation process.

Duration of lactation. Local and cultural patterns of infant feeding are of great significance in determining the duration of breast-feeding for a given mother. Although successful lactation can continue as long as sucking stimulation is maintained, a gradual fall in the amount of milk produced generally develops after twelve months. This drop in milk output largely relates to reduced demand and loss of recurrent nipple stimulation by the baby.

GENERAL NATURE OF MAMMALIAN MILK[1] ≋

Unique Species Variation

Many investigations during the past decade have defined the biochemical and nutritional properties of different types of mammalian milk. It is clear from these studies that each type of milk is unique and consists of a highly complex mixture of organic and inorganic compounds.

Mother-child relation and nature of milk. It is likely that the characteristics of mammalian milks relate directly to the variable mother-child relationships that take place in infancy. Shaul found support for this idea while examining five groups of wild animals.[2]

> *Group 1:* **Marsupials** and animals that bear their young while in hibernation. In these animals, the mother is available at all times, and the milk is dilute and low in fat.
>
> *Group 2:* Animals born in a relatively mature state that follow or are carried by their mothers at all times. The maternal attentiveness is high, and the milk produced is rather low in fat and dilute. The low fat content is often seen in the milk of animals that nurse frequently.
>
> *Group 3:* Animals that leave their young in a secluded place and return to them at widely spaced intervals. The lioness is a good example of this type. This group of animals has very concentrated milk that is high in fat.
>
> *Group 4:* Animals born in a relatively immature state and that remain for a considerable time in nests or burrows. The mother must leave for several hours at a time, and nursing is more "on schedule" rather than "on demand."
>
> *Group 5:* Animals that spend much time in cold water or when on land are frequently made wet by the mother returning from the water. In these cases, the milk is very concentrated and has an extremely high fat content.

Marsupial
(L *marsupium,* a pouch) Member of the animal class of mammals that bear undeveloped young, which they carry and nourish in an abdominal pouch until their development is complete; includes such animals as kangaroos and koala bears.

Comparison of human milk. Human milk is dilute and thus resembles the milk of the marsupials and hibernating bears, whose offspring feed constantly. It is therefore not surprising that the human baby demands to be fed frequently (table 6-1). For this reason, in many parts of the world the mother carries the baby where she goes at all times.

The Nature of Human Milk

Variable basic content. Reports during the past twenty years on the biochemical composition of human milk have included over 1,000 publications. Large numbers of new components continue to be characterized such that more than a hundred constituents are now recognized. Basically, human milk consists of a solution of protein, sugar, and salts

TABLE 6-1   *Nutrient Content of Mature Human Milk*

Constituents (per Liter)	Human Milk	Constituents (per Liter)	Human Milk
Energy (kcal)	680.00	Minerals	
Protein (g)	10.50	Calcium (mg)	280.00
Fat (g)	39.00	Phosphorus (mg)	140.00
Lactose (g)	72.00	Sodium (mg)	180.00
Vitamins		Potassium (mg)	525.00
Vitamin A (RE)*	670.00	Chloride (mg)	420.00
Vitamin D (μg)	0.55	Magnesium (mg)	35.00
Vitamin E (mg)	2.30	Iron (mg)	0.30
Vitamin K (μg)	2.10	Iodine (μg)	110.00
Thiamin (mg)	0.21	Manganese (μg)	6.00
Riboflavin (mg)	0.35	Copper (mg)	0.25
Niacin (mg)	1.50	Zinc (mg)	1.20
Pyridoxine (μg)	93.00	Selenium (μg)	20.00
Folic acid (μg)	85.00	Fluoride (μg)	16.00
Cobalamine (μg)	0.97	Chromium (μg)	50.00
Ascorbin acid (mg)	40.00		

Data from Institute of Medicine. 1991. *Nutrition during lactation.* Washington DC: National Academy Press.
*RE, retinol equivalents

Gestational age

(L *gestare,* to bear) Period of embryonic-fetal growth and development from ovum fertilization to birth; varying with degree of preterm development to full-term mature newborn.

in which a variety of fatty compounds are suspended (table 6-2). The composition varies from one human to another, from one period of lactation to the next, and even hourly during the day. The composition of a given milk sample is related not only to the amount secreted and the stage of the lactation but also to the timing of the withdrawal and to individual variations among lactating mothers. These latter individual variations may be affected by such variables as maternal age, parity, health, and social class. **Gestational age** of the infant also makes a difference.

Milk volume. Observations of completely breast-fed babies who appear to be thriving suggest that daily volume of breast consumption ranges from 340 to over 1,000 ml/day. The mean falls between 600 and 900 ml/day, at least for representative North American women.[3] Mothers of twins may show an enhanced capacity for milk production (fig. 6-6). Hartmann, in western Australia, compared milk outputs of mothers of single infants with that of mothers of twins.[4] The obvious difference in milk production is demonstrated in fig. 6-6. Severe food restriction may limit the volume of milk production.[3] A lifestyle involving vigorous exercise, however, does not have a detrimental impact on milk output.[5]

Relation to maternal nutrition. Although many data have been recorded on the differences in samples of human milk, the general picture is the same throughout the world. Except for vitamin and fat content, the composition of human milk appears to be largely independent of the state of the mother's nutrition, at least until malnutrition becomes severe. Even after prolonged lactation for two years or more, the quality of the milk produced by Indian and African women appears to be relatively well maintained, although the quantity may be small. Also, it is well known that severely undernourished women during time of famine often manage to feed their babies reasonably well.[3]

Colostrum

In the first few days after birth, the mammary glands secrete a small amount of opaque fluid called colostrum. The volume varies between 2 and 10 ml per feeding per day during the first three days, related in part to the parity of the mother. Women who have had

TABLE 6-2 *Classes of Constituents in Human Milk*

Protein and Nonprotein Nitrogen Compounds	Carbohydrates
Proteins	Lactose
Caseins	Oligosaccharides
α-Lactalbumin	Bifidus factors
Lactoferrin	Glycopeptides
Secretory IgA and other immunoglobulins	
β-Lactoglobulin	**Lipids**
Lysozyme	
Enzymes	Triglycerides
Hormones	Fatty acids
Growth factors	Phospholipids
	Sterols and hydrocarbons
Nonprotein nitrogen compounds	Fat-soluble vitamins
Urea	A and carotene
Creatine	D
Creatinine	E
Uric acid	K
Glucosamine	
α-Amino nitrogen	**Minerals**
Nucleic acids	
Nucleotides	**Macronutrient elements**
Polyamines	Calcium
	Phosphorus
Water-Soluble Vitamins	Magnesium
	Potassium
Thiamin	Sodium
Riboflavin	Chlorine
Niacin	Sulfur
Pantothenic acid	
Biotin	**Trace elements**
Folate	Iodine
Vitamin B_6	Iron
Vitamin B_{12}	Copper
Vitamin C	Zinc
Inositol	Manganese
Choline	Selenium
	Chromium
Cells	Cobalt
Leukocytes	
Epithelial cells	

Modified from National Academy of Sciences. 1991. *Nutrition during lactation.* Washington, DC: National Academy Press.

other pregnancies, particularly those who have nursed babies previously, usually demonstrate colostrum output sooner and in greater volume than other women. Colostrum is typically yellow, a feature associated with its relatively high carotene content. Also, it contains more protein and less sugar and fat than milk produced thereafter. As might be expected from these composition differences, it is lower in kilocalories than mature milk—67 versus 75 kcal/100 ml. The ash content of colostrum is high, and concentrations of

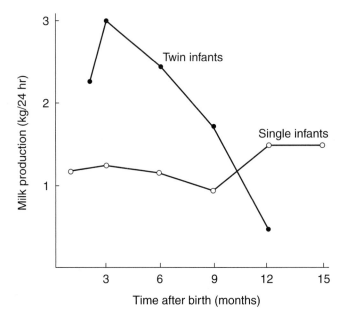

FIG. 6-6 Milk outputs of western Australian women breast-feeding twins and exclusively breast-feeding single babies.

Based on data from Hartmann, P.E., et al. 1981. Breast-feeding and reproduction in women in western Australia—a review. *Birth Fam J* 8:215.

sodium, potassium, and chloride are greater than in mature milk. The few composition analyses of human colostrum that have been reported show striking variability during any one day and from day to day. It is likely that these differences partially reflect the unstable secretory patterns that exist in the mammary apparatus as it begins the active production, secretion, and ejection of milk.

Transitional Milk

Colostrum changes to transitional milk between the third and sixth day, at which time the protein content is still rather high. By the tenth day, the major changes have been completed, and, by the end of the first month, the protein content has reached a consistent level that does not fall significantly thereafter. As the content of protein falls, the content of lactose progressively rises. This is also the case for fat, which increases to typical levels as lactation becomes more firmly established.

Preterm Milk

Preterm milk
Milk produced by mothers of premature infants.

With the renewed interest in the feeding of human milk to preterm infants, substantial attention has been focused on the composition of milk produced by mothers who deliver prematurely.[6] Early reports suggested that the protein and nonprotein nitrogen content of **preterm milk** was higher than that of term milk. Additional observations revealed that preterm milk might also have been higher in its concentration of calcium, IgA, sodium, potassium, chloride, phosphorus, magnesium, medium chain and polyunsaturated long-chain fatty acids, and total lipids, but lower in its lactose level than term milk. Thus, the opinion developed that premature infants who are fed their mother's milk might demonstrate growth and development superior to that observed in premature infants fed banked human milk. In general, this suspicion has proved to be true for very low birth weight infants, as reported by researchers who have completed appropriate comparisons. It appears, however, that commercial infant formulas designed for low birth weight infants may also be superior to banked human milk in supporting growth of these babies.

The controversy surrounding the nutritional adequacy of human milk for very low birth weight infants still exists. Although recent observations suggest that premature infants can thrive on milk from their own mothers, it is known that protein and sodium concentrations are marginal and calcium and phosphate levels are too low to support optimum development of the skeleton. In the face of immature gastrointestinal and renal function and poor nutrient stores, the very low birth weight infant who is provided human milk will often profit from an organized supplementation program.

It is even possible to supplement human milk with a powdered or liquid product designed to improve nutritional adequacy for very low birth weight infants.* The powdered fortifier contains protein and carbohydrate and increases the caloric density of breast milk to about 24 kilocalories per ounce. The product is sold in premeasured packets; one packet is designed for addition to 25 ml of human milk. The liquid fortifier is similar in composition and is designed to be mixed with human milk or to be fed alternately with human milk.

COMPOSITION OF MATURE HUMAN MILK [1] ≋

Protein

Amount and types of protein. It is well known that different animals show different rates of growth. This fact appears to be related to their milk. The slowest rate of growth is found in humans, and human milk contains the least protein. The major proteins found in breast milk are caseins and whey proteins. Caseins are phosphorus-containing proteins that occur only in milk. The **whey** proteins, such as lactalbumin and lactoferrin, are synthesized in the mammary gland. Other proteins, including protein hormones and serum albumin, are transported to the milk from the plasma. The concentration of protein found in human milk is lower than the previously accepted value of 1.5 g/100 ml that was calculated from analyzed nitrogen content. Since human milk has been found to contain 25% of its nitrogen in nonprotein compounds, the lower protein concentration (0.8 to 0.9 g/100 ml) is now accepted as the true amount.

Initial changes. The protein content of human milk, like that of other mammals, falls rapidly over the first few days of lactation and reflects a relatively higher loss of the proteins important in immune functions. Colostrum averages about 2% protein; transitional and mature milk average 1.5% and 1.0%, respectively.

Relation to maternal diet. Observations of many women in a variety of countries have shown that the protein content of human milk is not reduced in mothers consuming a diet low in protein or poor in protein quality. A study in Pakistan supports this idea.[7] The protein quality and quantity of milk collected from women of a very low socioeconomic group in Karachi were similar to those of well-nourished women there and in other parts of the world. Of interest, however, was the observation that the concentration of lysine and methionine in the free amino acid content of milk samples from malnourished women was reduced when compared with milk from healthy, well-nourished mothers. The investigators suggest that this finding could imply a reduction in nutritional *quality* of the protein in these samples. It is important to recognize, however, that dietary amino acid deficits may be readily subsidized from maternal tissues as long as reserves are available from which to draw in order to maintain protein homeostasis. Temporary fluctuations in free amino acid levels may be apparent, but alterations in quantity or quality of intact milk proteins are much less likely to occur until maternal protein stores are severely depleted.

Effect of chronic maternal protein deficit. With chronic protein undernutrition, breast milk composition may change. One study was carried out to assess the effects of prolonged lactation on the quantity of protein and patterns of amino acids in breast milk obtained from Thai women at various times during lactation.[8] Protein levels decreased from 1.56% during the first week to a low of about 0.6% from 180 to 270 days and then rose to about 0.7%. Using these data, one can calculate that a three-month-old infant in the 50th percentile for weight would require about 1,250 ml of milk per day to meet protein needs. Since few infants in developing countries would receive this volume of milk daily and since supplemental sources of protein are scarce, the protein status of such infants could be significantly compromised.

Whey
The thin liquid of milk remaining after the curd, containing the mild protein casein, and the cream have been removed; contains other milk proteins, lactalbumin and lactoferrin.

*Human Milk Fortifier (powdered), Mead Johnson Laboratories; Similac Natural Care (liquid), Ross Laboratories.

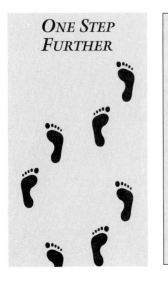

Genetic Engineering: Possible Future "Magic" of Recombinant Human Milk Proteins

Rapid developments in biotechnology have made it possible to modify the composition of many foods to an unprecedented extent. Biologically active proteins can be produced, including those derived from human milk. Since many of these proteins are known or believed to provide beneficial effects on the growth, development, and health of human infants, the production of these proteins for addition to infant foods is under study. It is unlikely that any infant-feeding product developed in the future will duplicate human milk. There may be justifiable uses for such products, but none will replace the "near-perfection" of the lactating woman's milk.

Lonnerdal, B. et al. 1998. Genetic engineering—Opportunities and challenges in infant nutrition. *Am J Clin Nutr* (suppl) 63:621S–662S.

TABLE 6-3   *Significant Features About the Amino Acid Composition of Human Milk*

Characteristics	Explanation
Lower in methionine and rich in cystine	An enzyme, cystathionase, is late to develop in the fetus; this impairs optimal conversion of methionine to cystine, which is needed for growth and development; methionine may increase in the bloodstream of an infant fed cow's milk but not one fed human milk; hypermethioninemia may damage the central nervous system.
Lower in phenylalanine and tyrosine	The enzymes tyrosine aminotransferase and parahydroxyphenyl pyruviate oxidase are late in developing: babies fed cow's milk may develop hyperphenylalaninemia and hypertyrosinemia, which may adversely affect development of the central nervous system, especially in the premature infant; breast milk offers much less chance of a problem.
Rich in taurine	Breast milk provides taurine for bile acid conjugation, and it *may* also be a neurotransmitter or neuromodulator in the brain and retina; humans cannot synthesize taurine well; cow's milk contains little taurine; the requirement for taurine in the developing neonate is uncertain.

Amino acids. The amino acid content of human milk is recognized as ideal for the human infant. Human milk is relatively low in several amino acids that are known to be detrimental if found in the blood at high levels—for example, in the genetic disease phenylalanine; on the other hand, it is high in other amino acids that the infant cannot synthesize well, such as cystine and taurine. Some of the positive features of the amino acid composition of human milk are summarized in table 6-3. These characteristics are especially useful to infants whose biochemical capabilities are underdeveloped at birth.

Nonprotein nitrogen. The total amount of nonprotein nitrogen in human milk averages nearly 25% of all nitrogen and is significantly higher than that found in cow's milk (about 5%). The importance of this to infant nutrition and health is unknown. Nonprotein nitrogen sources consist of a variety of organic, and trace amounts of inorganic, com-

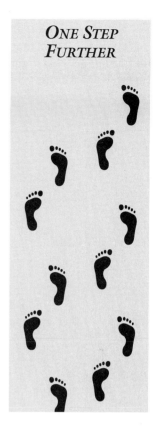

The Fatty Acid Pattern of Human Milk May Optimize Infant Development

Much effort has been made to evaluate the growth and development of breast-fed vs. formula-fed infants. Neurological differences have been reported in favor of the breast-fed babies. The roles played by long-chain highly unsaturated fatty acids in the development of brain tissues have received increasing attention. This exciting research may lead to the conclusion that the unique fatty acid pattern of human milk improves a child's chance of optimal development of the nervous system.

Birch, D.G., E.E. Birch, D.R. Hoffman, and R. Uauy. 1992. Dietary essential fatty acid supply and visual acuity development. *Invest Opthamol Vis Sci* 33:3242.

Birch, E., D. Birch, D. Hoffman et al. Breast feeding and optimal visual development. *J Pediatr Opthamol Strabis* 30:33.

Decsi, T., I. Thiel, and B. Koletzko. 1995. Essential fatty acids in full term infants fed breast milk or formula. *Arch/Dis Child* 72:F23.

Lanting, C.I., V. Fidler, M. Huisman et al. 1994. Neurological differences between 9-year-old children fed breast milk or formula milk as babies. *Lancet* 344:1319.

Lucas, A., R. Morley, T. Cole et al. 1992. Breast milk and subsequent intelligence quotient in children born preterm. *Lancet* 39:261.

Makrides, M., M.A. Neumann, R.W. Byard et al. 1994. Fatty acid composition of brain, retina and erythrocytes in breast- and formula-fed infants. *Am J Clin Nutr* 60:189.

Makrides, M., K. Simmer, M. Goggin, and R.A. Gibson. 1993. Erythrocyte docosahexaenoic acid correlates with visual response of healthy term infants. *Pediatr Res* 33:425.

Makrides, M., K. Simmer, M. Neumann, and R. Gibson. 1995. Changes in the polyunsaturated fatty acids of breast milk from mothers of full term infants over 30 weeks of lactation. *Am J Clin Nutr* 61:1231.

pounds shed into the milk supply. Among these compounds are peptides and free amino acids, the latter of which may provide a nutritional advantage to the infant. Nonprotein nitrogen sources also include urea, creatinine, and sugar amines. Scientists have speculated that it is of nutritional significance that each species of mammal seems to carry a characteristic pattern of free amino acids in its nonprotein nitrogen pool.

Taurine. Much recent discussion has centered on the amino acid taurine. Since taurine is found in particularly high levels in fetal brain tissue, it has been proposed that it may play a role in the development of the brain. In addition, taurine is associated with bile acid and thus plays an important role in digestion and may function in the management of cholesterol in the body. Since human milk contains much more taurine than does cow's milk, it has been speculated that the breast-fed infant might profit significantly from the higher taurine intake. Interestingly, however, observations have shown that breast-fed babies maintain plasma taurine levels that are similar to those of formula-fed infants. It would therefore appear that taurine is not an essential amino acid for infants. However, the general consensus is that taurine is a conditionally essential nutrient for human infants and children, especially those born prematurely.[9]

Lipids

Amount. The total lipid content of human milk varies considerably from one woman to another and is even affected by parity and season of the year. Separate observations by different investigators around the world give the following average levels of fat in human milk: 2.02%, 3.1%, 3.2%, 3.27%, 3.95%, 4.5%, and 5.3%. Sampling methods may affect fat content, since the first milk (fore-milk) is low in fat, and the last milk (hind-milk) shows about a threefold increase in the fat content.

Types. Nearly 90% of the lipid in human milk is present in the form of triglycerides, but small amounts of phospholipids, cholesterol, diglycerides, monoglycerides, glycolipids, sterol esters, and free fatty acids are also found. The fatty acid composition of human milk

TABLE 6-4 *Mean Breast Milk Fatty Acid Concentration in Vegetarians (Vegans) and Nonvegetarians (Controls)*

Methyl Esters	Vegans*	Controls*
Lauric ($C_{12:0}$)	39	33
Myristic ($C_{14:0}$)	68	80
Palmitic ($C_{16:0}$)	166	276
Stearic ($C_{18:0}$)	52	108
Palmitoleic ($C_{16:1}$)	12	36
Oleic ($C_{18:1}$)	313	353
Linoleic ($C_{18:2}$)	317	69
Linolenic ($C_{18:3}$)	15	8

Modified from Sanders, T.A.B. et al. 1978. *Am J Clin Nutr* 31:805. Studies of vegans: the fatty acid composition of plasma cholinephosphosphycerides, erythrocytes, adipose tissue, and breast milk and some indicators of susceptibility to ischemic heart disease in vegans and omnivore controls.
*Mean values expressed as milligrams per gram total methyl esters detected for four vegans and four controls (nonvegetarians)

Myelin
The fatty coating of nerve fibers.

Eicosapentanoic acid (EPA)
(Gr *eicosa*, twenty; *penta*, five) Long-chain polyunsaturated fatty acid composed of a chain of twenty carbon atoms with five double (unsaturated) bonds; one of the omega-3 fatty acids found in fatty fish and fish oils.

Docasahexanoic acid (DHA)
(Gr *docosa*, twenty-two; *hexa*, six) Long-chain polyunsaturated omega-3 fatty acid having a twenty-two-carbon chain with six double (unsaturated) bonds; metabolic product of omega-3 EPA, found in fatty fish and fish oils. The body synthesizes both EPA and DHA from the essential fatty acids linoleic and linolenic acids.

Omega-3 fatty acids
Group of long-chain polyunsaturated fatty acids having important precursor roles in producing highly active hormone-like substances, the *eicosanoids*, involved in critical metabolic activities such as vascular muscle tone and blood clotting.

Depot fat
Body fat stored in adipose tissue.

differs greatly from that of cow's milk. The content of the essential fatty acid linoleic acid is considerably greater in human milk than in cow's milk. The content of short-chain saturated fatty acids (C4 to C8) is greater in cow's milk. Of equal interest is the observation that human milk contains more cholesterol than cow's milk and much more cholesterol than commercial infant formulas. A beneficial effect of this higher cholesterol level has been suggested on grounds that 1) it is needed by the rapidly growing central nervous system for **myelin** synthesis, and 2) in early life it stimulates the development of enzymes necessary for cholesterol degradation.

Recent research has demonstrated that human milk contains not only linoleic acid and linolenic acid but also **eicosapentanoic acid (EPA)** and **docosahexanoic acid (DHA)**. Interestingly, infant formula does not contain the longer-chain forms EPA and DHA. Since animal experiments have provided evidence that these **omega-3 fatty acids** may be essential for the normal prenatal and postnatal development of the brain and retina, the contribution that human milk makes to this developmental process is receiving much attention.[10]

Maternal diet effect on composition. The composition of the fat in human milk varies significantly with the diet of the mother. Lactating women fed a diet rich in polyunsaturated fats, such as corn and cottonseed oils, produce milk with an increased content of polyunsaturated fats. This is best seen by comparing total vegetarians with nonvegetarians, as seen in table 6-4. Over the years, as dietary unsaturated fat intake has increased in the United States, the fatty acid composition of breast milk samples has reflected this change (table 6-5).

When maternal energy intake is severely restricted, fatty acid composition of human milk resembles that of **depot fat.** This effect is to be expected; it represents fat mobilization in response to the reduction in energy intake. A substantial increase in the proportion of dietary kilocalories from carbohydrates will result in an increase in milk content of fatty acids with carbon chain lengths less than sixteen. The significance of this latter observation is unknown.

As far as cholesterol is concerned, there is no evidence that its concentration in human milk is altered by the maternal diet. In fact, milk cholesterol level stays between 100 and 150 mg/L even in hypercholesterolemic women and increases only in severe cases of pathologic hypercholesterolemia.

Fat-digesting enzymes. Human milk contains several lipases. One is a serum-stimulated lipase (lipoprotein lipase) that may appear in the milk as a result of leakage from the mammary tissue. Another fat-digesting milk enzyme has an activity similar to that of pancreatic lipase, breaking down triglycerides to free fatty acids and glycerol. This enzyme is present in the fat fraction and appears to be inhibited by bile salts. It probably is re-

TABLE 6-5 *Reports of Fatty Acid Composition of Human Milk*

Fatty Acid	Breast Milk Content (Percent of Total Fatty Acid)	
	1953*	1977†
Lauric ($C_{12:0}$)	5.5	3.8
Myristic ($C_{14:0}$)	8.5	5.2
Palmitic ($C_{16:0}$)	23.2	22.5
Palmitoleic ($C_{16:1}$)	3.0	4.1
Stearic ($C_{18:0}$)	6.9	8.7
Oleic ($C_{18:1}$)	36.5	39.5
Linoleic ($C_{18:2}$)	7.8	14.4
Linolenic ($C_{18:3}$)	———	2.0

*Based on data from Macy, I.G. et al. 1958. *The composition of milks,* Pub. No. 254. Washington, DC: National Research Council.
†Based on data from Guthrie, H.A., M.E. Picciano, and D. Sheehe. 1977. *J Pediatr* 90:39. Fatty acid pattern of human milk

sponsible for **lipolysis** of milk refrigerated or frozen for later use. Additional lipases in the skim milk fraction are inactive until they encounter bile. These lipases, the bile salt–stimulated lipases, are believed to be present only in the milk of primates and are thought to serve a useful purpose for this species. Since the bile salt–stimulated lipases have been clearly shown to be stable and active in the intestines of infants, they can contribute significantly to the hydrolysis of milk triglycerides and partly account for the greater ease in fat digestion that is commonly demonstrated by breast-fed babies.

Carnitine. Both human milk and cow's milk contain **carnitine,** which plays an important role in the oxidation of long-chain fatty acids by facilitating their transport across the **mitochondrial** membrane. The body's supply of carnitine is derived in part through ingestion of dietary carnitine and in part through endogenous synthesis from the essential amino acids lysine and methionine. Newborns are especially in need of carnitine, since fat provides a major source of energy. It has been suggested that carnitine may be an essential nutrient for the newborn, since infants may have a limited synthetic capacity, especially those born prematurely.[11] Human milk contains about 50 to 100 **nmol** of carnitine per milliliter; formula products based on milk or beef contain 50 to 656 nmol/ml. Those formulas prepared from soy isolate, and specialized formulations from egg white and casein, carry an amount equal to or less than 4 nmol/ml. For this reason, most manufacturers of soy-based infant formulas now add carnitine to their products. Whether or not infants using any of these formulas or provided human milk require additional carnitine has been the subject of much debate. At this point, it appears that supplemental carnitine is unnecessary for the vast majority of neonates.

Carbohydrates

Lactose. Lactose, a disaccharide composed of glucose and galactose, is the main carbohydrate in human milk. In all species of mammals studied, milk is isotonic with plasma, which helps keep the cost of milk secretion low. Lactose exerts 60–70% of the total osmotic pressure of milk. The concentrations of lactose in human milk are remarkably similar among women, and there is no good evidence that they can be influenced by maternal dietary factors.

Lactose is relatively insoluble and is slowly digested and absorbed in the small intestine. The presence of lactose in the gut of the infant stimulates the growth of microorganisms that produce organic acids and synthesize many of the B vitamins. It is believed that the acid milieu that is created helps check the growth of undesirable bacteria in the infant's gut and improve the absorption of calcium, phosphorus, magnesium, and other

Lipolysis
(Gr *lipos,* fat; *lysis,* dissolution) Fat digestion or breakdown.

Carnitine
A naturally occurring amino acid ($C_7H_{15}NO_3$) formed from methionine and lysine, required for transport of long-chain fatty acids across the mitochondrial membrane where they are oxidized as fuel substrate for metabolic energy.

Mitochondrion
(Gr *mitos,* thread; *chondrion,* granule) Cell's "powerhouse," small elongated organelle located in the cell cytoplasm; principal site of energy generation (ATP synthesis); contains enzymes of the final energy cycle (citric acid cycle) and cell respiratory chains, as well as ribonucleic acid (RNA) and deoxyribonucleic acid (DNA) for some synthesis of protein.

Nanomole (nmol)
(Gr *nanos,* dwarf; *molekul,* molecule) Metric system unit for measuring extremely small amounts. Prefix *nano-* used in naming units of measurement to indicate one-billionth of the unit with which it is combined. *Mole* is the chemical term for the molecular weight of a substance expressed in grams-gram molecular weight.

minerals. Since human milk contains much more lactose than cow's milk (7% and 4.8%, respectively), these gut-associated benefits of lactose are more significant in the breast-fed than in the bottle-fed infant.

Other carbohydrates. Chromatographic processing of human milk samples has revealed trace amounts of glucose and galactose and an array of moderate-chain-length carbohydrates (oligosaccharides). Some of these appear to be protective, even though they are present in low concentrations. Nitrogen-containing sugars promote the growth of lactobacilli, the dominant acid-producing bacteria in the lower intestinal tract of breast-fed infants. Specialized oligosaccharides inhibit the binding of selected bacterial pathogens or their toxins to epithelial cells by acting as "trapping receptors."

Amylase. Although human milk does not contain much complex carbohydrate, it does contain a starch-splitting enzyme, amylase, which is quite stable at pH levels found in the stomach and small bowel.[12] This enzyme may provide an alternative pathway for the digestion of glucose **polymers** and starches in early infancy when pancreatic amylase is low or absent in duodenal fluid. The physiologic importance of mammary amylase may be analogous to that of the bile salt–stimulated lipase found in human milk.

Polymers
(Gr *poly-*, many; *meros*, part) Large compounds formed by chains of simple repeating molecules—such as glucose polymer oligosaccharide.

Minerals

Comparison with cow's milk. One of the most striking differences between human and cow's milk lies in the mineral composition. As with protein, it is believed that this difference may be related to the rate of growth of the species for which the milk was intended. According to typical estimates, there is six times more phosphorus, four times more calcium, three times more total ash, and three times more protein in cow's milk than in human milk. The high mineral and protein composition of cow's milk distinctly affects the amount of mineral and protein waste products provided to the kidney. One might speculate that the kidney of the newborn infant is prepared to handle the "waste" derived from breast milk but is stressed unduly by the requirements placed on it when cow's milk, especially nonfat milk, is selected as an alternative.

Major and trace minerals. The major minerals found in mature human milk are potassium, calcium, phosphorus, chlorine, and sodium. Iron, copper, and manganese are found in only trace amounts, and, since these elements are required for normal red blood cell synthesis, infants fed too long on milk alone become anemic. Minute amounts of zinc, magnesium, aluminum, iodine, chromium, selenium, and fluoride are also found in breast milk. Infants who are not provided with fluoridated water in addition to breast milk may benefit from a daily oral fluoride supplement of regulated dosage predetermined by the physician or pharmacist. Providing the lactating woman with a fluoride supplement does not significantly alter her milk output of fluoride (fig. 6-7).

Varying mineral composition. The total mineral content of human milk is fairly constant, but the specific amounts of individual minerals may vary with the status of the mother and the stage of lactation. Observations from a number of laboratories have shown declining concentrations of several minerals over the weeks and months following the onset of lactation (fig. 6-8). Of substantial interest are other reports in which the dietary intake and supplementation habits of mothers have been compared with the mineral composition of their milk. In most situations, little relationship has been found between maternal mineral intake and mineral content of milk. However, since the adequacy of maternal intake of some minerals has been questioned, this may place the mother at risk.

Iron and zinc bioavailability. Some minerals are more easily absorbed from breast milk than from cow's milk or commercial formulas. McMillan and others reported that nearly 50% of the iron in human milk is absorbed, whereas availability of iron from cow's milk and iron-fortified formulas is only 10% and 4%, respectively[13,14] More recently, Garry and associates found that iron absorption from human milk may be much higher than 50% during the first three months of life.[15] An explanation for this improved absorption has not been found.

Whether or not breast-fed infants should receive iron supplements is still the subject of much debate.[1,16] Several studies suggest that infants who are breast-fed during the first six months of life and receive little or no dietary iron other than that in human milk appear to be iron sufficient at age six months. However, based on changes in total body iron deter-

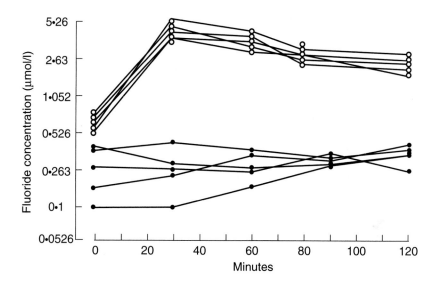

FIG. 6-7   Plasma *(open symbols)* and breast milk *(closed symbols)* fluoride concentrations in mothers after oral dose of 1.5 mg fluoride as sodium fluoride solution (conversion: fluoride − 1 mol/L ≈ 19 ng/ml).

From Ekstrand, J. 1981. No evidence of transfer of fluoride from plasma to breast milk. *Br Med J* 283:761.

mined by body weights and hemoglobin and Ferritin concentrations, others have concluded that some nonsupplemented breast-fed infants are in negative iron balance between ages three and six months. One might suggest that human milk alone cannot provide sufficient iron for optimum infant nutrition after five or six months of life.

Like that of iron, the **bioavailability** of zinc is substantially better from human milk than from alternative preparations.[17] In one study, the bioavailability of zinc fed to rats in various milk solutions was 59.2% for human milk, 42% for cow's milk, and 26.8–39% for commercial formulas. In other work, human subjects demonstrated better absorption of zinc from human milk than from cow's milk or selected infant formulas (fig. 6-9). An explanation for the better absorption of zinc from human milk is still being sought. It has been suggested, however, that the unique distribution and binding of zinc, and some other elements, to high and low molecular weight fractions of milk very likely are related to the differences in bioavailability that have now been demonstrated by a number of investigators.

Calcium.   The calcium content of human milk is low when compared with that of cow's milk. This low level is maintained no matter what the maternal diet contains. However, since the only storage site for calcium is found in the bones, one might suspect that maternal bone loss would occur if dietary calcium were low during lactation. Research into calcium homeostasis and bone dynamics during lactation has been active during the past decade. To date, it appears that bone loss occurs during lactation but that bone is renewed after weaning. Adaptation in the maternal hormonal pattern may allow for overall maintenance of bone health in the face of marginal calcium intake.[18–23]

Fat-Soluble Vitamins

General vitamin content.   All the vitamins, both fat- and water-soluble, required for good nutrition and health are supplied in breast milk, but the amounts vary markedly from one person to another. The major factor influencing the vitamin content of human milk is the mother's vitamin status. In general, when maternal intakes of a vitamin are chronically low, the levels of that vitamin in human milk are also low. As maternal intakes of the vitamin increase, levels in milk also increase. For many vitamins, however, a plateau develops that is not exceeded in the face of further augmentation in vitamin intake through diet or supplement. As a general rule, milk concentrations of water-soluble vitamins are more responsive to maternal dietary intake than are the concentrations of fat-soluble vitamins.

Bioavailability

Amount of a nutrient ingested in food that is absorbed and thus available to the body for metabolic use.

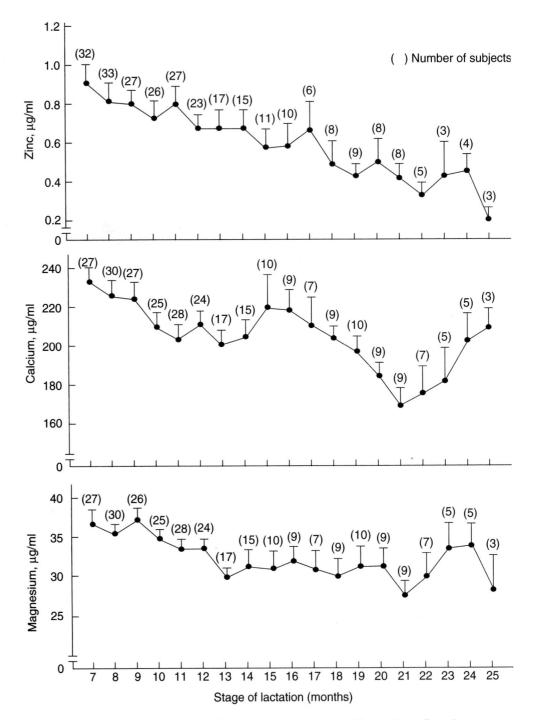

FIG. 6-8 Concentrations of zinc, calcium, and magnesium in milk samples collected at a morning feeding from seven to twenty-five months of lactation. *Vertical bars* represent SEM. Based on data from Karra, M.V., et al., 1986. *Am J Clin Nutr* 43:495.

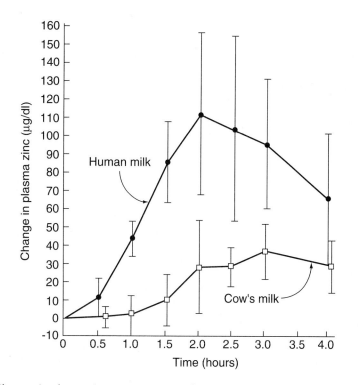

FIG. 6-9   Changes in plasma zinc concentration after ingestion of 25 mg of zinc with human milk (five subjects) and cow's milk (seven subjects). Points represent means ± SD variation from baseline value.

From Casey, C.E., P.A. Walravens, and K.M. Hambidge. 1981. Availability of zinc: Loading tests with human milk, cow's milk, and infant formulas. *Pediatrics* 68:394.

Vitamin D.   The amount of biologically active vitamin D in human milk has been found to be low (0.5 to 1.5 μg/L). However, maternal sunshine exposure and dietary intake affect infant vitamin D status through their effects on breast milk vitamin D content. This is supported by the finding that a short course of oral vitamin D (60 μg/day) supplementation or exposure to ultraviolet phototherapy quickly raised the levels of **antirachitic** (vitamin D) sterols in the plasma and milk of lactating women.[24] There was a peak effect in one week with oral vitamin D supplementation and two to three days after ultraviolet irradiation. The levels then rapidly returned to baseline. Other reports show a direct relationship between maternal and infant levels of 25-hydroxyvitamin D, implying that maternal vitamin D intake directly affects the vitamin D concentration in breast milk.

A question remains regarding the need for vitamin D supplementation in the term infant who is exclusively breast-fed. Although some clinicians do not believe it is necessary, the bulk of data support the practice. Greer and associates found low serum 25-hydroxyvitamin D concentrations and early decreases in bone mineral content in breast-fed infants not receiving supplemental vitamin D.[25,26] Ozsoylu and Hasanoglu reported low serum 25-hydroxyvitamin D levels at one month of age in breast-fed infants not supplemented with vitamin D.[27] In some of the sunniest parts of the world, such as the Middle East, rickets is common in certain breast-fed infants because cultural practices keep the babies well clothed and indoors for the first year.[28] Even in the United States, reports of resurgence in rickets among breast-fed infants provoke considerable concern.[29–32] Since no harm is associated with vitamin D supplementation at 10 μg/day and since expense and inconvenience are trivial, support of this practice seems justifiable. For light-skinned suburban populations in sunny regions and seasons, one may worry less about compliance with this recommendation.

Antirachitic
(Gr *anti-*, against; *rachitis*, a spinal disorder) Agent that is therapeutically effective against rickets, a nutritional deficiency disease affecting childhood bone development in which vitamin D is lacking.

Vitamin A. Milk is a good source of vitamin A and its precursors. Its concentration in human milk is influenced by the quality and quantity of the dietary elements consumed by the mother. The vitamin A content of breast milk is reportedly much lower in some developing countries than in the West. Maternal serum vitamin A levels in these same regions are also typically low. Vitamin A or carotene intake of some Western mothers is higher in the spring and summer months because of greater supplies of green leafy and yellow vegetables. Modern methods of preservation, however, have extended the length of seasons for many vegetables and fruits, so that dietary differences from season to season may be minimal for many women with access to supermarkets, home freezers, and other such luxuries of modern society.

Vitamin E. Levels of vitamin E in human milk are substantially greater than those in cow's milk. As might be expected, serum levels of vitamin E rise quickly in breast-fed infants and are maintained at normal levels without much fluctuation. Cow's milk–fed babies demonstrate depressed circulating levels of vitamin E unless supplemented. Fortunately, manufacturers of infant formulas have increased their levels of vitamin E fortification to avoid potential deficiency.

Vitamin K. In mature human milk, vitamin K is present at a level of 2 µg/L. Cow's milk contains much more than this amount, with a typical reported value of 60 µg/L. Vitamin K is produced by the intestinal flora, but it takes several days for the sterile infant gut to establish an effective microbe population. Even then, onset of hemorrhagic disease with bleeding as late as four weeks after delivery has been associated with breast-feeding if no vitamin K had been given at birth. It is recommended, therefore, that all newborn infants receive vitamin K.

Water-Soluble Vitamins

Effect of maternal intake. The levels of water-soluble vitamins in human milk are more likely to reflect maternal diet or supplement intake more than most other ingested compounds. Maternal dietary supplements with most of these vitamins have been shown to increase their content in breast milk. This is especially true in women whose dietary patterns or nutritional status are suboptimum. It appears that with some of these vitamins a plateau may be reached where increased intake has no further impact on milk composition. This idea was demonstrated when varying levels of supplemental ascorbic acid were provided to lactating women.[33] With comparable diets, women consuming either 90 mg or 250 mg per day of ascorbic acid produced milk with similar concentration of this vitamin. Women taking 1,000 mg of ascorbic acid per day produced milk that was only slightly higher in its ascorbic acid content.

Vitamin B_6. Felice and Kirksey have provided evidence that milk concentration of vitamin B_6 may be a sensitive indicator of vitamin B_6 status of the mother.[34] They further suggest that the majority of lactating women produce milk with a vitamin B_6 content that is substantially less than that recommended for good health and growth of infants. These researchers observed that mothers receiving 2.5 mg/day of supplemental vitamin B_6 failed to supply their breast-feeding infants with 0.3 mg of vitamin B_6 per day, which is the RDA for young infants.[35]

Vitamin B_{12}. The vitamin B_{12} content of human milk has been found to range from 0.33 to 3.2 ng/ml (mean 0.97 ng/ml), and ingestion of supplemental B_{12} does not significantly affect milk content.[36] Human milk from well-fed mothers was found to contain adequate amounts of B_{12}. Its bioavailability, however, depends on the sufficiency of **proteolytic enzymes** to release it from its bound form. Infantile neurologic disorders related to vitamin B_{12} deficiency have been reported in breast-fed infants of strictly vegetarian women.[37,38]

Resistance Factors

A thorough discussion of the composition of breast milk must include mention of the beneficial components of human milk that are not classified as nutrients (table 6-6).

Bifidus factor. One of the earliest resistance factors to be described in human milk was the bifidus factor, which may be a nitrogen-containing polysaccharide that favors the growth of *Lactobacillus bifidus*. Its uniqueness to human milk has been confirmed.[39] *L. bifidus* confers a protective effect against invasive enteropathogenic organisms.

Nanogram (ng)
(Gr *nano-,* dwarf) One billionth gram; also called millimicrogram.
Proteolytic enzymes
(Gr *protos,* first; *lysis,* dissolution) Series of enzymes that progressively split proteins, large molecular compounds, into their respective individual amino acids.
Lactobacillus bifidus
(L *bifidus*) Predominant fermentative lactobacillus in the intestinal flora of breast-fed infants.

CASE STUDY

Vitamin K Deficiency in Breast-fed Infants

Case 1

A five-week-old infant had seizures and apnea following twenty-four hours of increasing irritability and poor eating. Birth weight was 3.9 kg following a forty-two-week uncomplicated pregnancy; a self-trained midwife assisted at the home delivery. Neither vitamin K nor prophylaxis for eye infection was given. *Jaundice* was treated with a "grow light" and supplements of vitamins A and E. The infant was breast-fed; there was no history of illness or trauma. His mother took no medications, ate a regular diet, and took vitamin supplements.

On physical examination, jaundice, a bulging fontanelle, right-sided seizures, and a discharge from the left eye were observed. Weight was 4.6 kg (75th percentile); length, 53 cm (25th percentile); and head circumference, 38.5 cm (75th percentile). Persistent bleeding was noted following **venipuncture** and **intubation.** Cerebrospinal fluid was grossly bloody. Laboratory results were consistent with internal bleeding; **prothrombin time (PT)** and **partial thromboplastin time (PTT)** were greater than 200 seconds. A **subdural hematoma,** with obliteration of the right ventricle, was shown by **computed tomography** of the head.

Treatment consisted of 5 mg phytonadione (vitamin K), antibiotics, plasma, and phenobarbital salt. Laboratory studies, repeated following transfer to a hospital, showed significant decreases in clotting time indexes; PT and PTT were reduced to 11.6/11.6 (subject/control) and 35.4 seconds, respectively.

Case 2

A four-week-old, breast-fed infant was seen following three days of vomiting. She was treated with 250 ml of normal saline in each thigh. When needles were removed, bleeding was noted at the injection site. Tests on hospitalization showed indexes consistent with hemorrhaging, including a PT of 37.4/11.8 (patient/control) and a PTT of 107.5 seconds. Blood factors VII and X were both significantly decreased. Treatment began with 2 mg phytonadione; bleeding ceased within one hour of vitamin K administration and before the fresh frozen plasma had been infused. Repeat studies showed normalization of both clotting times and blood factors.

The patient had been born at home after an uncomplicated gestation to a gravida 5, para 4 mother. She received no vitamin K or prophylaxis for eye infection at birth. Her mother ate a regular diet and took vitamin supplements; penicillin had been taken for a possible uterine infection for two weeks following delivery.

Questions for Analysis
1. Describe why a newborn breast-fed baby needs to be given vitamin K.
2. Why can't vitamin K be given to the mother during the third trimester for protection of the newborn?

Venipuncture
A technique in which a vein is punctured through the skin by a sharp, rigid stylet or cannula carrying a flexible plastic catheter or by a steel needle attached to a syringe or catheter.

Intubation
Passage of a tube into a body hole—specifically, the insertion of a breathing tube through the mouth or nose or into the trachea to ensure a patent airway for the delivery of an anesthetic gas or oxygen.

Prothrombin time (PT)
A method of detecting specific coagulation defects.

Partial thromboplastin time (PTT)
A more specific way of detecting coagulation defects than PT.

Subdural hematoma
A collection of blood trapped under the outside layers of the skull, usually resulting from trauma.

Computed tomography
An x-ray technique that produces a film representing a detailed cross-section of tissue structure.

Immunoglobulins. Various **immunoglobulins** are present in human milk, including IgA, IgG, IgD, and IgE. Although IgG appears to migrate from maternal serum into milk, evidence suggests that IgA, IgD, and IgE are produced locally in mammary tissue. A variety of studies support the idea of the migration of **lymphoblasts** from maternal gut-associated lymphoid tissue to the mammary glands followed by local production of immunoglobulins at this site and secretion of them into the milk. This mechanism allows maternal lymphoblasts to obtain antigenic exposure from distant sites and to carry this experience to the mammary tissue, where synthesis of appropriate antibodies can occur for protection of the suckling infant.

Secretory IgA (sIgA) is the predominant immunoglobulin in human milk. It is found in large amounts in colostrum and in smaller, but still significant, levels in ma-

Immunoglobulins
Special components of the body's immune system, proteins synthesized by lymphocytes and plasm cells that have specific antibody activity.

Lymphoblasts
The immature stage of the mature lymphocyte.

TABLE 6-6   *Antiinfectious Factors in Human Milk*

Factors	Functions
Bifidus factor	Stimulates growth of bifidobacteria, which antagonizes the survival of enterobacteria
Secretory IgA (sIgA), IgM, IgE, IgD, and IgG	Act against bacterial invasion of the mucosa and/or colonization of the gut (show bacterial and viral neutralizing capacity; activate alternative complement pathway)
Antistaphylococcus factor	Inhibits systemic staphylococcal infection
Lactoferrin	Binds iron and inhibits bacterial multiplication
Lactoperoxidase	Kills streptococci and enteric bacteria
Complement (C_3, C_1)	Promotes opsonization (the rendering of bacteria and other cells susceptible to phagocytosis)
Interferon	Inhibits intracellular viral replication
Lysozyme	Lyses bacteria through destruction of the cell wall
B_{12}-binding protein	Renders vitamin B_{12} unavailable for bacterial growth
Lymphocytes	Synthesize secretory IgA; may have other roles
Macrophages	Synthesize complement, lactoferrin, lysozyme, and other factors; carry out phagocytosis and probably other functions

Lactoferrin
(L *lac,* milk; *ferrum,* iron) An iron-binding protein found in human milk.

Candida albicans
(L *candidus,* glowing, white) Most frequent agent of *candidiasis,* a yeast-like fungus infecting moist tissue areas of the body, involving skin, vagina, and oral mucosa.

Lactoperoxidase
An enzyme found in human milk that catalyzes the oxidation of organic substrate, including harmful microorganisms, thereby protecting the infant.

Prostaglandins
Potent hormone-like unsaturated fatty acids that act in extremely low concentrations on local target organs.

Lymphocytes
Mature leukocytes, special lymphoid white blood cells, T cells and B cells, forming major components of the body's immune system; also found in human milk.

Macrophages
(Fr *makros,* large; *phagein,* to eat) Large phagocytes, cells of the immune system that engulf and consume microorganisms, other cells, and foreign particles and that interact with T cells and B cells to produce inflammatory process and antibodies.

Complement
Series of enzymatic serum proteins that interact with an antigen-antibody complex to promote phagocyte activity and destroy other cells.

ture breast milk. Secretory immunoglobulins have been shown to be a major host resistance factor against organisms that infect the gastrointestinal tract—in particular, *E. coli* and the enteroviruses. Also, a protective effect against other organisms has been demonstrated. Human milk clearly exhibits a prophylactic effect against septicemia of the newborn.

Other host resistance factors. Some of the other host resistance factors in breast milk are also worthy of mention. Lysozyme, an antimicrobial enzyme, occurs in breast milk at 300 times the concentration found in cow's milk. **Lactoferrin** has been described as a compound with a "monilia-static" effect against *Candida albicans.* It inhibits the growth of staphylococci and *E. coli* by binding iron, which the bacteria require to proliferate. **Lactoperoxidase,** which has been shown in vitro to act with other substances in combatting streptococci, is also found in human milk. Specific **prostaglandins** have also been defined, and these may protect the integrity of the gastrointestinal tract epithelium against noxious substances.[40]

Lymphocyte-macrophage activities. Of additional interest is the discovery that the **lymphocytes** in human milk produce the antiviral substance interferon. **Macrophages** are also found in colostrum and mature milk; 21,000/mm reportedly are present in a typical colostrum specimen. Macrophages are motile and phagocytic and have been shown to produce **complement,** lactoferrin, lysozyme, and other factors. The full role of the macrophages is still under investigation, but they undoubtedly have a protective function, both within the mammary lacteals and subsequently within the baby. A number of investigators have studied the activities of lymphocytes in human milk. Milk samples from lactating mothers have been collected at various times postpartum and examined for cell types present and in vitro activities of the various identified cells. The greatest number of cells appear in colostrum, with numbers dropping significantly during the following eight weeks.

Effect of maternal malnutrition. As one might expect, maternal malnutrition adversely affects not only the nutritional composition of human milk but also its content of immunologic substances. Observations of malnourished Columbian women showed that colostrum contained only one-third the normal concentration of IgG and less than half the normal level of albumin. Significant reductions in colostrum levels of IgA and the fourth component of complement (C_4) were also observed.[41] These differences tended to disappear in mature milk, accompanied by improvement in the nutritional status of the malnourished mothers during the first several weeks postpartum. Therefore, the protec-

TABLE 6-7   *Drugs That Are Contraindicated During Breastfeeding*

Drugs	Reported Signs or Symptoms in Infant or Effects on Lactation
Amphetamine	Irritability, poor sleep pattern
Bromocriptine	Lactation suppression
Cocaine	Cocaine intoxication
Cyclophosphamide	Possible immunosuppression; unknown effect on growth or association with carcinogenesis; neutropenia
Cyclosporine	Possible immunosuppression; unknown effect on growth or association with carcinogenesis
Doxorubicin*	Possible immunosuppression: unknown effect on growth or association with carcinogenesis
Ergotamine	Vomiting, diarrhea, convulsions (doses used in migraine medications)
Heroin	Tremors, restlessness, vomiting, poor feeding
Lithium	⅓ to ½ therapeutic blood concentration in infants
Marijuana	Only one report in literature: no effect mentioned
Methotrexate	Possible immunosuppression: unknown effect on growth or association with carcinogenesis, neutropenia
Nicotine (smoking)	Shock, vomiting, diarrhea, rapid heart rate, restlessness; decreased milk production
Phencyclidine (PCP)	Hallucinations
Phenindione	Anticoagulant; increased prothrombin and partial thromboplastin time in one infant (not used in United States)

*Drug is concentrated in human milk.
From American Academy of Pediatrics, Committee on Drugs. 1994. The transfer of drugs and other chemicals into human breast milk. *Pediatrics* 93:137.

tive qualities of colostrum and milk may be significantly influenced by maternal nutritional status.

Contaminants

The lactating woman is often exposed to a variety of nonnutritional substances that may be transferred to her milk. Such substances include drugs, environmental pollutants, viruses, caffeine, alcohol, and food allergens. Although moderate amounts of many of these agents are believed to pose no risk to nursing infants, some substances provoke concern because of known or suspected adverse reactions.

Drugs. Much research has focused on the release of drugs into the milk of lactating women. Whether the mother drinks it, eats it, sniffs it, inserts it as an anal or a vaginal suppository, or injects it, some level of the active agents in the drug enters the maternal tissues and blood and finally migrates to the breast milk. The difference in method of administration determines the amount of drug that finally enters the blood and the speed with which it reaches the capillaries of the breast. In general, the amount of a drug excreted in milk is not more than 1–2% of the maternal dose. Although concern exists about the amount of a given drug in the breast milk, of greater concern is the amount that actually reaches the infant's bloodstream. Unfortunately, there is no accurate way to measure this, because other factors also affect the level in the infant's bloodstream. The tolerance of the chemical to the pH of the stomach and the enzymatic activity of the intestinal tract is significant. The volume of milk consumed by the infant is a factor as well.

Some drugs appear in human milk in sufficient quantities to be harmful to the infant (table 6-7).[42] Sedatives used to relieve tension may produce drowsiness in the baby as well as the mother. Lithium and reserpine produce a bluish tint to the skin, along with other disorders. Valium residuals in mother's milk induce lethargy in breast-fed babies. Lithium carbonate, a drug prescribed for relief of manic depression, may induce lowered body temperature, loss of muscle tone, and bluish skin in the nursing infant. Both cyclophosphamide

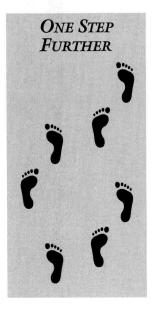

ONE STEP FURTHER

Barriers to Postpartum Treatment for Drug and Alcohol Addiction

- Negative attitudes toward this population may generate resistance to treating the women.
- The trend toward legal intervention in the pregnancies of women with alcohol and other drug problems discourages many from seeking care. Women fear criminal prosecution or loss of their children to foster care.
- Nationwide, substance-abuse treatment services are insufficient and inadequate to meet the needs of pregnant women and women who need child care while they are in treatment.
- Cultural insensitivity exists in treatment programs.
- Transportation to treatment is lacking or difficult to arrange.
- There is a lack of residential programs that accept women and their children.
- There are long intervals between locating and being admitted to a program.
- Community outreach providing information about programs is not available.
- Alcohol and other drug problems often are not diagnosed because physicians and other clinicians lack adequate training in the identification of substance abuse and the consequences of drug use during pregnancy.

and methotrexate cause bone marrow depression when ingested by infants. A variety of disorders follow intake by infants of breast milk contaminated with antimicrobial agents. Penicillin in breast milk may produce an allergic reaction in a sensitive infant. Other antibiotics may produce similar reactions, as well as sleepiness, vomiting, and refusal to eat. Radioactive thyroid medications may damage the thyroid gland. Bowel problems in infants may result from maternal consumption of some laxatives, such as anthraquinone, aloes, cascara, emodin, and rheum (rhubarb). Safe laxatives include magnesia, castor oil, mineral oil, bisacodyl (Ducolax), senna phenophthalein or nonprescription Ex-Lax, and fecal softeners. Heroin or the painkiller dextropropoxyphene (Darvon) can lead to infant addiction. Treatment of the heroin-addicted mother with methadone is problematic, since one infant death has been reported during maternal methadone therapy.

If a mother needs a specific medication and the hazards to the infant are believed to be minimal, the following important adjustments can be made to minimize the effects.

1. *Action time.* Do not use the long-acting form of the drug, because the infant has even more difficulty in excreting the agent, which usually requires detoxification in the liver. Accumulation in the infant is then a genuine concern.
2. *Dose schedule.* Schedule the doses so the least amount of the drug gets into the milk. Given the usual absorption rates and peak blood levels of most drugs, having the mother take the medication immediately after breast-feeding is the safest time for the infant.
3. *Observations.* Watch the infant for any unusual signs or symptoms, such as change in feeding pattern or sleeping habits, fussiness, or rash.
4. *Drug amount in milk.* When possible, choose the drug that produces the least amount in the milk.

One of the best sources of information on drugs in relation to human milk and infant health is the family pharmacist. It is also wise to read the product label to evaluate product composition and precautionary statements. Effective December 26, 1979, all drug manufacturers in the United States are required to provide relevant information on the labels of new drugs developed and marketed since that date. Whatever is known about excretion of the drug into milk and whatever is known of the effect on the infant are indicated on the label. If nothing is known, the label must state that fact. In such a case, and in all use of drugs, the prudent mother will exercise due caution.

Environmental contaminants. The current concern over pesticide residues, industrial wastes, and other environmental contaminants is not without cause. Many of these compounds have accidentally contaminated food and water supplies around the world. In general, the chemical contaminants that appear in breast milk have high lipid solubility, re-

TABLE 6-8   *"Typical" Levels, FDA Action Levels, Allowable Daily Intake, and Calculated Daily Intake of Representative Breast-fed Infants*

Substances	Typical Levels* (ppb)	FDA Action Levels for Cow's Milk† (ppb)	Allowable Daily Intake (μg/kg)	Daily Intake of Breast-fed Infants‡ (μg/kg)
Dieldrin	1-6	7.5	0.1	0.8
Heptachlor epoxide	8-30	7.5	0.5	4
PCBs	40-100	62.5	1	14
DDT (including metabolites)	50-200	50	5	28

Modified from Rogan, W.J., A. Bagniewska, and T. Damstra. 1980. *N Engl J Med* 302:1450. Pollutants in breast milk.

*Levels considered typical in whole milk in the United States

†Assuming 2.5% fat. FDA action levels represent the limit at or above which the FDA will take legal action against a product to remove it from the market.

‡Intake of a 5 kg infant drinking 700 ml of milk per day; levels are based on high values given under typical levels.

sistance to physical degradation or biologic metabolism, wide distribution in the environment, and slow or absent excretion rates. Of greatest concern among such chemicals are the **organohalides,** such as polychlorinated biphenyls (PCBs) and dichlorodiphenyl trichloroethane (DDT).[43] Long-term low-level exposure to the organohalides results in a gradual accumulation of residues in fat, including the fat of breast milk. Lactation is the only way in which large amounts of such residues can be excreted.

Savage and associates conducted a study of environmental contaminants that focused on levels of chlorinated hydrocarbon insecticide residues in nearly 1,500 human milk samples around the United States.[44] Most of the samples showed low but detectable levels of most of these insecticides or their metabolites, but significant differences were found among the five geographic regions. The southeastern United States had the highest mean residue levels, whereas the Northwest had the lowest levels. Although nursing infants around the United States would generally receive low levels of some of these residues, a small number could be exposed to fairly high amounts.

It is clear that human milk is a variable source of contaminants, but it is difficult to define a "safe" level of exposure to these compounds. However, both the World Health Organization and the U.S. Food and Drug Administration have set "regulatory," or "allowable," levels for daily intake of several organohalides (table 6-8). These standards provide a large margin of safety, so the fact that a given infant exceeds the level does not mean that such exposure is toxic. Much remains to be learned about the chemical contamination of human milk. Meanwhile, it is heartening to know that very few cases of illness caused by transmission of environmental chemicals through breast milk have appeared.[45]

Heavy metals. Lead and mercury, both heavy metals, are transferred placentally to the fetus and to the infant via maternal milk. Rat studies have shown that lactation increases lead absorption from the gut, which leads ultimately to an increased level of lead excretion via the milk. The exact mechanism for this phenomenon is not known. However, lactose may play a dominant role, since it is known to facilitate the absorption of calcium, other trace elements, and lead.

Nicotine. Nicotine enters human milk and can cause nicotine "poisoning" of the breast-fed infant. Infants three to four days of age whose mothers smoked six to sixteen cigarettes a day were reported to refuse to suckle, become apathetic, vomit, and retain urine and feces. In a chain-smoking mother, the nicotine content of milk may reach 75 μg/L. In the case of mothers who smoke very little, it is likely that the amount of nicotine the infant would get from breathing cigarette smoke in the immediate environment would be more significant than that obtained from milk. The long-term impact of such exposure is unknown.[1]

Organohalides
(Gr *organon*, organ; Chem *halides*, compounds of fluorine, chlorine, bromine, or iodine) Chemical compounds used as pesticides or in industrial processes—e.g., DDT and PCBs.

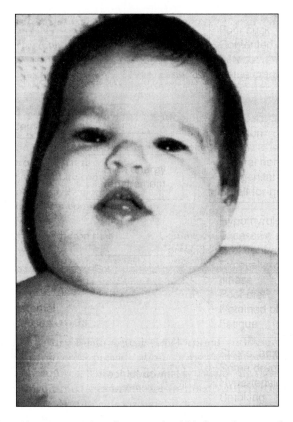

FIG. 6-10 Cushingoid appearance in a four-month-old infant whose mother consumed at least fifty cans of beer weekly plus generous portions of other, more concentrated alcoholic beverages.

From Binkiewiez, A., M.J. Robinson, and B. Senior. 1978. Pseudo-Cushing syndrome caused by alcohol in breast milk. *J Pediatr* 93:965.

Caffeine. Caffeine passes from the maternal bloodstream into breast milk. Although a small dose of caffeine comparable to that obtained from a cup of coffee is transported at low levels from the mother to her milk (1%), caffeine reaches the infant, where it can accumulate over time.[46] Wakeful, hyperactive infants sometimes are victims of caffeine stimulation. A mother who drinks more than six to eight cups of any caffeine-containing beverage in a day's time might expect her infant to demonstrate "coffee nerves." Such an infant does not require hospitalization, and verification of blood caffeine levels is not mandatory, although it might be helpful. An elimination trial should suffice to evaluate the role of maternal caffeine ingestion, and subsequent elimination, on infant behavior.

Alcohol. Beverage alcohol also passes from the mother's bloodstream into her breast milk. **Ethanol** has been shown to reach human milk in a similar concentration to that in maternal blood. Interestingly, however, the major breakdown product of ethanol, acetaldehyde, does not appear in human milk, even though significant amounts may have been measured in maternal blood.

The role of the mammary gland in eliminating acetaldehyde may be similar to that of the placenta. If human milk contains large amounts of ethanol, the nursing infant may develop a pseudo-**Cushing's syndrome,** as described (fig 6-10) by Binkiewica, Robinaon, and Senior.[47] The four-month-old infant they describe was breast-fed by a mother who consumed at least fifty 12-oz cans of beer weekly, plus generous amounts of other, more concentrated alcoholic drinks. When the mother stopped drinking but continued to nurse, the infant's growth rate promptly increased, and her appearance gradually returned to normal. The mother also noted that the infant did not sleep as much as she did before.

Observations of lactating women consuming various levels of alcohol suggest that regular consumption of several drinks per day is associated with delayed psychomotor development at one year of age.[48] Whether this adverse result indicates permanent damage is

Ethanol
Chemical name for beverage alcohol.

Cushing's syndrome
Condition first described by Boston surgeon Harvey Cushing (1869–1939), due to hypersecretion of adrenal corticotropic hormone (ACTH) or excessive intake of glucocorticoids, with rapidly developing fat deposits of face, neck, and trunk, giving a characteristic cushing–old "moon face" appearance.

SMOKING DURING PREGNANCY AND LACTATION AND ITS EFFECTS ON BREAST MILK VOLUME

Ten smoking and ten nonsmoking mothers were studied with regard to volume of milk production and growth of their infants. The nonsmoking mothers had significantly greater breast milk production (961 g per day) than the smoking mothers (693 g per day). The babies of the smoking mothers showed significantly reduced rates of growth. These results indicate that cigarette smoking has a negative influence on breast milk volume; the lower growth rates of the infants of the smokers suggest also that the smokers' breast milk output was insufficient to support the energy requirements of their infants.

Recommendations About Breastfeeding When Carrying the AIDS Virus

- *Centers for Disease Control and Prevention (CDC) (United States).* Infected women should be advised against breast-feeding to avoid postnatal transmission to a child who may not be infected.
- *World Health Organization (WHO).* This group contends that there is insufficient evidence to conclude that breast-feeding is an *important* mode of HIV transmission. It is noted that breast-feeding is of special importance in the Third World, where safe, effective substitutes are not accessible to most women. It also notes that more uninfected than infected breast-fed babies of HIV-positive mothers have been reported. It also points out that women who become infected via postpartum transfusions seem to be a special subset of infected mothers; the more common situation seems to involve women who are infected before or during pregnancy. WHO therefore recommends continued promotion, support, and protection of breast-feeding in both developed and developing countries and in the case of women known to be HIV-infected, that careful consideration be given to the availability of safe, effective use of alternatives before advising against breast-feeding.

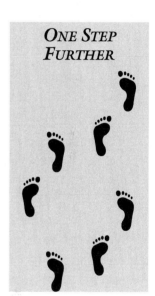

ONE STEP FURTHER

---

unknown. Until more information is available, lactating women are well advised to limit their consumption of alcoholic beverages.

The AIDS virus. Evidence suggests that the AIDS virus can be transmitted from mother to infant through breast milk. This finding has provoked much concern from the standpoint of providing appropriate advice about infant feeding to high-risk women. Should one encourage or discourage breast-feeding for such women? The current thinking in the United States is that breast-feeding should be discouraged when a woman is known to carry this virus. The World Health Organization, however, supports the concept that infants in many developing countries run greater risks of dying of diarrheal disease if they are not breast-fed than of developing AIDS from the breast milk exposure (see the box on p. 157). Debate on this issue continues around the world. In the meantime, breast milk banks are taking special precautions to screen out donors who potentially could contribute virus-contaminated specimens. Samples are also pasteurized sufficiently to destroy viruses that might be present.[49–52]

DIET FOR THE NURSING MOTHER ≈

General Recommendations

The optimal diet for the lactating woman should be one that supplies somewhat more of each nutrient than that recommended for the nonpregnant female (table 6-9). Obviously, the needs of specific women relate directly to the volume of milk they produce daily. The self-selected diets of lactating women often fail to meet dietary recommendations.[53]

CASE STUDY

Aids and Breast Milk

In 1986, Ziegler et al. reported a case in which a newborn infant apparently contracted the acquired immunodeficiency syndrome (AIDS) virus through breast milk from his mother. The child was delivered by cesarean section, and the mother contracted the AIDS virus after a blood transfusion given in conjunction with her cesarean section. In this case, the blood transfusion was given after delivery, and the baby was breast-fed for six weeks. Thirteen months later, AIDS developed in the donor of one of the units of blood used for the transfusion, resulting in testing of the mother and the child. Both the mother and the child were found to be positive for the virus. The mother had AIDS-related complex. The baby had a transient episode of failure to thrive and then developed lymphadenopathy and eczema but was otherwise well. The spouse and siblings were seronegative.

A subsequent study conducted in Kigali, Rwanda, involved observation of 212 mother-infant pairs who were negative for human immunodeficiency virus Type I (HIV-1) at delivery. All of the infants were breast-fed. The mothers were followed for 3 months; those who became positive for HIV-1 were compared with those who did not; comparisons were completed after 16.6 months of further evaluation. Results indicated that HIV-1 infection can be transmitted from mother to infant during the postnatal period. Colostrum and breast milk were considered to be efficient routes for the transmission of HIV-1 from recently infected mothers to their infants.

Questions for Analysis
1. In the United States, what advice should be given to an HIV-positive woman who wishes to breast feed?
2. How might this advice be different if you are talking with a similar woman in underdeveloped parts of the world?

From Wasserberger, J., Ordog, G.J. and J.J. Stroh. 1986. AIDS in breast milk. *JAMA* 255:464; and Van de Perre, P. et al. 1991. Postnatal transmission of human immunodeficiency virus Type I from mother to infant. *N Engl J Med* 325:593.

Energy

Prenatal storage. During pregnancy, most women store approximately 2 to 4 kg of body fat, which can be mobilized to supply a portion of the additional energy for lactation. It is estimated that stored fat provides 200 to 300 kcal per day during a lactation period of three months. This amount of energy represents only part of the energy needed to produce milk. The remainder of the energy needs should derive from the daily diet the first three months of lactation. During this time, lactation can be successfully supported and readjustment of maternal fat stores can take place. If lactation continues beyond the initial three months or if maternal weight falls below the ideal weight for height, the daily extra energy allowance may need to be increased accordingly. If more than one infant is being nursed during the first few months of life, maternal kilocalorie stores will be more quickly used, and daily supplemental energy needs may double when maternal stores are depleted.

Efficiency of milk production. The efficiency of milk production has been estimated by several researchers by the observation of energy intake and energy utilization of breast-feeding and nonbreast-feeding mothers. English and Hitchcock compared the energy intake of sixteen nursing mothers and ten nonnursing mothers and found that the energy intake of the breast-feeders in the sixth and eighth postpartum week was 2,460 kcal/day.[54]

TABLE 6-9   *Recommended Daily Dietary Allowances for Lactation*

	First Six Months	Second Six Months
Energy (kcal)	+500.0	+500.0
Protein (g)	65.0	62.0
Vitamin A (RE*)	1,300.0	1,200.0
Vitamin D (μg)	10.0	10.0
Vitamin E activity (mg αTE)†	12.0	11.0
Ascorbic acid (mg)	95.0	90.0
Folacin (μg)	280.0	260.0
Niacin (mg‡)	20.0	20.0
Riboflavin (mg)	1.8	1.7
Thiamin (mg)	1.6	1.6
Vitamin B_6 (mg)	2.1	2.1
Vitamin B_{12} (μg)	2.6	2.6
Calcium (mg)	1,200.0	1,200.0
Phosphorus (mg)	1,200.0	1,200.0
Iodine (μg)	200.0	200.0
Iron (mg)	15.0	15.0
Magnesium (mg)	355.0	340.0
Zinc (mg)	19.0	16.0

Modified from Food and Nutrition Board, National Research Council, National Academy of Sciences. 1989. *Recommended dietary allowances*, 10th ed. Washington, DC: U.S. Government Printing Office.

*RE, Retinol equivalents

†α-Tocopheral equivalents; 1 mg d-α-tocopheral = 1 αTE

‡Although allowances are expressed as niacin, it is recognized that, on the average, 1 mg of niacin is derived from each 60 mg of dietary tryptophan.

The energy intake of the nonnursing mothers during the same postpartum period was 1,800 kcal/day—a difference of 580 kcal. In a later study, lactating women were found to take in 2,716 kcal/day and nonnursing mothers 2,125 kcal/day—a difference of 590 kcal. By adding the assumed energy equivalents of body weight being lost, total energy available to the two groups was about 2,977 and 2,364 kcal/day, respectively. If one assumes that the energy requirements for basal metabolism and activity are equivalent for the two groups, the energy needed for daily milk production is close to 560 kcal. The production efficiency of human milk is therefore about 90%.[3]

Energy needs. Successful lactation is compatible with gradual weight reduction and attainable with energy intakes less than current recommendations (+500 kcal/day).[55] Manning-Dalton and Allen evaluated the postpartum weight loss patterns, breast-feeding completeness, and daily kilocalorie intakes of well-nourished North American women.[56] In spite of low mean kilocalorie intakes (2,178 kcal/day), breast-feeding was successful, and weight loss during the twelve to ninety days postpartum averaged only 2.0 kg for the entire sample and 1.6 kg for the solely breast-feeding women. These authors emphasize that almost every aspect of maternal energy balance in lactation needs further investigation. In the meantime, it should be recognized that the suggested intake for energy in lactation is probably higher than necessary, especially for the well-nourished woman with a sedentary lifestyle. It is also apparent that the commonly held belief that breast-feeding helps the mother lose weight cannot be substantiated.[57]

Postpartum maternal weight concerns. For many women, the usual slow rate of weight loss after childbirth may not satisfy their desires for immediate return to prepregnancy body weight. It is therefore likely that dietary restriction may be self-imposed, even though it is discouraged by health professionals. Suggested measures for improving the nutrient intake of women with restrictive eating patterns can be found in the box on p. 160. It is important to recognize that a moderate to severe restriction of caloric intake

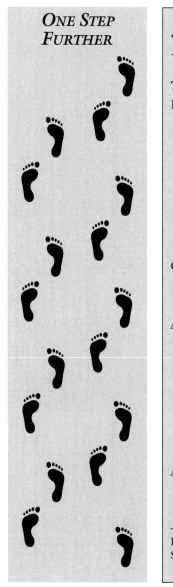

Suggested Measures for Improving the Nutrient Intake of Women with Restrictive Eating Patterns

Type of restrictive eating pattern	Corrective measures
Excessive restriction of food intake—i.e., ingestion of <1,800 kcal of energy per day, which ordinarily leads to unsatisfactory intake of nutrients compared with the amounts needed by lactating women.	Encourage increased intake of nutrient-rich foods to achieve an energy intake of at least 1,800 kcal per day; if the mother insists on curbing food intake sharply, promote substitution of foods rich in vitamins, minerals, and protein for those lower in nutritive value; in individual cases, it may be advisable to recommend a balanced multivitamin-mineral supplement; discourage use of liquid weight loss diets and appetite suppressants.
Complete vegetarianism—i.e., avoidance of all animal foods, including meat, fish, dairy products, and eggs.	Advise intake of a regular source of vitamin B_{12}, such as special vitamin B_{12}–containing plant food products or a 2.6 µg vitamin B_{12} supplement daily.
Avoidance of milk, cheese, or other calcium-rich dairy products.	Encourage increased intake of other culturally appropriate dietary calcium sources, such as collard greens for people from the southeastern United States; provide information on the appropriate use of low-lactose dairy products if milk is being avoided because of lactose intolerance; if correction by diet cannot be achieved, it may be advisable to recommend 600 mg of elemental calcium per day taken with meals.
Avoidance of vitamin D–fortified foods, such as fortified milk or cereal, combined with limited exposure to ultraviolet light.	Recommend 10 µg of supplemental vitamin D per day.

From Institute of Medicine. 1991. *Nutrition during lactation.* Washington, DC: National Academy of Sciences.

during lactation will compromise the woman's ability to synthesize milk. This is especially significant in the early weeks of lactation initiation before the process is firmly established. As a result of this effect of caloric restriction on milk production, lactating women should be advised to accept a gradual rate of weight loss in the first six months after childbirth. Otherwise, lactation success may be limited, and the infant may suffer from insufficient milk supply to meet growth needs.

Protein

Along with the recommended energy increment, a 15 to 20 g increase in daily protein intake is advised for lactating women. The extra protein is believed to be necessary to cover the requirement for milk production with an allowance of 70% efficiency of protein utilization.

The increased needs for protein, as well as energy, can be met easily by consuming three to four extra cups of milk per day. Although this will provide the needed protein and energy, it will not cover the increased recommendations for other nutrients—ascorbic acid, vitamin E, and folic acid. Thus, other foods such as citrus fruits, vegetable oils, and leafy green vegetables will also need to be added to the daily diet to supply these nutrients.

Vegetarian Diets

Maintenance of lactation while consuming a vegetarian diet can be managed well, providing all the basic principles of sensible vegetarian eating are followed carefully. The nutritional needs of the lactating vegetarian woman are the same as those of the lactating woman with a more traditional diet. Appropriate extra sources of kilocalories and protein must be clearly defined. If dairy products are acceptable in the chosen dietary regimen, extra milk can be used as indicated. If dairy products are not included in the accepted list of foods, extra energy and high-quality protein must be obtained from appropriately combined vegetables, legumes, grains, nuts, and other such food sources in larger amounts. Calcium needs can be met by eating large quantities of some green leafy vegetables (for example, kale), calcium-fortified foods, and other significant sources of vegetable calcium. Dietary supplements may be unacceptable. Thus, intelligent daily diet planning is essential for maintenance of successful lactation and health of the vegetarian mother.

Supplementation

Although lactation increases a woman's requirement for nearly all nutrients, these increased needs can be provided by a well-balanced diet as outlined. For this reason, nutritional supplements are generally unnecessary, except when there is a deficient intake of one or more nutrients. It is true, for example, if the lactating woman does not tolerate milk, calcium supplementation as well as alternative energy and protein sources are suggested to help prevent unnecessary calcium withdrawal from bones.

Cost of Nutritional Support for Lactation

The cost of providing adequate nutritional support for the lactating mother depends heavily on what foods she selects to meet her nutritional needs. Some older studies suggest that human milk costs more than bottle-feeding because of the extra nutrients the mother must consume. It is clear, however, in examining the costs of appropriate extra foods for the lactating mother that human milk is cheaper than proprietary cow's milk formulas if economical food choices are made. Beyond the price consideration, however, it is hard to justify "wastage" of human milk and the resultant unnecessary draw on the precious supply of other animal protein available to the world's population. Human milk represents a vital national resource that, if used to its fullest extent, could markedly improve not only the health and nutritional status of today's children but also the "natural resource base" of many underdeveloped countries.

Summary

Mammals produce milk for their babies through a process that demands nutritional support. However, production of high-quality milk is a high priority for the maternal organism such that her own nutritional well-being may be adversely affected in order to assure "good milk." Human milk is designed to meet the needs of a growing human infant. This is true for its nutrients as well as for its protective factors. Unfortunately, potentially harmful substances to which the mother is exposed may appear in her milk. Control of her diet and environment aids in the maintenance of a healthful milk supply and a healthy mother.

Review Questions

1. Describe the development of human mammary glands.
2. Outline the processes of milk production and let-down.
3. Compare the nutritional needs of the lactating woman with those of the normal woman of reproductive age.
4. Consider the impact that breast reduction surgery might have on lactation.
5. Define several ways in which human milk is truly unique when compared with commercial infant formulas.
6. In your community, is it appropriate to recommend that breast-fed babies receive vitamin D supplements?

LACTATION: BREAST-FEEDING IS A DESIRABLE OPTION*

Bonnie S. Worthington-Roberts

≋≋ ≋ ≋ ≋ ≋ ≋ ≋ ≋ ≋ ≋ ≋

Basic Concepts

☐ *The advantages of breast-feeding are numerous.*

☐ *Incidence of breast-feeding varies around the world and within segments of developed countries.*

☐ *Prenatal and postpartum counseling of new mothers (and their partners) aids choice making and lactation success.*

☐ *Lactating women have concerns that can be addressed.*

☐ *Lactation failure does occur but is rare.*

*T*oday's mother usually has the option to breast-feed or to provide a commercially available infant formula to her offspring. Under ideal circumstances, the mother makes her decision after learning about the advantages and disadvantages of both. The responsibility of the health care provider is to provide information about each alternative and to support the mother and her family when the choice is made. However, it is the consensus of the pediatric community that the weight of evidence favors breast-feeding.[1,2]

ADVANTAGES OF BREAST-FEEDING ≋

Human milk was designed for human infants. The process of lactation is normal for mammals. It is therefore not surprising that a number of advantages have been defined for mothers and infants who participate in the breast-feeding experience (see the box on p. 163). The degree of advantage varies among mother-infant pairs, since availability of alternative foods, environmental conditions, and lifestyle characteristics are markedly different from one setting to another. Reviewing the issue with an open mind, however, leaves no doubt that, in most situations, breast-feeding provides distinct benefits for both child and family.

---

*Excerpts from Jacobi, A.M., and M.L. Levin. 1997. Promotion and support of breast-feeding. In *Nutrition in Pregnancy and Lactation,* 6th ed. Dubuque, Ia: McGraw-Hill.

Benefits of Breast-feeding

Best for baby

- Designed exclusively for human infants.
- Nutritionally superior to any alternative.
- Bacteriologically safe and always fresh.
- Provides immunity to viral and bacterial diseases.
- Stimulates the infant's own immunologic defenses.
- Decreases risk of respiratory and diarrheal diseases.
- Prevents or reduces the risk of allergy.
- Promotes correct development of jaws, teeth, and speech patterns.
- Decreases tendency toward childhood obesity.
- Promotes frequent tender physical contact with mother.
- Facilitates maternal-infant attachment.

Best for mother

- Promotes physiologic recovery from pregnancy:
    Promotes uterine involution.
    Decreases risk of postpartum hemorrhage.
    Increases period of postpartum anovulation.
- Promotes psychologic attachment.
- Facilitates positive self-esteem in maternal role.
- Allows for daily rest periods.
- Eliminates need to mix, prepare, use, and wash feeding equipment.
- Saves money not spent on formula and equipment.
- Decreases risk of breast cancer and ovarian cancer.

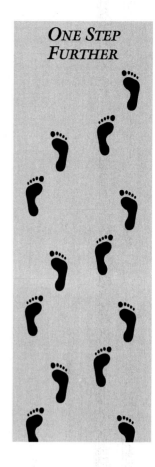

ONE STEP FURTHER

Antiinfective Properties

Around the turn of the century, there was little knowledge of microbiology or of immunology, and bottle-fed infants suffered from a much higher incidence of diarrhea and acute gastrointestinal tract infection. They also experienced higher mortality rates than breast-fed infants. Throughout much of the United States and the industrialized West, techniques for microbial control of the artificial diet have lessened the differences in mortality between bottle-fed and breast-fed infants. However, small differences are still apparent in the number and severity of illnesses contracted by bottle-fed and breast-fed infants.[3]

Gastrointestinal Benefits

Severe diarrhea is one of the major causes of morbidity and mortality worldwide. Infants and young children are the most significant victims. Breast-feeding has long been associated with reduced risk of gastrointestinal distress. Popkin et al.[4] have suggested that "global promotion of breastfeeding could reduce diarrheal morbidity rates 8% to 20% for infants up to the age of 6 months." The reason for less diarrhea in exclusively breast-fed babies remains unclear. Compounds above and beyond the protective factors may play a role.[5]

Reduced Risk of Allergies

There is some controversy about how breast-feeding is protective against allergies. Available evidence confirms, however, that breast-feeding at least delays the onset of allergies and reduces their severity in children for whom there is a family history of allergies.[6,7] The

Antigen

(*antibody* + Gr *genan*, to produce) Any disease agent, such as toxins, bacteria, viruses, and other foreign substances, that stimulates the production of *antibodies* to combat and destroy them.

presence of secretory lgA (slgA), an antibody, in breast milk is believed to decrease **antigen** entry across the gastrointestinal mucosa while the newborn's mucosal barrier is maturing. However, other mechanisms may be involved.

Optimum Nutrition

A main advantage of breast-feeding is freedom from "formulogenic disease." The complications of improper dilutions, such as incorrect caloric density and excessive renal solute load, are not concerns for breast-fed babies. Colostrum and breast milk contain factors whose functions are unclear, as well as micronutrients whose value to the newborn become apparent only when they are omitted from infant formulas. Human milk appears to have a fat composition and protein content ideally suited to the growth rate of the human infant; it is the standard by which formulas are measured.

Appropriate Growth

Bottle-fed and breast-fed infants follow similar growth curves from birth until the third or fourth month of age. From the fourth month on, the bottle-fed infant gains weight at a faster rate, especially beyond the sixth month of life. A sizable number of pediatric specialists feel that the slower rate of growth among older breast-fed infants represents the ideal pattern for optimum health. It has even been suggested that the National Center for Health Statistics[7] standards are not appropriate for evaluating the growth performance of breast-fed infants and that growth curves based exclusively on breast-fed infants should be used for that purpose. Thus far, such curves are not available, and agreement about what represents optimum growth in infancy has not yet been reached.

Cognitive Development

To say that breast-feeding will make a child more intelligent is bound to be controversial. However, there have been a few studies attempting to compare the IQ of artificially fed children vs. that of breast-fed children.

Data by Lucas seemed to show that a cohort of breast-fed children had higher developmental scores at 18 months.[8] This study attempted to measure neurodevelopment. The authors followed the same children and reported similar results for children ages 7 1/2 to 8 years old. In this study, 300 children were tested with an abbreviated version of the Weschler Intelligence Scale for Children (revised Anglicized). Those who had been given breast milk in the early weeks of life had a significantly higher IQ at this age than those who had received no breast milk. The babies in this study had been born preterm. The author acknowledges that social class and the mother's education may have been a factor in the decision to provide breast milk and might also have contributed to the difference in the IQ scores. However, he also found that the children of mothers who had planned to provide breast milk, but then had failed to do so, had scores nearly the same as those of the mothers who never intended to provide breast milk. The IQ advantage also was seen in babies who received breast milk only through a nasogastric tube while hospitalized, but not later, so mother-child interaction while nursing was ruled out as a factor. Lucas noted that the benefit found was larger than in similar studies done with infants born at full term. This finding has important implications for promoting breast milk for preterm infants who are less likely to be breast-fed because of the extended separation from their mothers resulting from their long hospitalization.

Other Protective Benefits

An array of other advantages for babies have been proposed to be associated with breast-feeding. Two studies, one done in Finland and one in Galway County, Ireland, seem to show that breast-feeding at least delays the onset of symptoms of coeliac disease.[9] Studies of the effect of breast milk on preterm infants are beginning to show some evidence that it may protect against necrotizing enterocolitis, which causes a significant amount of morbidity in this group of babies.[10]

There is some evidence that exclusive breast-feeding for at least six months confers protection from certain types of childhood cancer.[11] In a case-control study to assess whether inadequate exposure to the immunologic benefits of human milk affects infants' responses to infection and makes them more susceptible to childhood malignancies, a group from the National Institutes of Health (NIH) found higher risk for childhood cancers in children who were breast-fed less than six months or who were artificially fed. Some studies have related artificial feeding and early introduction of solid foods with obesity in later life. One study showed that exclusive breast-feeding seemed to keep infants in a normal weight range through the first six months of life.[12] However, the results were inconclusive for older infants and children.

Research is beginning to indicate a protective effect against Crohn's disease and insulin-dependent diabetes mellitus. Support for these and other hypotheses is limited, but future observations may confirm their validity.

Mothers start breast-feeding because they believe it is good for the baby, but they continue because they like it. Nature fixed it that way to ensure the continuation of the species and tucked in some benefits for the mother. The most obvious one is the tender physical contact, which helps form a special attachment between mother and child.

This attachment also is the basis for a long and important relationship, allowing the mother to recognize and respond to subtle behavior cues quickly. In addition, the closeness allows the newborn to feel secure in the warm, loving arms of its mother.

Breast-feeding may also contribute to maternal security. Virden studied sixty first-time mothers from a large urban area in California.[13] She found that, at one-month postpartum, the breast-feeding mothers had less anxiety and more mother-infant harmony than the women who were bottle-feeding their infants. Further analysis showed that the mothers who breast-fed patterned their touch and talking to the infant's activity more than did the bottle-feeding mothers. Virden found that "during feeding, the breastfeeding mother was more engrossed in the interaction than the bottle-feeding mother." Dr. Ashley Montague emphasized the importance of this in his book *Touching:*

> What is established in the breast-feeding relationship constitutes the foundation for the development of all human social relationships, and the communications the infant receives through the warmth of the mother's skin constitute the first of the socializing experiences of life.[14]

The onset of lactation is a spontaneous part of the "fourth trimester of pregnancy." There is a sense of harmony to the idea that the gradual rise of the hormones of pregnancy should, as a corollary, gradually reduce over the period of lactation. To prevent a newly delivered woman from lactating is like trying to hold back a sneeze. Each is a normal physiologic process that serves a useful purpose to the body and that must be forcibly repressed or it will proceed spontaneously. The urge to lactate is strong, just as is the urge to sneeze.

Breast-feeding immediately after birth has more immediate physical advantages for the mother than for the infant. The infant's suckling stimulates the release of oxytocin, which, in turn, stimulates uterine contractions, helping both expel the placenta and reduce maternal blood loss. Continued breast-feeding also helps the uterus return to its nonpregnant state.

There is some evidence that breast-feeding reduces the risk of later breast cancer in the mother. One study found lower levels of estrogens in the breast fluids of women who had nursed at least one child, which the researchers theorized may provide some protection.[15] A study of Chinese women in Shanghai, who normally nurse for prolonged periods, showed a clear beneficial effect on breast cancer risk.[16] The study showed a lower incidence of breast cancer in the women who had breast-fed, independent of age and menopausal status.

In addition, research on ovarian cancer showed a lower risk for women who had breast-fed than for those who had not.[17] Human lactation has long been cited as a way of inducing prolonged **anovulation** and, thus, as an important way to space pregnancies. In other words, breast-feeding can be used as a form of birth control—and is in many countries. However, the duration of anovulation varies with the mother and with other factors and can range from three months to twenty to twenty-four months. Prolonged cessation of ovulation occurs most often when the infants suckle frequently, and small amounts of solid foods are not introduced until the babies are at least six months old.[18] Although breast-feeding should not be relied on as the sole source of contraception, there is evidence that, if the baby is breast-fed on demand day and night for the first six months without the

Anovulation
Lack of ovulation or egg release from the ovaries.

Amenorrhea
Temporary cessation of menstruation.

use of pacifiers or supplemental feedings, if solid or other foods are gradually introduced in small amounts beginning at six months, and if nursing continues as the primary food source for the first year, there will be a longer instance of **amenorrhea** and possibly anovulation in the mother.

Many women are worried about the weight they gain during pregnancy. Breast-feeding may play an integral part here too. A few small studies seem to indicate that breast-feeding a baby for six to twelve months can help a mother reduce fat stores, including those on her thighs, better than if she chooses to bottle-feed.

Breast milk itself may have some curative powers. There is anecdotal evidence that mothers in some countries routinely apply breast milk to minor eye infections in their children. A study in Great Britain showed that, when nursing mothers applied breast milk to their cracked nipples, it promoted healing.[19] The women were on a postpartum ward and were instructed to apply expressed breast milk to their nipples and to let it air dry following each feeding.

INCIDENCE OF BREAST-FEEDING ≈

In spite of the recognized benefits of breast-feeding for the child and the mother, the number of babies in the United States who were formula-fed rose to an estimated 82% in the two decades before 1970. Comparable statistics were reported from England and France in the period following World War II.

More recent reports indicate that this prior trend reversed in the early 1970s and reached a peak in the early 1980s (fig. 7-1).[20] More mothers are not only breast-feeding but also are continuing to do so for a longer period of time throughout the months of their infants' most rapid growth and high nutritional demands. It is also apparent that the increased incidence of breast-feeding has not been limited to higher income, better-educated mothers. From 1971 to 1981, the incidence at two months postpartum more than tripled among mothers in lower-income families. The incidence of breast-feeding increased five times among mothers whose education did not extend beyond elementary or high school. Incidence of breast-feeding among mothers on the WIC program has increased. As might be expected, breast-feeding in any one year, especially long term, is much more common among mothers who have successfully breast-fed a previous child. Even mothers of preterm infants, however, may nurse for long periods of time.

Several surveys have considered the employment status of the mother as it relates to choices about infant feeding.[21,22] One report involved a large population of women in the Baltimore area. These women were interviewed twice during the first three months postpartum. Planning to be employed during the first six months of the postpartum period did not affect the choice to initiate breast-feeding. However, actually being employed was sig-

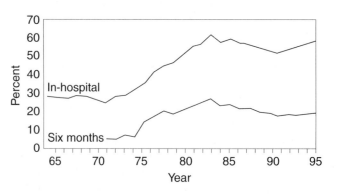

FIG. 7-1   Trends in breast-feeding in the United States, 1965–1995.

From Lawrence, R., et al. 1991. Recent declines in breastfeeding in the United States, 1984 through 1989. *Pediatrics* 88:719; American Dietetic Association. 1997. Position of the ADA: Promotion of breastfeeding. *J Am Diet Assoc* 97:662.

nificantly associated with cessation of breast-feeding as early as two or three months postpartum. Less than one-half of the mothers who were employed were still breast-feeding at the second postpartum interview, whereas two-thirds of those who were not employed were still breast-feeding. Among employed mothers, working no more than twenty hours/week appeared to be associated with continued breast-feeding.

Regional differences have been reported in the current incidence of breast-feeding. The highest rates of initiating breast-feeding in the hospital and at five or six months postpartum are found in the mountain and Pacific regions. Rates in the east south central region are the lowest. Ethnic differences within census regions are the same as those seen in national data.

One of the greatest influences on the current trend toward breast-feeding is the change in medical attitude. Today the American Academy of Pediatrics (AAP) actively recommends breast-feeding, as indicated by its Committee on Nutrition. Beginning with its 1978 report, the AAP has recommended that all physicians encourage mothers to breast-feed their infants.[23,24] The AAP Committee on Nutrition declared:

1. Despite technologic advances in infant formulas, breast milk is "the best food for every newborn infant."
2. All physicians need to become "much more knowledgeable" about infant nutrition in general and breast-feeding in particular.
3. Attitudes, practices, and instruction in prenatal clinics and maternity wards should be changed to encourage breast-feeding.
4. In hospitals, mothers and infants should be kept together after birth so babies can be fed on demand.
5. Not only should information about breast-feeding be supplied to all schoolchildren, but nursing should also be portrayed as natural on television and other media.
6. To prevent conflict between breast-feeding and employment, legislation should mandate three to four months' postdelivery leaves, so that working mothers can breast-feed.

This hearty endorsement was followed in 1982 by a critical evaluation of how and why breast-feeding should be encouraged.[24] The AAP again voiced its support for the promotion of breast-feeding but made note of the maternal characteristics and family circumstances that may need attention when deciding on infant feeding strategies.

To reinforce the needed changes in health care practices, the AAP, in 1982, provided specific guidelines for activities to support breast-feeding. The final recommendations of the AAP include the following practices:

- Education about breast-feeding in school for boys as well as girls, since later support by the father helps breast-feeding succeed.
- Public education through television, newspapers, magazines, and radio to enhance the acceptability of breast-feeding.
- Improved education about breast-feeding techniques in medical and nursing schools, as well as residency programs in obstetrics, pediatrics, and family practice.
- Factual educational material designed to present the advantages of breast-feeding.
- Encouragement not to use breast-feeding alternatives for relief, vacation, or night feeding until nursing is well established.
- Breast-feeding information provided in prenatal classes and at any prenatal contact.
- Decreased sedation of the mother for labor and birth.
- Extended contact between mother and infant in the first twenty-four hours.
- Rooming-in encouraged, except when specifically contraindicated.
- Avoidance of routine supplemental feeding.
- Lactation suppressants not given unless requested by the mother.
- Discharge packs of formula given only at the discretion of the physician or at the request of the mother, not as a routine hospital practice.
- Development of day nurseries adjacent to school or workplaces to encourage and support working and school-aged mothers to breast-feed.
- Use of lay support groups, such as La Leche League.
- Encouragement of continued breast-feeding of the hospitalized child.
- Relactation instruction when necessary[24].

THE DECISION TO BREAST-FEED ≋

The decision to breast-feed is a significant one for the parents and is usually made relatively early in the pregnancy. The factors that influence this decision are complex and interrelated.

Where parents have not yet made a decision or have not been exposed to the advantages of breast-feeding, it is the responsibility of health care professionals to support lactation as the optimum method of infant feeding. Although health professionals must support the parents' ultimate decision regarding feeding method, they often fail to take a positive stand in support of lactation early enough in the prenatal period to influence the decision-making process. It has long been recognized that physicians who support lactation have higher percentages of breast-feeding mothers.

Involving other family members often is a good promotional tool. A study of 1,525 women showed that, if the woman is married, her husband's opinion is a strong influence on her decision to breast-feed. There also is a strong association between the child's grandmother's method of feeding.

Outside influence can be subtle too. Encouraging clinic and hospital staff to wear pro-breast-feeding buttons, use breast-feeding slogans, and integrate such conveniences as a private breast-feeding or pumping room into the regular scheme of things sends a powerful message: WE SUPPORT THE BREAST-FEEDING FAMILY.

Historically, health professionals have been taught to be neutral in discussions of infant feeding. The notion was that, if health care workers were to support breast-feeding, it might make bottle-feeding mothers feel guilty. However, some lactation advocates feel that bottle-feeding mothers are not feeling guilty but, rather, very angry with health professionals for not having disclosed the facts that would have given them a stronger motivation to begin or to continue breast-feeding. An opinion held by many is that women fail to breast-feed because professional personnel have failed to take this major physiologic process seriously and, so, frequently provide inaccurate diagnosis and inappropriate advice.

There are a few breast-feeding concerns that most prospective mothers have; treating them seriously, honestly, and respectfully, can go a long way toward promoting breast-feeding. These concerns include:

1. How does it feel?
2. Does it hurt?
3. How long should I breast-feed?
4. What if the baby gets hungry in public?
5. What happens when I return to work?
6. What about sex?

There are some concepts that apply to all mother-baby couples; these can be shared with prospective parents, so that they are prepared to breast-feed. These concepts lay the foundation on which individual differences between mother-baby couples can be built. Techniques that work for one mother may not work for another; the same can be said for differences between siblings who were breast-fed. What worked for the first or second baby may not work for the third. Sticking with the basics in the prenatal period is therefore important. These basics include the following:

1. Benefits of breast-feeding for mother and baby.
2. Prenatal assessment and preparation of nipple.
3. How breast-feeding works.
4. Assessing a "baby friendly" hospital (see the box on p. 170).

Experienced breast-feeding educators maintain that preparation for breast-feeding takes place 99% in the head and 1% in the nipples. Every prenatal contact is an opportunity to reinforce the choice to breast-feed.

When the decision has been made to breast-feed, an individual or small-group instruction session is indicated. Simply handing out pamphlets is not very effective. These sessions may be held early in the second trimester. Both parents should be included in the instruction session if possible. Fathers tend to be more supportive if they know what to expect and understand the difficulties they may encounter. The prenatal visit provides the opportunity to get to know the parents, to find out how much they know about breast-

Initiation and Duration of Breast-feeding:
Benefits of Home Support Visits

Public health nutritionists and dietitians agree that breast-feeding is best for both mother and baby. *Healthy People 2000: National Health Promotion and Disease Prevention Objectives* has set the goal that 75% of all mothers will breast-feed and 50% will continue breast-feeding for at least five to six months. Current practices fall well below those goals, and breast-feeding is lowest among low-income, less-well-educated, and African American and Hispanic mothers. Many new mothers do not have a relative or another support person nearby to answer questions about breast-feeding or to help with problems that may arise after they have left the hospital. This lack of support after returning home appears to be critical to the decision to discontinue breast-feeding. Intervention programs that provide home support by trained lactation counselors have resulted in about a twofold increase in the number of mothers who are continuing to breast-feed after two months.

Schedule for visits

It is important to visit the nursing mother within one to two days after she leaves the hospital and as often as needed during the first two weeks until breast-feeding is established. At that time, it can be determined if further visits are necessary or if the process is moving along smoothly. Mothers should be provided with the telephone number of their counselors, so they can obtain answers to questions as they arise.

Activities for visits

Information provided in early visits might include the frequency of feeding, relaxation techniques, and how to determine if intake is adequate in the breast-fed infant. The lactation counselor might also observe the breast-feeding process and make suggestions regarding the positioning of the infant and nipple care to avoid the development of sore nipples. Concerns relating to the adequacy of breast milk and the development of sore, cracked nipples are major factors leading to the discontinuation of breast-feeding.

Selection and training of lactation counselors

Lactation counselors providing home support might include public health nutritionists, dietitians, or nurses sponsored by a local hospital, visiting nurse association, or WIC (Supplemental Food Program for Women, Infants, and Children) program. To reduce the costs of a home support program, trained paraprofessionals supervised by a home health agency or the Expanded Food and Nutrition Education Program (EFNEP) might provide lactation counseling. Factors to be considered in the recruiting and training of lactation counselors include:
• Workshops to develop a strong knowledge base on lactation.
• Hands-on experience with breast-feeding mothers in a supervised clinic situation.
• Ability to be at ease when observing breast-feeding and offering assistance.
• Nonjudgmental approach to the attitudes and decisions of others.

Serafino-Cross, P., and P.R. Donovan. 1992. Effectiveness of professional breastfeeding home support. *J Nutr Educ* 24:117.
U.S. Department of Health and Human Services. 1991. *Healthy people 2000: National health promotion and disease prevention objectives.* DHHS Pub. No. (PHS) 91-50213. Washington, DC: U.S. Government Printing Office.

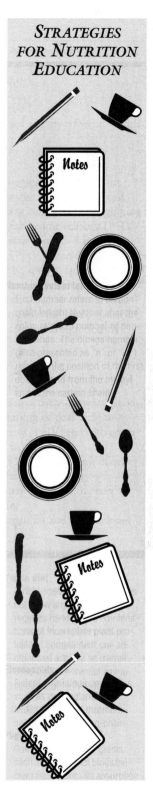

STRATEGIES FOR NUTRITION EDUCATION

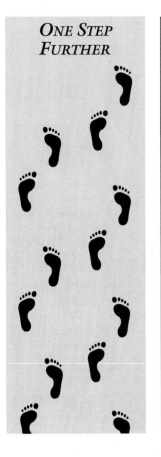

ONE STEP FURTHER

Is Your Hospital "Baby Friendly?"

WHO/UNICEF has jointly launched an initiative aimed at promoting breast-feeding through the creation of "baby friendly" hospitals. Institutions that adopt and apply the ten steps to successful breast-feeding will be designated as "baby friendly" and will receive a plaque or another award of public recognition.

Every health facility providing maternity services and care for newborn infants should:

1. Have a written breast-feeding policy that is routinely communicated to all health care staff.
2. Train all health care staff in the skills necessary to implement this policy.
3. Inform all pregnant women about the benefits and management of breast-feeding.
4. Help mothers initiate breast-feeding within a half-hour of birth.
5. Show mothers how to breast-feed and how to maintain lactation, even if they are separated from their infants.
6. Give newborn infants no food or drink other than breast milk, unless medically indicated.
7. Practice rooming-in—allow mothers and infants to remain together twenty-four hours a day.
8. Encourage breast-feeding on demand.
9. Give no artificial teats or pacifiers (also called dummies or soothers) to breast-feeding infants.
10. Foster the establishment of breast-feeding support groups and refer mothers to them on discharge from the hospital or clinic.

Representatives of the International Pediatric Association, at whose meeting the "baby friendly" campaign was introduced, ask for the assistance of all health professionals as partners in this initiative. The UNICEF resolution also calls on "manufacturers and distributors of breast milk substitutes to end free and low-cost supplies of infant formula to maternity wards and hospitals by December 1992," to reduce their detrimental effect on breastfeeding.

feeding, to determine what apprehensions they may have, and to estimate how much help and support the mother is likely to need in the early weeks of breast-feeding. It is important to remember that there is a typical breast-feeding personality. Women who appear to be "nervous" can learn to breast-feed successfully if they cultivate a relaxed and confident attitude. This is best accomplished by adequate instruction, along with professional and family support.

PRENATAL PREPARATION FOR BREAST-FEEDING ≋

Breast-feeding information is only part of the overall preparation for the baby's arrival. As such, it should be integrated into all prenatal care and education. Every prenatal contact is an opportunity to reinforce the choice to breast-feed.

Health care providers should assess the breasts and nipples at the first prenatal visit. This is another opportune moment to ask how the client plans to feed her baby. It also is a good time to encourage breast-feeding. Breast assessment should begin with a visual inspection. Assure the client that any minor size differences are normal. Anyone with palpable lumps or cysts should be referred for evaluation. Anyone with a history of breast augmentation or reduction surgery should also be referred to a lactation specialist for follow-up after delivery, since the extent of lactation function can be evaluated only after the baby is nursing. Significant breast size discrepancies may also indicate the need for postpartum follow-up for lactation adequacy.

Everted
Protruding.

Next, the nipples should be inspected. Overtly **everted** nipples are ready for breast-feeding. Less than fully everted nipples should be monitored for spontaneous eversion, which usually occurs during pregnancy (fig. 7-2).

Before stimulation After stimulation

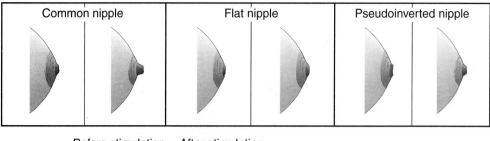

Before stimulation   After stimulation

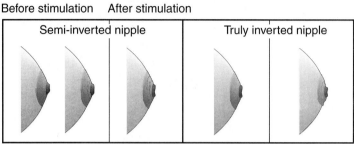

FIG. 7-2   Five types of nipples and their responses to stimulation.

From Lauwers, J. and C. Woessner. 1989. *Counseling the nursing mother: A reference handbook for health care providers and lay counselors.* Garden City Park, NY: Avery. Reprinted with permission.

Moderate manipulation of the breasts and nipples as a natural part of lovemaking can assist in everting the nipples. In addition, the mother can use gentle outward manipulation of the nipples or the Hoffman technique to help nipples turn outward. Nipples that remain inverted into the third trimester can be helped by wearing breast cups during the day (fig. 7-3). There is one contraindication to nipple stimulation during pregnancy: women who are at risk for preterm labor are advised to refrain from any form of nipple stimulation, as this could cause the onset of contractions leading to preterm labor and preterm birth.

Prenatal breast care has become simplified as more has been learned about successful lactation. The old techniques designed to "toughen" the nipples were not only unnecessary but also counterproductive and have given way to a more gentle approach. The Montgomery glands of the areola secrete lanolin, which lubricates the nipple and areola, to keep them soft and pliable. Therefore, soap should be avoided, since it will remove the lanolin.

Tangible ongoing support in the form of accessible prenatal classes on breast-feeding, as well as referrals to dietitians and lactation consultants, are an important part of prenatal breast-feeding promotion efforts. Appropriate pamphlets, posters, and videos posted at the office will give clients a clear message that the health professional supports breast-feeding.

However, the strongest message that can be given in support of breast-feeding is to provide a clean, quiet, comfortable place for mothers to nurse and pump while at the health care facility. To the mother, this not only shows support for breast-feeding during pregnancy but also proves that the facility and staff will assist her in it after the baby arrives.

BREAST-FEEDING IN THE POSTPARTUM PERIOD ≋

Breast-feeding is often a new experience for the mother as well as for the baby. The new mother may be apprehensive and unsure of herself and may need help and guidance in handling the infant. The clinician who is to instruct the mother at the first feeding should try to make her feel as much at ease as possible. The father should be encouraged to be

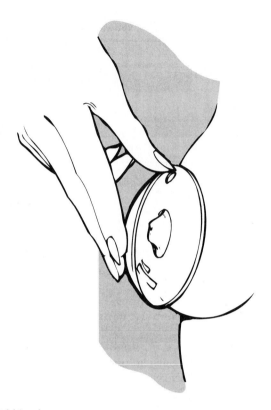

FIG. 7-3   Breast shield in place.

present at feedings and during instruction if the hospital permits it and if the mother is comfortable with his presence. The father's support, knowledge, and understanding will be valuable later on. He may remember techniques and advice the mother has forgotten.

There are two basic breast-feeding positions, each of which is subject to a wide variety of individual adaptations. The chief requirements are 1) the comfort of the mother throughout the feeding and 2) the positioning of the baby so that the process of swallowing is not impaired.

Episiotomy
A surgical procedure in a woman's perineum to enlarge her vaginal opening for delivery.

If the mother has had an **episiotomy** or operative delivery (cesarean section), she may be more comfortable breast-feeding lying down. She should position herself comfortably on her side, using pillows for additional support as required. The baby should be placed on his or her side with the mouth parallel to the nipple. A roll of receiving blankets makes a good support for the baby's back. This position is illustrated in fig. 7-4. The baby can then feed comfortably from the lower breast without undue nipple traction or unnecessary distortion of the infant's alimentary tract. Both baby and mother will probably need help in repositioning to feed from the other breast.

The second common position for breast-feeding is that in which the mother sits in a comfortable chair that provides good back support, arm rests, and, if possible, foot and leg support. She cradles the baby in her arm, placing the baby's head over her elbow so that the mouth is adjacent to the nipple. A pillow may be required on her lap to support the baby's body and under her elbow to prevent her arm from becoming too tired while holding the baby's head in the proper position for feeding. This position is illustrated in fig. 7-5 and must be reversed for feeding on the opposite breast. This position can be modified for use in the hospital bed (fig. 7-6). If this is to be successful, the head of the bed should be raised fully and the foot adjusted to provide leg support. Pillows are required to support the arm holding the baby's head. An additional blanket roll or pillow under the mother's knees may make the position more comfortable. After feeding has begun, the

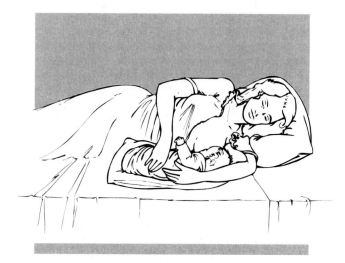

FIG. 7-4 Recommended recumbent position for breast-feeding.

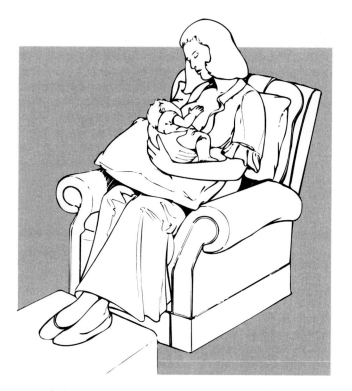

FIG. 7-5 Recommended positioning for breast-feeding while sitting in a comfortable chair.

position should be checked to make sure that nipple traction and distortion of the infant's alimentary tract are at a minimum.

Another popular position, especially with small babies or twins, is the "football hold." The baby's head is held in the palm of the hand while the forearm is used to support the baby's torso (fig. 7-7). This allows the mother to move the baby easily to achieve the proper position of the baby's mouth relative to the nipple. The "football hold" can be used while "tailor" sitting in bed with the mother's back supported. It is especially comfortable for mothers who have had cesarean deliveries.

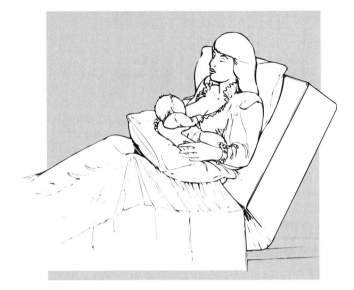

FIG. 7-6 Modified positioning for breast-feeding while sitting in a hospital bed.

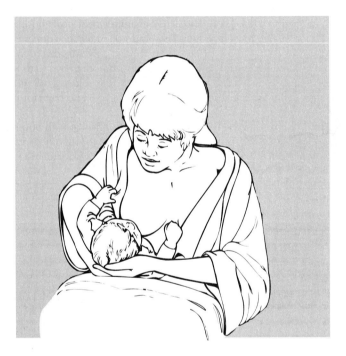

FIG. 7-7 Baby is tucked under right arm, like a football, and is nursing on right breast.

IMPORTANCE OF CORRECT LATCHING ON ≋

The mother should tickle the baby's upper lip lightly with her nipple until the baby opens his or her mouth very wide to teach it how to open wide enough to engage both the nipple and the areola. This activity may take a considerable amount of time and patience. Most babies should know what to do intuitively. Some babies respond to gentle training in a matter of a few minutes. However, if they are sleepy from medication given during labor or a difficult birth or are not hungry because hospital policy requires that they be given a feeding, the process may take more time and patience. This is where a lactation consult-

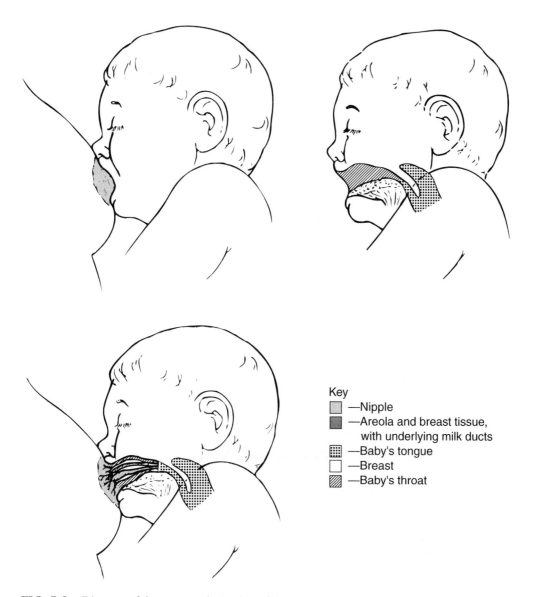

Key

- —Nipple
- —Areola and breast tissue, with underlying milk ducts
- —Baby's tongue
- —Breast
- —Baby's throat

FIG. 7-8 Diagram of the proper relationship of the nipple to the baby's mouth.

From Worthington-Roberts, B., and S.R. Williams. 1997. *Nutrition in pregnancy and lactation,* 6th ed. Dubuque, IA: WCB/McGraw-Hill.

ant or maternity nurse who is experienced with proper breast-feeding management is invaluable. The result of these efforts should be a well-latched baby. Only recently have studies investigated what the baby's mouth is doing during breast-feeding. Older diagrams were inaccurate and led to erroneous ideas about what the baby's tongue does during breast-feeding (fig. 7-8).

Some babies are able to go easily to the breast within the first day of life. Other babies need more practice to learn the correct movements of lips and tongue. When a baby is having trouble, it is essential to consult a professional who can correctly assess the problem and recommend techniques to overcome it. Lactation consultants and specialized physical and occupational therapists are able to assess sucking problems and suggest ways to get the baby to latch on.

It is vital to teach both the mother and her baby correct techniques for positioning and latching on from the beginning. So much of the dissatisfaction and early abandonment of breast-feeding that occurs because of sore nipples and other problems could be avoided if every feeding were initiated properly, so that correct techniques were reinforced and problems avoided. The responsibility for modeling the correct techniques is clearly the responsibility of the nursing staff who care for the mother and baby during the intrapartum period. However, the lack of breast-feeding knowledge on the part of medical and nursing staff in United States hospitals is an unfortunate reality. Furthermore, current short hospital stays, outdated hospital policies mandating complementary water/formula before or after nursing, extended delays between birth and initiation of first feeding, time limitations at breast, and commercial formula discharge packs all contribute to early weaning from breast to bottle. Hospital policies that support early initiation of breast-feeding after birth, feeding on demand, rooming-in, prohibition of complements or supplements unless ordered by the physician for a specific reason, and encouragement from a lactation consultant can contribute to increased breast-feeding duration.

FEEDING FREQUENCY ≋

The baby needs frequent access to the breast, so the mother will be able to build a milk supply that will provide the fluids and kilocalories needed for the infant's growth. For almost this entire century, instructions from physicians and nurses on all infant feeding, but especially breast-feeding, has included regimented timing of feedings. This attempt to schedule breast-feeding was motivated, in part, by a wish to prevent nipple damage. What it has done, in fact, is untold damage to the willingness of mothers to continue breast-feeding. It is now known that human newborns need to nurse a minimum of ten to twelve times in twenty-four hours for at least the first month of life to receive adequate nutrition. This means the infant must nurse about every two to three hours around the clock.

Demand feeding
Feeding baby when signs of hunger appear.

This is a departure from the concept of **demand feeding,** which represents the opposite end of the spectrum from scheduled feeding. Nursing every two to three hours around the clock represents a reasonable compromise, which allows the baby to meet its nutritional needs while the mother meets her comfort needs by moving milk through her breasts frequently. For new parents, this translates into a departure from clock watching to baby watching, the bottom line of which is "When in doubt, feed the baby."

New parents need guidelines, not rules. They need to know that not all feedings will last the same length of time, nor will the baby nurse an equal number of minutes from each breast at each feeding. Generally speaking, though, both breasts should be offered at each feeding to facilitate the mother's comfort with her milk supply. Encouraging frequent unlimited breast-feeding produces increased milk output, which leads to greater infant weight gain, decreased nipple and breast problems, and increased duration of breast-feeding. The mother needs to be assured that, as the baby grows older, the time between feedings will lengthen. This is especially important for mothers who are hesitant to begin breast-feeding because of limited maternity leave policies and for mothers who fear that breast-feeding will prevent them from pursuing other activities.

Growth spurt
A period of rapid growth.

Finally, new parents can be told that, after a while, they will begin to observe a pattern to their baby's feedings. The baby will then have a **growth spurt,** and the pattern will change. Growth spurts occur at regular intervals during the first year of life and can be identified by a day when all the baby wants to do is nurse. If the baby is allowed to nurse liberally for the next twenty-four hours or more, the mother's milk supply will increase and the baby will settle down into a new pattern. However, if the mother gives formula to "fill the baby up," she will start a pattern of insufficient milk supply that can be devastating to her continued breast-feeding.

ASSESSMENT OF THE ADEQUACY OF BREAST-FEEDING ≋

Performance and outcome are the breast-feeding concepts that are most important to the mother and baby in the postpartum period. First, the mother may need to be shown basic breast-feeding techniques. She may need a hands-on demonstration to feel comfortable with correct positioning for herself and the baby. She may need assistance with helping the baby latch on over the nipple to the areola for correct suckling and nipple comfort. Some babies do this without help; some do not. These mothers need extra support and instruction.

The mother should also be provided with some tools to evaluate the outcome, such as does she hear swallowing? Is the baby having six to eight wet diapers in a twenty-four-hour period? Is her baby alert when awake? Unfortunately, she also needs this information toward against well-meaning but ill-informed doctors, nurses, dietitians, husbands, mothers, in-laws, neighbors, friends, and others. Many individuals say and do things to undermine the mother's confidence in her ability to breast-feed. As in the prenatal period, these breast-feeding concepts need to be kept to a minimum, so that the mother can focus on what is important and not be confused or turned off by a rigid, extensive list of do's and don'ts. The most important concepts to be shared in the immediate postpartum period are assessment of feeding adequacy, positioning of mother and baby, latching on, and nursing frequency.

The clinician should instruct the mother to listen to her baby. This helps her tune in to her infant, which is sometimes difficult for the first-time breast-feeding mother to do. Television, roommates, telephones, and various hospital personnel are distractions to the first-time breast-feeding mother. There is also the general excitement and disorientation that comes with being hospitalized. The experience of having just gone through a vaginal or cesarean delivery is usually accompanied by both relief and elation, along with the discomforts of intravenous (IV) lines, stitches, fatigue, and bruising. The effect of medications can sedate or decrease the mother's ability to focus. Finally, there is the gradual realization that the baby is truly here, real, and in need of attention.

Listening to the baby provides a mother with an opportunity to learn about the normal variety of infant reflexes that make noise, such as breathing, swallowing, hiccupping, and sneezing. Many new parents are so unfamiliar with babies that they think that the only noise a baby makes is crying.

The most important reason to tell a mother to listen to audible breathing and swallowing is to give her immediate feedback about breathing and feeding. For instance, contrary to breast-feeding instruction in the past, it is not necessary for the mother to press her breast away from the baby's nose for it to breathe, and, if she learns to listen to her baby, she will be able to hear that. The infant nose was designed to stick out just enough to push the breast back to create an adequate air passage. When the mother listens for swallowing sounds, she hears her milk going into the baby's esophagus. It tells her that there is something in her breast. Far too many women have been told there is no milk, that the milk does not "come in" for a certain number of days, or, worst of all, that they do not have enough milk. This negative thinking is often reinforced by the size of the infant formula bottles used in the hospital. The formula industry packages newborn formula in 3 oz bottles because it is convenient and cost-efficient for the manufacturer to do so. This volume is too much for any newborn to consume. However, for inexperienced parents, it is a measure of feeding need. If the baby nurses frequently, both his or her fluid and nutritional requirements will be met by the breast milk alone. Folding the baby's hand into a fist demonstrates to the parents the size of their baby's stomach and provides them with a better understanding of the small volume needed to satisfy the baby's needs at a given feeding.

All mothers will experience let-down, but some mothers may not feel it physically. As discussed in chapter 6, *let-down* is a term borrowed from the dairy industry and used to describe the process by which milk from sinuses higher up in the breast is moved down to those surrounding the areola and nipple, where the baby can milk it out. As the baby's mouth massages the areolar tissue around the nipple, it stimulates the mother's body to release oxytocin, which in turn stimulates the muscles surrounding the alveoli and milk ducts to contract. This sends the milk forward in the breast. Sometimes the only way a mother knows her milk is letting down is when she hears her baby swallowing faster. Other mothers feel a tingling sensation or pressure inside of the breast. Mothers with a particularly strong let-down may notice the baby rearing his or her head back until the initial gush subsides. All of these activities are normal.

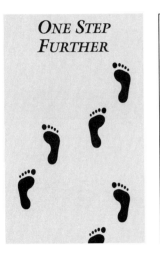

Calculation of Newborn Caloric Requirements

To calculate the number of ounces of breast milk needed per day by the baby, use the following calculation:

$$\frac{\text{Weight (kg)} \times 110 \text{ kcal/kg}}{20 \text{ kcal/oz}} = \frac{\text{Total}}{\text{oz/day}}$$

Fluid requirements must also be calculated to ensure adequate hydration. The baby needs about 150 ml/kg (70 ml/lb) of fluid per day. This is calculated as follows:

$$\text{Weight (kg)} \times 150 \text{ ml} = \text{Total oz/day}$$

To convert milliliters to ounces, divide by 30 (30 ml = 1 oz). Therefore, a 3 kg (6 lb 5 oz) baby requires 16.5 oz of milk and fluid.

ASSESSMENT OF OUTPUT AS A MEASURE OF ADEQUACY ≋

If the baby is exclusively breast-feeding, then everything the baby excretes will be the end products of breast milk metabolism. Generally, new parents have equally unrealistic ideas about the output as they do about the input. Television commercials for disposable diapers go to great lengths to explain the need to control wetness. The children used for these commercials are not newborns, so parents have no idea how much to expect in a newborn's diaper. However, urine and stool output are good measures of breast milk input.

For a newborn who is nursing every two to three hours around the clock, parents can expect about six to eight wet diapers and a minimum of one stool per day for the first few weeks. The measurement of "wetness" can be problematic for new parents. Total urine excretion is about 200 to 300 ml per twenty-four hours in the first weeks of life. The newborn bladder involuntarily empties when filled by approximately 15 ml. This can result in fifteen to twenty voidings per day.

To help parents assess these small amounts of wetness in diapers, a tissue or paper towel can be placed inside the diaper. The tissue or towel will be wet, while the paper diaper, which is so absorbent, will not. This proves that the baby is urinating. Breast-fed babies are known to pass stools often. A normal breast-fed baby's stool is very liquid. This pattern should not be mistaken for diarrhea. Normal stool frequency in a breast-fed baby varies widely. A minimum of one to three stools a day in the first month of life is considered a baseline indicator of minimal intake. Conversely, many newborns have a bowel movement with each feeding. However, older infants can pass a stool either more or less often and still be normal. Some older babies even go days between bowel movements. The color of the stools of breast-fed babies is also important information for the new parents. Newborn stool goes through several color changes in the first few days of life as the colostrum pushes the meconium stool out of the body and the infant's bowels adapt to oral feeding. The normal stool changes are from black to greenish to bright yellow. A yellow, mushy stool is normal for a totally breast-fed baby. Finally, the baby should begin to show readily visible signs of growth. A return to birth weight by about two weeks of age and the outgrowing of newborn sleepers are considered good measures. Over the long term, a gain of 4 oz per week or 1 lb per month is considered satisfactory growth for a breast-feeding baby.

Pediatrician Ruth Lawrence has reiterated the American Academy of Pediatrics guidelines, which state that all infants should be seen by their practitioner within seven days of discharge from the hospital, because all infants are at risk for complications in the early weeks regardless of feeding mode. She goes on to say that, in the event of early discharge from the hospital (twenty-four hours after delivery or less) the pediatrician should provide within three days of discharge in the office or in the home a weight check and observation of the infant for physical status, jaundice, hydration, and successful breast-feeding. She lists the following criteria for a healthy infant.

By the third day, the infant should:
• Stop losing weight
• Have lost no more than 7% of birth weight
• Be passing milk stool (yellow)
• Have at least three stools (minimum) per day
• Wet at least six diapers per day (cloth diapers are preferred for accurate assessment in the first six weeks)
• Latch on to the breast well

The mother should:
• Experience some breast engorgement
• Notice dripping of milk from opposite breast
• Expect the infant to feed every three hours or a minimum of eight times a day[25]

MOST FREQUENT BREAST-FEEDING CONCERNS ≋

Self-Care for Mother

One of the most important things a new mother can do to get breast-feeding to work for her is to take care of herself. This is not easy under the current system of health care and life in America. Information about and access to prenatal care are not as available to American women as they are to women in the rest of the Western world. Hospital care during the intrapartum period is brief, and more than half of all new mothers must return to employment outside the home within six to eight weeks after delivery. Furthermore, routine home visiting and well-baby care are also not available to many American children, resulting in morbidity and mortality statistics that compare unfavorably in a study of ten European countries.[26]

Time to provide guidance for the new breast-feeding mother is limited. Therefore, it is important to emphasize the basics before she returns home from the hospital: to continue to eat a well-balanced diet, to drink fluids to satisfy thirst, and to sleep when the baby sleeps.

New mothers also usually are unaware that life with a new baby will be tiring for at least the first month, regardless of how they are fed. The idea of napping during the day sounds foreign to modern women, who think they are going to bounce right back from delivery to their usual routine.

As for nutritional counseling, the adage that she can "eat anything in moderation" serves the new mother well. Reports of breast-fed infants becoming **colicky** from ingestion of certain gas-forming foods have been largely disproved. However, repeated references to such outdated ideas in grocery store tabloids and other lay literature perpetuate such mythology. The limited number of foods that remain exceptions because they seem to have a proven relation to colicky behavior are caffeine, chocolate, and cow's milk.[27,28] That does not mean an individual newborn might not react to other foods that the mother eats, but this seems to be the exception. The cycle of feeding, fussing, and crying in babies is part of a larger picture of accepted childrearing practices in a multicultural society and within each family.

Colicky
Fussy; irritable.

Perceived Insufficient Milk Supply

One of the main reasons mothers cite for giving up breast-feeding is a perception of insufficient milk. Insufficient milk supply is defined as a mother's perception that the quantity or quality of her milk is unable to satisfy the baby or not adequate for anticipated weight gain.[29] This is a complex phenomenon, which is receiving increased attention by researchers. A mother's perception of insufficient milk involves such factors as maternal confidence, paternal support, maternal health, mother-in-law disapproval, infant birth weight, baby behavior, solid foods, and formula. The reasons stated most often by mothers for believing they have insufficient milk are a fussy baby, crying after a feeding, and poor weight gain. As a result, mothers begin to believe that their breast milk is inadequate to satisfy their infant's needs. In an attempt to satisfy their infants, the mothers turn to artificial baby milk, which begins a cycle of less demand for the breast, which leads to less frequent nursing, which leads to decreased supply and a self-fulfilling prophecy of insufficient milk for the baby. This cycle is very real and prevalent in U.S. culture. It is reported as the main reason mothers abandon breast-feeding for bottle-feeding.[30,31] Successful intervention to change this pattern of premature weaning to artificial baby milk involves teaching the mother how successful lactation works. The concept of frequent nursing (every two to three hours around the clock for the first month) should be reinforced as a way to balance infant need and maternal supply. Increased support for breast-feeding in the early postpartum period must come from family and friends who are committed to supporting breast-feeding. Health care providers must make a commitment to learn about correct breast-feeding management techniques, so that new mothers who turn to them for advice and support are given accurate information.

PHYSICAL DISCOMFORTS WHEN BEGINNING BREAST-FEEDING ≋

Nipple Problems

Among the many concerns new mothers have about breast-feeding, one of the most distressing is the fear of pain. Breast-feeding instruction in nursing textbooks and many infant care books would be incomplete without a discussion of sore nipples, cracked nipples, and mastitis. These concepts are so thoroughly ingrained in the medical, nursing, and lay childbirth literature that they have come to be considered an expected part of breast-feeding. However, many of the initial problems mothers have with breast-feeding are iatrogenic, stemming from hospital policies and myths, resulting in practices harmful to the successful initiation of breast-feeding.

The great majority of these problems can be prevented by prenatal nipple assessment, intervention to evert nipples when necessary, and correct instruction in breast-feeding techniques that suit each mother-baby couple.

Despite these interventions, some mothers still experience nipple problems. The old techniques, such as prenatal nipple "toughening," limiting time at the breast, and the use of soaps, nipple creams, and nipple shields, must be abandoned in favor of techniques that have proved to provide relief and healing to damaged nipple tissue.[32]

Using soaps, creams, and ointments on the nipple is of particular concern for a number of reasons. Current management of nipple trauma is best treated by air drying of the nipples, with or without the use of breast shells. As previously mentioned, this treatment should be accompanied by applying the mother's own breast milk, which contains natural lanolin as well as antibodies to fight infection and promote healing.[32] Also, of the nine most commonly recommended nipple creams, five are listed as "for external use only," and the others contain instructions to remove the product before nursing. However, these preparations are routinely recommended, without regard for the implications for feeding this chemical cocktail to newborn babies.

Mothers also need to know that a certain amount of tenderness may occur when beginning breast-feeding. This is related to the compression of the infant's mouth on the breast tissue. Most mothers report that the sensation passes as soon as the milk is flowing and the baby settles at breast. This can take from thirty to sixty seconds or longer for new mothers, and it disappears as the baby gets older.

Two other frequently used breast-feeding products can be hazardous for the mother— breast pads and nipple shields. Wearing breast pads is akin to leaving a bandage on while taking a shower. The moisture collects under the pad, making an already jeopardized breast-feeding experience all the more likely to fail. A far better tool for treating nipple problems is breast shells with ample holes for air circulation. Breast shells also serve as an acceptable alternative tool for nurses who feel the need to use a piece of equipment to relieve the mother's problem.

Breast Problems

New mothers also fear **engorgement.** This is another example of antiquated practices creating a problem. In breast-feeding situations in which the baby has unlimited access to the breast from birth, engorgement is a rare or nonexistent problem. The baby stimulates milk production and is able to move the milk freely through the breast so that the mother's supply and infant need are in harmony.[32] This is the ideal. It is certainly attainable in situations of normal birth with rooming-in and even early discharge from the hospital. However, engorgement can become a problem when breast-feeding initiation is delayed or early feedings are irregular. When engorgement occurs, there are several interventions that can minimize the problem before it leads the mother to abandon breast-feeding out of frustration. Initial engorgement should be an indicator that the baby needs to go to breast more often. If that is not possible, then the milk needs to be moved before tension in the breast becomes so severe that the baby cannot latch on.[32]

Sometimes just manually expressing milk from the areolar area of the breast makes enough room for the baby to latch on. If the baby is unavailable, then the mother should use a breast pump to relieve the congestion, move the milk, and maintain the milk supply.

Applying warm moist compresses to the breast before nursing or pumping can help ease the problem. Another technique is for the mother to shower, letting warm water run over her breasts while she either manually expresses or pumps the milk. Another technique is to use warm, moist compresses before nursing or pumping, and cold compresses afterward. The cold eases discomfort and reduces swelling.

Finally, Australian midwives report good results with the application of fresh washed cabbage leaves directly on the engorged breasts, under the bra. The history and mechanism for how and why it works is unknown, but both the Australians and Chinese are familiar with the use of cabbage leaves for sprains and other wounds. The treatment provides rapid relief; sometimes just one two-hour application relieves the congestion. The treatment can also be used to suppress lactation completely when rapid delactation is necessary, as in the case of the death of a premature infant for whom the mother was pumping. The only identified contraindications for the use of cabbage leaves in this way would be history of cabbage allergy and maternal objection to the idea.[33] The technique has been used by American lactation consultants with encouraging results. However, further reports and scientific studies need to be conducted to validate the use of cabbage leaves as a treatment for engorgement.

Infections in the Breast: Mastitis, Herpes, Candidiasis

Any time there is nipple trauma, there is a rise of infection. Therefore, it is hoped that a reduction in initial nipple trauma would lead to a reduction in nipple and breast infections. One study puts the incidence of mastitis at under 3%.[34] However, regardless of its low incidence, it is a serious complication of breast-feeding that needs immediate attention to prevent unnecessary weaning to bottle-feeding. The rule of thumb with mastitis is that influenza-like symptoms in a breast-feeding mother should be considered mastitis until proven otherwise. The immediate treatment is to increase the frequency of movement of the milk, either by nursing or by pumping more often. The mother should also be counseled to increase her intake of fluids and go to bed. If the symptoms are not improved in two to four hours, a physician must be consulted for a course of antibiotics. Mastitis is not dangerous to the baby; the milk is not infected and breast-feeding should not be stopped—the breasts can become abscessed.[32] A plugged milk duct frequently precedes a case of mastitis and can be treated in the same manner as for mastitis. Other infections seen during breast-feeding include herpes and candidiasis (thrush). These infections involve the nursing couple, because the infectious agent can go back and forth from mother to baby and may even include other family members. Infections of this nature need consultation with a lactation consultant and physician to recommend modifications of the nursing techniques as well as medications.

Engorgement
Swelling (edema) of mammary tissue in early lactation.

MAINTENANCE OF LACTATION DURING SEPARATION AND ILLNESS ≋

Maintenance of Milk Supply

If the mother and baby will be separated for any reason, steps should be taken to keep the milk moving, or the supply will diminish. This can be done by hand or pump expression. There is no one method of expressing milk that is right for everyone. Some women prefer **manual expression,** whereas others prefer a particular type of pump. Many women accept and use whatever is made available to them, regardless of whether it is convenient, because they are motivated to provide milk for their babies.

Manual expression
Gentle stroking of the breast with the hands to stimulate milk release.

When counseling a mother about pumping, a clinician should first assess the mother's goals and the baby's needs. This will help determine the techniques best suited to the situation. For a long separation, she should be provided with the best pump she can afford. The mother of a hospitalized or premature infant has very little time or emotional energy for pumping, so the most effective and least stressful option is to rent a double-electric pump. The same is true for a sick or hospitalized mother.

Babies usually are older by the time their mothers return to work or school, and pumping need be done only once or twice per separation. In this situation, the mother usually has more time to weigh price vs. convenience and can choose among a variety of battery or hand pumps or manual expression.

Pumping for a Premature or Sick Baby

Providing breast milk is something tangible that the mother of a premature or sick baby can do. Ideally, a mother should receive extra support from the lactation consultant from whom she rents the electric breast pump, as well as the nurses at the hospital. Even if the mother is recovering from a high-risk pregnancy or cesarean birth, pumping should begin as soon as the mother is physically able. Ideally, she should pump every two to three hours during the day and at least once a night. This should total a minimum of seven or eight pumpings in twenty-four hours, each of which should last ten to fifteen minutes.

Guidelines vary for the timing and frequency of pumping; however, the rule of supply and need still applies. The more the mother pumps, the more she will stimulate her prolactin levels, which will help keep up her milk supply. A falling milk supply can be helped in a number of ways, not the least of which is support from family, friends, and health care providers.

Mothers can use a variety of techniques to enhance milk production. Sipping water or juice, pumping in a quiet place, using gentle breast massage, looking at a picture of the baby, using deep breathing and relaxation techniques, and listening to music have all been known to help milk production. Pumping instructions for the mother of a hospitalized newborn may be more stringent than those for a working mother of an older, healthy baby. It is important for the mother to follow the instructions supplied by the hospital about washing and sterilizing the pump equipment and storing, transporting, and freezing the milk.

Breast milk can be stored in nursing bags, glass or plastic bottles, or hospital-provided containers. One study suggests that, ideally, expressed breast milk should be used within seven hours of refrigerator storage for maximum antibody and cellular function. This research also suggests that glass containers offer a slight advantage over other containers for cellular integrity and efficiency.[35]

Breast milk that will not be fed to the baby within twenty-four to forty-eight hours should be frozen. Frozen breast milk can be kept frozen for weeks or months. Since breast milk changes as the baby grows, the frozen milk should be dated, so the first pumped is used first. Breast milk should be defrosted using tap water; it should not be boiled or heated in the microwave.

Neonatologists' opinions differ about the merits of adding artificial milk fortifiers to the breast milk given to very low birth weight babies. This subject is controversial and deserves further study by dietitians and neonatologists with expertise in the care of these extremely premature infants. Most important for the mother and premature or sick newborn is that the baby be given the opportunity to go directly to breast as soon as he or she is

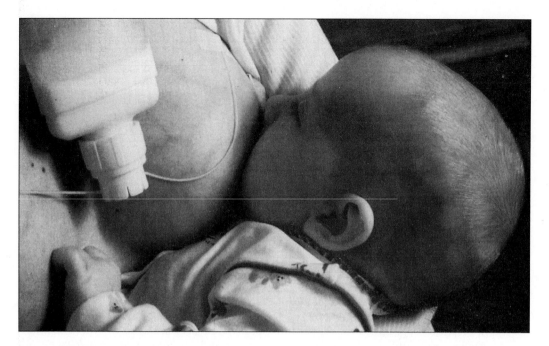

FIG. 7-9   Mother and infant using nursing supplementer, which helps keep baby nursing when supplementation is needed. These devices are useful in relactation situations, for weak or ineffective nursers, for premature babies, for inducing lactation, and for mothers whose milk supply is low.

From Medela Breast Pump Company, McHenry, Illinois.

physically able to do so. Research studies show that premature infants stay warmer and suck better at a breast than on a rubber nipple. They also have better oxygenation during breast-feeding and grow well on breast milk at an earlier age and size than was formerly thought possible.[36]

Other Medical or Surgical Conditions in the Baby

Early initiation or resumption of breast-feeding is just as important when the breast-feeding has been delayed or interrupted by a medical or surgical condition in the baby. A study conducted by Weatherly-White et al. of early repair of cleft lips with breast-feeding in the immediate postoperative period demonstrates advantages, not only for babies who have undergone cleft repair but also for babies receiving general anesthesia for other surgeries.[37] The stresses to both the mother and baby who must experience a hospitalization during infancy are ameliorated to a great extent by staff support for maintaining a milk supply and resuming breast-feeding as soon as possible. It is important to use a team approach to identifying appropriate feeding techniques for infants with craniofacial defects, keeping provision of breast milk in the foreground. Physicians, dietitians, lactation consultants, and physical or occupational therapists can provide essential input to clinical case conferences on the management of hospitalized breast-fed infants.

Nursing Supplementers

Infants with medical conditions that cause them to be poor feeders can be assisted with a nursing supplementer—a feeding-tube device that can be used to give supplemental feedings at the breast. These devices can be valuable when dealing with premature infants, infants with Down syndrome, weak or ineffective nursers, babies who tire easily (such as those with congenital heart defects), low-weight-gain babies, and those with failure to thrive. Nursing supplementers are easy for the mother to use but should be used only under the supervision of a lactation consultant who is familiar with their use (fig. 7-9). A team of specialists may be needed to evaluate and support neurologically impaired breast-feeding infants.

Neurodevelopmental and occupational therapists, who are trained to assess sucking disorders, can often assist the lactation consultant and dietitian to help a mother continue breast-feeding a baby who previously would have been tube-fed. These babies especially can benefit from the closeness and comfort afforded by breast-feeding, as well as from the immunologic benefits of the breast milk.

Nursing supplementers also can be useful in breast-feeding adopted babies and in relactation. Relactation is a situation in which there has been a fall in milk production and the mother wishes to resume breast-feeding. Lactation consultants are useful resources in both situations.

Maternal Illness

Maternal illness can delay breast-feeding initiation. Three major medical problems account for most cases of maternal perinatal morbidity: hemorrhage, infection, and hypertensive disorders of pregnancy. These complications can occur with either vaginal or cesarean birth. Recovery from any of these complications is compounded when the mother is recovering from surgery as well. Historically, hospital policies kept these mothers and babies separated. Certainly, if a mother is too ill to care for her baby, it is appropriate that the baby be cared for by the nursing staff. However, babies should be brought in for visits, and infant care can be performed in the mother's room by family members if they wish. Initiating breast-feeding or pumping as soon as the mother is able to sit up is important to begin to stimulate her milk supply. The decision as to whether the infant can consume the milk is a secondary consideration and should not be used as an excuse to delay the initiation of pumping to build a supply. The milk can be frozen in the nursery freezer for later use by the baby if there is a question about the safety of the milk because of the prescription of an unusual medication or because of the nature of the maternal illness.

There are very few situations in which an ill mother cannot maintain a milk supply. Many mothers with chronic illnesses have successfully breast-fed a baby, due, in no small part, to their courage in insisting they want to breast-feed. They have actively encouraged the health care community to research the safety of doing so. Historically, women with physically debilitating conditions or chronic diseases that required extensive medication were told not to bear children. However, with improved treatment regimens, not only are these women having children, but they also are breast-feeding them. Women can breast-feed with a variety of conditions, including diabetes, systemic lupus erythematosus, and multiple sclerosis. Certainly, mothers with these conditions and their infants need to be monitored closely, but these motivated mothers and babies can breast-feed. Maternal cystic fibrosis and maternal phenylketonuria, although reported in the literature as being compatible with breast-feeding, need to be carefully monitored for milk composition and infant well-being. The nature of these diseases leads to altered milk composition, which may affect growth and development as the baby gets older.

The question of whether the baby can consume the milk during other maternal illnesses remains controversial but is open to case conferences and consultation to see if breast-feeding is compatible with the mother's treatment. Maternal postpartum depression is a good example. There is considerable controversy over the role played by maternal hormones in the onset and severity of postpartum depression. One school of thought believes lactation would prolong the effect and production of the offending hormones; the other school believes the chance to maintain a mother-baby connection is therapeutic. In postpartum depression, there is also the question of home management or hospitalization. Again, a team approach in evaluating the mother's condition and safety of the milk is important. A pharmacologist skilled in drug evaluation, in consultation with the baby's pediatrician, is best able to answer questions about maternal milk contamination by medication.

In summary, when it comes to a separation of the mother and baby through illness or surgery, increasingly consultations with physicians, surgeons, anesthesiologists, nursing staff, lactation consultants, dietitians, pharmacists, and patients have reached an amicable, workable resolution to the problem of separation for a breast-feeding mother and baby.

These situations have included instances of maternal surgery for a variety of conditions, such as emergency appendectomy, knee arthroscopy, thyroidectomy, cholecystectomy, heart surgery for correction of a maternal ventricular defect, and lobectomy to remove a cancerous lung. Progressive medical centers make electric breast pumps available immediately after surgery for the mother's comfort. Provisions for visiting-in by the baby under the supervision of a family member, who also handles infant care such as diaper changing, have been allowed, provided the mother is in a private room. Families respond positively when these needs are met. There are even reports in the literature of successful breast-feeding after extensive surgical procedures, such as maternal renal transplantation. The maternal immunosuppressive drugs were not found to be problematic, and two babies were breast-fed for three to four months each by mothers who had undergone transplantation. Mothers on renal dialysis are also breast-feeding with extensive support and encouragement from the dietitians at a dialysis center in Chicago.

Nutritional problems, such as a history of anorexia or bulimia, also have been overcome, and these women have gone on to become pregnant and breast-feed well.[38] A Danish study that involved a long-term follow-up of fifty women with a history of anorexia, reported pregnancy rates the same as those of the general population, an unexplained elevated rate of prematurity, and breast-feeding rates and durations similar to those of the country as a whole.[39]

SPECIAL BREAST-FEEDING CIRCUMSTANCES ≈

Multiple Births

It is possible to nurse more than one infant, and many case reports support this fact. Historical observations of wet nurses indicate that the support of six babies simultaneously is within the realm of physiologic capability. The key deterrent to nursing twins or triplets is not usually the milk supply but the time. Nursing two infants at the same time is clearly more efficient. A number of tricks have been proposed to accommodate more than one infant, but, as they become larger and more active, it may be a challenge to keep them simultaneously nursing without assistance from the father or a friend. The nursing mother of more than one infant needs to attend conscientiously to her own rest and nourishment.

Working During Lactation

Many women believe that breast-feeding conflicts with working outside the home. This is a myth, since the two can go nicely together. The reduced incidence and severity of illness in the breast-feeding infant may actually reduce the days the mother misses from work. It is desirable for the working mother to have a minimum of four to six weeks at home with her nursing infant before returning to a full-time job. This time will allow for the successful establishment of lactation and the development of a close mother-child relationship. This strong foundation will provide the mother with substantial motivation to continue breast-feeding as her work commitments increase and her time with the infant decreases. The dedicated working mother will want to learn to express her milk, so that she can provide it to her infant and maintain her lactation capacity for the days she has to work.

Pregnancy During Lactation

Occasionally, a mother may wish to nurse an infant after she becomes pregnant again. This circumstance is physiologically possible, but the nutritional and psychologic demands on the mother are substantial. Some women may even experience uterine contractions while nursing and in some cases may need to consider weaning to avoid the possibility of spontaneous abortion. The child may become discouraged from nursing because of the changing composition and taste of the milk produced as the pregnancy proceeds. The mother's milk supply may also decrease, and this may cause her child to lose interest in nursing.

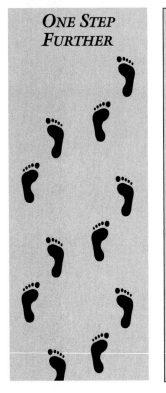

How Long Should I Nurse My Baby?

The tradition in most parts of the world is to breast-feed for two to three years. Weaning is rather natural at this age, since the child can now feed him- or herself and eat a full adult diet. The child also has teeth and can walk and talk a little and thus express wishes and disagreements. The mother, too, may again become pregnant at this time, so that her attention will need to be directed toward the new infant.

Many young children spontaneously give up breast-feeding at about one year of age or soon thereafter, especially if they are receiving adequate supplementary foods. Some mothers feel much relief, and others feel sad or rejected. Some children cling to the breast for years, and again maternal response to this behavior is mixed. There are also a few children who cling to the breast and refuse to eat solid foods. These are usually one-year-old children who have had solids introduced too late. It is essential that these children be trained to eat solid food; the sooner the training takes place, the easier it will be for the parent.

Each mother-child couple must determine their own ideal duration of breast-feeding. Factors to consider include the following:
1. Convenience of the mother.
2. Needs of the child, both psychologic and physiologic.
3. Availability of satisfactory alternative or supplemental feeds.
4. Custom in the community.

Whether a mother breast-feeds her child for two months or two years, the main goals of the health care provider is to support the mother in her decision and to help her avoid cessation of breast-feeding against her wishes.

Tandem Nursing

With sufficient sucking stimulus, most mothers can produce enough milk to successfully nurse a young infant, as well as an older child. It is important, however, to consider the emotional needs of the older sibling and the physical well-being of the mother. If the mother feels that the older child may satisfy his or her sucking needs and may benefit emotionally from the breast-feeding experience, she may decide to continue nursing both children. However, if she feels that this undertaking is too demanding or she resents the older child nursing, she is well advised to wean the older child as soon as possible.

If the mother decides to wean the toddler, she should go about it gradually. It may be rather difficult while she is nursing the young baby, since the older one may want to nurse when he or she sees the younger sibling at the breast. An obvious solution is to nurse the baby at the times when the older child is not around or is happily occupied with other things. The mother will need to decide on alternative activities and snacks to take the place of breast-feeding, so that the transition from nursing to total weaning will go smoothly.

Relactation

As previously mentioned, relactation is the resumption of lactation after it has been stopped some time beyond the immediate postpartum period. This process may be attempted by women who, for various reasons, have not nursed their infant for a while or by women who change their minds about lactation after weaning has taken place. Reactivating the lactation process requires that appropriate stimuli be provided to the breasts. The baby's sucking or manual stimulation may be accompanied by the use of medications or hormones. Success generally depends on the mother's determination and the baby's willingness to suckle at the less than satisfying breast. The longer the interlude between initial lactation and relactation, the more likely the effort is to fail.

A mother needs to decide if she really wishes to attempt relactation. Considerable motivation is required, and initially the effort may be very time consuming. It should be clear to the mother that she may not be able to produce an adequate milk supply to meet all the infant's nutritional requirements. In fact, such a goal may be unrealistic and undesirable. The majority of mothers who express great pleasure in their relactation experience indicate that the mother-infant relationship is of far greater short- and long-term importance than the act of the breast-feeding alone. They emphasize that breast-feeding is as much *nurturing at* the breast as it is *nutrition from* the breast. In many instances, undue emphasis on a complete milk supply actually hinders the mother's ability to achieve it.

Nursing the Adopted Infant

It is extremely time consuming, and sometimes impossible, to induce lactation without having been pregnant. Even when a pregnancy has been carried out in the past, great motivation is required to nurse an adopted infant. Chances increase if the mother has given birth or has nursed another baby. If she is currently nursing another baby or has recently weaned one, her chances for success are good. A mother embarking on this nursing experience should have realistic motives and goals. She should not expect to provide all the infant's nutrition through lactation but should look forward to a satisfying emotional experience.

The nipple preparation and relactation techniques previously described apply also to the adoptive mother. In addition, it is useful for the mother to pump her breasts to stimulate milk production. She can gradually increase the frequency and duration of this activity until it reaches a level of about twenty minutes every two hours when the baby's arrival is near. The mother should realize that it may be quite a while before she sees any results from her pumping and that even a small amount of milk means success. The milk supply will increase rapidly when the baby begins suckling. If the mother is not able to obtain her baby soon after birth, however, her chances of success may decline, since the baby will have been bottle-fed and may suffer from nipple confusion.

The fact that some women have succeeded in nursing their adoptive infants does not mean that all adoptive mothers can nurse or should attempt to do so. This point was well made by a physician whose family had adopted a young infant.[40] He pointed out that adoptive parents often have decided to adopt a child after a long period of reproductive failure and a trying experience with an adoptive agency. When the adopted infant finally arrives, the parents have to cope with a considerable role handicap. In view of the substantial time commitment of induced lactation and the stress and frustration that can be associated with it, one must ask whether the advantages outweigh the disadvantages. Attempting lactation may set up the mother for another failure of physical function and loss of self-esteem; in addition, it requires much time and energy that could be devoted to more significant areas of social adjustment. *No pressure should ever be put on the adoptive mother to breast-feed.* If she wishes to try, she should have support and guidance. However, if she finds that she and her family are frustrated and exhausted, she should immediately reevaluate her intentions and should not be encouraged to continue.

Teenage Mothers

Most teenage mothers elect to keep their babies even when their home environments are neither supportive nor conducive to successful lactation. The self-image of the teenager may be poor, and she may have much doubt about her self-worth. She frequently feels uncomfortable in her new role as a mother. If the young mother expresses some interest in breast-feeding, effort should be made to determine her motives, and advantages and disadvantages should be discussed. It should be determined whether or not breast-feeding would significantly compromise her ability to continue in school or to provide for the infant's other needs. Physiologically, teenagers are entirely capable of breast-feeding, although some have less functional breast tissue than adult women. Teenage mothers are capable of satisfactory milk production and experience the same difficulties as other women. When problems arise, however, teenagers are less likely to overcome them and continue breast-feeding. They require much support. Those with good support systems often breast-feed for the same amount of time as older mothers.

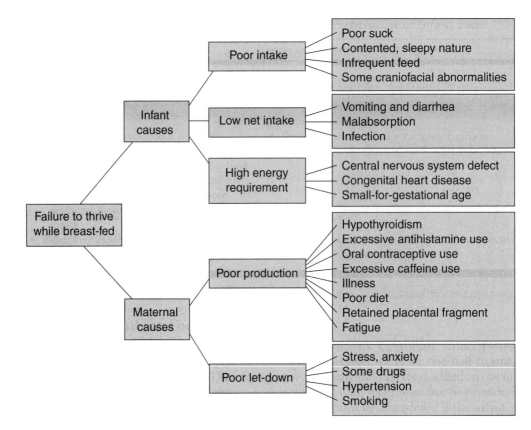

FIG. 7-10 Diagnostic flowchart for failure to thrive.

Modified from Lawrence, R. 1989. *Breastfeeding: A guide for the medical profession,* 3d ed. St. Louis: Mosby.

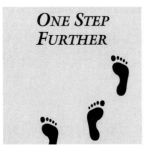

ONE STEP FURTHER

How to Tell If the Infant Is Getting Enough to Eat

1. Urination six or eight times a day. Most breast-fed infants have at least one or two stools a day during the first few weeks and may have as many as one every feeding.
2. Adequate weight gain.
3. Good color and skin tone.
4. Feeding every $1\frac{1}{2}$ to 3 hours, after which baby seems content.

Failure to Thrive

Causes. The failure of some breast-fed infants to thrive has been reported for several decades and in many respects is no less puzzling today than when it was first described. A flow chart summarizing possible maternal and infant causes of the problem is provided in fig. 7-10. In some cases, there is no history of excessive crying or dissatisfaction. The infant takes the breast well, nurses for a sufficient length of time, and sleeps well. There may be nothing to indicate abnormal nutrition or whether the infant is getting enough to eat (see the box on p. 188), until marked signs of dehydration and even marasmus appear.

Suckling process. According to Frantz and Fleiss, a major cause of failure to thrive in the totally breast-fed infant is a weak or ineffective suck.[41] As these clinicians have repeatedly observed, the baby who is gaining weight poorly often has a rapid, flutter-type chewing suckle

---

🍎	*CASE STUDY*

A Breast-feeding Infant's Early Growth Pattern

A young mother and her three-month-old infant appear in the clinic for routine well-baby care. The infant appears to be healthy but small. The body measurements reveal that weight falls on the 5th percentile and height plots on the 40th percentile. The mother reports that she is breast-feeding her baby, that things are going well but she is very tired, and that the baby is well behaved and rarely cries.

Questions for analysis
1. Define appropriate questions for the mother.
2. Outline a strategy to determine if the infant is receiving sufficient nutritional support through breast milk.
3. Propose an acceptable monitoring protocol.
4. Suggest solutions to the various problems that might be identified.

---

that does not seem to have any drawing pause between the jaw motions, and swallowing occurs only every three to fifteen suckles. On the other hand, they have noted that the babies who gain weight well also have a chew action to their jaw motions but display a slight pause in their cheeks between each suckle, and they appear to swallow with every suckle. The quality of the suckle often improves when an effort is made to hold the tongue down at the start of the feed and the tongue position is periodically checked. It also helps to have the mother switch breasts frequently, switching when inappropriate suckling begins to develop.

Evaluation of growth rate.   The breast-fed infant should be evaluated regularly to determine if growth is proceeding normally. If the infant fails to thrive, even after using techniques to enhance let-down and improve milk supply, and then improves when placed on a formula, either breast-feeding should be abandoned or a regular program of supplementary feeding should be established. The important point is to monitor growth closely enough that a life-threatening emergency and panic-weaning to bottle can be avoided. In some cases of failure to thrive at the breast, the mother should receive additional support to allay feelings of guilt and failure that will inevitably arise. Breast-feeding of a subsequent child is not necessarily contraindicated.

COMMON REASONS FOR FAILURE OF LACTATION ≋

Poor Maternal Attitude

Probably the chief reason for the failure of breast-feeding is a poor maternal attitude toward lactation in the first place. The mother who does not sincerely want to breast-feed her infant but agrees to do so to placate her family, friends, or nurse will have a very difficult time. Fear, worry, distraction, anger, and other such emotions have a potent effect on the let-down reflex. When this reflex functions poorly, the infant receives only a portion of the milk supply, because the bulk of the milk stored in the alveoli is not released. The infant cries from hunger and eventually fails to gain weight. This provides negative feedback to the mother, and a vicious cycle begins.

Inadequate Milk Supply

Failure to establish adequate milk supply by frequent feeding on demand is a great deterrent to successful lactation. Before breast-feeding is abandoned, the clinician should check to see if caloric intake has been adequate to support lactation. Are there anxieties and distractions to nursing that can be eliminated? Is the mother getting enough rest? Is she taking oral contraceptives or other medication that suppresses lactation? The problem may be inhibition of the let-down reflex rather than failure of milk production. Is the hospital routine nonsupportive? Other problems can stem from the use of supplements too soon and too frequently, as well as from early introduction of solid foods.

Lack of Information and Support

Another common reason for failure of lactation is lack of information and support for the mother. Many women do not have the support of friends or relatives who have successfully breast-fed infants. These women are often poorly informed about the physiology of lactation and about the virtually fool-proof method of meeting the infant's nutritional needs. New breast-feeding mothers may have fears of the milk supply being too low in quality or quantity to support the infant's growth requirements. They may become discouraged when the infant does not feed well because he or she has been sedated during labor and delivery. They may be discouraged by nipple discomfort or engorgement, common complaints during the first few days of breast-feeding. Often a new mother feels mildly depressed around the fourth or fifth day postpartum, and any initial lactation problems will be magnified out of proportion. This is particularly true if the mother does not see these occurrences as normal. If the parents have had adequate prenatal instruction and good counseling during the hospital stay, the chances of weathering these storms are greatly increased. If the breast-feeding mother has the support of her partner and understanding professionals who can provide kind words to bolster her confidence even when things are going fine, she will feel she has a place to which to turn for help and advice when things go badly. Under these circumstances, problems that cannot be avoided can be more easily overcome.

CONTRAINDICATIONS TO BREAST-FEEDING ≈

Galactosemia
Rare inherited disease in newborns caused by a missing enzyme (galactose-1-phosphate uridyl transferase—G-1-PUT), required for conversion of galactose (from lactose) to glucose. Untreated galactose accumulation in the blood causes extensive tissue damage and potential death. Normal growth and development now follows newborn screening and immediate initiation of a galactose-free diet with a special soy-base formula.

Phenylketonuria (PKU)
Genetic disease caused by a missing enzyme, phenylalanine hydroxylase, required for the metabolic conversion of the essential amino acid phenylalanine to the amino acid tyrosine. Untreated, profound mental retardation occurs. Normal growth and development now follow current mandatory newborn screening and immediate initiation of a low phenylalanine diet with special "low-phe" formula, such as Lofenalac.

Although each case must be evaluated on its own merit, there are very few conditions that automatically preclude breast-feeding. The genetic disease **galactosemia** is one *absolute* contraindication to breast-feeding. Breast milk is a rich source of lactose, and the very survival of infants with galactosemia depends on their receiving a nonlactose-containing formula. Galactosemia is a rare disorder, occurring in approximately 1 in every 60,000 births. Another genetic disease, **phenylketonuria (PKU),** is also often mentioned as a contraindication to breast-feeding. However, breast milk has relatively low levels of phenylalanine. In fact, infants who are exclusively breast-fed may receive a phenylalanine intake near the amount recommended for treating PKU. Total or partial nursing can therefore be used, although close monitoring of the infant's blood phenylalanine levels is required.

Mothers with a known transmissible viral disease, such as acquired immunodeficiency syndrome (AIDS) should probably not breast-feed (see chapter 6). Breast-feeding is also inappropriate in cases of alcoholism, heroin addiction, malaria, or severe chronic disease resulting in maternal malnutrition. Patients with active tuberculosis should not breast-feed. However, if the mother is being treated with an antituberculosis drug and is culture negative, breast-feeding is allowed. In such cases, careful checks of mother and infant are necessary, because an accumulation of the antituberculin drug Isoniazid can cause liver damage. Women with diagnosed breast cancer are usually advised not to breast-feed, so that the needed treatment can be given immediately. Maternal chemotherapy and radiation are incompatible with breast-feeding.

Mothers requiring drug therapy for management of chronic medical conditions may not be able to breast-feed if the only drug of choice is contraindicated during lactation. Recommendations of the American Academy of Pediatrics related to lactation and drug use are periodically updated (table 6-7).

Mothers who are active substance abusers should not breast-feed, out of a concern both for infant safety while a mother is under the influence of drugs and for the drug effects themselves. Cocaine is particularly dangerous, not only when ingested by the mother but also in the case of direct application of cocaine to sore nipples.

The use of diagnostic radioisotopes for use in one-time procedures, such as a thyroid scan or lung scan, should be evaluated on a case-by-case basis. Radiologists can often find an alternative isotope, or the dosage can be controlled, so that breast-feeding need be suspended for only a short time. Furthermore, with planning, a mother can pump and store her milk in advance of the test for the time during which she cannot nurse and can resume nursing when it is safe again. The other option when time is of the essence is for the mother to "pump and dump" her milk until the contamination period has passed. The baby will need to be fed either artificial baby milk or donated breast milk during the interim.

Contamination of breast milk by various toxins in the environment has also raised safety questions. These situations are also best evaluated on a case-by-case basis. Research into the aftereffects of the Chernobyl nuclear accident has yet to pick up levels of radioactivity in breast milk that exceed those in the environment in general, and no warnings have been noted in the literature coming out of Europe. The consensus among radiation oncologists in Chicago is that there is no radiation danger from the breast milk to infants born to mothers who have immigrated from the Chernobyl area to Chicago. However, cases of cerebral palsy in Minamata, Japan, from contaminated fish and in Iraq from contaminated seed have been documented. Cases have also been documented of fish contamination in Sweden, which has adopted a policy of discouraging breast-feeding in women from contaminated areas, despite the researchers' inability to identify a clear link between methylmercury and cerebral palsy.

WEANING ≋

Weaning signals the end of one phase and the beginning of another. Ideally, it should be a nonevent. Many cultures and the La Leche League support the idea of baby-led weaning. Actually, the minute the baby begins eating something other than breast milk, weaning has begun, even if nursing continues for months or years after that. *Weaning* is a term that connotes a certain maturity on the baby's part, which allows him or her to move from the breast to other foods and beverages. This is rarely the case in current American culture. Far too often, the mother weans prematurely for any of the reasons discussed in this chapter. Certainly, there comes a time when a baby needs to move on to other foods for proper growth and development, but all in good time. The U.S. surgeon general, the American Academy of Pediatrics, the American Dietetic Association, and others recommend that babies be breast-fed exclusively for the first six months of life, after which weaning should begin with the introduction of solids. How weaning progresses should be up to each mother-baby couple in consultation with their pediatrician and with correct information from dietitians.

Summary

An abundance of data support the concept that the advantages of breast-feeding far outweigh the disadvantages. Almost all women have the capacity to breast-feed in the postpartum period. A successful and enjoyable breast-feeding experience often depends largely on the early support of knowledgeable health care providers and the ongoing encouragement of significant family members, friends, and employers. Difficulties encountered along the way are usually manageable. Contraindications are few. Failures are rare. It is a desirable goal that all new mothers comprehend the importance of breast-feeding, for their infants as well as for themselves. In the end, however, the ultimate choice as to the mode of infant feeding is up to the mother and her family.

Review Questions

1. List six benefits of breast-feeding for the infant.
2. Define means by which a mother can determine if her infant is getting enough to eat.
3. Describe several reasons breast-feeding fails when it should not.
4. Are there any contraindications to breast-feeding?
5. List six sources of support for the woman who chooses to breast-feed her infant.
6. How long should a mother breast-feed her baby?

NUTRITION IN INFANCY: PHYSIOLOGY, DEVELOPMENT, AND NUTRITIONAL RECOMMENDATIONS

Donna B. Johnson

≋ ≋ ≋ ≋ ≋ ≋ ≋ ≋ ≋

Basic Concepts

❑ *Nutritional support of early physical growth and development provides the foundation for a healthy, productive life.*

❑ *Infants are born with the ability to digest and absorb nutrients from human milk or formula. The digestive system matures during infancy, so that a wide variety of foods can be used by the end of the first year.*

❑ *Individual energy and nutrient needs reflect rapid growth demands for fuel, building materials, and basal metabolism.*

❑ *Infant feeding behavior follows a defined developmental sequence.*

❑ *Maturing oral structures and function determine developing infant eating skills and appropriate textures of food.*

*T*he first year after birth is one of dramatic change for human infants. Growth is more rapid during infancy than at any other time in life. Infants progress from being newborns with no head control to being babies who pull themselves up to a standing position and begin to take steps. They move from securing their nourishment with a reflexive suck while they are held snuggly in the caregiver's arms to joining the family at the table and feeding themselves with a precise pincer grasp.

GROWTH AND MATURATION ≋

From birth to one year of age, normal human infants triple their weight and increase their length by 50%. Throughout this important first year of life, infant feeding and nutrition influence both physical and psychosocial growth and development. Growth and maturation can be either compromised or accelerated by undernutrition or overnutrition. The first six months of life are a critical period for brain growth, which is promoted by overall physical growth.[1] The stage of maturation determines the infant's developmental readiness to progress in the acceptance of foods, texture, and self-feeding. Through feeding and other interactions, parents and infants establish secure and trusting relationships.

The rate of growth in the first four months of life is faster than at any other time. A young infant uses a substantial portion of his or her energy intake to meet growth needs.

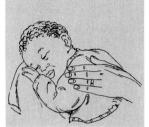

TABLE 8-1   *Weight Gain (g/day) in One-Month Increments*

Girls			
Age	10th percentile	50th percentile	90th percentile
Up to 1 month	16	26	36
1–2 months	20	29	39
2–3 months	14	23	32
4–5 months	13	16	20
5–6 months	11	14	18

Boys			
Age	10th percentile	50th percentile	90th percentile
Up to 1 month	18	30	42
1–2 months	25	35	46
2–3 months	18	26	36
3–4 months	16	20	24
4–5 months	14	17	21
5–6 months	12	15	19

Adapted from Guo, S.M., A.F. Roche, S.J. Foman. 1991. *Reference data on gains in weight and length during the first two years of life.* J. Pediatr, 119:355–62.

The period of four to eight months is a time of transition to a slower growth pattern, and by eight months the growth pattern is similar to that of a two-year-old. Assessment of physical growth is the primary method of determining infant nutritional status.

Weight and Length

Birth weight is determined by the mother's medical history, her nutritional status before and during pregnancy, the health-related events that occur during pregnancy, and fetal characteristics. Maternal prepregnancy weight and weight gain during pregnancy are especially important determinants of infant birth weight. After parturition, genetics, environment, and nutrition determine rates of gains in weight and height. Immediately after birth, there is a weight loss due to a loss of fluid and some catabolism of tissue. This loss averages 6% of body weight but occasionally exceeds 10%. Birth weight is usually regained by the tenth day; thereafter, weight gain during infancy proceeds at a rapid but decelerating rate. Average weight gains for the first six months of life are shown in table 8-1. The rate of growth slows substantially in the second half of the first year of life. By four months of age, most infants weigh twice their birth weight, and by twelve months they usually weigh three times what they weighed at birth. Males double their birth weight earlier than do females, and smaller newborns may double their birth weight sooner than do heavier neonates.

Length usually increases by 50% during the first year of life. The average length gain is 25 to 30 cm (10 to 12 in), but a period of "catch-up" or "lag-down" growth may occur. Most infants who are born small but are genetically destined to be longer shift percentiles on growth grids during the first three to six months. However, larger infants at birth whose genotypes are for smaller size tend to grow at their fetal rates for several months before the lag-down in growth becomes evident. During this lag-down period, length drops from a higher to a lower percentile rating on the growth chart. Often, a new percentile rating is not apparent until the child is thirteen months old.[2] Racial differences have been noted in rates of growth. African American males and females are smaller than Caucasians at birth, but they grow more rapidly during the first two years.[3,4,5]

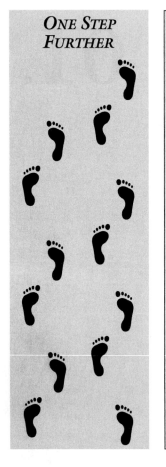

NCHS Charts

The most commonly used growth grids in North America are those prepared by an expert committee of the National Center for Health Statistics (NCHS). These charts have recently been revised and are soon scheduled to be available on the NCHS web site at **http://www.cdc.gov/nchswww.**

Previous growth grids were based on data collected from 1929 through 1975 on 867 white, mostly bottle-fed infants. The DARLING study of healthy, full-term breast-fed and formula-fed babies found that the growth of the breast-fed infants differed from both the NCHS standards and the growth of the formula-fed infants.* Mean weight of these breast-fed infants fell below the median on the former NCHS charts from six to eighteen months. Length gain was similar between the two groups, so the breast-fed infants were leaner than the formula-fed infants between four and eighteen months. There were no adverse consequences of this pattern of growth in breast-fed infants.

The new charts are based on a representative sample of U.S. infants that includes both breast-fed and bottle-fed infants. Infants are assessed using charts that go from birth to thirty-six months. Growth grids are provided for weight for age, length for age, head circumference for age, and weight for length. The grids are prepared so that age values lie along the axis, and height or weight values are plotted along the abscissa. Measurements at one age rank the baby's height or weight in relation to 100 other infants of the same age. Height-weight percentiles rank the baby's weight in relation to 100 other babies of the same length. Sequential measurements plotted on the growth grid indicate if the baby is maintaining, reducing, or increasing the percentile rating as growth proceeds.

*Reference only applies to study on breast-fed babies **not** new growth charts or growth assessment. K.G. Dewey, M.J. Heinig, L.A. Nommsen, I.M. Peerson, and B. Lonerdal. 1992. Growth of breast-fed and formula-fed infants from 0 to 18 months: The Darling Study. *Pediatrics,* 89:1035–41.

Growth acceleration
Period of increased speed of growth at different points of childhood development.

Growth deceleration
Period of decreased speed of growth at different points of childhood development.

Growth velocity
Rapidity of motion or movement; rate of childhood growth over normal periods of development, as compared with a population standard; also referred to as incremental growth.

Lean body mass
Collective fat-free mass of body composition; most metabolically active portion of body tissues.

Extracellular water
Water found in fluids outside of cells.

Intracellular water
Water found in fluids inside of cells; in body composition, this reflects lean body mass.

Growth Assessment

Growth is expected in a healthy infant, and physical growth is an indicator of the health and nutritional status of infants and children. Height, weight, and head circumference data are plotted on growth charts to assess how growth is proceeding. Measurements must be accurately obtained and accurately recorded, so that **growth acceleration** or **growth deceleration** can be monitored.

Assessment of incremental growth, or **growth velocity,** is an additional method of determining if growth is appropriate. This method is especially useful in assessing short-term growth and the growth of infants who are at high risk of growth problems.

Changes in Body Composition

Changes during growth occur not only in height and weight but also in the components of the tissue. Increases in height and weight and skeletal maturation are accompanied by changes in water, **lean body mass,** and fat.

Total body water as a percentage of body weight decreases throughout infancy from approximately 70% at birth to 60% at one year of age. Reduction of body water is almost entirely extracellular. **Extracellular water** decreases from about 42% of body weight at birth to 32% at one year of age. At the same time, **intracellular water** increases with the rapid growth of lean body mass toward the end of the first year.

The fat content of the body develops slowly during fetal life. Fat accounts for 0.5% of body weight at the fifth month of fetal growth and 16% at term. After birth, fat accumulates rapidly until approximately nine months of age. Between two and six months of age,

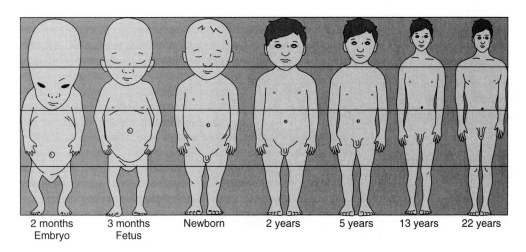

| 2 months Embryo | 3 months Fetus | Newborn | 2 years | 5 years | 13 years | 22 years |

FIG. 8-1   Changes in body proportions from second fetal month to adulthood.

the increase in **adipose tissue** is more than twice as great as the increase in the volume of muscle. Sex-related differences appear in infancy; females deposit a greater percentage of weight as fat than do males.

Adipose tissue
Loose connective tissue in which fat cells (adipocytes) accumulate and are stored.

Changes in Body Proportions

Increases in height and weight are accompanied by dramatic changes in body proportions. The head proportion decreases as the torso and leg proportion increases. At birth, the head accounts for approximately one-fourth of total body weight. When growth has ceased, the head accounts for one-eighth of total body length (Fig. 8-1). Between birth and adulthood, leg length increases from approximately three-eighths of the newborn's birth length to one-half of the adult's total body height.

Psychosocial Development

Feeding is the fundamental interaction from which the relationship between parents and infants evolves and the infant's psychosocial development proceeds. A parent's responsiveness to the infant's cues of hunger and satiation and the close physical contact during a feeding facilitate healthy development. For optimal development in early infancy, babies need to be fed as soon as they express hunger, so that they learn that their needs will be met. As they grow older and learn to trust that their needs will be met, they can wait longer for the initiation of the meal. All babies need to be held and cuddled while they are fed. Propping the bottle is unsafe and developmentally unsound in the first months of life.

Parents' ability to interpret cues and negotiate the feeding experience with their babies fosters healthy parent-child interactions and a sense of parental competency. Infants are born with characteristics that contribute to their overall **temperament.** Some infants are more irritable and less easily soothed. Some infants adapt easily to a regular schedule, whereas others continue to be unpredictable and irregular for several months. Parents may benefit from the opportunity to learn about temperamental characteristics to understand their infants better and to prevent the development of problematic feeding interactions.

Ideally, the infant should be in a quiet, wakeful **state** when feeding is initiated. An infant who is distressed and crying may find it difficult to feed appropriately. The quiet, wakeful state facilitates caregiver-infant interactions during feeding. The identification of the infant's cues of hunger and satiation is basic to developing a strong caregiver-infant feeding relationship. Cues change rapidly as development proceeds during the early years. The observant parent will recognize the changes and respond appropriately as the baby grows and develops.

Temperament
Inherited pattern of physiologic and behavioral reactions to situations. Components commonly include activity level, rhythmicity, approach, adaptability, intensity, mood, persistence, distractibility, and threshold.

State
The infant's condition. State is important in understanding an infant's response to environment. May be thought of as a continuum that includes quiet sleep, active sleep, drowsy, quiet alert, active alert, and crying.

DIGESTION AND ABSORPTION ≋

The physiologic development of the gastrointestinal (GI) tract is influenced by several factors. In utero, the fetal GI tract is exposed to amniotic fluid, which contains physiologically active factors, such as growth factors, hormones, enzymes, and immunoglobulins. As discussed in chapter 6, human milk provides epithelial growth factors and hormones, as well as digestive enzymes, to enhance the newborn's ability to digest and absorb feedings. These play a role in mucosal differentiation and GI development, as well as the development of swallowing and intestinal motility. Digestion and absorption in the newborn require:

- Coordinated sucking and swallowing.
- Gastric emptying.
- Intestinal motility.
- Salivary, gastric, pancreatic, and hepatobiliary secretions.
- Intestinal cell function to synthesize enzymes, absorb nutrients, and offer mucosal protection.
- Expulsion of undigested waste products.

The full-term newborn is prepared to digest and absorb an adequate supply of nutrients for normal growth and development from breast milk or formula. The infant's digestive capacity matures and increases during the first year of life. Feeding stimulates the release of several hormones that are related to GI motility, intestinal development, and pancreatic cell function. The developing stomach and intestines provide an increasing ability to handle various nutrients and textures provided by food. See Table 8-2.

GI Functions

Esophageal motility is decreased in the newborn, compared with that of older infants and children. In addition, the lower esophageal sphincter (LES) is primarily above the diaphragm, and LES pressure is less for the first months of life. Gastric emptying may be delayed in early infancy, and intestinal motility is more disorganized. Due to these physiologic realities, infants commonly experience regurgitation, or "spitting up." Stomach capacity at birth, 10 to 12 ml, increases to 200 ml by twelve months. Thus, newborns require small, frequent feeds.

Transit time through the small intestine is slower for infants than for adults. This may help assure the adequate digestion and absorption of nutrients. Passage through the large intestine is more rapid. Infants are at increased risk of dehydration if water and electrolyte resorption in the large intestine are further compromised.

Enzymes. Enzymatic secretions allow infants to digest and absorb the milk and food they consume. Quantitative information about exactly the amounts of these enzymes at each stage of infancy is lacking, but some relative findings have been established as summarized in the following paragraphs.[6]

Proteins. Protein digestion and absorption are limited by several factors in infancy. **Gastric pH** may limit digestion, although not as much as previously thought. Concentrations of **chymotrypsin** and carboxypeptidase in the duodenum are at only 10–60% of adult levels. Babies can digest adequate protein, even though the quantity of enzymes is limited. Newborns can completely digest about 1.95 g/kg/day of protein; four-month-old babies, about 3.75 g/kg/day. In other words, a 3.5 kg newborn would be expected to digest 6.75 g of protein. An intake of 12.5 oz (369.6 ml) of human milk meets the suggested energy intake and provides approximately 4.0 g protein. A formula-fed infant who consumes the same quantity receives 5.54 g protein; either protein intake is adequately digested by the infant.

Fats. Pancreatic lipase activity is low in the newborn, but other lipases from breast milk, the tongue (lingual lipase), and the stomach (gastric lipase) offer compensatory mechanisms for fat digestion. Human milk and colostrum have bile salt–stimulated lipase (BSSL), and the fat in human milk is more easily absorbed than that of infant formula.[7] The newborn bile acid pool, although present, is about half that of an adult on the basis of body surface area.

Gastric pH
Chemical symbol relating to H+ concentration or activity in a solution; expressed numerically as the negative logarithm of H+ concentration: pH 7.0 is neutral—above it, alkalinity increases and below it acidity increases. The hydrochloric acid (MCI) gastric secretions make gastric pH about 2.0.

Chymotrypsin
One of the protein-splitting and milk-curdling pancreatic enzymes, activated in the intestines from precursor chymotrypsinogen; breaks peptide linkages of the amino acids phenylalanine and tyrosine.

TABLE 8-2   *Summary of Digestive Factors in Early Infancy*

Factors	In Early Infancy Compared with Adult Levels	Compensating Mechanisms
Protein		
Gastric acid	Lower production: rapid fall in pH after a meal	
Trypsin	Reduced activity	
Chymotrypsin	Low levels	
Pancreatic proteases	Low levels	
Intestinal mucosal peptidases	Adequate	
Fats		
Pancreatic lipase	Very low levels	Lingual, gastric, and breast
Bile acids	Low levels	milk bile salt–stimulated lipase
Carbohydrates		
Salivary amylase	Low levels	Stays active in stomach
Pancreatic amylase	Very low levels	Breast milk amylase
Disaccharidases	Adequate levels	Fermentation and absorption in large intestine

Hamosh, M. 1996. Digestion in the newborn. Clin Perinatal 238:191–206.

Trypsin
Protein-splitting enzyme formed in the intestines by action of enterokinase on inactive precursor trypsinogen.

Carbohydrates. Sugars are well utilized. Maltase, isomaltase, and sucrase activity reach adult levels by twenty-eight to thirty-two weeks' gestation. Lactase, present in low levels at twenty-eight weeks' gestation, increases near term. True lactase deficiency in infancy is very rare, even in populations that have high rates of lactase insufficiency in adulthood. Pancreatic amylases are low or absent up to four months of age. Salivary amylase, present at birth, rises to adult concentrations between six months and one year of age. Even though a large percentage of the salivary amylase is suspected of being inactivated by hydrochloric acid in the stomach, young infants do digest some starch. This is thought to be due to the presence of glycosidase and glucoamylase present in the brush border of the small intestines. These enzymes hydrolyze starch to glucose.

Renal Function

The newborn has immature kidneys and can maintain water and electrolyte balance only within a fairly narrow range of intakes and losses. The functional development of the nephron is not complete until one month of age. The tubules are short and narrow and do not reach mature proportions until approximately five months. In addition, the pituitary gland produces only limited quantities of the antidiuretic hormone (ADH) vasopressin, which normally inhibits diuresis. These factors limit the newborn's ability to concentrate urine and to cope with fluid and electrolyte stress—that is, caused by electrolyte-dense formula, limited fluid intake, and diarrhea.

The major percentage of solutes presented to the kidneys for excretion are the nitrogenous end products of protein metabolism, sodium, potassium, phosphorus, and chloride. If none of these elements were utilized in new body mass or lost by nonrenal routes, such as perspiration, they would need to be excreted in the urine. They are therefore referred to as the potential **renal solute load.** The potential renal solute load can be calculated by assuming all nitrogen is excreted, dividing dietary nitrogen by 28, and adding sodium, potassium, chloride, and phosphorus in the feed expressed as **milliosmoles,** abbreviated **mOsm.**[8] Most healthy adults are able to achieve urine concentrations of 1,300 to 1,400 mOsm/L. A healthy newborn may be able to concentrate urine to 900 or even 1,100 mOsm/L, but an isotonic urine of 280 to 310 mOsm/L is the goal.

Renal solute load
Collective number and concentration of solute particles in solution, carried by the blood to the kidney nephrons for excretion in the urine, usually nitrogenous products from protein metabolism, and the electrolytes Na+, K+, Cl−, and HPO4.

Milliosmoles (mOsm/L)
Standard unit of osmotic pressure; equal to the gram molecular weight of solute divided by the number of particles (ions) into which a substance dissociates in solution. The term *osmolality* refers to this concentration of solutes per unit of solvent.

TABLE 8-3   *Potential Renal Solute Load of Representative Milks and Formulas*

Feeding	Potential Renal Solute Load, mOsm/L
Human milk	93
Cow's milk–based formula	135
Soy-based formula	165
Whole cow's milk	308

Difficulties with the renal solute load are unlikely in normal infants fed human milk or a correctly prepared formula (table 8-3). Problems may occur, however, when elevated environmental temperature or fever increases evaporative loss, when diarrhea occurs, or when infants reduce the volume of fluids they consume.

NUTRIENT NEEDS OF INFANTS ≋

Estimates of energy and nutrient needs in infancy have been made from intakes of infants growing normally and from the nutrient content of human milk. These are only guidelines, and each infant has requirements at different stages of infancy. The Food and Nutrition Board of the National Academy of Sciences has adopted new policies for establishing nutrient recommendations. The new recommendations are called **Dietary Reference Intakes.** Recommendations for individual nutrients are currently being phased in. New nutrient recommendations for vitamins and minerals listed in table 8 have not yet been established and these recommendations continue to be **Recommended Dietary Allowances.** The Academy has made new recommendations for nutrients listed in tables 7 and 9 but there was insufficient evidence to establish an **Estimated Average Requirement.** These have been established as **Adequate Intake** levels. Because of the declining growth rates during the latter part of the first year, recommended intakes have been set for two six-month periods, from birth to six months and from six months to one year.[9]

Energy

The current RDA for **energy intake** in infancy is 108 kcal/kg/day from birth through six months of age, and 98 kcal/kg/day for the second half of the first year.[9] These values were estimated from WHO data on intakes from healthy infants, with an additional 5% allowance for underestimation of intake. Energy requirement is higher in the first weeks of life, but it was determined that the data were insufficient to establish more precise breakdowns. A recent review of studies of well-nourished infants found that current recommendations are significantly higher than actual energy requirements and could lead to overfeeding if closely adhered to.[10] Breast-fed infants have lower requirements for total energy expenditure and energy cost of growth than do formula-fed infants (table 8-4).

The energy requirement in infancy is determined primarily by body size, physical activity, and growth rate. Since large variations in these variables are seen among infants at any age and in any one infant from month to month, ranges of energy needs are large. Total energy needs (kcal/day) rise during the first year, but energy needs per unit of body size decline in response to changes in growth rates. Energy expended for growth declines from approximately 32.8% of intake during the first four months to 7.4% of intake from four to twelve months.[11] The contribution of physical activity to total energy expenditure is quite variable but can be expected to increase with age as motor skills develop. Some infants are quiet and cuddly, while others spend a considerable amount of time crying, kicking, or just exploring with motor skills they have acquired. The most appropriate way to judge the adequacy of babies' energy intake is to monitor the adequacy of their linear growth and weight gain.

Dietary Reference Intakes (DRIs)
Nutrient recommendations established by the Food and Nutrition Board of the National Academy of Sciences.

Recommended Dietary Allowances (RDAs)
Intakes that meet the nutrient needs of almost all (97–98%) individuals in a group.

Estimated Average Requirement (EAR)
Daily intake value that is estimated to meet the requirement, as defined by the specified indicator of adequacy in 50% of individuals.

Adequate intake (AI)
Observed or experimentally set intake by a defined population or subgroup that appears to sustain a defined nutritional status, such as growth rate, normal circulating nutrient values, or other functional indicators of health. AI is used if sufficient scientific evidence is not available to derive an Estimated Average Requirement. AI is not equivalent to RDA.

Energy intake
Energy value of carbohydrates, fat, and protein in food, measured in kilocalories per kilogram.

TABLE 8-4   *Recommended Energy and Protein Intake for Infants*

Age in Months	Reference Weight (kg)	Energy Recommendations (kcal/kg/day)	Protein Recommendations (g/kg/day)
0–6	6	108	2.2
6–12	9	98	1.6

From National Academy of Sciences: 1989. *Recommended dietary allowances,* 10th ed. Washington, DC: National Academy Press.

TABLE 8-5   *Estimated Amino Acid Requirements of Infants Three to Four Months of Age*

Amino Acids	mg/kg/day
Histidine	28
Isoleucine	70
Leucine	161
Lysine	103
Methionine plus cystine	58
Phenylalanine plus tyrosine	125
Threonine	87
Tryptophan	17
Valine	93

From Energy and Protein Requirements, Report of a Joint FAD/WHO Ad Hoc Committee, World Health Organization technical report series No. 522, FAO Meeting Report No. 52, Geneva, 1973, World Health Organization.

Protein and Amino Acids

Infants require protein for synthesis of new body tissue during growth, as well as synthesis of enzymes, hormones, and other physiologically important compounds. Increases in body protein are estimated to average about 3.5 g/day for the first four months and 3.1 g/day for the next eight months.[11] The body content of protein increases from about 11.0% to 15.0% over the first year. The recommended intake is 2.2 g/kg for the first six months and 1.6 g/kg from six to twelve months.[9] The American Academy of Pediatrics has set minimum protein standards for infant formula of 1.8 g/100 kcal, with a protein efficiency ratio equal to that of casein.[12,13]

Nine amino acids are dietary essentials in infancy (see table 8-5). The subcommittee responsible for determining the amino acid requirements for infancy for the Recommended Dietary Allowances has concluded that the composition of human milk should be used as a reference pattern for amino acid requirements in infancy.[9]

Lipids

Fat. Fat, the most calorically concentrated energy nutrient, supplies between 40% and 50% of the energy consumed in infancy. The energy provided by fat spares protein for tissue synthesis. Its caloric concentration is an asset during periods of rapid growth, when energy demands are great. Fat provides about 50% of the energy when human milk or commercial infant formulas are the only source of nutrients, and it provides 47–49% of the energy content of commercial formula and about 52% of the energy content of human milk.

In the second half of infancy, as foods become increasingly important in the diet, the nutrient and energy content of those foods must be considered. Excessive consumption of traditional, high-carbohydrate weaning foods, such as cereal, vegetables, and fruits, may

CASE STUDY

Is My Baby Doing OK?

Mindy is a female Caucasian baby who was born at thirty-nine weeks' gestation with a weight of 3,000 g. She is the first child in her family, and her parents are seeking advice and reassurance about Mindy's nutritional situation. Mindy is now two months old. Two weeks ago, she weighed 4,000 g, and today she weighs 4,406 g.

There is a strong history of heart disease in Mindy's family, and her parents are very concerned about Mindy gaining extra weight and eating too much fat. Mindy's thighs and arms appear to be "filling out," and this is concerning her parents.

Mindy is being fed a low-iron commercial formula that provides 20 kilocalories per ounce. She usually takes six 4 oz bottles in a twenty-four-hour period. Her mother has given her some bites of infant cereal on the advice of an older family member. Mindy did not appear to like the cereal. She pushed it out with her tongue and turned her head away from the spoon. When her parents persisted, Mindy started to cry vigorously. Mindy's parents are concerned about her food refusal, and the older relative has insisted that they should "make" Mindy eat the cereal, even if she is crying. Mindy's parents are asking for advice about this practice. Her parents are also asking for advice about a vitamin or mineral supplement with fluoride.

Questions for analysis
1. Is Mindy's weight gain over the past two weeks appropriate?
2. When would you expect Mindy to double her birth weight? When would you expect her to triple her birth weight?
3. What can you tell Mindy's parents about fat deposition and body composition in the first months of life?
4. What can you tell Mindy's parents about nutrition and growth in infancy and adult chronic diseases?
5. Does Mindy's energy intake appear to be adequate?
6. How many kilocalories would the RDA suggest that Mindy needs?
7. How many kilocalories are being provided by her formula?
8. What might you counsel Mindy's parents about her iron intake?
9. What would you say about the need for a vitamin-mineral supplement with fluoride?
10. What are some reasons that cereal might not be appropriate for a two-month-old infant?
11. What advice can you offer about infant feeding cues and the possible consequences of "force feeding"?

Essential fatty acids
Fatty acids that must be provided in the diet because humans do not have the enzymes capable of forming the omega-3 or omega-6 double bonds. These include **linoleic acid** (18:2, omega-6), **arachidonic acid** (20:2, omega-6), and **α-linolenic acid** (18:3, omega-3). Important fatty acids formed from essential fatty acids are Docosatetraenoic acid (22:4 omega-6), Eicosapentaenoic acid (EPA)(20:5 omega-3), and Docosahexaenoic acid (DHA) (22:6 omega-3).

compromise both energy and nutrient intake for some infants. It is common for the percentage of energy from fat to drop precipitously between six and nine months of age and then to rise again as infants begin to eat more high-fat family foods.[14] This pattern of food and energy consumption may pose a problem for children with health or developmental problems that interfere with the ability to eat or digest foods or for children from vegan or health-conscious families who do not consume higher-fat, nutrient-dense foods. Growth failure has been reported in some infants and toddlers when fat intake has been inadequate.[14]

Long-term effects of lipid intake in infancy. Lipid and cholesterol intakes in infancy may establish metabolic programming that influences health throughout the life span. Research in this area is preliminary, but there are indications that feeding choices in infancy influence such factors as bile acid metabolism, cholesterol metabolism, and obesity.

Fatty acids. Major considerations of fatty acids in the infant diet include the adequacy of **essential fatty acids** to prevent essential fatty acid deficiency and the assurance of adequate long-chain fatty acids to promote growth and neurological development.

TABLE 8-6   *Range of Average Water Requirements of Infants and Children Under Ordinary Circumstances*

Ages	Amount of Water (ml/kg/day)
Three days	80–100
Ten days	125–150
Three months	140–160
Six months	130–155
Nine months	125–145
One year	120–135
Two years	115–125

Modified from Behrman, R.E, and R.M Khegman, eds. 1992. Nekon textbook of pediatrics, 14th ed. Philadelphia: W.B. Saunders.

Linoleic and **α-linolenic** fatty acids are the essential fatty acids for humans.[12] **Arachidonic** is sometimes considered essential as well, because it can prevent fatty acid deficiency when linoleic acid is inadequate. Linoleic is the 18-carbon fatty acid from the omega-6 family. α-linolenic is the 18-carbon fatty acid from the omega-3 family. A deficiency of linoleic or arachidonic (20 carbon, omega-6 fatty acid) acids results in the traditional fatty acid symptoms of scaly skin, hair loss, diarrhea, and impaired wound healing. Human milk contains 3–7% of kilocalories as linoleic acid. The American Academy of Pediatrics and the Food and Drug Administration specify that infant formula should contain at least 300 mg of linoleate per 100 kilocalories, or 2.7% of total kilocalories, as linoleate.

These essential fatty acids serve as precursors for the longer-chain fatty acids that are required for normal cell function. Humans have the capacity to make these longer-chain fatty acids if the essential fatty acids are present. However, this process is limited, especially in preterm infants. Considerable recent interest has focused on the importance of dietary sources of preformed long-chain fatty acids of the omega-6 and -3 families.

Human milk provides both parent and longer-chain essential n-3 and n-6 fatty acids. The brain and other neural tissue preferentially accumulate the omega-3 long-chain fatty acid **Docosahexaenoic** acid (DHA) in utero and in the first months after birth. Human infants have limited capacity to synthesize DHA from the parent omega-3, linolenic acid, and the availability of preformed DHA from the diet has been proposed as one possible explanation for higher intelligence quotients for breast-fed children.[15,16] Improved visual function has been reported in many, but not all, studies of infants who received formula with DHA, compared with controls fed nonsupplemented formula. However, some studies of DHA supplementation have found that the addition of DHA to formulas for preterm infants lowers growth rates. A balance of both omega-3 and omega-6 fatty acids appears to be the key factor.[17]

The dietary ratio of n-6 to n-3 fatty acids is critical, as these fatty acids compete for enzymatic pathways, and each can be metabolized to potent **eicosanoids.** In the United States, there are currently no commercially available infant formulas with DHA, and the addition of DHA and arachidonic acid (AA) to infant formulas is under discussion.[18] The case for adding DHA and AA to preterm infant formula is thought to be stronger than that for including long-chain polyunsaturated fatty acids (LC-PUFA) in all formulas. Preterm infants have very low LC-PUFA stores at birth. The appropriate commercial ingredient source for these fatty acids for infant formulas is not clear at this point.

Water

Infants require more water per unit of body size than do adults (table 8-6). A larger percentage of water is located in the extracellular spaces. As previously noted, young infants have immature kidneys. These two factors make the infant vulnerable to water imbalance. The water requirement is determined by water loss, water required for growth, and solutes derived from the diet.

Naming system for fatty acids
First number refers to carbon chain length. Number after the colon refers to number of double bonds. The omega number (also presented as "n" or "ω") refers to the position of the first double bond from the methyl end of the carbon chain.

Eicosanoids
Potent physiologic mediators such as prostaglandins, leukotrienes, and thromboxanes made from long-chain fatty acids.

TABLE 8-7 *Infant Dietary Reference Intakes for Calcium, Phosphorus, Magnesium, Vitamin D, and Fluoride, 1997*

Age	Calcium (AI) (mg/day)	Phosphorus (AI) (mg/day)	Magnesium (AI) (mg/day)	Vitamin D (AI) (μg/day)	Fluoride (AI) (μg/day)
0–6 months	210	110	30	5	0.01
6–12 months	270	275	75	5	0.50

Food and Nutrition Board. 1998. *Dietary reference intakes for calcium, phosphants, magnesium, vitamin D, and fluoride.* Washington, DC: National Academy Press.
AI: Adequate intake

Insensible water loss
Daily water loss through the skin and respiration, so-named because a person is not aware of it. An additional smaller amount is lost in normal perspiration, the amount varying with the surrounding temperature.

Hyponatremia
Abnormally low levels of sodium (Na+) in the blood; can be easily caused by excess water intake to point of water intoxication, with resulting dilution of the major electrolyte (Na+) in extracellular circulating fluids.

Water is lost by evaporation through the skin and respiratory tract (**insensible water loss**), through perspiration when the environmental temperature is elevated, and by elimination in urine and feces. During growth, additional water is necessary, since water is needed as a constituent of tissue and for increases in the volume of body fluids. The amount of water required for growth, however, is very small.

Water lost by evaporation in infancy and early childhood accounts for more than 60% of water intake needed to maintain homeostasis, as compared with 40–50% in adults. At all ages, approximately 24% of basal heat loss is by evaporation of water through the skin and respiratory tract. This amounts to 45 ml of insensible water loss per 100 kcal expended. Fomon estimates evaporative water loss at one month of age to average 210 ml/day and, at age one year, 500 ml/day.[11] Evaporative losses increase with fever and increased environmental temperature. Increases in humidity decrease respiratory loss. Loss of water in the feces averages 10 ml/kg/day in infancy.

The National Research Council recommends an intake of 1.5 ml/kcal of energy expenditure for infants.[9] Water intoxication resulting in **hyponatremia**, irritability, and coma can result if infants are fed too much water. This has been reported to occur when families do not have the resources to obtain adequate infant formula.[19] Under normal conditions, infants fed breast milk or infant formulas do not need additional water.

Minerals and Vitamins

The need for minerals and vitamins is influenced by growth rates, the mineralization of bone, increases in bone length and blood volume, and energy, protein, and fat intakes. Recommended intakes have been established for nutrients for which there is adequate information. Starting in 1997, the Food and Nutrition Board of the National Research Council began to publish the results of a new approach to nutrient recommendations. New Dietary Reference Intakes (DRIs) have been established for thiamin, riboflavin, niacin, vitamin B_6, folate, vitamin B_{12}, pantothenic acid, biotin, and choline,[20] as well as for calcium, phosphorus, magnesium, vitamin D, and fluoride (table 8-7)[21]. Current nutrient intake recommendations are listed in tables 7, 8, and 9. New DRIs for antioxidant vitamins and minerals are under consideration. In general, with the exception of vitamin K and possibly vitamin D, healthy infants who receive human milk or commercial infant formula do not need vitamin supplements.[12]

Calcium and phosphorus. The recommended intakes of calcium and phosphorus are based on the adequate intake that is observed in infants fed primarily with human milk. Calcium is well absorbed from human milk. About 61% of the calcium in human milk is absorbed, compared with 38% of the calcium in formula.[11,22] Commercial infant formulas have higher calcium content than human milk to compensate for decreased rates of absorption.

In the past, a great deal of attention has been given to the ratio of calcium to phosphorus in the diet. Healthy full-term infants can adjust to a range of phosphorus intakes, and phosphorus levels that are found in commercial infant formulas and from food in the infant's diet are unlikely to be a cause of concern.[23]

TABLE 8-8   **Infant Recommended Dietary Intakes for Fat-Soluble Vitamins, Vitamin C, and Minerals, 1989**

Age	Vitamin A (μg RE)	Vitamin D (μg)	Vitamin E (mg α-TE)	Vitamin K (μg)	Vitamin C (mg)	Iron (mg)	Zinc (mg)	Iodine (μg)	Selenium (μg)
0–6 months	375	7.5	3	5	30	6	5	40	10
6–12 months	375	10.0	4	10	35	10	5	50	15

From Food and Nutrition Board. 1989. From *Recommended dietary allowances,* 10th ed. Washington, DC: National Academy Press.
TE: Tocopherol equivalents
RE: Retinol equivalents

TABLE 8-9   **Infant Dietary Reference Intakes for Thiamin, Riboflavin, Niacin, Vitamin B$_6$, Folate, Vitamin B$_{12}$, Pantothenic Acid, Biotin, and Choline**

Age	Thiamin (AI) (mg)	Riboflavin (AI) (mg)	Niacin (AI) (mg)	B$_6$ (AI) (mg)	Folate (AI) (μg)	B$_{12}$ (AI) (mg)	Pantothenic Acid (AI) (mg)	Biotin (AI) (μg)	Choline (AI) (mg)
0–5 months	0.2	0.3	2	0.1	65	0.4	1.7	5	125
6–11 months	0.3	0.4	3	0.3	80	0.5	1.8	6	150

Food and Nutrition Board. 1998. *Dietary reference intakes for thiamin, riboflavin, niacin, vitamin B$_6$, folate, vitamin B$_{12}$, pantathenic acid, biotin, and choline.* (proposed) Washington, DC: National Academy Press.
AI: Adequate Intake

Iron. Rates of iron deficiency in U.S. infants have declined with increased breast-feeding prevalence and the consumption of iron-fortified formulas. However, iron deficiency anemia remains a concern for infants who do not receive breast milk, iron-fortified formulas, or foods with adequate iron in the second half of the first year of life. Iron deficiency in infancy may have long-term developmental consequences.

Infant iron needs are supplied from two sources, prenatal reserves and food sources. Before birth, the fetus accumulates iron in the last trimester of pregnancy. Premature infants have limited reserves, which are quickly depleted. Even with the advantage of full-term iron stores, the rapidly growing infant is at risk for iron deficiency because of the increase in blood volume as the baby grows larger. The concentration of hemoglobin at birth averages 17 to 19 g/100 ml of blood. During the first six to eight weeks of life, the concentration decreases to approximately 10 to 11 g/100 ml because of the shortened life span and decreased formation of fetal red blood cells. After this age, there is a gradual increase in hemoglobin concentration to 13 g/100 ml to two years of age.

Iron absorption is highly variable. See table 8-10. Two levels of **ferrous sulfate** fortification are available in commercial infant formulas—very-low-iron formulas and iron-fortified formulas. Iron-fortified commercial infant cereals are fortified with electrolytically reduced iron. Absorption of iron from infant cereal averages 5%. Many have recommended mixing this cereal with a fruit juice containing vitamin C to enhance the iron absorption. Healthy, full-term, breast-fed infants can maintain satisfactory hemoglobin levels without supplemental iron in early infancy. However, if they continue to be fed only breast milk after six to seven months, they are at risk of negative iron balance and may deplete reserves in the latter half of infancy.[24,25]

Zinc. Zinc deficiency is unlikely in healthy, full-term infants fed breast milk or a commercial infant formula in developed countries, but it is frequently reported in developing countries and in infants with failure to thrive. Compared with iron, relatively little is known about true zinc requirements and zinc absorption in infancy. It appears that infants

Iron absorption
Degree of iron absorption, relatively small at best, depends on the form of the iron (heme or non-heme) and its acid reduction either by accompanying food, such as orange juice, or by the gastric HCl secretions, from the ferric form (Fe+++) in foods to the ferrous form (Fe++) required for absorption.

Ferrous sulfate
Iron fortification compound in infant formulas; has been shown to be effective in prevention of iron deficiency anemia.

TABLE 8-10   *Iron Absorption in Infancy*

Feeding	Percent Reported Absorbed
Human milk*	48
Human milk—in 5- to 7-month-olds who are also eating solid foods†	21
Iron-fortified cow's milk–based formula‡	6.7
Infant cereals**	4–5

*Hallberg, L., Hutton L. Rossander, Brune, N., 1992. *Bioavailability in man of iron in human milk and cow's milk in relation to their calcium content.* Pediatr. Res. 31:S24–27.

†Abrams, S.A., Wen, J., and Stuff, J.E. 1997. *Absorption of calcium, zinc, and iron from breastmilk by five- to seven-month-old infants.* Pediat. Res. 41:384–90.

‡Hurrel, R.F., Davidsson, L., Reddy, M., Kastenmayer, P., and Cook, J.D. 1998. *A comparison of iron absorption in adults and infants consuming identical infant formulas.* Br. J. Nutr. 79:31–36.

‡Foman, S.J., Reigler, E.E, and Rogers, D.R. 1989. *Iron absorption from infant foods.* Pediatr. Res. 26:250–54.

TABLE 8-11   *Fluoride Supplementation Schedule*

Age	Fluoride Concentration in Local Water Supply (ppm)		
	<0.3	0.3–0.6	>0.6
6 months to 3 years	0.25	0.00	0.00
3–6 years	0.50	0.25	0.00
6 years to at least 16 years	1.00	0.50	0.00

American Academy of Pediatrics, 1998. Pediatric Nutrition Handbook, 4th ed. American Academy of Pediatrics. Elk Grove Village, IL.

Fluorosis

Effects of excess fluoride on dental enamel. Fluorosis can be classified on a continuum from "questionable" (slight aberrations from the normal glossy translucency of enamel) to "severe" (all surfaces affected with pitting and widespread brown stains).

Retinol

Chemical name for vitamin A, derived from its function relating to the retina of the eye and light-dark adaptation. Daily RDA standards are stated in retinol equivalents (RE) to account for sources of the preformed vitamin and its precursor, beta-carotene.

adapt to varied zinc intakes by increasing or decreasing absorption rates. Rates of absorption from formula have been reported to range from 41% when total zinc intake was low to 17% when total intake was high.[26]

Fluoride. Adequate fluoride intake is an essential component of preventive dental health care. On the other hand, excessive fluoride intake can cause **fluorosis.** Fluoride adequacy should be assessed when infants are six months old. Dietary fluoride supplements are recommended for infants who have low fluoride intakes (table 8-11).

Breast milk has a very low fluoride content.[27] Fluoride content of commercial formulas has been reduced to about 0.2 to 0.3 mg/L to reflect concern about fluorosis.[28] Fluorosis is likely to develop with intakes of 0.1 mg/kg or more.[28] Formulas mixed with water reflect the fluoride content of the water supply. The Food and Drug Administration does not require manufacturers of beverages to determine or disclose the fluoride content of their products.

Vitamin A. In the United States, excess vitamin A is more of a health risk in infancy than is inadequate vitamin A.[12,29] Human milk, commercial infant formula, and cow's milk are good sources of vitamin A. Vitamin A activity in foods is stated in **retinol** equivalents. In developing countries, low vitamin A intakes are associated with infectious diseases. These relationships are under study in more developed countries. At this time, the American Academy of Pediatrics recommends vitamin A supplementation under two circumstances in infants and toddlers who have complications of measles: supplements are recommended for infants between six and twenty-four months of age who are hospitalized with serious complications and for those older than six months who have risk factors, such as opthalmologic evidence of vitamin A deficiency, immunodeficiency, impaired absorption, moderate to severe malnutrition, and recent immigration from areas with high mortality from measles.[12]

Vitamin D. Vitamin D acts in concert with other nutrients—principally, calcium, phosphorus, and protein—to promote bone mineralization. Vitamin D requirements are dependent on the amount of exposure to sunlight. Rickets has been reported in some high-risk U.S. infants with dark skin,[30] and the American Academy of Pediatrics recommends supplements of 10 μg (400 IU) per day for breast-fed infants. On the other hand, the *Pediatric Nutrition Handbook*[12] states that, for white infants, adequate exposure to sunlight to produce vitamin D is thirty minutes per week, clothed only in a diaper, or two hours per week, fully clothed with no hat. These exposures are mediated by time of year as well as latitude.

Vitamin E. Defining appropriate intakes for vitamin E is complicated by large variations in the susceptibility to peroxidation of fatty acids in the diet and tissues. The recommended intake during infancy reflects the **tocopherol** concentration of human milk in which 6% of the kilocalories are provided by polyunsaturated fatty acid.

Vitamin K. Vitamin K is necessary for blood coagulation and other physiologic processes. Infants have low vitamin K stores at birth and are at risk for hemorrhagic disease of the newborn, which usually occurs two to ten days after birth. Breast-fed infants are at higher risk of this condition, which develops in 1 in 200–400 infants who do not receive prophylactic vitamin K soon after birth. Late-onset vitamin K–responsive bleeding is less common, but it has been reported in breast-fed infants who do not receive vitamin K therapy early in life. Since 1961, the Committee on Nutrition of the American Academy of Pediatrics has recommended a prophylactic intramuscular dose of vitamin K at birth. A Canadian committee recently revisited this recommendation and recommended a 1 mg dose of vitamin K shortly after birth.[31] Oral doses may also be given, but these are not as effective in maintaining adequate vitamin K status for the first months of life.

Water-soluble vitamins. In 1998, Dietary Reference Intakes were established for nine water-soluble vitamins (see table 8). In general, the Committee on the Scientific Evaluation of Dietary Reference Intakes found insufficient evidence to establish an RDA for these vitamins during infancy. Instead, the committee established a level of adequate intake (AI). For young infants, the AI is based on the daily mean nutrient intake supplied by human milk. The following are major considerations for each water-soluble vitamin:

- Requirements for thiamin and riboflavin are related to energy intake, since they function as coenzyme factors in energy metabolism.
- The fact that the amino acid tryptophan can be converted to niacin makes the basic requirements for niacin difficult to determine. Human milk contains 1.5 mg of niacin and 210 mg of tryptophan per liter.
- Vitamin B_6 (pyridoxine) functions as an essential coenzyme factor in the metabolism of amino acids and lipids, as well as nucleic acid, a key component of the genetic structure in the cell nucleus deoxyribonucleic acid (DNA). The requirement for this vitamin increases as protein intake increases.
- Vitamin B_{12} (cobalamin) is found primarily in foods of animal origins. Symptoms of B_{12} deficiency have been found in a few breast-fed infants whose mothers followed a strict vegan diet or had pernicious anemia.
- Body stores of folate at birth are small and rapidly depleted. Serum and erythrocyte levels fall below adult levels by two weeks of age and remain there during the first year of life. The folate needs of infants are adequately met by both human milk and commercial infant formulas. Goat's milk is folate deficient for human infants.
- Newborn infants consuming 7 to 12 mg/day of vitamin C (ascorbic acid) are protected from scurvy. An intake of 30 mg/day, based on the amount provided by human milk, is recommended during the first six months of life. Infants who are fed human milk or commercial infant formula receive adequate vitamin C.

Tocopherol
Chemical name for vitamin E, so-named by early investigators because their initial work with rats indicated a reproductive function, which did not turn out later to be the case with humans, in whom it functions as a strong antioxidant to preserve structural membranes, such as cell walls.

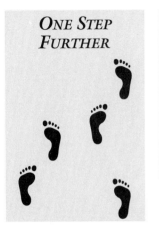

What About Supplements?

After initial supplements of vitamin K, full-term infants who receive milk from a well-nourished lactating mother will receive all the vitamins they need, with the possible exception of vitamin D and fluoride. The American Academy of Pediatrics recommends a supplement of 400 IU of vitamin D per day for breast-fed infants, especially African American infants and others with darker skin. Fluoride supplement decisions are based on the fluoride content of the water supply. Infants who receive a commercially available formula prepared with fluoridated water do not need a vitamin supplement. The need for supplemental iron depends on the composition of the diet consumed. Solely breast-fed infants should receive a source of iron by six months of age. Those who receive iron-fortified cereals probably do not need additional iron supplements. Infants receiving iron-fortified formula need no supplemental iron.

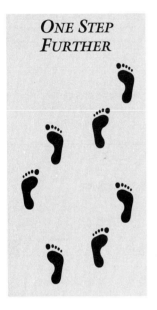

American Academy of Pediatrics Iron Recommendations for Full-Term Infants

- Breast-fed infants need an adequate source of iron by four to six months, preferably from a supplementary food. Iron-fortified infant cereal is a good source of iron.
- If a breast-fed infant is unable to consume sufficient iron from dietary sources, an elemental iron supplement may be used.
- For infants less than twelve months, only iron-fortified formula should be used for weaning or supplementing breast milk.
- Introduce iron-fortified cereal by four to six months or when the infant is developmentally ready.
- For infants, a good dietary iron source beyond fortified cereal is strained meal. This can be introduced after six months of age.
- Avoid the use of regular cow's, goat's, or soy milk before twelve months of age.

American Academy of Pediatrics. 1998. American Academy of Pediatrics. Elk Grove Village, IL.

DEVELOPMENT OF ORAL STRUCTURES AND FUNCTIONS ≋

Cineradiographic techniques
Fluoroscopic motion film records of internal structures and their functions.

In 1937, Gesell and Ilg published their now classic observations made during extensive studies of infant feeding behavior.[32] Their observations are as valid today as they were then. **Cineradiographic techniques** developed since then have permitted more detailed descriptions of the actions involved in sucking, suckling, and swallowing.

Even though the normal neonate is well prepared to suck and swallow at birth, the physical and motor maturation during the first year alters both the form of the oral structures and the methods by which the infant extracts milk from a nipple. Each of these changes influences the infant's eating skills. At birth, the tongue is disproportionately large in comparison with the lower jaw and essentially fills the oral cavity. The lower jaw is moved back relative to the upper jaw, which protrudes over the lower by approximately 2 mm. When the mouth is closed, the jaws do not rest on top of each other; the tip of the tongue lies between the upper and lower jaws. There is a "fat pad" in each of the cheeks. It is thought that these pads serve as a prop for the muscles in the cheek, maintaining rigidity of the cheeks during suckling. The lips of the neonate are also instrumental in suckling and have characteristics appropriate for their function at this age. A mucosal fold disappears by the third or fourth month, when the lips have developed muscular control to seal the oral cavity. The newborn infant sucks reflexively; the young infant suckles beginning at two or three weeks of age; and, as infants grow older, they learn mature sucking.

Suckling

The processes of breast and bottle suckling are similar, but there are subtle differences that make it difficult for some infants to go easily from bottle-feeding to breast-feeding once bottle-feedings have been established. The nipple of the breast becomes elongated during breast-feeding, so that it resembles a rubber nipple in shape, and both assume a similar position in the infant's mouth. The infant grasps the nipple in the mouth. The oral cavity is sealed off by pressure from the middle portions of the lips, assisted by the mucosal folds of the jaws. The nipple is held in the infant's mouth, with the tip located close to the junction of the hard and soft **palates.** During the first stage of suckling, the lower jaw and tongue are lowered while the mouth is closed, thus creating a negative pressure. The tip of the tongue moves forward. Next, the lower jaw and tongue are raised, compressing the beginning base of the nipple. The compression is moved from the beginning base to the tip of the nipple as the tip of the tongue withdraws, thus stroking or milking the liquid from the nipple. The moved-back position of the lower jaw maximizes the efficiency of the stroking action. As the tongue moves back, it comes into contact with the tensed soft palate, thus causing liquid to squirt into the side food channels. The location of the **larynx** is further elevated by the muscular contractions during swallowing. As the liquid is squirted back in the mouth, the epiglottis is positioned so that it parts the stream of liquid, passing it to the sides of the larynx instead of over it. Thus, liquid does not pass over the laryngeal entrance during early infancy because of the relatively higher position of the larynx and the parting of the stream of liquid by the epiglottis.

Sucking

Mature sucking is an acquired feature of the **orofacial muscles.** It is not a continuous process. On accumulation of sufficient fluid in the mouth, a swallowing movement interrupts sucking and breathing. The closure of the **nasopharyngeal** and laryngeal sphincters in response to the presence of food in the **pharynx** is responsible for the interruption of nasal breathing.

Swallowing

During swallowing, the food lies in the swallow preparation position on the groove of the tongue. The farther back portion of the soft palate is raised toward the **adenoidal pad** in the roof of the **epipharynx.** The tongue presses upward against the nipple, so that the swallow of milk follows gravity down the sloping tongue and reaches the pharynx. As the milk in the mouth moves downward, the rear wall of the pharynx comes forward to displace the soft palate toward the back surface of the tongue, and the larynx is elevated and arched backward. The accumulated milk is expressed from the pharynx by peristaltic movements of the pharyngeal wall toward the back of the tongue and the larynx. The milk spills over the joining folds of the pharynx, and epiglottis folds into the side food channels and then into the esophagus. The tonsils and **lymphoid tissue** play an important role as infants swallow. They help keep the airway open and the food away from the rear pharyngeal wall as the infant is held in a reclining position, thus delaying nasopharyngeal closure until food has reached the pharynx.

Mature Feeding

As the infant grows older, the oral cavity enlarges so that the tongue no longer fills the mouth. The tongue grows differentially at the tip and attains motility in the larger oral cavity. The elongated tongue can be protruded to receive and pass solids between the gum pads and erupting teeth for mastication. Mature feeding is characterized by separate movements of the lip, tongue, and gum pads or teeth.

Sequence of Development of Feeding Behavior

Newborn. The "rooting reflex" caused by stroking of the perioral skin including the cheeks and lips causes an infant to turn toward the stimulus, so that the mouth comes into contact with it. A stimulus placed on the lip causes involuntary movements toward it, closure, and pouting in preparation for sucking. These reflexes, thus, enable the infant to

Palate
Partition separating the nasal and oral cavities, with a hard, bony front section and a soft, fleshy back section.

Larynx
Structure of muscle and cartilage lined with mucous membrane, connected to the top part of the trachea and the pharynx; essential sphincter muscle guarding the entrance to the trachea and functioning secondarily as the organ of the voice.

Orofacial muscles
Adjoining muscles of the mouth and face.

Nasopharyngeal
Definition to come?

Pharynx
Muscular membranous passage between the mouth and posterior nasal passages and the larynx and esophagus.

Adenoidal pad
Normal lymphoid tissue in the nasopharynx of children.

Epipharynx
Nasopharynx; part of the pharynx that lies above the level of the soft palate.

Lymphoid tissue
Tissue related to the body system of lymphatic fluids.

suck and receive nourishment. Both rooting and suckling can be elicited when the infant is hungry but are absent when the infant is satiated. During feeding, the neonate assumes a tonic position, the head rotated to one side and the arm on that side fisted. The infant seeks the nipple by touch and obtains milk from the nipple with a rhythmic suckle.[32] Semi-solid foods, introduced by spoon at an early age into the diets of many infants, are secured in the same manner as milk, by stroking movements of the tongue with the tongue projecting as the spoon is withdrawn. Frequently, the food is expelled from the mouth.

Age four to six months. By four months of age, the more mature suckling pattern becomes evident, with the tongue moving back and forth as opposed to the earlier up-and-down motions. Spoon feeding is easier, because the infant can draw in the lower lip as the spoon is removed. The tonic neck position has faded, and the infant assumes a more symmetric position, with the head at midline. The hands close over the bottle. By five months of age, the infant can grasp on tactile contact with a palmar squeeze. By six months, the infant can reach for and grasp an object on sight. In almost every instance, the object goes into the mouth.

Age six to seven months. Between six and seven months of age, chewing movement, an up-and-down movement of the jaws, begins. This movement, coupled with the ability to grasp and the hand-to-mouth route of grasped objects as well as sitting posture, indicates the infant's readiness to finger feed. Infants at this age grasp with a **palmar grasp.** Therefore, the shape of the food presented to the child is important. Cookies, melba toast, crackers, and teething biscuits are frequently introduced at this stage.

Age seven months to one year. Between seven and eight months of age, the infant gains control of the trunk and can sit alone without support. The sitting infant has greater mobility of the shoulders and arms and is better able to reach and grasp. The grasp is more digital than the earlier palmar grasp. The infant is able to transfer items from one hand to the other and learns to release and resecure objects voluntarily. The tongue shows more maturity in spoon feeding than in drinking. Food is received from the spoon by pressing the lips against

Palmar grasp
Grasp of the young infant, clasping an object in the palm and wrapping the whole hand around it.

TABLE 8-12 *Sequence of Development of Feeding Behavior*

Age	Reflexes	Oral, Fine, Gross Motor Development
1–3 months	Rooting and suck and swallow reflexes are present at birth. Tonic neck reflex is present.	Head control is poor. Infant secures milk with suckling pattern, the tongue projecting during a swallow. By the end of the third month, head control is developed.
4–6 months	Rooting reflex fades. Bit reflex fades. Tonic neck reflex fades by four months.	Suckling pattern changes to a mature suck with liquids. Sucking strength increases. Munching pattern begins. Infant grasps with a palmar grasp. Infant grasps, brings objects to mouth, and bites them.
7–9 months	Gag reflex is less strong as chewing of solids begins and normal gag is developing. Choking reflex can be inhibited.	Munching movements begin when solid foods are eaten. Rotary chewing begins. Infant sits alone. Infant has power of voluntary release and resecural. Infant holds bottle alone. Infant develops an inferior pincer grasp.
10–12 months		Infant bites nipples, spoons, and crunchy foods. Infant grasps bottle and foods and brings them to the mouth. Infant can drink from a cup that is held. Infant uses the tongue to lick food morsels off the lower lip. Infant finger feeds with a refined pincer grasp.

Modified from Gessell, A., and F.L. Ilg. 1937. *Feeding behavior of infants.* Philadelphia: J.B. Lippincott.

the spoon, drawing the head away, and drawing in the lower lip. The infant is aware of a cup and can suck from it. Milk leaks frequently from the corners of the mouth, as the tongue is projected before swallowing. By seven months of age, infants are able to help themselves to their bottle in sitting postures, although they are not able to tip the bottle adaptively as it empties. By the end of the first year, they can completely manage bottle-feeding alone. By eight months of age, infants bring their heads forward to receive the spoon as it is presented to them. The tongue shows increased motility and allows for considerable increased manipulation of food in the mouth before swallowing. At the end of the first year, infants are able to manipulate food in the mouth with definite chewing movements.

During the fourth quarter of the first year, the child develops an increasingly precise **pincer grasp.** The bottle can be managed alone and can be rescued if lost. The child can drink from a cup if help is provided. Infants at this age are increasingly conscious of what others do and often imitate the models set for them.[32] By one year of age, eating patterns have changed from sucking to beginning rotary chewing movements. Children understand the concept of the container and the contained, have voluntary hand-to-mouth movements and a precise pincer grasp, and can voluntarily release and rescue objects. They are thus prepared to learn to feed themselves, a behavior they learn and refine in the second year. The development of feeding behavior is summarized in table 8-12 and is shown in the sequence of illustrations in figure 8-2.

Pincer grasp
Digital grasp of the older infant, usually picking up smaller objects with a precise grip between thumb and forefinger.

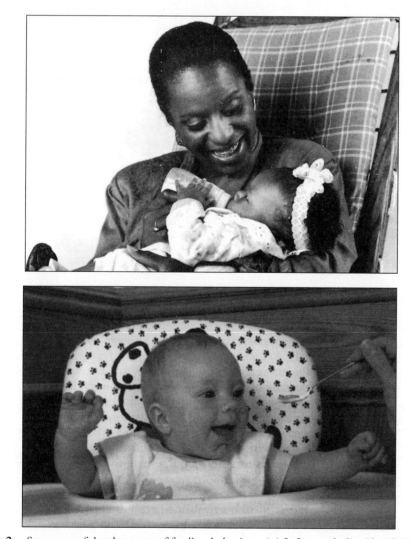

a

b

FIG. 8-2 Sequence of development of feeding behaviors. (*a*) Infant sucks liquids. (*b*) Eight-month-old infant is fed table food.

Continued

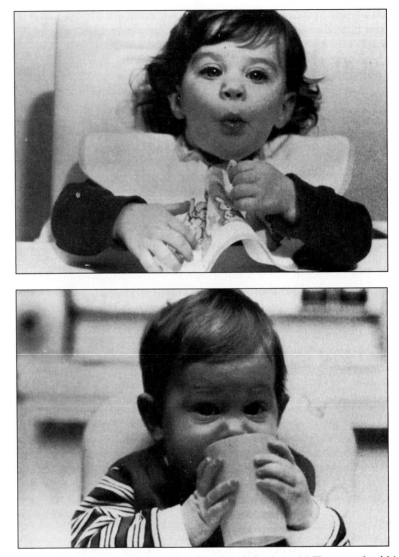

c

d

FIG. 8-2 cont'd.   Sequence of development of feeding behaviors. (*c*) Ten-month-old infant purses her lips. (*d*) Twelve-month-old infant drinks from a cup.

Summary

Like infants of all species, the human baby proceeds through a sequence of development that affects its nutritional requirements and the appropriate forms that foods should take to be "processed" adequately. The rapid growth of infants is supported largely by liquid nutrition. This source of nutrition must be highly nutritious, providing sufficient energy, protein, and micronutrients in a volume that can be taken easily. The quality of the infant diet can be judged to a large extent by monitoring physical growth.

Review Questions

1. Define the critical period for brain growth.
2. By one year of age, how much has a normal infant changed in weight and length?
3. How do body proportions of an infant change during the first year?
4. What is the difference between suckling and sucking?
5. Describe the "rooting reflex."

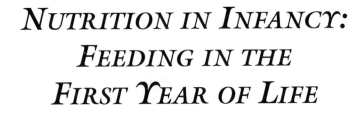

NUTRITION IN INFANCY: FEEDING IN THE FIRST YEAR OF LIFE

Donna B. Johnson

≈≈≈ ≈≈ ≈≈ ≈≈ ≈≈ ≈≈ ≈≈ ≈≈ ≈≈

Basic Concepts

❏ *The caregiver-infant feeding relationship is a key factor both in establishing long-term feeding behaviors and enhancing psychological development.*

❏ *The ideal food for the first months of life is breast milk. If breast milk is not available, a commercial infant formula is recommended for the first twelve months of life.*

❏ *Gradual introduction of solid foods in the second half of the first year of life supports both nutritional and developmental needs.*

❏ *Consequences of infant-feeding decisions may extend into adulthood.*

This chapter stresses the importance of feeding as a way to achieve an adequate energy and nutrient intake in a loving and supportive environment. Breast milk, or a substitute commercial formula if human milk is not available, can be the baby's sole source of nutrients and energy for the first six months.[1] Most healthy, full-term infants can regulate their intake to consume the amount they need to grow appropriately when they are fed on demand. The addition of semisolid foods, progressing to "table foods" in the latter half of the first year, provides energy and nutrients as well as support for oral and fine motor development. Feeding infants in a loving and nurturing environment helps them develop a sense of security and trust.

The discussions in this chapter are directed at the feeding of healthy, full-term infants in developed areas of the world where malnutrition in infancy is rare. In developing countries, breast-feeding and careful selection of weaning foods are the only safe and economically feasible approaches to infant feeding.

INFANT FORMULAS ≈≈≈

Breast-feeding is the preferred feeding method for human infants for the first year of life (see chapters 6 and 7). If human milk is not available, cow's milk–based infant formula should be substituted for the first twelve months of life. Infants who do not tolerate cow's milk may receive a soy or hydrolyzed casein formula, but these are indicated only in relatively few circumstances.[2]

The differences between human and cow's milk were discussed in chapter 6. From such comparisons, it soon becomes apparent that, if cow's milk is offered to infants, it

TABLE 9-1   *Nutrient Content of Human Milk and Representative Cow's Milk–Based Formulas*

Products	Protein		Fat		Carbohydrates	
	g/100 ml	Sources	g/100 ml	Sources	g/100 ml	Sources
Human milk	~1.0	Human milk	~3.9	Human milk	~7.2	Human milk lactose
Enfamil	1.4	Reduced mineral whey, nonfat milk	3.6	Palm olein, soy, coconut, high-oleic sunflower	7.4	Lactose
Gerber	1.5	Nonfat milk	3.7	Palm olein, soy, coconut, high-oleic sunflower	7.3	Lactose
Good Start	1.6	Hydrolyzed reduced mineral whey	3.5	Palm olein, soy, coconut, high-oleic sunflower	7.4	Lactose, corn maltodextrine
Similac (improved)	1.4	Nonfat milk, whey protein concentrate	3.7	High oleic safflower, coconut, and soy oil	7.2	Lactose
Lactofree	1.5	Milk protein isolate	3.6	Palm olein, soy, coconut, and high oleic sunflower oils	6.9	Corn syrup solids

must be modified to be more like human milk. Commercial formula ingredients have changed through the years to reflect current knowledge about optimal infant feeding. It is likely that this process will continue as the beneficial constituents of human milk continue to be identified. Antiallergenic factors, immunity-enhancing antibodies or antigens, growth-promoting factors, and biologically active factors that increase nutrient absorption have all been proposed as possible future additions to commercial infant formulas. In general, nutrients are offered in higher amounts in formula than in breast milk because of the lower bioavailability of nutrients from formula.

Formulas are usually categorized by the source and form of protein. In addition to the formulas discussed in the following sections, infant formulas are available for several special populations, such as infants born prematurely, those with severe problems of digestion and absorption, and those with special metabolic needs.

In the United States, regulations regarding the composition of infant formula have been recommended by the American Academy of Pediatrics Committee on Nutrition Task Force[3] and adopted by the Food and Drug Administration.[4] Laws and regulations set minimum levels for twenty-nine nutrients and maximum levels for nine nutrients, as well as labeling and quality-assurance requirements. For many years, the number of commercial infant formula choices was very limited, but formula brands have proliferated in the past few years. Some manufacturers now make brands that are marketed under different store labels.

Modified Cow's Milk Formulas

The American Academy of Pediatrics states that "standard cow's milk–based formula is the feeding of choice when breast-feeding is not used or is stopped before one year of age."[3] Table 9-1 lists approximate composition of major milk–based commercial infant formulas used in the United States. One difference between brands of formula is the relative content of cow's milk proteins, whey and casein. The predominant protein of human milk is whey, and the predominant protein in cow's milk is casein. Some formulas provide more whey proteins than do others. However, the whey proteins of human and cow's milk are of different composition. Infants appear to thrive equally well with either a whey- or casein-predominant formula. The proteins in **whey hydrolysate formulas** have been modified to have smaller peptides and to be less allergenic. However, they may still cause serious allergic responses in some infants. The butterfat of cow's milk is replaced with

Whey hydrolysate formulas
Cow's milk–based formulas in which the protein is provided as whey proteins that have been hydrolyzed to smaller protein fractions—primarily, peptides. This formula may provoke an allergic response in infants with cow's milk protein allergy.

TABLE 9-2 *Nutrient Content of Representative Soy Formulas and Other Milk Substitutes for Infants*

Products	Protein		Fat		Carbohydrates	
	g/100 ml	Sources	g/100 ml	Sources	g/100 ml	Sources
Prosobee	2.0	Soy protein isolate, L-methionine	3.6	Palm olein, soy, coconut, high oleic sunflower oils	6.8	Corn syrup solids
Isomil	1.7	Soy protein isolate, L-methionine	3.7	High oleic safflower, coconut and soy oils	7.0	Corn syrup, sucrose, modified corn starch
Nutramigen	1.9	Casein hydrolysate, L-cystine, L-tyrosine, L-tryptophan, taurine	2.7	Palm olein, soy, coconut, high oleic sunflower oils	9.1	Corn syrup solids, modified corn starch
Pregestimil	1.9	Casein hydrolysate, L-cystine, L-tyrosine, L-tryptophan, taurine	3.8	55% MCT,* corn, soy, high oleic safflower oils	6.9	Corn syrup solids, dextrose, corn starch
Alimentum	1.9	Casein hydrolysate, L-cystine, L-tyrosine, L-tryptophan	3.8	50% MCT, safflower and soy oils	6.9	Sucrose, modified tapioca starch

*Medium chain triglycerides

vegetable fat sources to make the fatty acid profile of cow's milk formulas more like those of human milk and to increase the proportion of essential fatty acids. Lactose is the major carbohydrate in most cow's milk–based formulas. Cow's milk–based formulas come in both a low-iron ($\leq$4.5 mg/L) and a more highly iron-fortified form (10–12 mg/L). The use of formula with iron is strongly encouraged to prevent iron deficiency anemia. True intolerance of iron-fortified formula is found to be low when placebo-controlled and blinded trials are used to assess the effects of iron in formula.

Soy Protein–Based Formulas

In the United States, formulas that provide protein in the form of soy protein isolate with added methionine account for about 25% of the formulas fed to infants. While they are a safe and nutritionally equivalent alternative to cow's milk formulas, soy formulas are not really needed by 25% of formula-fed infants. Approximate compositions of major commercial soy protein–based formulas are presented in table 9-2. Soy-based formulas are indicated primarily in the case of vegetarian families and for the very small number of infants with galactosemia and hereditary lactase deficiency.[2] They are often used inappropriately as a solution to feeding-associated problems due to physiologic immaturities, such as spitting, colic, and soft stools. Many infants with true protein milk allergy also develop allergy to soy proteins. These formulas are contraindicated in preterm infants, because they may provide inadequate bone mineralization. They are also inappropriate for infants with cow's milk protein–induced enteropathy or enterocolitis, for most previously well infants with acute gastroenteritis, and for the prevention of colic or allergy.[2]

Casein Hydrolysate Formulas

Casein hydrolysate formulas have been developed primarily for infants who cannot digest and absorb nutrients from other formulas and for those who have severe milk protein allergies. Proteins for these formulas are hydrolyzed to form free amino acids and small peptides. Most casein hydrolysate formulas are lactose free. Formulas may also contain varying amounts of **medium chain triglycerides (MCT)** to enhance digestion and absorption of fatty acids. These formulas are expensive and have a strong taste, and they should be used only for infants who truly need them.

Casein hydrolysate formulas
Infant formulas based on hydrolyzed casein protein, produced by partially breaking down the casein into smaller peptide fragments and amino acids.

Medium chain triglycerides (MCT)
Form of fat composed of fatty acids with carbon chain lengths of six to twelve carbon atoms. Compared with fats with long-chain fatty acids, MCTs are more easily digested and absorbed.

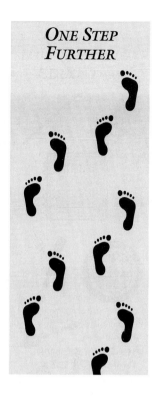

Remember Sterilization?

Sterilization of bottles and formula is no longer recommended if water supplies are safe and caregivers observe clean techniques. Commercially prepared liquid formulas are sterile before they are opened, and powdered formulas are free of viable microorganisms of public health significance. To prepare formula by clean technique, the hands of the person preparing the formula should be washed carefully. All equipment to be used during preparation, including the cans that contain the milk, the can openers, the bottles, and the nipples, must be thoroughly washed and rinsed. Once opened, cans of formula must be covered and refrigerated. After the formula has been heated and the infant has been fed, any remaining milk should be discarded; warm milk is an excellent medium for bacterial growth. Formula from bottles that have been partially finished should be discarded.

The microwaving of formula bottles is generally discouraged. Serious burns have resulted from this practice.* Safe techniques have been proposed, as parents are known to use the microwave for warming bottles despite advice to do otherwise. Recommended techniques include heating only 4 ounces at a time in an 8-ounce, uncovered bottle, heating for no more than thirty seconds, inverting the bottle ten times after heating, and testing the formula on the caregiver's tongue or top of the hand.

---

*Dixon, J.J., Burd, D.A., and Roberts, D.G. 1997. *Severe burns resulting from an exploding teat on a bottle of infant formula milk heated in a microwave oven.* Burns, 23: 268–69.

Formula and Milk for Older Infants

Follow-up formulas have been developed for older infants and toddlers. These products have a higher protein and mineral content than standard formulas. They have been developed to complement the high-carbohydrate diet that results when weaning foods, such as cereals, fruits, and vegetables, are added to the diet. Follow-up formulas have the advantage of being higher in iron than cow's milk, but they offer no clear advantage when weaning foods are chosen carefully.[3]

The use of whole, 2%, 1%, or nonfat cow's milk, goat's milk, or evaporated milk in the first year is strongly discouraged. Use of these products may lead to iron deficiency anemia. These milks have high solute loads and limited levels of essential fatty acids, vitamin E, zinc, and other nutrients, and goat's milk has inadequate folate.

Substitute and Imitation Milks

Feeding infants formulas made from recipes, substitute milks, or imitation milks that have not been proven to support adequate nutrition is strongly discouraged. Substitute milk is defined by the U.S. Food and Drug Administration as nutritionally equivalent to whole or nonfat milk, based on the content of only fourteen or fifteen nutrients. It does not include all nutrients and could pose significant problems for infants who have no other source of nutrients in the diet. Malnutrition was observed in infants fed a barley water, corn syrup, and whole milk formula suggested in a magazine for mothers.[5] Kwashiorkor, an advanced protein-deficiency state of malnutrition, has been reported in infants fed a nondairy creamer as a substitute for milk.[6] Substitute or imitation milks should not be offered to infants.

Formula Preparation

Standard infant formula provides 20 kcal/oz if prepared according to manufacturers' directions. Manufacturers market three basic types of formulas, each of which is prepared according to its form: 1) liquid concentrate prepared for feeding by mixing equal amounts of the liquid and water; 2) ready-to-feed formulas available in an assortment of sizes (4, 6, and 8 oz bottles and 32 oz containers); and 3) powdered formulas prepared by mixing them with a prescribed amount of water. All of these formulas, when properly prepared, provide the nutrients important for the infant in an appropriate caloric concentration and present a solute load reasonable for the full-term infant.

Errors in dilution caused by lack of understanding of the proper method of preparation, improper measurements, extra water added to make the formula last longer, and parents' belief that their child should have greater amounts of nutritious food can lead to problems. Feeding dilute formula over time can lead to undernutrition and water intoxication, with symptoms of hyponatremia, irritability, and, in severe cases, coma.[7] Feedings that are too highly concentrated increase kilocalories, protein, and solutes presented to the kidneys for excretion and may predispose the young infant to hypernatremia, dehydration, and tetany, as well as obesity.[8,9] Problems of improper formula preparation have been reported most frequently with the use of powdered formula and occur most often when an increased need for water caused by a fever or an infection is superimposed on consumption of an already high-solute formula. Infants fed concentrated formula during such illnesses may become thirsty, demand more to drink, or refuse to consume more liquid because of anorexia secondary to the illness. When presented with more milk concentrated in the protein and solutes, the **osmolality** of the blood increases, and **hypernatremic dehydration** may result. Cases of cerebral damage and gangrene of the extremities have been reported to be the result of **hypernatremic dehydration** and **metabolic acidosis.**

A DEVELOPMENTAL APPROACH TO INFANT FEEDING ≈≈

Infancy is a time of rapid physical and psychosocial development. Recommendations for infant feeding reflect understandings about the best way to support optimal development. Illingworth and Lister have defined a "critical or sensitive" period of development in relation to eating.[10] For example, they point out that infants learn to chew at about six or seven months of age; thus, at this point they are developmentally ready to consume food. If solid foods are withheld until a later age, the child will have considerably more difficulty in accepting them.

Between six and twelve months of age, the infant gradually progresses from pureed and strained to mashed and chopped foods. Foods should be carefully selected and modified, so that they are presented in a form that can be manipulated in the mouth without the potential for choking and aspirating. Family foods such as well-cooked ground meats, mashed beans and peas, flaked tuna, tofu, and family casseroles can be added gradually at the end of the first year.

It is important to note that not all infants develop at the same rate and that temperamental characteristics and the temperamental match between caregivers and infants influence the feeding situation. Children who are overly sensitive to their environment may not want to explore food in the same way as other children. Some children are more **neophobic** when they encounter new foods and will take longer to warm up to them. Parents may need support and guidance as they seek the best approach to feeding their children. Disturbed feeding interactions that result from a lack of understanding and/or insistence on inappropriate parental control may result in persistent feeding problems and eating disorders.

The American Academy of Pediatrics states that newborns should be fed whenever they show signs of hunger, such as increased alertness or activity, mouthing, or rooting. By the time an infant is crying from hunger, earlier cues have usually been missed. Newborn infants initially feed eight to twelve times a day at intervals of two to four hours. Formula-fed infants usually consume 2 to 3 ounces at a feeding. Formula-fed infants may go longer between feedings than do breast-fed infants. There is wide variation in the age at which young infants are capable of sleeping through the night without waking for feedings. Although it is easier on parents, going through the night without a feeding is not necessarily best for quiet and undemanding infants in the first weeks of life, especially if they are growing slowly.

To avoid both under- or overfeeding, infant caregivers should attend to the infant's feeding cues (see table 9-3). Infant cues for hunger and satiety range from subtle to obvious. A young infant who is hungry usually suckles vigorously. Older infants lean forward

Osmolality
Property of a solution that depends on the concentration of the particles (solutes) in solution per unit of solvent base; measured as milliosmoles per liter (mOsm/L).

Hypernatremic dehydration
Abnormally high sodium ion concentration in the extracellular fluid, due to water loss or restriction, drawing cell water to restore osmotic balance, causing dangerous cell dehydration.

Metabolic acidosis
Abnormal rise in acid partner of the carbonic acid-base bicarbonate buffer system by excess of organic acids, which displace part of the base bicarbonate in the buffer system and cause the H+ concentration to rise.

Neophobic
Fear of new and unfamiliar foods.

TABLE 9-3   *Hunger and Satiety Behaviors of Infants*

Age Behaviors Established	Hunger	Satiety
Early infancy	Fusses and cries, mouths the nipple.	Draws away from nipple, falls asleep.
16–24 weeks	Actively approaches breast or bottle, leans forward to spoon.	Releases nipple and withdraws head, fusses or cries, bites nipple, increases attention to surroundings.
28–36 weeks	Vocalizes eagerness for bottle or food.	Changes position, shakes head, keeps mouth tightly closed, hands become more active.
40–52 weeks	Points or touches spoon or feeder's hand.	Behaviors as above, sputters with tongue and lips, hands bottle or cup to feeder.

Are We Born with a Sweet Tooth?

Newborn infants demonstrate a preference for sugar solutions over water and formula and show adverse responses to sour and bitter tastes. Many other food-related likes and dislikes appear to be learned. Infants may require repeated exposures before they accept a new food. Sullivan and Birch found that most of the infants they studied increased their intake of vegetables when they had been exposed to them at least five to ten times.* This study also found that the breast-fed infants accepted new foods more readily than did those fed with bottles. One explanation for this finding may be that the passage of flavors from the mother's diet through her milk programs the infant to be more accepting of new tastes. Young children learn their food habits from their families. Anticipatory guidance about optimizing family food habits may be helpful.

---

*Sullivan, S.A. and Birch, L.L. 1994. *Infant dietary experience and acceptance of solid foods.* Pediatrics. 93: 271–77.

ONE STEP FURTHER

toward the food or reach out for the breast, bottle, or spoon. To demonstrate satiety, a young infant may fall asleep or stop suckling at the breast. An infant who is being fed in a high chair or on a caregiver's lap may avert his or her eyes, wave his or her arm in a "halt" hand, turn away from the caregiver, start playing with the eating utensils, refuse to open his or her mouth, or push the dish away.

Both bottle- and breast-feeding parents benefit from basic feeding information in the newborn period. Lawrence[11] calls attention to the importance of positioning and interactions during feedings and recommends the following:

1. All infants should be fed in a semiupright position, with the infant's head held securely in the crook of the elbow of the caregiver. Semi-upright feeding has been associated with reduced incidence of entrance of milk into the middle ear during feedings.[12]

2. The rooting reflex should be elicited by stimulating the central portion of the lower lip.

3. The bottle should be positioned so that the nipple and neck remain filled with milk until the end of the feeding.

4. Bottle-feeding, like breast-feeding should be a social event.

Experience with "problem eaters" in later infancy and early childhood suggests that parents can also benefit from anticipatory guidance about approaches to feeding[13]:

1. It is important to introduce foods with differing tastes and textures in the second half of the first year of life.
2. "Neophobia" is normal, and most infants benefit from repeated exposure to new foods.
3. Food should not be used as a reward or bribe.
4. Force feeding and excessive coaxing are counterproductive, and parents should pay attention to the infant's satiety cues.

SEMISOLID FOODS IN THE INFANT'S DIET ≋

Introduction of Foods

Recommendations to introduce nonmilk feedings between four and six months of age have been in place since the 1960s, but many families have chosen to give foods before four months. Data from the 1988 National Maternal and Infant Health Survey found that many Caucasian and African American infants had received foods earlier than recommended.[14] In both groups, more than a quarter of the infants had received solid foods by 2 months, and intakes rapidly increased after 2 months. The African American infants had been offered both a greater quantity of solid foods and more variety of solid foods than the Caucasian infants from 1 month until 5 months of age. See tables 9-4 and 9-5.

Recommendations for the lower age limit for the introduction of nonmilk feedings are based primarily on the achievement of indicators of physiologic and developmental readi-

TABLE 9-4 *Suggested Ages for the Introduction of Semisolid Foods and Table Food*

	Age		
Foods	**Four to Six Months**	**Six to Eight Months**	**Nine to Twelve Months**
Iron-fortified cereals for infants	May begin to add but are not necessary	Add	
Vegetables		Add strained	Mashed and chopped, progressing to table foods
Fruits		Add strained	Mashed and chopped, progressing to table foods
High-protein foods		Add strained or finely chopped table meats, mashed legumes (prepared dried beans and lentils), tofu	Decrease the use of strained products, increase texture
Finger foods, such as arrow-root biscuits and oven-dried toast		Add those that can be secured with a palmar grasp	Increase the use of safe, small finger foods as the pincer grasp develops
Well-cooked mashed or chopped table foods, prepared without added salt or sugar			Add
Juice by cup			Add small amounts if desired

ness. These include adequate head and truck motor control to indicate desire for food or satiety by leaning forward or backing away, as well as the disappearance of the extrusion reflux. Most infants are developmentally ready for an introduction to pureed foods between four and six months of age.

Several concerns have been raised about the introduction of foods in infancy before four months of age. In the first weeks of life, immaturity of the kidneys precludes large osmolar loads of protein and electrolytes, and the digestion of some fats, proteins, and carbohydrates is compromised. At age three to five months, infants are able to digest and absorb cereal, but, at age one to two months, carbohydrate and protein digestion and absorption are compromised by cereal ingestion.[15] In the first months of life, poorly developed swallowing skills may lead to aspiration. Increased respiratory illness and persistent cough have been reported in infants given solids early,[16] and coughing may increase following the ingestion of formula thickened with infant cereal.[17] Early introduction of a variety of solid foods may increase risk of atopic and immunological disease in susceptible children.[18,19]

If the introduction of nonmilk feedings is delayed past age six or seven months, nutritional status may be compromised. Breast milk alone may not provide sufficient nutrients or energy for the rapidly growing infant. The growth of breast-fed infants may be compromised if supplemental feedings are not initiated in the second half of the first year, but there seems to be a great deal of individual variability in response to the delay in introduction of foods.

Food Choices

First foods for infants may be prepared from family foods or may be purchased as commercially available infant foods. Most families use a combination of food sources (see table 9-6). Few infants require specialized infant foods beyond the first year. If feeding of semisolid foods is delayed until the infant is developmentally ready, the period of time that modified infant foods are required is fairly short. Foods should be introduced one at a time to assure that any adverse reactions can be pinpointed. Within general categories, the order of food introduction is not important.

TABLE 9-5 *Sample Menus for Infants at Various Ages*

Age	Weight (kg)	Energy Needs (kcal/kg)	Menu
2 months	5.00	540	26–28 oz human milk or infant formula
6–8 months	7.75	775	30 oz human milk or infant formula
			1/4 cup mashed or strained carrots
			1/2 cup iron-fortified infant cereal
			1/4 cup mashed or strained pears
			1 piece dry toast
10 months	9.50	925	24–30 oz formula or human milk
			1/2 cup iron-fortified cereal
			1/4 cup applesauce
			1/4 frozen bagel
			1 oz finely chopped chicken
			1/4 cup mashed baked potato
			1/4 cup mashed peas
			1/4 oz cheese strip
			1/2 cup soft noodles mixed with ground meat
			2 tbsp well-cooked broccoli
			1/2 banana
			1/4 cup Cheerios

TABLE 9-6 *Advantages of Commercial and Home Preparation of Infant Foods*

Home Preparation	Commercial Infant Foods
• Prepares infant for transition to family foods.	• Easily and safely transported for meals away from home.
• Usually less expensive.	• Low in sodium (although salt is added to some commercial products).
• Mixed "dinner"-type foods usually higher in protein and more nutrient-dense than commercial products that may have higher water and carbohydrate content.	• Fast and easy to prepare for busy families.
• Meats and protein foods usually more aesthetically acceptable than commercial meats.	• Some vegetables have lower levels of nitrites.
• Infant cereals are fortified with iron that is easily absorbed by infants.	• Commercial companies make an effort to secure pesticide-free foods.

Commercial Infant Foods

Cereals. Ready-to-serve dry infant cereals are fortified with electrically reduced iron. Three level tablespoons of cereal provide about 5 mg of iron, or from one-half to one-third of what the infant requires. Therefore, cereal is usually the first food added to the infant's diet. Cereal and fruit mixtures in jars are fortified with ferrous sulfate to provide 7 to 9 mg of iron per 4.5 oz jar. Other sources of iron should be considered if the infant is not offered commercial infant cereals.

Fruits and vegetables. Strained and junior fruits and vegetables provide carbohydrates and variable amounts of vitamins A and C. Vitamin C is added to a number of the fruits and all of the fruit juices. Several fruits, including apricots, have sugar added and are marketed as fruit desserts. Tapioca is added to a number of the fruits. Milk is added to creamed vegetables, and wheat is incorporated into mixed vegetables. Commercial infant juices are convenient but expensive and unnecessary; most regular fruit juices may be used for infants. Juice should never be given in a bottle, and intakes over 4 ounces a day present a risk for oral health.

Meats and combination foods. Strained and junior meats are prepared with only water, except for lamb, which has lemon juice added. Strained meats, which have the highest caloric density of any of the commercial baby foods, are an excellent source of high-quality protein and heme iron. Water is the most abundant ingredient in meat and vegetable combinations and high-meat dinners, and these products are generally low in protein and other nutrients. The introduction of these products should be delayed until it has been determined that the infant has no allergic reactions to any of the wide variety of ingredients they contain.

Desserts. Infant puddings and fruit desserts are also available. The nutrient composition of commercial desserts varies, but all contain sugar and modified corn or tapioca starch. These products should be used in moderation. See table 9-7.

Home Preparation of Infant Foods

There are two overarching considerations in the preparation of foods for infants at home: 1) food safety and 2) preservation of nutrients. The following procedures should be followed:

- Foods should be carefully selected from high-quality fresh, frozen, or canned (without added salt or sugar) fruits, vegetables, and meats and prepared so that nutrients are retained.
- The preparation area and all utensils should be well cleaned. Salt and sugar should be used sparingly, if at all.

TABLE 9-7   *Ranges of Selected Nutrients per Ounce in Commercially Prepared Infant Foods*

Foods	Energy (kcal)	Protein (mg)	Iron (mg)	Vitamin A (RE)	Vitamin C (mg)
Dry cereal	120	2.0–10.0	14.3	*	*
1st Foods, 2nd Foods, and 3rd Foods fruits	12–29	0.0–0.3	0.0–0.1	0.3–34	*–6.3
1st Foods, 2nd Foods and 3rd Foods vegetables	9–20	0.2–0.9	0.0–0.3	0.3–440	0.0–2.2
2nd Foods and 3rd Foods meats	28–37	3.0–4.4	0.2–0.4	*	*
2nd Foods and 3rd Foods dinners	12–22.4	0.5–1.1	0.1–0.2	0.3–341	*–5.3
2nd Foods and 3rd Foods desserts	19–25	0.0–0.5	0.0–0.1	*–10.5	*–4.0

From 1995 Gerber Products Company: Nutrient Values, Fremont, MI, Rev l2/94. 1st Foods, 2nd Foods, and 3rd Foods are trademarks of Gerber Products Company.
*Quantity insignificant

- Fruits and vegetables should be cooked in minimal amounts of water or steamed until tender.
- Depending on the infant's readiness for texture, food can be pureed or strained with a food processor, blender, grinder, or fork.
- Foods can be moistened with water, cooking water, or milk.
- If food is being prepared for future meals, it should be packaged in individual portions and refrigerated or frozen, so that a single portion can be heated and fed without compromising the quality and bacterial content of the entire batch.
- Individual portions of frozen foods should not be thawed at room temperature but should be thawed in the refrigerator or gently heated.

Food from the family menu is introduced at an early age in the diets of many infants. The age of infants at introduction and type of food offered reflect cultural practice. Although it has been common to offer bland foods to infants in the United States, many older infants enjoy highly flavored foods, which reflect the family's culture, with no apparent adverse effects. Examples include crumbled cornbread mixed with pot liquor (the liquid from cooked vegetables), traditionally fed to African American infants, and mashed beans with some of the cooking liquid, fed to Mexican American infants.

By the end of the first year, the diets of most infants should be similar to that of the family, and dietary guidelines for older infants are similar to those for the general population. Older infants need a variety of foods from all the pyramid food groups and adequate energy to support growth. Moderation is key in food choices. There is little room in the infant's diet for large servings of foods that are low in nutrients and high in fat or sugar. On the other hand, excessive intakes of low-energy/low-fat foods have been associated with growth failure. Adequate intakes of fiber normalize digestive and absorption processes. A target of 5 grams of fiber per day is suggested for the second six months of life;[20] this can be achieved easily with a daily total of $\frac{1}{2}$ cup each of fruits and vegetables and $\frac{1}{2}$ cup of infant cereal.

Feeding Infants: Safety Issues

Form and texture. Semisolid foods offered to infants should be in a form easily masticated and not in small pieces. Choking and aspiration can occur if small pieces of hot dogs, grapes, hard candy, nuts, and other food are consumed.

Honey. Sometimes honey is used as a sweetener for home-prepared infant foods and formulas. In the past, honey has also been recommended for use on pacifiers to promote

Botulism
Serious, often fatal form of food poisoning from ingesting food contaminated with the powerful toxins of the bacterium *Clostridium botulinum*. The toxin blocks transmission of neural impulses at the nerve terminals, causing gradual paralysis and death when affecting respiratory muscles. Most cases result from eating carelessly home-canned food, so all such food should be boiled at least ten minutes before eating. Cases reported in infants have been related to eating spore-containing honey, so honey should not be used.

sucking in hypotonic infants. However, honey has been implicated as a source of spores of *Clostridium botulinum* during infancy. These spores are extremely resistant to heat and are not destroyed by present methods of honey processing. **Botulism** in infancy is caused by ingestion of the spores, which germinate into the toxin in the lumen of the bowel. Honey should not be fed to infants less than one year old.[3]

Microwaving. Microwaving of infant foods, like that of infant formulas, is potentially dangerous. Microwave ovens heat in an uneven pattern, and some infants have been seriously burned. If microwaves are used, the food should be removed from the jar, heated only to a warm temperature, and thoroughly stirred before giving it to the infant.

SPECIAL CONSIDERATIONS ≋

Spitting Up

During the early months of life, some otherwise healthy infants spit up a small amount of any milk or food digested at each feeding. If an infant is growing well and appears to suffer no distress associated with feeding, this can be interpreted as a normal event. When growth is inadequate or the spitting up appears to be associated with pain or feeding aversions, further evaluation is warranted.

Colic

Colic is described as persistent, unexplained crying in infants.[21] Colic affects 10–30% of infants throughout the world, and it affects breast-fed infants at the same rate as those fed formula. For the most part, most infants with colic outgrow the problem with no adverse consequences, and treatment consists of comforting measures for both the infant and the parent. Most infants with colic do not respond to nutritional therapies. Cow's milk proteins in mother's milk may be associated with higher rates of colic for some infants. If nursing mothers choose to decrease dairy products in their diet, an adequate intake of calcium should be assured.[22] Some infants have been found to respond favorably to a protein hydrolysate formula in some studies, but other studies have not reached this conclusion.[23]

Screening for Infants with Special Health Care Needs

During observations of feeding and assessment of physical growth, infants with problems may be identified. A poor suck and poor weight gain may be indicative of abnormalities of muscle tone, which may be diagnosed later as cerebral palsy. Stiffening and arching during a feed may precede the diagnosis of spasticity. Delays in achieving the developmental landmarks may be indicative of generalized developmental delays. Short stature and poor weight gain may result from physical or neurological difficulties. Assessment and intervention for babies who have these symptoms will require an interdisciplinary team that will include physicians, therapists skilled in oral motor intervention, nurses, and dietitians.

Early Childhood Caries

Early childhood caries (also known as nursing bottle syndrome and baby bottle tooth decay) is a condition of rampant infant caries that develops between one and three years of age (fig. 9-1). The cause of this condition is not entirely clear, but there are at least two components: 1) the presence of carbohydrates in the mouth, with bacterial fermentation of carbohydrates, which leads to the production of acids and the demineralization of tooth structure, and 2) the presence of bacteria in the mouth.

The development of early childhood caries often proceeds rapidly once it has started. It usually begins with the development of spots on the primary maxillary incisors. These decalcified lesions may progress to frank caries within six to twelve months in infants and young children, because the enamel layer on new teeth is thin.

The risk of developing early childhood caries is associated with lack of water fluoridation, ethnicity (American Indian, Alaska native, and Mexican American children are at especially high risk), maternal dental health, later weaning from the bottle, and bottle-feeding in bed. Children who develop early childhood caries often require extensive dental work, and their secondary teeth are at risk of caries as well. Anticipatory guidance to

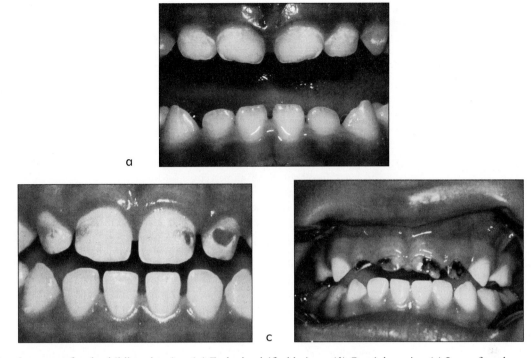

FIG. 9-1 Development of early childhood caries. (*a*) Early decalcified lesions; (*b*) Outright caries; (*c*) Loss of teeth. Pediactric Dentistry, University of Washington.

prevent early childhood caries is important. Parents can benefit from information about the importance of primary teeth, the early use of cups for liquids, the problems associated with putting a child to bed with a bottle, and the use of fluoride.

CHRONIC DISEASE AND DIET IN INFANCY ≈

The etiology of chronic disease is usually multifactorial, and the ability to establish a relationship between disease prevalence and early nutritional experiences is limited. Nevertheless, some provocative reports have been published. Bergstrom[24] found that early introduction of formula feeding and short duration of breast-feeding were associated with higher total cholesterol and other adverse lipid levels in adolescents. Low anthropological measurements both at birth and at one year have been associated with increased risk of later cardiovascular disease. Animal models provide support for a role of nutritional programming in utero and early in life in the establishment of metabolic pathways that eventually influence health outcomes in later adulthood.[24]

Obesity

In the past, there has been speculation that formula feeding and the early introduction of semisolid foods might be factors in excessive intakes of energy and the development of infant obesity and that obese infants very often become obese adults. Breast-feeding and delayed introduction of solids may be protective against childhood obesity.[25] The association between weight for length and the development of obesity later in life is very limited.

Diabetes

A relationship between infant diet and insulin-dependent diabetes mellitus (IDDM) has received great interest in the past few years.[19] The American Academy of Pediatrics has recommended that intact cow's milk protein should be avoided in the diets of infants who are genetically susceptible to developing IDDM, and breast-feeding is strongly recommended for infants with a family history of diabetes. Initial investigations focused on the

CASE STUDY

What Is Best for This Baby?

Michael is an African American baby who was born at forty-one weeks' gestation to a mother with insulin-dependent diabetes. He weighed 4,400 g at birth (the 95th percentile for weight) and was 55 cm in length (the 75th percentile). Both of Michael's parents are fairly short. His mother is 5 ft 2 in and his father is 5 ft 5 in. Since birth, Michael's weight has remained at the 95th percentile. Today he is six months old and weighs 9.5 kg. His length for age has declined in the first months of his life, and today his length is 69 cm (the 50th percentile for his age).

Michael is breast-fed when he is with his mother. He nurses once during the night, once before his mother leaves for work, and twice in the evening. When he is well, he is given three 8 oz bottles of iron-fortified Similac during the day at the family day care home that he attends. The day care provider has several other children under her care. At day care, Michael spends most of his time in a crib. He cries a lot, and the provider tries to feed him whenever he cries by propping a bottle in his crib. Several days out of the month, Michael is congested or irritable, and he frequently gets ear infections. When this happens, the day care provider gives him juice or sweetened lemon tea throughout the day, instead of formula.

Michael shows a strong interest in food. When the family eats, Michael reaches out for the foods they are eating. Since he was about three months old, he has been given "bits and pieces" of family foods, such things as french fries, ground meats with gravy, and ice cream. At day care, he also seems to want the foods the other children are eating. Other than these exposures to family foods, Michael has not been given other foods.

Questions for analysis
1. What are the positive aspects of Michael's nutritional status?
2. What might be going on with Michael's length growth pattern?
3. What might be going on with Michael's weight growth pattern?
4. What would you counsel this family in terms of the relation of foods to Michael's risk of developing diabetes?
5. What anticipatory guidance would you give in terms of early childhood caries?
6. What might you counsel about the relationship between Michael's positioning for feedings at day care and his frequent ear infections?
7. What kind of feeding plan would you like to be able to work out with Michael's family and day care provider?

diabetogenicity of bovine serum albumin in infancy. It now appears that several plant proteins, including soy and wheat, may also be diabetogenic for some individuals and that the critical period for exposure to diabetogenic foods may extend beyond infancy. Early introduction of nonmilk feedings has been associated with the development of IDDM in high-risk infants. Data from epidemiological and animal studies are inconclusive, but it appears prudent to recommend breast-feeding and a delay in introduction of nonmilk feedings until at least six months of age for infants who are known to have genetic susceptibility to IDDM.

Food Allergies

Avoidance of potential allergens in infancy has been suggested as a way to prevent or delay symptoms of IgE-mediated diseases, such as eczema, allergic rhinitis, gastrointestinal symptoms, and chronic wheezing or asthma in families with genetic susceptibility.[18] In children with high genetic risk, careful attention to maternal diet in pregnancy and lactation, as well as a strict hypoallergenic diet in infancy, appears to reduce IgE-mediated reactions in infancy and early childhood but not to affect prevalence of atopic disease in later childhood.[18] A complete avoidance of potential allergens may be burdensome to families, but, for high-risk families who are willing to make significant changes, it is reasonable to suggest avoidance of highly allergenic foods during pregnancy, lactation, infancy, and early childhood with ongoing dietary guidance to assure nutrient adequacy. All infants from families with a history of allergy will benefit from breast-feeding, avoidance of cow's milk in the first year of life, and delay in nonmilk feedings until six months.

Summary

Feeding is an important component in the development of parent-child relationships. Long-term feeding behaviors and overall psychologic development relate directly to these early interactive processes. The ideal source of nutrition for the infant is breast milk; ideally, this breast milk derives from the infant's mother. When breast milk will not or cannot be provided to the infant, commercial infant formulas provide a high-quality alternative. Unmodified milks and other foods are inappropriate for the first few months of life. Gradual introduction of solid foods should occur in most cases during the second six months of the first year. Decisions regarding the choice of foods and their consistency/texture should depend on the developmental progress the infant demonstrates. Inappropriate feeding choices during infancy may have lasting adverse consequences.

Review Questions

1. Why is breast milk considered to be the superior feed for human infants?
2. How is cow's milk changed so that it resembles human milk?
3. Identify the three forms of commercial infant formula, and specify the advantages of each.
4. Why is microwaving of infant formula discouraged?
5. Outline an appropriate sequence for introducing solid foods into the diet of a normal infant.
6. Define basic feeding guidelines for parents of an infant with a strong family history of allergy.

CHAPTER

10

NUTRITION IN CHILDHOOD

Christine M. Trahms
Peggy Pipes

≋ ≋ ≋ ≋ ≋ ≋ ≋ ≋ ≋ ≋ ≋ ≋

Basic Concepts

❏ *Nutrient requirements are affected by a generally slowed and erratic growth rate between infancy and adolescence and a child's individual needs.*

❏ *A child's food choices are determined by numerous family and community factors.*

❏ *Nutrient intake and developing food patterns in young children are governed by food availability and food choices.*

❏ *Considerations in feeding young children are guided by meeting physical and psychosocial needs.*

❏ *Nutrition concerns during childhood relate to growth and development needs for positive health.*

*A*fter the infant's first year of rapid growth, the interval between infancy and adolescence is a period of slower growth. This interval is a time for the acquisition of skills that permit independence in eating and feeding and the development of individual food preferences. The development of gross motor skills makes increased activity possible. Preschool children learn to control body functions, to interact with others, and to behave in a socially acceptable manner. School-age children attempt to develop personal independence and establish a scale of values. Individual variations in children become more noticeable in such areas as rates of growth, activity patterns, nutrient requirements, personality development, and food intakes.

There is a wide range of nutrient requirements of children at any age during this period. Body size and composition, activity patterns, and rates of growth influence basic needs. The foods available to and accepted by the child are determined not only by parental food selection but also by the mealtime environment, peer pressures, advertising, and the child's previous food experiences. If appropriate support is provided by parents, food patterns can be established that support appropriate growth in height and weight, that ensure good dental hygiene, and that prevent nutritional deficiencies, including iron-deficiency anemia.

I. PHYSICAL GROWTH DURING CHILDHOOD ≋

A. Growth Rate

The rapid rate of growth during infancy is followed by a deceleration during the preschool and school-age years. Weight gain approximates 4 to 6 lb (1.8 to 2.7 kg) per year. Length increases approximately 3 inches (7.6 cm) per year between one year and seven to eight years of age, then increases 2 inches (5.1 cm) per year until the pubertal growth spurt. Between six years of age and the adolescent growth spurt, gender differences can be noted. At age six, boys are taller and heavier than girls. By age nine, the height of the average female is the same as that of the nine-year-old male, and her weight is slightly more.

Racial differences have been noted in rates of growth. African American infants are smaller than American white infants at birth. However, they grow more rapidly during the first two years of life and, from two years of age through adolescence, are taller than American white children of the same age. Asian children tend to be smaller than black children and white children.[1] Recent assessments of growth of specific populations of children indicate that Mexican American children, regardless of family income, tend to be shorter and heavier than either African American or white children of the same age.[2] A longitudinal survey of Southeast Asian refugee children indicated a marked improvement in growth status of those children and eventual achievement of growth curves much like those of children of similar ethnic backgrounds.[3]

B. Body Composition

Muscle mass accounts for an increasingly greater percentage of body weight during the preschool years. Children become leaner as they grow older. Skinfold measurements decrease. Females, however, have more subcutaneous fat than males.

Brain growth is 75% complete by the end of the second year; by six to ten years of age, brain growth is complete. This results in a decrease in head size in relation to body size.

Body fluid proportion is similar to that of an adult by the time the child is two to three years of age. Rapid shifts in fluid between intracellular and extracellular compartments are less likely. The child is less vulnerable to dehydration than the infant because of a decreased ratio of body surface area to body mass. The extracellular fluid continues to decrease while intracellular fluid increases because of the growth of new cells. The approximate percentage of total body fluid is 59% in the toddler, compared with 64% in the adult male.

Bone growth results in increased stature. Bone is an active tissue and is constantly being remodeled by the destruction and renewal of collagen and the addition and loss of mineral. Increases in skeletal length are achieved by this process of dissolution and reshaping of bone. The school-age child with longer legs appears more graceful and slimmer than the preschooler.

C. Assessment of Growth

Growth differences in individual children become apparent in the percentile channel of growth followed by each child. Once the percentile ranking is established on the growth chart, children can be expected to maintain **growth channels** when sequential measurements over time are recorded. It is more important to know that a child is maintaining his or her length or height and weight in relation to other children and in the weight-height percentile than it is to know that the child is tall or short for age.

The current infant growth charts, as described in chapter 8 (p. 192), are constructed to thirty-six months of age and should be used until the child is at least twenty-four months old. The growth charts for children from two to eighteen years of age were prepared from data from the National Health and Nutrition Examination Surveys (NHANES).[4] It should be noted that length measurements on the infant chart are recumbent lengths and those on the children's chart are standing height measurements. Children should be weighed in stocking feet and standard examination clothing on a beam balance scale. Standing height is measured using a hard board while the heels, buttocks, and shoulders touch a flat wall (see chapter 8). It is not unusual for small changes to occur in percentile ratings on growth charts when changing from recumbent to upright measurement.

Interpretation of growth or body size measurements and calculations of body composition estimates depend on the accuracy of the measurement of the individual. Accurate measurements require reliable, standardized anthropometry equipment and trained anthropometrists. For validity of interpretation, measurements must be performed in the same manner as the measurements used for the growth charts.

Growth channels
The progressive regular growth patterns of children, guided along individual genetically controlled channels, influenced by nutritional and health status.

Because individual children typically grow in a narrow range of percentiles, growth can be assessed using the growth charts in a general manner. Children whose growth channels for weight and length or height are between the 25th and 75th percentiles are considered to be growing appropriately. Children whose weight and length or height channels are consistently greater than the 75th to 90th percentiles or less than the 10th to 25th percentiles may be growing appropriately but warrant a closer evaluation of growth velocity and energy intake. Children whose growth channels for weight and length or height are consistently greater than the 90th percentile or less than the 10th percentile may also be growing appropriately but are considered to be at risk for overgrowth or growth failure and warrant a closer evaluation of general health, activity, growth velocity, and nutrient intake.

Excesses or inadequacies in energy and nutrient intakes, as well as the genetic potential for growth, are reflected in patterns of growth. The child who is not eating sufficient food will show a decrease in channel of weight gain charts (fig. 10-1). Changes in height or weight channel may also be a reflection of genetic potential for growth. If food deprivation is severe enough and lasts long enough, rates of linear growth will be reduced or growth will cease. Intakes of energy in excess of expenditure will be noted by increases in weight percentile (fig. 10-2).[5,6]

Newer growth charts are being prepared. The base population for the new growth charts is a comprehensive national sample that includes more minorities and is considered to be representative of infants, children, and adolescents in the United States. This set of growth charts is appropriately used for full-term breast-fed and formula-fed infants and persons of ethnicity. Size percentiles will be defined as the 3rd to the 97th percentiles. The age parameters and weight for length will remain the same for infants. The age range on the charts for individuals from age two will be increased to age twenty. Body mass index (BMI) will be used for individuals from age six to twenty years to replace the current weight-for-height estimation of body composition. It is assumed that BMI is a more reliable index of overweight than skinfold measurements. The 85th percentile for BMI has been added to help identify children at risk for overweight.[7,8]

The NHANES III data has shown an increase in weight in children six years and older in the past twenty years; this increase is not reflected in the new charts. The charts no longer exactly describe the American population of children and adolescents but, for the first time, make judgments about reasonable growth channels. The main concern is overweight, not poor growth of children.

Feeding Skills

The child's rate of physical growth is also reflected in the development of self-feeding skills. Children learn to feed themselves independently during the second year of life. The fifteen-month-old child will have difficulty scooping food into the spoon and bringing food to the mouth without turning the spoon upside down and spilling its contents because of lack of wrist control. By two years of age, spilling seldom occurs.

By sixteen to seventeen months of age, a well-defined **ulnar deviation** of the wrist occurs, and the contents of the spoon may be transferred more steadily to the mouth. By eighteen months of age, the child lifts the elbow as the spoon is raised and flexes the wrist as the spoon reaches the mouth, so that only moderate spilling occurs, in contrast to earlier stages of self-feeding.

Handedness is not established at one year of age. Children may grasp the spoon with either hand and, when they try to fill the spoon, find that the bowl is upside down.

A refined pincer grasp is developed in the first year. Finger feeding is easy and often preferred. Foods that provide opportunities for finger feeding should be provided at each meal (table 10-1), avoiding inappropriate ones that may cause choking. Young children, especially preschoolers, are at risk of choking on food. Death from asphyxiation resulting from intakes of small pieces of food has been described primarily among children less than two years of age. Foods most often responsible include hot dogs, hard candy, nuts, and grapes. Foods that are hard, round, and do not readily dissolve in saliva are those that are involved in choking episodes of young children. Choking may also be caused by too much

Ulnar deviation
Turning and articulation of the *ulna* (inner and larger bone of the forearm on the side opposite the thumb) with the wrist joint to accomplish coordinated movement of the wrist and hand.

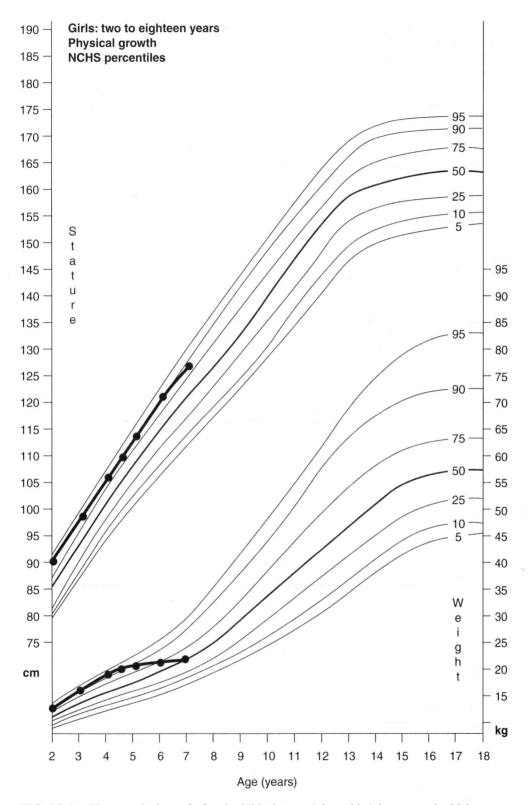

FIG. 10-1   The growth chart of a female child whose weight and height were at the 90th percentile from age 2 until age 4 1/2 years; she continued at the 90th percentile for height but crossed channels downward from the 90th to the 50th percentile for weight. Her energy intake decreased because of decreased appetite, and she did not consume enough food to support continued weight gain.

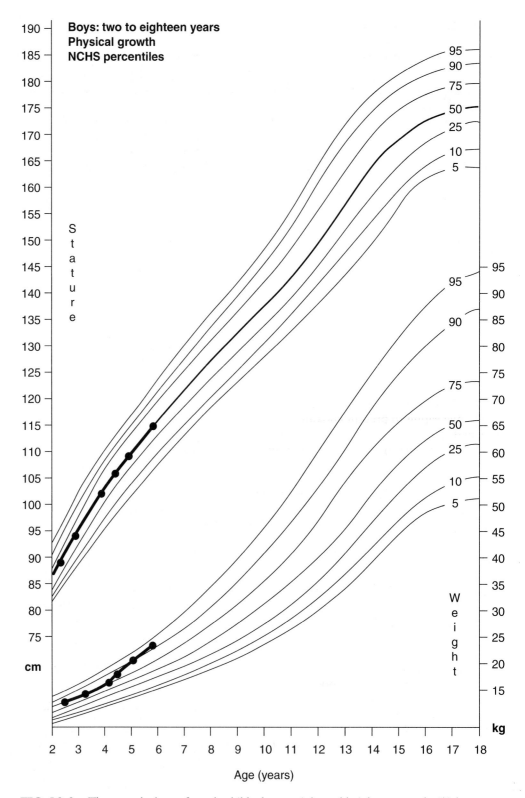

Boys: two to eighteen years
Physical growth
NCHS percentiles

FIG. 10-2 The growth chart of a male child whose weight and height were at the 50th percentile from 2 1/2 to 4 1/2 years of age; he continued at the 50th percentile for height but crossed channels upward in weight from the 50th to the 90th percentile. His energy intake increased because of consumption of high energy density food, and his rate weight gain increased.

TABLE 10-1   *Appropriate Finger Foods for Young Children with a Refined Pincer Grasp*

Appropriate Foods (No Skins or Peeling)	Inappropriate Foods (May Cause Choking or Gagging)
Dry cereal: Cheerios, Kix	
Banana slices	Dried fruits: Raisins, coconut, dates
Soft, cut-up fruit	Small fruit with skin or peel: grapes
Mealy apple	Raw vegetables
Canned or well-cooked vegetables (green beans, broccoli, carrots)	Processed American cheese
	Hot dogs
Cheese sticks, hard cheese (cheddar, Monterey Jack)	Nuts, including peanuts
	Peanut butter
Large-curd cottage cheese	Popcorn
Small pieces tender meats (small meatballs, chicken)	Potato chips
	Corn chips
Scrambled eggs	Tortilla chips
Fish sticks (no bones)	
Oven-dried toast	
Zwieback toast	
Arrowroot biscuits	
Graham crackers	

food in the mouth or running while eating. It is important that young children be supervised while eating to prevent choking.

Children often place food in the spoon with their fingers and may finger feed foods that are commonly spoon-fed, such as vegetables and pudding.

By fifteen months of age, children can manage a cup but have difficulty in lifting, tilting, and lowering it. The cup is tilted, using the palm, often too rapidly. By eighteen to twenty-four months of age, the cup is tilted by manipulation of the fingers.

Children refine the rotary chewing movements that began at one year of age. The ability to chew hard and fibrous foods increases through the school years.

II. NUTRIENT NEEDS OF CHILDREN ≋

Recommendations for energy intakes for children have been derived from intakes of healthy children growing satisfactorily. Recommendations for nutrient intakes are based on a few balance studies, mostly extrapolated from requirements for infants and adults. It is important to remember that the range of adequate intakes of nutrients is quite wide among groups of children. The Recommended Dietary Allowances (RDAs) provide guidelines for studying groups of children, but not for evaluating diets of individual children.[9]

As discussed earlier in this book, the National Academy of Sciences Food and Nutrition Board is in the process of reevaluating the recommended intakes of all nutrients for infants, children, and adolescents. The new reference data are called the Dietary Reference Intakes (DRIs). The board has established a category of recommendations called Adequate Intake (AI) for some nutrients, which is defined as the nutrient intakes needed for optimal health.

A. Energy

Individual needs. The energy requirements for individual children are determined by resting energy expenditure (REE), rate of growth, and activity. REE varies with the amount and composition of **metabolically active** tissue, which varies with age and gender. However, gender differences are relatively small until children reach ten years of age, and no gender differences have been made in recommended energy intakes before this age.

Metabolic activity
Sum of biochemical actions and reactions in the body that build and maintain tissue, regulate body functions, and require a constant energy source. The most metabolically active body tissue is the lean body mass.

TABLE 10-2 *Recommended Energy Intakes for Children*

Age (Years)	Weight (kg)	Height (cm)	Energy Allowances/Day (kcal)	Energy Allowances/kg/Day (kcal)
1–3	13	90	1,300	102
4–6	20	112	1,800	90
7–10	28	132	2,000	70

From National Academy of Sciences. 1989. *Recommended dietary allowances,* 10th ed. Washington, DC: National Academy Press.

The average energy cost of growth after infancy is small, about 5 kcal/g of tissue gained. The energy needs of individual children of the same age, gender, and size vary. Reasons for these differences remain unexplained. Differences in physical activity, in the metabolic cost of minimal and excessive protein intakes at equivalent levels of energy intake, and in the efficiency with which individuals utilize energy have all been hypothesized to exert an influence. The RDA guidelines established by the Food and Nutrition Board of the National Research Council are given in table 10-2.[10,11]

Physical activity. The contribution of physical activity to total energy expenditure is quite variable among children and in individual children from day to day. At all ages, activity patterns among children show wide ranges, both in the time spent in the various activities and in the intensity of the activities. Some children may engage in sedentary activities, such as looking at books or watching television, whereas their peers may be engaged in physical activities that demand running, jumping, and general body movements. The energy expenditure for physical activity of fourth- and fifth-grade schoolchildren, for example, was estimated to be 31.2% and 25.3% of total energy expenditure for males and females, respectively.[11]

Studies indicate that the actual energy intakes of children agree with the recommended intakes. However, wide-ranging intakes of energy will be noted among individual children. The most appropriate evaluation of adequacy of a child's energy intake is based on observation of rates of growth as depicted on growth charts and on measurements of body fat.

Catch-up growth. During a period of catch-up growth, such as recovery from illness or injury, the requirements for energy and nutrients is increased. During periods of catch-up growth, daily intakes of 150 to 250 kcal/kg of body weight have been recommended for children of preschool age. An intake of 200 kcal/kg/day should produce a weight gain of 20 g/day.[12]

B. Protein

Basis of need. The protein needs of children include those for maintenance of tissue, for changes in body composition, and for synthesis of new tissue. During growth, the protein content of the body increases from 14.6% at one year of age to 18% to 19%, which are adult values, by four years of age. Estimates of protein needs for growth range from 1 to 4 g/kg of tissue gained. As the rate of growth decreases, maintenance requirements gradually represent an increasing proportion of the total protein requirement.

Recommended intakes. The recommended protein intake—calculated on the maintenance requirements of the adult, growth rates, and body composition—gradually decreases from 1.3 g/kg at one year of age to 1.0 g/kg at ten years of age (table 10-3).[9,13] This intake approximates 4% to 5% of the total kilocalories of energy, less than most children consume. Protein provides 13% to 15% of the energy intake in the average child's diet.

An evaluation of a child's protein intake must be based on 1) the adequacy of growth rate, 2) the quality of protein in the foods eaten, 3) combinations of foods that provide **complementary amino acids** when consumed together, and 4) the adequacy of the in-

Complementary amino acids
Amino acids from a variety of combined protein foods that complement one another according to their relative amounts of the individual amino acids; used to meet growth requirements for the nine essential amino acids that the body does not sufficiently synthesize.

TABLE 10-3   *Recommended Dietary Allowances of Protein*

Age (Years)	Protein (g/kg)	Protein (g/day)
1–3	1.2	16
4–6	1.1	24
7–10	1.0	28

From National Academy of Sciences. 1989. *Recommended dietary allowances,* 10th ed. Washington, DC: National Academy Press.

TABLE 10-4   *Recommended Daily Dietary Allowances for Minerals*

Age (Years)	Phosphorus (mg)	Iodine (μg)	Iron (mg)	Magnesium (mg)	Zinc (mg)	Selenium (μg)
1–3	800	70	10	80	10	20
4–6	800	90	10	120	10	20
7–10	800	120	10	170	10	30

TABLE 10-5   *Current Recommendations for Adequate Calcium Intake (AI)*

Age (Years)	New AI (mg Calcium/Day)
1–3	500
4–10	800
11–18	1,300

take of vitamins, minerals, and energy. All the components are necessary for protein synthesis to proceed.

Inadequate protein intakes are rarely noted in North America. Some children have such limited energy intakes that part of the protein consumed must be used for body fuel and is not available for the synthesis of new tissue. Children who consume a **vegan diet** have been reported to be shorter and leaner than the average child.[5,14] This decreased growth is believed to be the result of an inadequate energy intake, rather than an overt inadequate protein intake.

C. Minerals and Vitamins

Minerals and vitamins are necessary for normal growth and development. Inadequate intakes are reflected in slow growth rates, inadequate mineralization of bones, insufficient iron stores, and anemia. The RDAs are shown in tables 10-4, 10-5, and 10-6.

Calcium. How much calcium does a child need to grow properly? Attempts to establish recommended intakes of calcium have caused considerable controversy for many years. Calcium is essential for bone growth and mineralization. More than 98% of body calcium is bone. Absorption of calcium fluctuates from 30% to 60% of intake. Lactose increases absorption, binders such as **phytic acid** and **oxalic acid** reduce absorption, and the level of dietary protein affects the urinary excretion of calcium. As levels of protein intake increase, levels of urinary calcium increase.

It is estimated that daily calcium accretion rates must average 150–200 mg calcium/day, with a peak of 400 mg/day during rapid growth. Recommendations for children are set at 800 mg/day, since growing children may need two to four times as much calcium per unit of body weight as adults require. It is suggested that low calcium intake

Vegan diet
Strict vegetarian diet that does not allow any animal protein; requires careful food combinations of incomplete plant proteins to complement one another and achieve an overall adequacy of essential amino acids for growth needs.

Phytic acid
Compound in certain grains, such as wheat, that binds calcium and hinders its absorption.
Oxalic acid
Compound in a variety of foods, including green leafy vegetables, corn, soy products such as tofu, and wheat germ, that binds calcium in the food mix and hinders its absorption.

TABLE 10-6   Recommended Levels of Vitamins per Day

	Age (Years)		
Vitamins	1–3	4–6	7–10
Fat-soluble*			
Vitamin A (μg RE)	400	500	700
Vitamin D (μg)	10	10	10
Vitamin E (mg α-TE)	6	7	7
Vitamin K (μg)	15	20	30
Water-soluble			
Thiamin (mg)	0.5	0.6	0.9
Riboflavin (mg)	0.5	0.6	0.9
Niacin (mg)	6.0	8.0	12.0
Vitamin B_6 (mg)	0.5	0.6	1.0
Folate (μg)	150.0	200.0	300.0
Vitamin B_{12} (μg)	0.9	1.2	1.8
Ascorbic acid (mg)*	40.0	45.0	45.0

*From National Academy of Sciences. 1989. *Recommended dietary allowances,* 10th ed. Washington, DC: National Academy Press.
All other values from *CNI Newsletter,* April 10, 1998.

limits linear growth and bone mineralization. There is also the likelihood that efficiency of absorption and conservation of calcium may, in fact, increase with low calcium intake and high biologic requirement.[15]

Milk and other dairy products are the primary sources of bioavailable calcium. Thus, children who consume limited amounts of these products risk a deficient calcium intake.
Zinc. The trace mineral zinc is essential for normal protein synthesis and growth. Variations in plasma zinc concentrations during growth reflect the continual use and depletion of body stores of zinc. Zinc deficiency has serious consequences; most notable are growth retardation, hypogeusia, and diarrhea, as well as impaired wound healing and cell-mediated immunity. Zinc intakes of children one to three years of age have been estimated to average 5 mg/day; those of children three to five years of age average 5 to 7 mg/day.[16]

There is speculation that poor linear growth in early childhood in some low-income populations may result from a growth-limiting zinc deficiency state. A study of Hispanic children two to six years of age who consumed 5 to 6 mg of zinc per day and whose linear growth was below the 10th percentile found low hair and plasma zinc levels. Increasing their zinc intake to 10 mg/day increased rates of linear growth.[17]

Small amounts of zinc are more efficiently absorbed than large amounts. Children in poor zinc status absorb zinc more efficiently than those in good status. High intakes of phytate and fiber depress zinc absorption. The bioavailability of zinc varies with the food source. Meats are a good source of available zinc; cereal grains contain a less available form. The average toddler in the United States consumes 8.5 mg of zinc per day.
Iron. Iron deficiency is the most common nutritional deficiency. It occurs most frequently in children four to twenty-four months of age, in adolescent males, and in females in their childbearing years. In a recent survey, it was demonstrated that iron deficiency and iron deficiency anemia are still significant public health problems. Nine percent of children one to two years of age were iron deficient and of these, 3% had iron deficiency anemia.[18] It may result from inadequate iron intake, impaired absorption, a large hemorrhage, or repeated small blood losses. Iron deficiency anemia in preschool children causes delayed mental and physical development and decreased resistance to infection.

TABLE 10-7 *Estimated Safe and Adequate Daily Dietary Intakes of Selected Trace Minerals for Children*

Age (Years)	Copper (mg)	Manganese (mg)	Fluoride (mg)	Chromium (μg)	Molybdenum (μg)
1–3	0.7–1.0	1.0–1.5	0.5–1.5	20–80	25–50
4–6	1.0–1.5	1.5–2.0	1.0–2.5	30–120	30–75
7–10	1.0–2.0	2.0–3.0	1.5–2.5	50–200	50–150
11+	1.5–2.5	2.0–5.0	1.5–2.5	50–200	75–250

From National Academy of Sciences. 1989. *Recommended dietary allowances,* 10th ed. Washington, DC: National Academy Press.

TABLE 10-8 **Estimated Minimum Requirements of Electrolytes**

Age (Years)	Sodium (mg)	Potassium (mg)	Chloride (mg)
2–5	300	1,400	500
6–9	400	1,600	600
10–18	500	2,000	750

From National Academy of Sciences. 1989. *Recommended dietary allowances,* 10th ed. Washington, DC: National Academy Press.

The RDA guidelines assume 10% iron absorption and are planned to meet variations of need in individuals.[9] Iron requirements of individual children vary with rates of growth and increasing total iron mass, iron stores, variations in menstrual losses of iron in adolescent females, and the timing of the growth spurt of adolescents. Larger, more rapidly growing children have the greatest requirements for iron, because they are increasing their blood volumes more rapidly.

Prevention of anemia. At ages two and three years, the best predictor of iron status was the iron status of the child at age one year.[19] Many younger preschoolers do not have the oral motor strength to masticate meat and prefer **nonheme** plant sources of **iron.** The consumption of foods or a supplement containing vitamin C along with the foods containing nonheme iron can help increase the amount of the iron absorbed. Absorption can also be increased by consuming meat when nonheme iron is ingested. Iron absorption is decreased by antacids, bran, and tea. Also, directing parents to use more foods containing heme iron that are easier to chew, such as ground beef, can increase iron intake. For children whose iron intake is limited, a supplemental maintenance dose of iron (10 mg/day) may be indicated. Children with diagnosed iron deficiency anemia receive therapeutic doses of iron, 3 mg/kg/day, for three months.

It is increasingly clear that iron deficiency anemia causes long-term developmental effects. The iron status of a group of infants in Costa Rica was reevaluated at age five years. The children all demonstrated reasonable growth and iron status at that time. The children who had demonstrated moderately severe iron deficiency anemia (hemoglobin < 10 mg/l) in infancy had lower mental and motor-functioning scores at age five.[20]

It has been suggested, based on a review of iron supplementation studies worldwide, that a weekly iron supplement to young children at risk for iron deficiency may improve weight gain, appetite, and psychomotor and mental development.[21]

Vitamins. The function of vitamins in metabolic processes means that their requirements are determined by intakes of energy, protein, and saturated fats. Exact needs are difficult to define. The RDA guidelines for most vitamins and for some trace minerals (table 10-7, 10-8) are interpolated from infant and adult allowances or calculated on the basis of energy and protein allowances.

Nonheme iron
The portion of dietary iron, including all of the plant food sources and 60% of the animal food sources, that lack the more easily absorbed and bioavailable heme iron.

Ethnic, geographic, and situation variation in nutrient intake and subsequent concerns about nutritional status and deficiency have been documented. Recent studies have documented the extent of hungry children in the United States. It is estimated that one out of three poor children (living in households at or below 50% of poverty level) does not obtain even two-thirds of the RDA for energy.[22]

III. NUTRITIONALLY VULNERABLE CHILDREN

In the United States there are several groups of children that are believed to be at greater risk for deficiencies in nutrient intakes. The nutritional vulnerability of these children is primarily related to poverty and may also be related to adverse family circumstances.

A. Vegetarian Children

Many families are vegetarian and are raising their children to choose nonmeat-containing food patterns. Children who are offered appropriately chosen vegetarian-style meals will grow and develop as expected. Children who ingest vegetarian or vegan food patterns and who demonstrate poor growth are those with inadequate intakes of energy, protein, calcium, and or other essential nutrients.

Older infants who are weaned from breast milk should receive an equivalent source of protein, calcium, and other nutrients. This source may be calcium-fortified soy milk or cow's milk. Additional protein sources, such as cheese, yogurt, peanut butter, and bean spreads, may also be introduced. Pasta, breads, rice, cereals, crackers, fruits, and vegetables prepared in a manner that the child can manage, depending on the child's skill level, are appropriate sources of energy and nutrients. Providing an adequate intake of iron may be problematic, however, depending on the foods offered and the child's willingness to accept them.

B. Mexican American Children

Mexican American children have been considered at high risk for inadequate nutrient intakes. Mexican American preschool children in San Diego demonstrated worrisome intakes (<2/3 of the RDA) for iron, zinc, vitamin D, vitamin C, and niacin. Mexican American girls also had a significantly lower calcium intake. The study participants were all lower income to lower-middle income families.[23] Another recent report suggests that these children consume vegetables less often than other groups of children. Twenty-five percent of the children consumed no vegetables.[24]

C. Native American Children

There has been long-term concern about the adequacy of nutrient intakes and growth for Native American children. Height and weight status of school-aged Native American children was assessed. The overall prevalence of overweight in this group was 40%, compared with the NHANES II reference population and about 29% compared with the HHANES-MA Mexican American population. Overweight is much more prevalent in Native American children than among other children in the United States at all ages and in both sexes.[25]

D. Children in Foster Care

There is little known of the nutritional intake of young children in foster care in the United States. These children are vulnerable for many reasons, including the crises in their lives and a high incidence of health problems. The chaotic social situation is considered to be a precursor for negative feeding behaviors and poor nutritional intake.[26]

E. Homeless Children

Unfortunately, homelessness is an all too common occurrence in the United States. Each night there are about 100,000 homeless children, and about half of these children are under six years of age. Efforts have been made to assess the nutrition and growth of young children without homes. Compared with children of similar ages and income level in homes, homeless children demonstrate a growth pattern compatible with moderate, chronic nutritional deprivation—that is, stunting without wasting. This indicates a dietary pattern that is not deficient in total energy but, rather, inadequate in some nutrients and composed primarily of cheaper carbohydrate-rich foods.[27]

Height-for-age and weight-for-age measurements of homeless children in Baltimore were generally comparable to other groups of low-income children.[28] Intakes of all nutrients except calcium (77% of the RDA) and zinc (79% of the RDA) met or exceeded the RDAs for preschool children. Nutrient-fortified ready-to-eat cereals were credited with providing many of the nutrients consumed, since fruits, vegetables, and dairy products were seldom available.

Calculated nutrient intakes of young children living in temporary shelters indicated very low iron and folic acid intakes, 40% and 30% of the RDA, respectively, and moderate intakes of all other nutrients (>60% RDA). The overall dietary adequacy score was low.[29]

In addition to nutritional inadequacies and the risk for poor growth, children who are hungry are at risk for poor ability to learn. Children who are hungry—that is, those who suffer prolonged periodic food insufficiency—are at high risk for development of psychosocial dysfunction and negative behaviors, such as fighting, stealing, and anxiety, that interfere with learning.[30]

IV. VITAMIN SUPPLEMENTATION

A. Dietary Evaluation

Vitamin supplementation of children's diets should be recommended only after careful evaluation of the child's food and nutrient intake. Diets of children who restrict their intake of milk because of documented or suspected allergies, lactose intolerance, or psychosocial reasons should be monitored for adequate intakes of calcium, riboflavin, and vitamin D. Diets of infants and children receiving goat's milk should be carefully monitored for food sources of folate. Diets of children who consume limited amounts of fruits and vegetables should be checked for sources of vitamins A and C.

B. Children at Risk

The Committee on Nutrition of the American Academy of Pediatrics has defined six groups of children at particular risk and for whom vitamin supplementation may be appropriate.[31]
1. Children from deprived families, especially those who suffer from parental neglect or abuse.
2. Children who have anorexia, poor and capricious appetites, or poor eating habits.
3. Children with chronic disease.
4. Children on dietary regimens to manage obesity.
5. Pregnant teenagers.
6. Children who consume vegan diets.

Children needing supplements can be determined by a nutritional assessment and, in addition to those in the preceding list, might include children with food allergies, limited food acceptance, or frequent illness. Any vitamin supplements, especially those that are colored and sugar-coated, should be stored in places inaccessible to young children so they are not mistaken for candy.

The importance of appropriate vitamin supplementation of breast-fed infants is discussed in chapter 8. After infancy, however, the percentage of toddlers who are given vitamin supplements declines, but over half of preschool and school-age children receive multivitamin/mineral preparations.

V. FACTORS THAT INFLUENCE FOOD CHOICES

Food acceptance and the development of food choice patterns are multifactorial and complex processes that are not fully understood. The adequacy of children's food intake and, consequently, their nutrient intake depends not only on the foods available to them but also on cultural, environmental, interactional, and societal factors. Most investigators who have studied food choices have focused on preschoolers, because it is at this stage of development that parents often become confused about children's food selections and become concerned that their children are not eating the kinds and amounts of foods they should.

Food Acceptance

Acceptance of food is affected by factors that include nutritional status, degree of satiation, taste, previous experiences, and beliefs about specific foods. Infants have a preference for sweetened water, a preference that can be extinguished by offering only beverages that are not sweetened.[32] Young infants seem to have an aversion to bitter tastes and an indifference to salty tastes. Tastes for salt change from neutral to preferred at four months of age, when the salt taste is combined with other tastes in food. Preschoolers reject salty beverages but prefer a higher level of salt in soup than do adults.[33]

Recently, research has focused on genetic factors that influence food preferences.[34] Monozygotic twin pairs demonstrated a greater similarity in food preferences than dizygotic twin pairs. Foods with similar preferences were orange juice, broccoli, cottage cheese, chicken, sweetened cereal, and hamburger. A strong genetic influence was demonstrated for phenylthiocarbamide (PTC). Individuals sensitive to the bitter taste of such compounds as PTC tended to have more food dislikes than those who were less sensitive. Foods identified as tasting bitter were turnips, broccoli, green beans, strawberries, bacon, grapefruit, orange, and apple, all of which contain some PTC. Sensitivity to bitter tastes, tested by sensitivity to 6-n-propylthiouracil (PROP), appears to have a genetic basis for influencing food preferences.[35] The role of the genetics of taste on day-to-day food choices and subsequent growth and health has not been determined.

Parental Influences

Parents have a profound influence on food-related behaviors of young children. Many research studies have documented that parents, with or without conscious effort, guide the food preferences of their young children and establish the style for where food is eaten, how it is eaten, with whom it is eaten, and how much is eaten.

Nutrition knowledge.   The nutrition knowledge of parents and other caregivers appears to be an important influence on children's food choices. The degree to which knowledge of nutrition is incorporated into family meal planning seems to be related to mothers' positive attitudes toward self, mothers' problem-solving skills, and family organization. All mothers interviewed expressed concern about the total diet offered to their young children and the importance of mealtime with children.[36] The ordinal position of the preschool child in the family appears to influence choices of specific foods, regardless of equivalent knowledge of nutrition between groups of mothers.[37] When a preschool child is the youngest child in the family, the mothers appear to be less susceptible to the child's requests for new products. Mothers are willing, however, to accommodate that preference when the preschooler is the oldest child in the family. In one study, parents of four- to seven-year-old children reported that the types of foods made available and eaten for meals were influenced by the likes and dislikes of the children. However, snack food availability and portion sizes were controlled by the adult that was present.[38]

Young children influence how families spend their food dollars. Research efforts have documented child-prompted purchases comprised about 14% of the family food budget. Over half of child-prompted food items were energy dense.[39] Mothers reported feeling a sense of guilt because they realized that their families, including the young children, ate foods they preferred rather than the foods she felt to be nutritious.[40]

Models.   The models set for children by their families—especially their parents—and other persons close to them exert a strong influence on their developing food patterns. Food habits of siblings exert an influence equal to that of parents. Parents report they know little about nutrition but think it is important.

Parent-child interactions.   Children's interactions with their parents influence their acceptance of foods and the food patterns they develop. If parents casually accept transient strong food preferences preschoolers develop, these passing food behaviors are soon for-

TABLE 10-9 *Factors That Influence the Food Choices of Young Children*

Food Acceptance Influences

Nutritional and hydration status of the child.
Health or illness state of the child.
Previous experiences with the offered food, such as familiarity, taste, texture.
Portion size; size of pieces of food.
Ease of handling the food based on age and motor skills.
Current degree of satiation.

Parent, Caregiver, and Sibling Influences

Food availability.
Nutrition knowledge.
Nourishing properties of foods that are offered.
Style and pace of eating.
Expectations and modeling of where, when, and with whom food is eaten.
Expectations and modeling of amount of food to be eaten.
Modeling of nonnourishment uses of foods.

Parent-Child Interaction Influences

Expectation about the child's pace and style of eating.
Establishment of contingencies about which foods and how much to be eaten.
Positive, neutral, or critical verbal interaction during mealtimes.
Establishment of a pattern of meals and snacks.

gotten. However, parents who find these behaviors difficult to accept and give much attention to them by trying to bribe or encourage the child to eat, discussing the children's dislikes in front of them, or providing a preferred food when they refuse to eat may pattern that behavior into a permanent food habit. A child's social-emotional environment is related to the adequacy of the child's dietary intake. Companionship at mealtime, a positive home atmosphere, and appropriate food-related parenting behaviors are strongly associated with improved quality of diet.[41]

The parent-child interaction also has an important influence on the amount of food consumed. There appear to be differences between the interactions of thinner children and their mothers and fatter children and their mothers, both in food and nonfood situations. Thinner children and their mothers talk more with each other and eat less food more slowly than do fatter children and their mothers.[42] Preferences for foods are enhanced when foods are offered as a reward or with a brief positive social interaction with adults.[43]

Contingencies. It is also a common practice for parents to use rewards such as "Clean your plate and you can have dessert" to achieve a child's acceptance of foods. While this practice often achieves its immediate goal, the long-term effects are often negative. Children understand that external pressure is usually applied to get them to eat a less preferred food. When the contingency is removed, they eat less of the food.[44] The child's ability to recognize hunger and satiation has also been studied by Birch.[45,46] Of all the children in the study, 95% ate less lunch after a high-energy density preload than a low-energy-density preload. Only 60% of the adults followed the same pattern. Parental monitoring (or threat of parental monitoring) decreased the number of nonnutritious foods chosen and thus the total energy content of the meal.[47]

Food choices are shaped by the child's physiology, activity, environment, and exposure to foods in a complex series of interactions. Table 10-9 summarizes the primary factors that influence food choices, as they are currently understood.

Quantities of food consumed. If normal, well-nourished children are offered a variety of nutritionally appropriate foods and are permitted to eat the foods they select in the amounts they wish, they consume an appropriate energy intake. Studies conducted in the 1920s and early 1930s on six-month-old to four-year-old foundlings in a Chicago hospital presented the children with ten unprocessed foods at each meal. The children were permitted to self-select the foods and amounts they ate at any meal. A more recent study by Birch with fifteen children in a day care center used the same menu for two days each week for three weeks in the day care center and at home. Foods included in the menu would provide appropriate nutrient intake. In both studies, there was considerable variability in the quantity of food each child consumed from one day to the next. However, the children self-selected an appropriate energy intake when the study days were averaged.[11,48] It is important to note that both researchers used a laboratory setting and controlled environment for a variety of parent-child interaction issues that influence food acceptance. These studies do, however, provide a model of an optimal method of achieving children's acceptance of a nutritionally appropriate diet.

Influence of Television on Children's Food and Activity Patterns

Sylvester et al.[49] have summarized the research on children and television over the past twenty years: "Children spend enough time in front of TV to warrant concern as to the content and effect of this medium." It would appear that the number hours of viewing television for young children has been fairly constant over the past two decades. Younger children continue to watch more Saturday morning television than older children.

Food attitudes and requests. In addition to the many familial, cultural, and psychosocial influences on children's food habits, mass media have an impact on children's attitudes toward food and their requests for particular products. Of all the forms of mass media, television has the greatest impact on children, because it reaches many children before they are capable of verbal communication and because it engages much of their time. Children spend more time watching television than they do in any other activity, except for sleeping. Children from low-income families watch more television than do children from moderate- to high-income families. It has been estimated that children watch television twenty-two to twenty-five hours per week.

Obesity. Extensive television viewing can be detrimental to growth and development by encouraging sedentary and passive activities, thus promoting a lifestyle that may lead to obesity. An association between obesity and time spent watching television has been documented in six- to eleven-year-old children and in adolescents.[50] "The amount of TV viewing may be a factor in development of obesity . . . insofar as it precludes other activities that require much greater energy expenditure."[49] Sylvester goes on to state, "The major impact of TV is not the behavior it produces, but the behavior it prevents." Children who watch more television and are less likely to participate in vigorous activity tend to have higher BMIs.[51]

Snacking. Television viewing by children is also correlated with between-meal snacking. The total amount of TV watched positively correlates with the act of snacking. Short-term consumption behaviors appear to be influenced by the content and amount of TV viewed.[49]

Advertisers attempt to use children to influence their parents' purchasing behavior. They present frequent cues for food and drink and often encourage consumption of a wide variety of sugared products. Television programs, as well as advertising, present models of behavior children may imitate.

Television advertising. Kindergarten children often are unable to separate commercials from the program and frequently explain them as part of the program. Younger school-age children five to ten years of age watch commercials more closely than do older children eleven to twelve years of age. Older children are more conscious of the concept of commercials, the purpose of selling, and the concept of sponsorship and are less likely to accept advertisers' claims without question. They perceive that television commercials are designed to sell products rather than entertain or educate. Children in the second grade have been found to have a concrete distrust of commercials based on experience with advertised products. Children in the sixth grade have been found to have global mistrust of all commercials.

TV and food choices. On Saturday morning TV programming for children, more than 56% of the advertisements were for food; of these, nearly 44% were for fats, oils, and sweet foods. The most frequently advertised foods were high-sugar cereals.

Certain attributes of food are promoted by television advertising as being superior to others. The main characteristics presented positively are "sweetness" and "richness." Many food manufacturers, in other words, deemphasize the physiologic need for nutrients and encourage selection on the basis of sweet flavor. Exposure to such messages may distort a child's natural curiosity toward other characteristics of food, such as the fresh crispness of apples or celery.

There has been ongoing concern about the influence of television on the growth and health of young children[50-52]. Dietz and Gortmaker outline aspects of television watching that are of concern: 1) the relationship between increased television watching and snacking, 2) the increased consumption of foods advertised on television as watching time increases, and 3) the direct association of increased viewing time with the number of attempts of the young child to influence the supermarket purchases of the parent. The foods advertised on weekend children's programs are usually ones of high-energy density—which, if purchased and consumed without an increase in activity, can lead to inappropriate weight gain and poor food habits. The larger intake of highly concentrated sweets and fat foods plus the decrease in activity that is associated with excess television watching have led to an increase in obesity among children in the United States.[51,52]

Parental response. Children are influenced by television commercials and attempt to influence their parents' buying practices. Commercials for food have the strongest influence, and mothers are more likely to yield to requests for food than for other products. Parents have a greater tendency to respond to requests from older children but certainly do not ignore those of younger children. Mothers of children aged three to eight years were interviewed to assess children's viewing habits and parental response to children's requests for food advertised on television. Children requested the foods they saw advertised on TV. The number of hours a week that a child watched TV correlated significantly with the reported number of requests for foods that were advertised and energy intake.[53] Highly child-centered mothers are less likely to buy children's favorite cereals than are mothers who are not as child-centered. The American Academy of Pediatrics has taken a strong stand on this issue, with the recommendation that televised advertising aimed at children be eliminated. The position paper states, "Parents rather than children should determine what children should eat."[31] Parents need support from many people, including immediate or extended family, health care providers, school personnel, and community program organizers, in their efforts to provide nourishing foods for their children while limiting access to TV and promoting exercise and other activities.

PRESCHOOL CHILDREN

Although clinical signs of malnutrition are rarely found in preschool children in the United States and many low-income families show good management of scarce economic resources for food, there is evidence that some children receive diets that are limited in some nutrients and energy.

Both longitudinal and cross-sectional studies of nutrient and energy intakes of children have shown large differences in intakes between individual children of the same age and gender. Some children consume two to three times as much energy as others.[11,49,54] After a rapid rise in intake of all nutrients during the first nine months of life, reductions can be expected in the intakes of some of the nutrients as increases occur in intakes of others. Several researchers have noted gender differences in intakes of energy and nutrients. In all studies, males consumed greater quantities of food, thus greater amounts of nutrients and energy.

The Preschool Years

During the preschool years, there is a decrease in intake of calcium, phosphorus, riboflavin, iron, and vitamin A because of discontinued use of iron-fortified infant cereals, a reduction in milk intakes, and a disinterest in vegetables. During this period, children increase their intake of carbohydrates and fat. Protein intakes may plateau or increase only slightly. Between three and eight years of age, there is a slow, steady, and relatively consistent increase in intake of all nutrients. Since intakes of vitamins A and C are unrelated to energy intakes, greater ranges of intakes of these nutrients have been noted.

Normal Food Behaviors of Preschool Children

Food rituals. Few children pass through the preschool years without creating concern about their food intake. Between nine and eighteen months of age, children display a disinterest in food that lasts from a few months to a few years. Strong preferences for specific foods are common. Likes and dislikes may change from day to day and week to week. For example, a child may demand only boiled eggs for snacks for a week and completely reject them for the next six months. Rituals become a part of food preparation and service. Some children, for example, accept sandwiches only when they are cut in half; when parents quarter the sandwich, the children may throw tantrums. Others demand that food have a particular arrangement on the plate or that dishes be placed only in certain locations on the table.

Appetites. During this period, appetites are usually erratic and unpredictable. The child may eat hungrily at one meal and completely refuse the next. The evening meal is generally the least well received and is of the most concern to most parents. It is possible that children who have consumed two meals and several snacks have already met their needs for energy and nutrients before dinnertime.

Food preferences. Parents report that preschool children enjoy meat, cereal grains, baked products, fruit, and sweets. They frequently ask for dairy products, cereal, and snack items, such as cookies, crackers, and fruit juice. Food preferences during the preschool years seem to be for the carbohydrate-rich foods that are easiest to masticate. Cereals, breads, and crackers are selected often in preference to meat and other protein-rich foods. The use of dry **fortified cereal** as a primary source of many nutrients is increasing. Yogurt and cheese appear to be increasing in popularity among young children. Young children express their pleasure when they are rested and hungry, when foods are offered at a temperature and in shapes and sizes they can manage, and when foods are offered without undue pressure from parents about eating style (fig. 10-3).

Fortified cereal
Cereal food products enriched by addition of minerals, such as iron and zinc, and vitamins, such as thiamin, riboflavin, niacin, folate, B_6, and B_{12}.

Frequency of Eating

Nearly 60% of children three to five years of age eat more than three times a day. They consume food on an average of five to seven times a day, although ranges of three to fourteen times a day have been noted. The frequency of food intakes appears to be unrelated to nutrient intakes, except when children consume food less than four or more than six times a day.[55] Children who consume food less than four times a day consume fewer kilocalories of energy and less calcium, protein, ascorbic acid, and iron than the average intakes of other children their age. Those who consume food more than six times a day consume more energy, calcium, and ascorbic acid than average intakes of children their age.

Appetite and Activity

In spite of the reduction of appetite and erratic consumption of food, preschool children enjoy well-prepared and attractively served food. If simply prepared foods are presented in a relaxed setting, children consume an appropriate nutrient intake. Meals and snacks should be timed to foster appetite. Intervals necessary between meals and snacks may vary from one child to another. Rarely can the clock be depended on to know appropriate intervals and times when it may be important for a child to eat. However, indiscriminate snacking dulls the appetite, and such patterns should be discouraged.

Foods for young children. Children accept simple, unmixed dishes more willingly than casseroles and prefer most of their food at room temperature, neither hot nor cold. Food preparation is important. Children recognize poorly prepared food and are likely to refuse it. Most children eat most easily the foods with which they are familiar. Small portions of new foods can be introduced with familiar and popular foods. Even if the child only looks at the new food or just feels or smells it at first, this is a part of learning about it and accepting it.

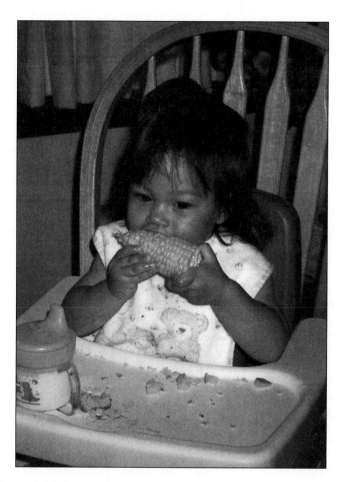

FIG. 10-3   Young children enjoy foods that they can manage at their developmental skill level.

Dry foods are especially hard for preschool children to eat. In planning a menu, a dry food should always be balanced with one or two moist foods. For example, it is wise to put a slice of meat loaf, relatively dry, with mashed potatoes and peas in a little cream sauce. Also, combinations of sharp, rather acid-flavored foods with mild-flavored foods are popular with young children, and they are pleased to find colorful foods, such as red tomatoes, green peppers, and carrot sticks, included in their meals.

Ease of manipulation. Foods eaten easily with the unskilled and seemingly clumsy hands of a young child are very important. Many small pieces of foods, such as cooked peas or beans, are difficult for a child to spoon up. Foods can be prepared so that a child can eat them with the fingers. Hard-cooked eggs may be served in quarters, cooked meat can be cut in small strips, and cooked green beans can be served as finger foods. Children like oranges that have been cut in wedges, skin and all, much better than peeled and diced oranges. Mixed-up salads, when there are layers of food to be eaten, are much more difficult to eat than are simple pieces of raw vegetables with no salad dressing. Cottage cheese or similar foods should be served separate from the lettuce leaf on the child's plate. Creamed foods served on tough toast are difficult for children to manage.

Relatively small pieces of food that can be handled with the child's eating tools are best for preschool children. The problem of handling silverware and conveying food to the mouth at this early age is a greater task than many adults realize. Pieces of carrots that slide across the plate and are too small to remain on the fork are frustrating. On the other hand, cubes of beets so large that they must be cut into smaller pieces before they can be eaten exhaust the patience of a two- or three-year-old child. Most foods for these children should be served in bite-size pieces. When the child is four years of age and older, the skills

TABLE 10-10 *Guidelines for Supporting a Child's Efforts at Self-feeding*

Offer:

Simply prepared foods.

Attractively served foods, such as variety in color and shape of foods.

Foods at a moderate temperature.

Moist rather than dry foods.

Finger foods, such as 1/4 sandwiches.

Bite-size pieces of fruits, vegetables, meats.

Familiar foods with a small amount of an unfamiliar food.

Soft and crisp foods at the same meal.

Small portions, depending on the age, motor skills, and appetite of the child.

Meals at three- to four-hour intervals, rather than chronic snacking.

Positive conversational interaction with the child.

to cut up some foods may have been developed. If, however, difficulty in managing food is noticed, small pieces should be served, with occasional encouragement to cut up some easier-to-manage foods. Canned pears and other soft fruits, for example, are usually easy to cut into bite-size pieces.

In general, the aim is to support the young child's early efforts at self-feeding, and many creative adaptations can be helpful. Stringy spinach or tomatoes, for example, are a trial for anyone to eat. Much can be done with food shears in the kitchen to make these foods easier to eat. Finger foods, such as pieces of lettuce or toast, can be used in meals in which some of the foods are difficult to handle. Small sandwiches—that is, a large one cut into four small squares—are popular with young children. As the young child matures, self-help skills become more sophisticated. In general, a two-year-old child uses arm muscles for tasks, a three-year-old child uses hand muscles, and a four-year-old child uses finger muscles. This maturation enables the child to wipe, scrub, pour, mix, and peel foods for eating.[56] These guidelines are summarized in table 10-10.

Food characteristics. Three general food characteristics affecting taste, acceptance, and self-feeding skills development are important considerations in early feeding of young children. These aspects are texture, flavor, and portion sizes.

Texture It is wise to serve one soft food for easy chewing, one crisp food for easy chewing and enjoyment of the sounds in the mouth, and one chewy food for emerging chewing skills without having too much to chew in each meal for young children. Pieces of meat seem to be hard for a young child to eat, which explains why many children prefer hamburgers to frankfurters. Most children's meat can be served as ground meat. Ground meat should be cooked only long enough for the color to change to brown and not be allowed to become dry and crusted, which makes it hard for a child to eat. Some children may prefer moderately rare meat, which is even more moist, but care must be taken that it is cooked sufficiently to be safe.

Flavor In general, young children reject strong flavors. Many children, however, seem to like pickles and some spicy sauces, which may seem to contradict this. In general, it has been found that children like food only mildly salted. Pepper and other sharp spices and acids, such as vinegar, should also be used sparingly on children's food.

Portion sizes Children are easily discouraged by large portions of food. The child should be offered less than the child usually eats and should be permitted seconds, rather than discouraged with portions that are too large. Appropriate portion sizes are shown in table 10-11.

Parental concerns. Occasionally, anxious or concerned parents need help with food sources of nutrients usually supplied by food refused or in establishing limits to the preschooler's food intakes and feeding behavior. Of the commonly expressed concerns, limited intakes of milk, refusal of meat and vegetables, too many sweets, and limited intakes of food appear to cause the most problems. Parental concerns about the type, variety, and quantity of foods their young children consume are often based on the sometimes

TABLE 10-11 *A Feeding Guide for Children*

This is a guide to a basic diet. Fats, desserts, and sauces will contribute additional kilocalories of energy to meet the needs of the growing child.

Foods	One-Year-Old		Two- to Three-Years-Old	
	Portion Sizes	No. of Servings	Portion Sizes	No. of Servings
Milk	½ cup	4–5	¼–¾ cup	4–5
Meat and meat equivalents	¼–1 oz 2–4 tbsp	1	1–2 oz	2
Fruit and vegetables		4–5		4–5
Vegetables				
Cooked	1–2 tbsp		2–3 tbsp	
Raw	1–2 tbsp		Few pieces	
Fruit				
Canned	2–4 tbsp		2–4 tbsp	
Raw	2–4 tbsp (chopped)		½–1 small	
Juice	2–4 oz		3–4 oz	
Grains and grain products	½ slice	3	¼–1 slice	3

Modified from Lownberg, M.E. 1997. The development of food patterns in young children. In *Nutrition in infancy and childhood,* ed. C.M. Trahms and P.L. Pipes. 6th ed. Dubuque, IA McGraw-Hill, 1997.

Continued

annoying and frequently time-consuming but developmentally appropriate behaviors the child demonstrates around food and feeding rather than on intake of nutrients to support nourishment.

If the child is growing appropriately in channel and an assessment of usual food intake patterns is reassuring that essential nutrients are ingested in reasonable amounts, then the parents can be reassured about the nourishment status of their child. They can be guided through the developmental milestones of independence in self-feeding in a positive manner. A developmental understanding of the child's view of food and meals plus guidelines for appropriate mealtime behavior can ease these tensions.

Milk It is important to recognize that 1 oz of milk supplies 36 mg of calcium, and many children receive 6 to 8 oz of milk on dry cereal daily. Although they consume only 1 to 2 oz at a time, their calcium intakes may be acceptable when they consume milk with meals and snacks. When abundant amounts of fruit juice or sweetened beverages are available, children may simply prefer to drink them instead of milk. Other dairy products can be offered when milk is rejected. Cheese and yogurt are usually accepted. Powdered milk can be used in recipes for soups, vegetables, and mixed dishes. Fruit juice may replace milk and, consequently, essential nutrients in the diets of young children. Excessive consumption of fruit juice has been implicated as the cause of chronic nonspecific diarrhea.

Meat Parents' perceptions of children's dislike of meat may need to be clarified, or an easier-to-chew form used. If, in fact, preschoolers do consistently refuse all food sources of heme iron, their daily intake of iron should be carefully monitored.

TABLE 10-11—cont'd

This is a guide to a basic diet. Fats, desserts, and sauces will contribute additional kilocalories of energy to meet the needs of the growing child.

| Four- to Six-Years-Old | | Seven Years to Puberty | | |
Portion Sizes	No. of Servings	Portion Sizes	No. of Servings	Comments
$\frac{1}{2}$–$\frac{3}{4}$ cup	3–4	1 cup	3	The following may be substituted for $\frac{1}{2}$ cup of liquid milk: $\frac{1}{2}$–$\frac{3}{4}$ oz cheese $\frac{1}{4}$–$\frac{1}{2}$ cup yogurt $2\frac{1}{2}$ tbsp nonfat dry milk powder
1–2 oz	2	2–3 oz	3	The following may be substituted for 1 oz of meat, fish, or poultry: 4–5 tbsp cooked legumes 1 egg 2 tbsp peanut butter
	4–5		4–5	Include 1 green leafy or yellow vegetable, such as spinach, broccoli, carrots, winter squash
3–4 tbsp		$\frac{1}{2}$ cup		
Few pieces		$\frac{1}{2}$ cup		
4–6 tbsp		$\frac{1}{2}$ cup		Include one vitamin C–rich fruit or juice per day
$\frac{1}{2}$–1 small				
4 oz		4 oz		
1 slice	4	1 slice	6	The following may be substituted for 1 slice of bread: $\frac{1}{2}$ cup cooked cereal $\frac{1}{2}$ cup spaghetti or other pasta $\frac{1}{2}$ cup rice 5 saltines Whole-grain products provide additional bulk to the diet.

Vegetables When vegetables are consistently refused, wars between parents and children should not be permitted to erupt. Small portions of 1 or 2 tsp should continue to be served without comment and should be discarded if the child does not eat them. Preschool behavior modification programs that include token rewards when children consume vegetables served at mealtime have been found to increase children's acceptance and intake of them.[54]

Sweets Parents concerned about children's excessive intakes of sweets may need help in setting limits on amounts of sweet foods they make available to their children. It may be important also to help parents convey their concerns about the need to set limits on the availability of these foods. Other family members, day care providers, and teachers may need to be involved in the plan for change.

Food intake If children's food intakes are so limited that their intakes of energy and nutrients are compromised, parents may need help in establishing guidelines so that the children develop appetites. They should provide food often enough so that children do not get so hungry that they lose their appetite, yet not so often that they are always satiated. Intervals of three to four hours are often successful. Very small portions of foods should be offered and second portions permitted when children consume the foods already served. Attention should always be focused on children when they eat, never when food is refused.

Group Feeding

Increasing numbers of mothers of young children are working outside the home. Over half of the three- to five-year-old children in the United States are in child care settings at least part-time each week. This has been estimated at 5.1 million preschool-aged children in child care centers and 4 million children in family day care homes. Children whose mothers work

CASE STUDY

A Preschooler's View of Milk and Vegetables

During a well-child clinic visit, the mother of a three-year-old boy expresses concern about his nutrient intake. She tells the clinical nutritionist, "He doesn't like to drink milk and refuses vegetables."

Questions for analysis
1. How does his food behavior compare with that of other preschool children?
2. What nutrients should be assessed in the food he does eat?
3. What nonfood parameters should be evaluated?

Response
This child demonstrates a seemingly typical pattern of three year old child food acceptance. First, establish that the child has no known chronic illness or condition that could affect his growth and appetite. Weight and height should be carefully measured and plotted along with weight for stature on the appropriate growth chart. If data points from previous measurements are available they should also be plotted to provide a view of his size over time. If his height and weight attainment are appropriately 'in channel', his mother can be reassured that his energy intake is adequate to support growth.

Mother should be asked to provide either a food frequency or a 24 hour recall of foods consumed. Intake of protein, calcium and vitamin D are of concern because of a reported lack of milk in his food pattern. Fruit juices or sodas as exclusive beverages are a concern because of the non-nutritive energy intake and risk for dental caries they provide. Iron nutriture is a concern for all young children. The B vitamins are a concern because he refuses to eat vegetables. However, if he enjoys fruits, these nutrients are provided to him. In conversation with mother, she should be asked to describe timing of meals and snacks, sleep and activity patterns and her sense of whether mealtimes are organized and relatively peaceful or chaotic.

A more detailed assessment should be undertaken if:
1. The child's height and or weight attainment are less than the 10th percentile or greater than the 90th percentile (without previous data for comparison);
2. There is no obvious source of protein, calcium, vitamin D, or B vitamins in his food pattern;
3. There is no pattern to meals and snacks or the child is able to demand and receive non-nourishing foods to replace milk and thus satisfy his appetite.

---

full-time are often in a child care facility for nine to ten hours five days a week and receive both meals and snacks in this setting. Kindergartens and preschools also offer snacks and meals along with food experiences that are often included as part of the learning activities.

Family day care homes and day care centers are licensed by state agencies that mandate the meal pattern and types of snacks to be provided for the children, as well as the percentage of the Recommended Dietary Allowances that must be included in the menus. In general, a child in day care for eight hours should receive at least one-third the RDA from food and snacks; a child in day care for more than eight hours should receive one-half to two-thirds of the RDA.

Breakfast should be provided for children who receive none at home. Snacks should be planned to complement the daily food intakes. Small portions of food should be served, and children should be permitted second servings of the foods they enjoy. Disliked or unfamiliar foods may be offered by the teaspoonful and the child's acceptance or rejection received without comment. Children who eat slowly will need to be served first and permitted to complete meals without being rushed to other activities. Teachers and caretakers should eat with the children without imposing their attitudes about food.

A new setting provides an opportunity for children to have exposure to many new foods. Day care centers, kindergartens, and preschools can provide an important educational setting for both children and their parents. Children learn how to prepare food, how food grows, how it smells, and what nutrients it contains. Parents learn through participation, observation, and conversation with the staff. An organized approach to feeding children must include parents, teachers, and other staff who offer food to children. Teachers and day care workers can provide important information to parents about how children successfully consume food, the nutrients children need, and the foods that provide these nutrients. Parents offer important information to the centers about their children's food acceptance and needs. Each needs to be reinforced positively by the other for their efforts to provide food for the children to be successful.

Day care providers are influential in the development of food choices and food patterns for young children. Providers need to be aware of the influence they have, as well as to have a basic understanding of the foods and nutrients required to support the growth and development of young children. The American Dietetic Association has taken a straightforward policy position on this issue. The association mandates dietitians and nutritionists to take a leadership role in providing technical assistance and training in nutrition and nutrition education to providers of programs for children, adolescents, and their families.[57]

SCHOOL-AGE CHILDREN ≋

School-age children, generally considered to be ages six to twelve years, have a consistent, slow rate of physical growth. They continue to gain in maturation of fine and gross motor skills and demonstrate significant gains in cognitive, social, and emotional skills. Many food habits, likes, and dislikes are established and form the basis for a lifetime of food and nutrient intake. Food choices are significantly and increasingly affected by peers and influences other than the family. Feeding programs at school and at day care continue to make a significant contribution to food intake. Opportunities for physical activity need to be available and supported by the community; this is a critical period for developing activity patterns that are maintained.

Studies of the school-age population have found that most children are adequately nourished. One will, however, find groups in which an inadequate food and nutrient intake is of concern. In a comparison of first-grade children in low- and high-poverty areas in Washington State, obesity was the most common growth deviance observed. Eighteen percent of the children from low-poverty areas and 12% from high-poverty areas had a weight-height ratio greater than the 90th percentile on the NCHS growth charts.[58] There have been several reports of failure to thrive and delayed onset of puberty because very zealous parents' efforts to prevent obesity and cardiovascular disease caused them to allow their children inadequate energy intake that was insufficient for normal growth.[59,60] It is clear that children who eat regular meals in preference to only snacking do better nutritionally. Studies have also revealed that currently the amount of fat in children's diets is the same as in the diets of adults, and these amounts are lower than they were several years ago.[61]

School entrance provides an opportunity to identify children whose growth parameters indicate nutrition concerns, such as growth failure, obesity, and underweight. Feeding programs, such as the school lunch and breakfast programs, contribute significantly to children's nutrient intake.

Patterns of Nutrient Intake

By school age, most children have established a particular pattern of food and nutrient intake relative to their peers. Although wide ranges of food intake, and thus of energy and nutrients, continue to be observed, those who consume the greatest amount of food consistently do so, whereas those consuming smaller amounts maintain these lesser intakes relative to their peers. Differences in intake between males and females gradually increase to age twelve and then become marked. Boys consume greater quantities of food—thus, energy and nutrients—than girls. Snacks contribute 33% of the daily energy, 20% of the protein, 33% of the fat, and 40% of the carbohydrates consumed each day by ten-year-old chil-

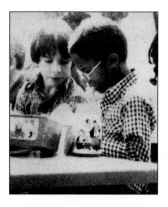

FIG. 10-4   Food habits are part of both physical and psychosocial development.
Steve Fritz.

dren.[62] School-age children eat less frequently than younger children, about four or five times a day on school days. They usually have a snack after school, which they often prepare themselves. These snacks contribute about one-third of their total energy intake.[63]

Physical and Social Development

The school-age period is one of few apparent feeding conflicts. A natural increase in appetite creates normal increases in food intake. Because children spend their days at school, they adjust to a more ordered routine. As they explore the environment of school and peers, children are influenced by these experiences (fig. 10-4). Often, the credibility of parents is questioned, in the face of advice from teachers, peers, or peers' parents. The school-age child has more access to money, grocery stores, and vending machines and, therefore, to foods with questionable nutrient value. Many school-age children have some responsibility for preparing their own breakfasts or sack lunches and arrive home from school hungry and ready for a snack.

Food Patterns

Although school-age children usually increase the amount they eat and the varieties of food they accept, many continue to reject vegetables and mixed dishes. The range of food they voluntarily accept may be small. Sugar contributes 24–25% of the total energy in the diets of many school-age children. Sweetened beverages, fruits, fruit juice, cakes, cookies, and other dessert items are significant sources of sugar in the diets of school-age children.

Food dislikes of older children consistently include cooked vegetables and mixed dishes. Children accept raw vegetables more readily than cooked ones but often ingest only a limited amount. Sweetness and familiarity are significant factors that influence food preferences in all children.

A common difficulty for parents is finding a time when school-age children are willing to sit down and eat a meal. Frequently, they are so involved with other activities that it is difficult to get them to take time to eat with the family. Often, they satisfy their initial hunger and rush back to their activities and television programs, returning later for a snack. The food patterns of second- and fifth-graders were assessed. Forty percent of the children did not eat vegetables, except for potatoes and tomato sauce; 20% did not eat fruit; 36% ate at least four types of snack foods daily. The fifth-graders ate significantly more snack foods than the second-graders and were also more likely to skip breakfast.[64]

Meal Patterns

Breakfast is an important meal. Even so, estimates of children who do not eat breakfast range from 8% to 29%. Children have to rise earlier to eat an unhurried and balanced meal and may have to prepare it themselves. Early morning school activities may make preplanning necessary. Some may find a glass of milk and fruit juice important before early sports activities. Studies have shown that, when breakfast is consumed, children have a better attitude and school record, compared with when it is omitted. Pollitt, Leibel, and Greenfield found that nine- to eleven-year-old well-nourished children who skipped breakfast showed a decrease in accuracy of response in problem solving but an increase in immediate memory in short-term accuracy.[65] The effect was attributed to a heightened arousal level, which in turn had a qualitative effect on cognitive function.

Actually, most children do eat breakfasts that contribute at least one-fourth of the RDA standard. A larger percentage of children in the lower grades eat breakfast than those in the middle and upper grades. Reasons for skipping breakfast include "not hungry," "no time," "on a diet," "no one to prepare food," "do not like food served for breakfast," and "foods are not available." Breakfast is noted as being an important contributor to overall dietary quality and adequacy in school-age children. Girls are more likely than boys to have breakfast at home (46%), and about 20% of all ten-year-old children skip breakfast entirely.[66]

The school-age child often participates in the National School Lunch Program administered by the Department of Agriculture, which provides cash reimbursement and supplemental foods to feeding programs that comply with federal regulations. Low-income children may receive reduced prices or free meals. Children who do not participate in the school lunch program generally bring a packed lunch from home. Studies have indicated that, compared with the school lunch, these meals provide significantly fewer nutrients but do supply energy. Little variety is seen in the lunches, since favorite foods tend to be packed and lack of refrigeration limits the kinds of foods that can be carried.

The evening meal provides an opportunity for family interaction and socialization, as well as one of food and nutrient intake. Children should be expected to participate in both activities. It is important that parents not cater to children's food idiosyncrasies but offer them the family menu of nourishing foods.

The emotional environment at the dinner table may influence nutrient intake. The evening meal is not an appropriate time for family battles or punitive action toward children. If eating is to be successful and enjoyable, it must occur in a setting that is comfortable and free from stress and unreasonable demands.

School Meals

School feeding and nutrition education programs, when adequately implemented, provide not only important nutrients for children but also an opportunity to learn to make responsible food choices. These feeding programs contribute significantly to the nutrient and energy intake of many low-income children. In fact, such feeding programs may provide motivation for children to go to school.

Since its inception in 1946, the National School Lunch Program has been administered by the U.S. Department of Agriculture. Federal regulations require that school lunches and breakfasts be sold at reduced prices or be given free to children whose families cannot afford to buy them. The breakfast and lunch menus must be planned to meet the guidelines established for the National School Lunch Program. Tables 10-12 and 10-13 show minimum quantities of food required for the various age groups in a school breakfast and lunch.

To provide variety and to enlist participation and consumption, schools are encouraged to provide a selection of foods. About half of the schools participating in the lunch program also serve breakfast. Breakfast must include liquid milk, fruit or vegetable juice, and bread or cereal. Schools are encouraged to keep fat, sugar, and salt at moderate levels.

Current regulations require that schools involve students and parents in planning the school lunch program. They may be included in such activities as menu planning, enhancement of the eating environment, program promotion, and related student community support activities.

Foods sold in competition with school lunch in snack bars and vending machines must provide at least 5% of the Recommended Dietary Allowances for one or more of the following nutrients: protein, vitamin A, vitamin C, niacin, riboflavin, thiamin, calcium, and iron. This regulation eliminates the sale of soda water, water ices, chewing gum, and some candies until after the last lunch period. It should also encourage the offering of more fruits, vegetables, and fruit and vegetable juices in places that compete with the school lunch. Concentrated sources of sucrose have been a concern of many interested in dental health, the control of obesity, and the development of sound food habits for all children.

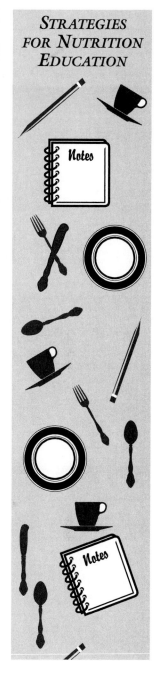

STRATEGIES FOR NUTRITION EDUCATION

School Meal Initiative for Healthy Children: Improving Nutritional Health

The National School Lunch Program was begun in 1946 and now serves about 25 million lunches every day. A school breakfast program was added in recent years to serve children who for socioeconomic or other reasons cannot eat breakfast at home. The National School Lunch Program has two important goals. First, this program strives to improve the dietary intake and nutritional health of the nation's children. Children who receive an appropriate supply of nutritious food and adequate energy throughout the day are more physically, mentally, and emotionally prepared for learning. A second major goal of the National School Lunch Program is to promote nutrition education and teach children to make appropriate food choices for a lifetime. School meals should provide examples of healthy meal patterns based on the Food Guide Pyramid. Food habits are shaped early in life, and the school nutrition program should introduce children to a wide variety of foods, which they may or may not have eaten at home. To maximize this effort, the food and nutrition education provided by the school breakfast and lunch program must be coordinated with education received in the classroom. Children must develop positive health attitudes and learn about the relationships of food, nutrition, and health. Some schools have developed a comprehensive curriculum in which food and nutrition concepts are introduced and reinforced from kindergarten through grade 12. Appropriate food and fitness behaviors can be integrated within all major subject areas in the school curriculum. Following are examples of appropriate learning activities.

Social studies: Studies of foods consumed by different ethnic or cultural groups, foods grown in different parts of the world, nutrition labeling regulations, and functions of the Food and Drug Administration.

Mathematics: Calculation of energy or total nutrients consumed by the student per meal or per day; calculation of the energy in a particular food based on the grams of fat, carbohydrates, and protein given on the label, calculation of the total cost of a meal and cost per person.

Physical and biological sciences: Studies of the process by which food is digested; how nutrients are used for growth and regulation of body functions; food tests for protein, carbohydrates, or starch; the classification and origin of fruits and vegetables; energy and muscle function.

Health and physical education: Exercise activities for lifelong enjoyment, exercise and weight management, components of a healthy diet, avoidance of addictive behaviors, and good food sources of particular nutrients.

Communication arts: Writing a story about a favorite food, writing and producing a class play about healthy food and activity behaviors, and making posters for the school lunch room about good food choices.

1994. ADA supports USDA School Meals Initiative for Healthy Children but recommends more improvements for child nutrition. *J Am Diet Assoc* 94:841.

Sufficient concern has been created in some school districts that only machines that provide fruit, milk, nuts, and seeds have been made available to students. Initially, sales have been found to decrease, but ultimately they increase. One school discovered that it made a greater profit on apples than on chocolate bars.

Many persons concerned about the prevention of atherosclerosis and obesity have made statements about the quantity and saturation of fats as well as the energy density of foods in these school lunches. Indeed, some schools have responded to these concerns and have provided low-fat menu options.

Although elementary schoolchildren are making more decisions regarding food selection, supervision and supportive guidelines may be necessary at lunchtime. Children may give priority to activities other than eating and rush through their meals. Some may refuse

TABLE 10-12   *School Breakfast Pattern—School Breakfast Program*

Food Components		Minimum Quantities		
		Age 1–2	Age 3–5	Age 6 and Older
Milk	Beverage, on cereal, or both	$\frac{1}{2}$ cup (4 fl oz)	$\frac{3}{4}$ cup (6 fl oz)	$\frac{1}{2}$ pt (8 fl oz)
Fruit/vegetable/juice*	Fruit or vegetable or both or full-strength fruit or vegetable juice	$\frac{1}{4}$ cup	$\frac{1}{2}$ cup	$\frac{1}{2}$ cup
Select *one* serving from each of the following components or *two* servings from one component				
Bread or bread alternate	Whole-grain or enriched bread	$\frac{1}{2}$ slice	$\frac{1}{2}$ slice	1 slice
	Whole-grain or enriched biscuit, roll, muffin	$\frac{1}{2}$ serving	$\frac{1}{2}$ serving	1 serving
	Whole-grain, enriched, or fortified cereal	$\frac{1}{4}$ cup or $\frac{1}{3}$ oz	$\frac{1}{3}$ cup or $\frac{1}{2}$ oz	$\frac{3}{4}$ cup or 1 oz
Meat or meat alternate	Lean meat, poultry, or fish	$\frac{1}{2}$ oz	$\frac{1}{2}$ oz	1 oz
	Cheese	$\frac{1}{2}$ oz	$\frac{1}{2}$ oz	1 oz
	Yogurt	$\frac{1}{4}$ cup	$\frac{1}{4}$ cup	$\frac{1}{2}$ cup
	Large eggs	$\frac{1}{2}$	$\frac{1}{2}$	$\frac{1}{2}$
	Peanut butter	1 tbsp	1 tbsp	2 tbsp
	Cooked dry beans or peas	2 tbsp	2 tbsp	4 tbsp
	Nuts or seeds or both	$\frac{1}{2}$ oz	$\frac{1}{2}$ oz	1 oz

From Food and Nutrition Service, USDA 1990. *Meal pattern requirements and offer versus serve manual.* FNS-265. Bethesda, MD.
*A citrus fruit or juice or a vegetable that is a good source of vitamin C is recommended daily.

to eat the food on the menu. Children who need therapeutic diets need guidance in the foods they should and should not eat. Model projects are underway to evaluate nutrient standard menu planning (NSMP)—that is, using the nutrient content of foods to plan menus rather than the more traditional meal pattern components menu planning system. It is hoped that the new system will facilitate greater variety of foods of lower fat and sodium content in school lunch menus.[67]

PREVENTION OF NUTRITION AND HEALTH PROBLEMS ≋

Nutrition concerns during childhood include iron deficiency anemia, overweight and obesity, and dental caries. In addition, some persons are worried about children's intakes of specific foods and food constituents, such as artificial flavors and colors and sugar, and their possible effect on behavior. Also, it is important to recognize that many risk factors for cardiovascular disease can be modified by changes in dietary patterns. Identifying children at risk and modifying fat and salt intakes, as well as other factors, are important health promotion actions.

The prevention of iron deficiency anemia was discussed earlier in this chapter (p. 234–35).

Weight Management

An excessive rate of weight gain and deposition of fat occurs when energy intake exceeds energy expenditure. Over time, this situation can lead to obesity. Between 1988 and 1994, 11% of children and adolescents in the United States were estimated to be overweight and

TABLE 10-13 *School Lunch Pattern—National School Lunch Program*

Food Components	Minimum Quantities				Recommended Quantities*
	Group I: Age 1–2; Preschool	Group II: Age 3–4; Preschool	Group III: Age 5–8; Gr. K–3	Group IV: Age 9 and Older; Gr. 4–12	Group V: Age 12 and Older; Gr. 7–12
Milk Whole and unflavored lowfat milk must be offered‡	¾ cup (6 fl oz)	¾ cup (6 fl oz)	½ pt (8 fl oz)	½ pt (8 fl oz)	½ pt (8 fl oz)
Meat or meat alternate (quantity of the edible portion as served)					
Lean meat, poultry, or fish	1 oz	1½ oz	1½ oz	2 oz	3 oz
Cheese	1 oz	1½ oz	1½ oz	2 oz	3 oz
Yogurt	¼ cup	¼ cup	½ cup	½ cup	½ cup
Large eggs	½	¾	¾	1	1½
Cooked dry beans or peas	¼ cup	⅜ cup	⅜ cup	½ cup	¾ cup
Peanut butter or an equivalent quantity of any combination of above	2 tbsp	3 tbsp	3 tbsp	4 tbsp	6 tbsp
Vegetable or fruit 2 or more servings of vegetable or fruit or both to total	½ cup	½ cup	½ cup	¾ cup	¾ cup
Bread or bread alternate (servings per week) Must be enriched or whole-grain—at least ½ serving‡ for group I or one serving‡ for groups II–V must be served daily	5	8	8	8	10

From Food and Nutrition Service, U.S. Department of Agriculture. 1990. *Meal pattern requirements and offer versus serve manual.* FNS-265. Bethesda, MD.

*The minimum portion sizes for these children are the portion sizes for group IV.

†This requirement does not prohibit offering other milk, such as flavored milk or skim milk, along with the above.

‡Serving, 1 slice of bread; or 1/2 cup of cooked rice, macaroni, noodles, other pasta products, other cereal products such as bulgur and corn grits; or 1 biscuit, roll, muffin, and similar products; or any combination of these.

an additional 14% had BMIs between the 85th and 95th percentiles. Alarmingly, there is an increase in the prevalence of overweight among preschool children in the United States.[68] Current estimates for overweight among preschool children are as high as 18–20%.[69,70] The possible influence of family factors in childhood on adult obesity has been debated for decades. A study in Denmark followed a cohort of school-aged children for ten years, from midchildhood to young adulthood. Parental neglect—that is, lack of emotional support and general hygiene—predicted a great risk of obesity in young adulthood, independent of age and body mass index in childhood, gender, and social background.[71] By monitoring rates of growth and deposition of adipose tissue, children who are accumulating more fat than would be anticipated can be identified, and measures to increase activity and decrease excessive energy intake can be taken.

Children with a BMI greater than the 85th percentile with the complications of obesity or with a BMI greater than the 95th percentile with or without complications should undergo evaluation and possible treatment. These complications include hypertension, sleep disorders, and insulin resistance.[72] The emphasis on obesity prevention and treatment in children and youth has been reinforced by the belief that body size affects the socialization of children and adolescents and may lead to the development of a negative body image, associated with subsequent eating disorders.[73]

Young children are increasingly concerned about their weight and are attempting to modify it. About 60% of fourth-grade girls, compared with about 39% of boys, report a desire to be thinner. Weight-related behaviors and concerns increase with increasing weight-for-age and body mass index. The most frequent weight-related behavior is increased consumption of diet soft drinks.[74]

Family attitudes. At increasingly younger ages, children make their own decisions about what and when they eat. However, parents can manage the food available to younger children, create the environment that influences their acceptance of food, and influence energy expenditure by the opportunities they create for physical activity for their children. Some parents may not recognize that their expectations for the quantity of food they encourage their children to consume are excessive and that the "chubby" child is not necessarily the healthy child.

Parents may need help in developing appropriate parenting skills. They may need to learn how to respond to hunger and other needs of their infants and how to interact with their children. Families with overweight or obese children may need help with task accomplishment and control, which are two functions involved in making changes.[75] They may need help in identifying ways to help their children develop initiative and to cultivate friends and outlets in the community.[76]

Physical activity. The activity pattern of both the child and the family should be explored. It may be important to help parents find ways of increasing their child's level of activity. Parents who live in apartments often reinforce sedentary activities to reduce the noise level and complaints from neighbors. Those who live in one-family dwellings may have limited space for children's activities. Many city park departments, preschools, and schools have programs that offer opportunities for increasing children's activities. All children are encouraged to participate in about thirty minutes of moderate-intensity activity on most days of the week. It is believed that only about 20% of U.S. children currently achieve this goal.

Appropriate energy intakes. It is important to remember that at any age the range of appropriate energy intakes is large. Overweight children and children with familial trends toward obesity may need fewer kilocalories of energy than do their peers. Families of children with a familial tendency toward obesity may require help in identifying the kinds and amounts of food that provide an energy intake that supports normal growth and weight gain.

Nutrition counseling. An increasing number of children in the United States are overweight, and overweight affects younger and younger children. Programs of nutrition counseling should be family-oriented and based on normal nutrition, emphasizing foods that provide a balance of nutrients as well as appropriate energy intakes. Families need to realize that these efforts are directed at reduction in rates of weight gain and are not intended to effect weight loss. They must recognize that the food available and the models set for their child will determine the child's response to efforts to control weight gain. Family meals may need to be modified to include fewer fried foods, less gravy, and fewer

CASE STUDY

Wise Weight Management for a School-Age Girl

At the regular pediatric clinic visit of a seven-year-old girl, the pediatrician and pediatric nutritionist found that the girl's BMI on the growth chart was above the 85th percentile. Her rate of weight gain had increased in the past year, crossing from the 50th to the 90th percentile.

Questions for analysis
1. What factors that influence her food intake and energy expenditure should be assessed?
2. What is a reasonable goal to correct her overweight status?
3. Outline a daily food plan to achieve this goal.

First, it should be established by the pediatrician that there are no organic causes for this increased rate of weight gain. The girl should be addressed directly in a low-key manner and asked to describe her usual daily food intake and activity pattern. Her mother will be asked to provide supportive information or to clarify food choices, portion size and activities. Mother should be asked to clarify the family mealtimes and patterns and any other careproviders who may be providing meals and snacks.

A food frequency or 24 hour recall will provide information to establish the basic patterns of the child and family and perhaps identify those conducive to immediate modification.

Generally, a reasonable expectation for a young child is to maintain the current weight rather than promote weight loss. Without 'counting calories', negotiate with the child and mother to establish a 'standard' meal pattern with a limited selection of food items. For example, breakfast might be unsweetened or lightly sweetened cereal, low fat milk, and fruit or juice. A packed lunch might be a sandwich of meat, cheese or peanut butter without added fat, fruit and beverage or a school lunch could be organized by the parents and child working together to pre-choose acceptable items and eliminate unacceptable ones from the school lunch menu. An afternoon snack might be a carbohydrate such as popcorn, $\frac{1}{2}$ bagel, or $\frac{1}{2}$ sandwich, low fat milk, and fruit. For dinner with the family an adult would prepare a simple meat, chicken, vegetable, pasta or rice meal without added fat or pre-selected food choices could be negotiated for a fast food meal. A list of acceptable low-energy snacks might be made available at home.

This is a one-step-at-a-time process which involves commitment of the child, mother, and the rest of the family. It is also a long-term process of 'learning by doing' and immediate and startling changes in food related behaviors are not expected.

---

rich desserts. Parents and siblings may have to modify their own eating practices to set appropriate examples. Teachers, baby-sitters, and day care providers should be alerted to and included in programs designed to maintain or control weight. Food experiences at school may need to be modified to exclude corn dripping with butter and chocolate cupcakes, so frequently provided for special occasions. Low-energy snacks, such as raw fruits and vegetables, can be provided instead of cookies, candy, and hot dogs.

It is important to recognize that school-age children are very concerned about size. In fact, many are on self-imposed diets because they worry about becoming overweight. Weight control programs should be planned carefully, so that they do not become the cause of an eating disorder in adolescence (see the box on p. 255).

Dental Caries

Dental caries, one of the most common nutritional diseases, affects children of all ages and family income levels. Schoolchildren in the United States have an average of 3.07 decayed, missing, or filled permanent tooth surfaces (DMFS). This rate increases to 8.04 DMFS by age 17.[77] It has been documented that 61% of African American and 55% of

Dental caries
(L *caries,* rottenness) Molecular decay or death of hard tissue; disease of the calcified tissue of the teeth resulting from action of microorganisms on carbohydrates, characterized by disintegration of hard outer enamel, followed by breakdown of softer inner dentin material, leaving cavities and exposed soft tissue.

Mexican American children exhibit tooth decay by age 8[78] and that 59% of all children aged two to four years old have never visited a dentist. As with other tissues, nutrition plays an important role during development in the acquisition of sound teeth and the surrounding structures that hold them and in the later susceptibility of the teeth to caries. Once the tooth has erupted, the composition of the diet, the presence of acid-producing bacteria, and the **buffering capacity** of the saliva interact and result in control or development of dental caries. Calcified dental tissues, unlike the long bones, which are subject to constant remodeling and repair, do not have the ability to repair themselves. Tooth destruction by decay is permanent.

Etiology. Dental plaque, a prerequisite for dental caries, has been described as a sticky, gelatinous mixture that contains water, salivary protein, **desquamated** cells, and bacteria. The plaque bacteria, using energy derived from the catabolism of dietary carbohydrate, synthesize several toxic substances, including enzymes that have the potential to degrade the **enamel** and **dentin** and are precursors of acidic fermentation products. *Streptococcus mutans* appears to be the primary bacterium. These acids and enzymes cause demineralization of the **hydroxyapatite** of the enamel, followed by **proteolytic** degradation and demineralization of the enamel and dentin. It has been proposed that, when the acidic environment falls below 5.5, cariogenic bacteria invade the tooth and caries results. The saliva, the **pH** of which is 6.5 to 7.0, acts as a buffer and provides mechanical cleansing of the teeth.

Sugar. The incidence of caries can be reduced when intakes of sugar are reduced. Glucose is thought to be the next most cariogenic sugar, and maltose, lactose, and fructose have been found to have equal effect. Starch can also cause the production of large amounts of plaque acid, because the carbohydrate, once attacked by salivary amylase, is broken down into sugar and attacked by plaque bacteria.

Frequency of eating. The presence of sucrose, or even the total amount of sucrose in the diet, may not be the determining factor in the incidence of dental caries. An often quoted study in an institution for the mentally handicapped in Sweden showed that the more important factors were the frequency with which the sugar was consumed and the food's adhesiveness to the teeth.[79] The researchers who conducted this five-year study showed that the consumption of sticky candy between meals produced a high increase in the incidence of dental caries, whereas the increase in incidence of caries from the addition of sugar-sweetened water at mealtime was small. When sucrose was fed in chocolate or bread, an intermediate increase in the incidence of caries was noted. Other studies have not supported these findings. Many researchers have found no difference between the meal-eating habits of caries-free and caries-prone individuals.

Snacking at bedtime is especially effective in increasing dental caries. Reduction of the flow of saliva, which occurs during sleep, reduces the natural cleansing mechanism and permits greater fermentation of cariogenic material. The ingestion of foods that alter the buffering capacity of the saliva—for example, milk and fats, which form a protective oily film on the tooth surface—may offer some protection for the teeth.

Control. The less frequently sucrose-containing foods are consumed and the less ability the foods have to adhere to the teeth, the more positive is the outlook for the control of dental caries.

Fluoride It has been proven that fluoride can reduce the incidence of dental caries. Fluoride suppresses sugar metabolism by bacteria, makes enamel more resistant to acid, and stimulates remineralization of the teeth. A fluoridated water supply is an important approach to the prevention of dental caries.

Diet: foods and frequency Dietary control continues to be a very important and effective approach to the control of dental caries. The frequency of eating breads, rolls, and cereals has not been associated with an increase in dental caries, whereas the frequency of eating candy and chewing gum has been shown to increase the number and incidence of dental caries. Cookies, cakes, pies, and candies have been shown to cause profound falls in pH levels of the plaque. It is interesting that more acid-carbonated beverages depress the pH less than apple and orange juice.[80] A study of 147 junior high school students' snacking patterns in relation to caries production showed chocolate

Buffering capacity
Function of the body's main buffer system of two balancing partners, an acid partner (carbonic acid) and a base partner (sodium bicarbonate), which act together to buffer, or neutralize, any incoming acid or base to maintain the necessary degree of acidity and alkalinity in the body fluids that is compatible with life and health.

Desquamation
(L *de-*; *squama*, scale). Shedding of epithelial tissue, mainly the skin and oral mucosa, in scales or small sheets.

Enamel
A hard white substance that covers the dentin of the crown of a tooth.

Dentin
The chief material of teeth inside the enamel. It is harder and denser than bone.

Hydroxyapatite
Inorganic compound of calcium and phosphorus found in the matrix of bones and teeth; gives rigidity and strength to the structure.

Proteolytic
Pertaining to any substance that promotes the break down of protein.

pH
Abbreviation for potential hydrogen which is a scale representing the relative acidity or alkalinity of a solution.

Nutritional Snacks for Dental Health

Protein foods*

Natural cheese (cheddar, jack, string)
Milk
Cooked turkey, chicken, beef, ham
Plain yogurt
Peanut butter
Cottage cheese
Unsalted nuts and seeds
Tuna
Hard-cooked egg

Breads and cereals[†]

Whole-grain breads
Whole-grain cereals
Whole-grain, low-fat crackers
Tortillas
English muffins
Rice crackers
Pita bread
Popcorn
Bagels

Fruits[†]

Apples
Bananas
Pears
Berries
Oranges, other citrus fruits
Melon
Grapes
Unsweetened canned fruit
Unsweetened fruit juices

Vegetables

Carrots
Celery
Green pepper
Radishes
Cucumbers
Cabbage
Cauliflower
Broccoli
Tomatoes
Jicama
Vegetable juices

Examples: Apple wedges with peanut butter; egg salad sandwich; raw vegetables with yogurt or cottage cheese dip; plain yogurt with unsweetened applesauce and cinnamon; tortilla with melted cheese; pita bread with tuna; popcorn with parmesan cheese; frozen banana rolled in plain yogurt and chopped nuts; rice cracker with peanut butter or cheese

---

Trahms, C.M., and P.L. Pipes. 1997. *Nutrition in infancy and childhood.* McGraw-Hill. Dubuque, IA.
*These foods may be protective against lowering plaque pH when eaten with foods that contain fermentable carbohydrate.
[†]Fruits, juices, and most cereal/bread products contain fermentable carbohydrate; limit to one serving in a snack.

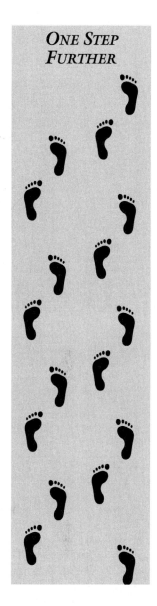

ONE STEP FURTHER

candy to be the most carious snack food selected. The children who consumed fruit drinks, cookies, or apples at bedtime and between meals had a significant caries increment during the year studied. No carious lesions developed in 47 children who had higher intakes of fruit juice and oranges and lesser use of sugar-sweetened chewing gum than in the other children.[81]

Plaque control Researchers have studied the cariogenicity of foods by noting changes in the plaque pH before and immediately after a food is eaten. Foods that cause the plaque pH to fall below 5.5 are considered to be cariogenic. Certain foods do not cause the plaque pH between the teeth to fall to levels at which demineralization occurs. These foods have a relatively high protein content with basic amino acids, a moderate fat content, a strong buffering capacity, a high mineral content including calcium and phosphorus, and a pH greater than 6.0. They also stimulate saliva flow. Meats, nuts, and cheese have been found to be noncariogenic. In fact, they have a beneficial effect when consumed with other foods. Cheddar cheese has been observed to block caries formation caused by sweet snacks when sweets and cheese have been eaten alternately. Nutritional snacks for dental health are shown in the box on p. 257.

Nutrition education Children should be taught to select foods that provide the essential nutrients and to limit their consumption of cariogenic foods. It is important that they learn to include noncariogenic protective foods in their snacking patterns, especially when sucrose-containing foods are included in the menu. The important between-meal snacks can be carefully planned to contribute nutrients without creating an oral environment conducive to tooth decay. Sweet foods, such as dessert items, should be consumed as infrequently as possible within the framework of acceptability to the child and the family.

Food and Behavior

There has been considerable speculation that certain additives and food constituents, such as sugar and caffeine, play a part in the etiology of hyperactivity in childhood. This condition is characterized by inattention, excess motor activity, impulsiveness, and poor tolerance for frustration; the onset of hyperactivity occurs before seven years of age. It affects 5–10% of school-age children.

Salicylates
Compound salts of salicylic acid, found in certain plants and in drugs such as common aspirin (acetylsalicylic acid—ASA).

Additives. In recent years, the hypothesis that artificial flavors and colors and naturally occurring **salicylates** cause hyperactivity in as many as 50% of children so affected has been popular. Many persons have felt that a diet that eliminated these constituents was indicated, but research has not supported this hypothesis. A very small percentage of children, however, have been identified to be "responders" to the additives.

Open clinical trials have indicated positive behavioral changes in as many as 50% of hyperactive children when food additive intake was restricted. They have also reported that diet improved behavior in nonhyperactive children, suggesting that behavioral changes may be due to changes in the parent-child interactions and family dynamics. A study using a total dietary replacement design looked at dietary manipulations in twenty-four hyperactive preschool boys. All children received both the experimental and control diets. Food dyes, food flavorings, preservatives, monosodium glutamate, chocolate, and caffeine were eliminated from the diet. Specific foods that the family felt to be detrimental to the child's behavior were also eliminated. Almost 50% of the boys showed some behavioral improvement using the accepted rating scales. Sleep patterns also were better.[82]

Sugar. Sugar has also been hypothesized to play a role in the etiology of behavioral difficulties in children. Most of the reports that have indicted sugar have been based on clinical assessment, with few on controlled studies.

Several double-blind challenge studies have not found sugar to contribute to hyperactivity even in children whose mothers felt they were responders. However, speculation that sugar is an offender in the etiologies of the disorder continues on the basis of observations of behavior and food intake. An association was suggested between destructive aggressive behavior and sugar intake of four- to seven-year-old hyperkinetic but not normal children on the basis of seven-day food diaries kept by the mothers and videotaped observations of behavior by trained observers.[83] Another study noted an inverse relationship in the percentage of sugar in the children's diets suggested by a one-day dietary recall and standardized measures of intelligence and school achievement.[84] It should be noted that none of these studies has shown a cause and effect relation between sugar and behavior.

Definitive evidence that sugar causes behavioral problems in children has not been found. However, there may be some children who are sensitive to sugar, and further investigation using a double-blind crossover design is appropriate.

Prevention of Atherosclerosis

Atherosclerosis
(Gr *athere,* gruel; *skleros,* hard) Condition characterized by gradual formation, beginning in childhood in genetically predisposed individuals, of fatty, cheese-like streaks then harder plaques in the intima, or inner lining, of major blood vessels such as coronary arteries, eventually in adulthood cutting off blood supply to the tissue served by the vessel; the underlying pathology of coronary heart disease.

Atherosclerotic lesions
Characteristic lesions, called *athromas;* the fatty, raised streaks and plaques that signal atherosclerosis, the underlying cardiovascular disease associated with elevated levels of serum lipids, especially cholesterol, and related risk factors, such as smoking, obesity, and hypertension.

Risk factors. Major risk factors associated with **atherosclerosis** and its resulting cardiovascular disease include obesity, a strong family history of heart disease, a sedentary lifestyle, hypertension, and elevated blood lipids, especially low-density lipoprotein (LDL) cholesterol. These risk factors are independent and continuous variables. Studies of adults have shown a significant relation between elevated serum cholesterol, blood pressure, and the extent of **atherosclerotic lesions.** The extent of the raised lesion is associated with total fat, saturated fat, cholesterol, and animal protein intakes.

Evidence that the atherosclerotic process leading to adult coronary heart disease begins in childhood includes 1) observations at autopsy of children and young adults who died of noncoronary events and 2) epidemiologic studies of adult relatives of children with elevated plasma cholesterol levels. Findings at autopsy have described fatty streaks in the **aorta** of preschool children and fibrous plaques in the coronary arteries of twenty- to twenty-two-year-old American soldiers who died in the Korean and Vietnam wars. Epidemiologic studies indicate that blood lipids and lipoproteins track from birth to the young adult years.[85-87] It is also known that food habits developed in childhood continue into the adult years.

Because of these findings, it is becoming increasingly clear that the origin of atherosclerosis, especially in genetically predisposed persons, is in early childhood. Several groups have recommended changing the diet of all children over two years of age. The recommendation includes reducing total dietary fat to less than 30% of the day's total energy, reducing saturated fat to less than 10% of the total kilocalories, and limiting cholesterol to 300 mg/day.[88] Many pediatricians disagree with this universal recommendation, feeling that such diets may not provide sufficient energy and essential nutrients for normal growth and development. In fact, children of some conscientious parents trying to implement the recommendations have been diagnosed with growth deficits and failure to thrive.[60,61] The American Academy of Pediatrics states that the recommendation should be followed with moderation.[31]

Panel report. A panel from the National Institutes of Health also recommends screening of high-risk children. Children, it indicated in its report, should be selected by their pediatricians for cholesterol screening if they have high-risk families with parents or grandparents with diagnosed cardiovascular heart disease or a cardiac event before age fifty-five or if one or both parents have had elevated serum cholesterol levels over 240 mg/dl. The panel recommended dietary intervention for children with borderline low-density lipoprotein (LDL) cholesterol levels of 110 to 129 mg/dl and drug therapy for children over ten years of age who have very high serum cholesterol levels over 200 mg/dl or an LDL cholesterol level above 130 mg/dl that does not respond to dietary intervention.[89]

The American Academy of Pediatrics recommends cholesterol testing only for children over age two who have a family history of **hyperlipidemia** or early **myocardial infarction.** If an elevated serum cholesterol is confirmed in the child, dietary counseling is advised. Drug therapy is advised only for children with serum cholesterol levels greater than 200 mg/dl and for those who do not respond to dietary intervention in a reasonable period of time.[90] The new guidelines in the National Cholesterol Education Program (NCEP) report for blood total cholesterol and LDL-cholesterol limits for children, shown in the box, are consistent with the American Academy of Pediatrics recommendations, as well as the national health guides and objectives of the American Heart Association, National Academy of Sciences, and U.S. surgeon general, and are supported by the American Dietetic Association.[91-96]

Aorta
Main large trunk blood vessel from the heart, leading down the center of the body through the chest and into the abdomen, from which the systemic arterial blood system proceeds.

Hyperlipidemia
(Gr *hyper,* above; *lipos,* fat; *haemia,* blood) General term for elevated concentrations of any or all of the lipids in the blood plasma.

Myocardial infarction
An occlusion of a coronary artery caused by atherosclerosis or an embolus.

NCEP Report:
Recommended Cholesterol Levels for Children and Adolescents

	Total Cholesterol		Low-Density Lipoprotein Cholesterol	
	mmol/L	mg/dl	mmol/L	mg/dl
Acceptable	<4.4	<170	<2.8	<110
Borderline	4.4–5.1	170–199	2.8–3.3	110–129
High	≥5.2	≥200	≥3.4	≥130

The National Cholesterol Education Program. 1991. *Report of the Expert Panel on Blood Cholesterol Levels in Children and Adolescents.* Bethesda, MD: National Heart, Lung and Blood Institute.

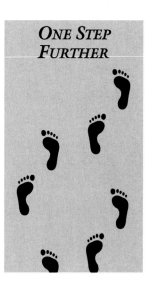

ONE STEP FURTHER

TABLE 10-14   *Healthy Children 2000 Objectives*

Reduce iron deficiency to less than 3% among children aged one to four years.

Reduce growth retardation among low-income children to less than 10% for children aged one to five years.

Reduce average dietary fat intake to less than 30% of total energy and saturated fat to less than 10% of total energy or less for individuals aged two years and older.

Maintain prevalence of obesity at no more than 15% among individuals aged twelve to nineteen years.

Increase calcium intake, so that at least 50% of individuals over age fourteen consume three or more servings of calcium-rich foods per day.

Increase to at least 50% the proportion of overweight individuals over age twelve who have adopted dietary practices to attain appropriate body weight.

Increase to at least 90% the proportion of school lunch and breakfast services with menus consistent with nutrition principles in *Dietary Guidelines for Americans.*

Increase to at least 75% the proportion of schools that provide nutrition education from preschool through grade 12.

Increase to at least 75% the proportion of children and adolescents who engage in vigorous physical activity at least three days per week for twenty minutes or more per occasion.

HEALTHY CHILDREN 2000 OBJECTIVES ≈

The goals for promoting nourishment and health of children in the United States are described in the Healthy Children 2000 Objectives.[97] These health promotion and disease prevention objectives are addressed by public health and clinical intervention programs for children; progress toward achievement of these goals in monitored and updated regularly. The current objectives related to children are shown in table 10-14. The objectives are being updated and revised as Healthy People 2012.

Summary

Children between one year and the onset of puberty grow at a steady rate. They acquire new skills, learn much about their environment, and test the limits of behavior the environment will accept. All of these factors influence the food they accept and the frequency with which they eat. As children grow older, their food intakes become more influenced by peers, activities, and stimuli in their environment.

Prevention of nutrition problems is important during childhood. Of particular concern is the prevention of iron deficiency anemia, obesity, and dental caries, as well as the reduction of later adult risks for cardiovascular coronary heart disease in identified children of high-risk families.

Review Questions

1. Why do energy needs of children vary so widely at any age?
2. What would you expect the progression of typical feeding skills to be from twelve to twenty-four months of age?
3. What factors influence food acceptance by children?
4. List food and feeding behavior concerns of most importance to mothers of preschool children.
5. List snack foods appropriate for children that are supportive of a program to prevent excessive weight gain and dental caries.
6. Describe the family history and blood lipid levels that would identify a child at risk for development of arteriosclerotic heart disease.

- Position papers and handbooks have been published to address the critical need for appropriate meal service in child care centers and educational programs. The components of nutrition education, appropriate food to provide needed nutrients, and a supportive physical and emotional environment are endorsed to protect and promote children's health and well-being.

1992. *Building for the future: Nutrition guidance for the child nutrition programs.* U.S. Department of Agriculture, Food and Nutrition Service, FNS-279.

Edelstein, S. 1992. *Nutrition and meal planning in child-care programs: A practical guide.* Chicago, IL: The American Dietetic Association.

1998. Carol Parkman Williams, ed. *Pediatric Manual of Clinical Dietetics,* Chicago, IL: The American Dietetic Association.

1995. Position of ADA, SNE, and ASFSA: School-based nutrition programs and services. *J Am Diet Assoc* 95:367.

Position paper of the American Dietetic Association. 1996. Child and adolescent food and nutrition programs. *J Am Diet Assoc* 96:913.

1993. Nutrition standards in child care programs: Technical support paper. *J Am Diet Assoc* 93:334.

- Several useful handbooks address the complex issues of child health.

1991. *Healthy children 2000: National health promotion and disease prevention objectives related to mothers, infants, children, adolescents and youth.* Department of Health and Human Services, Public Health Service, Health Resources and Service Administration, Maternal and Child Health Bureau.

Sharbaugh, C.O., ed. 1991. *Call to action: Better nutrition for mothers, children and families. Washington, D.C. National Center for Education in Maternal and Child Health.*

Green, M., ed. 1998. Bright futures: Guidelines for health supervision of infants, children, and adolescents. Arlington, VA: National Center for Education in Maternal and Child Health.

- An increasingly multicultural population requires that all health care providers have knowledge and skills in understanding the foodways of people in the United States.

Bronner, Y. 1994. Cultural sensitivity and nutrition counseling. *Top Clin Nutr* 9:13–19.

Bronner, Y. et al. 1994. African American/soul foodways and nutrition counseling. *Top Clin Nutr* 9:20–27.

Eliades, D.C., and C.W. Suitor. 1994. *Celebrating diversity: Approaching families through their food.* Arlington, VA: National Center for Education in Maternal and Child Health.

Lynch, E.W., and M.J. Johnson. 1994. *Developing cross-cultural competence: A guide for working with young children and their families.* Baltimore: Brookes.

Randall-David, E. 1989. *Strategies for working with culturally diverse communities and clients,* Bethesda, MD: Association for the Care of Children's Health.

Rodriguez, J. 1994. Diet, nutrition, and the Hispanic client. *Top Clin Nutr* 9:28–39.

Wu-Jung, C.J. 1994. Understanding food habits of Chinese Americans. *Top Clin Nutr* 9:40–44.

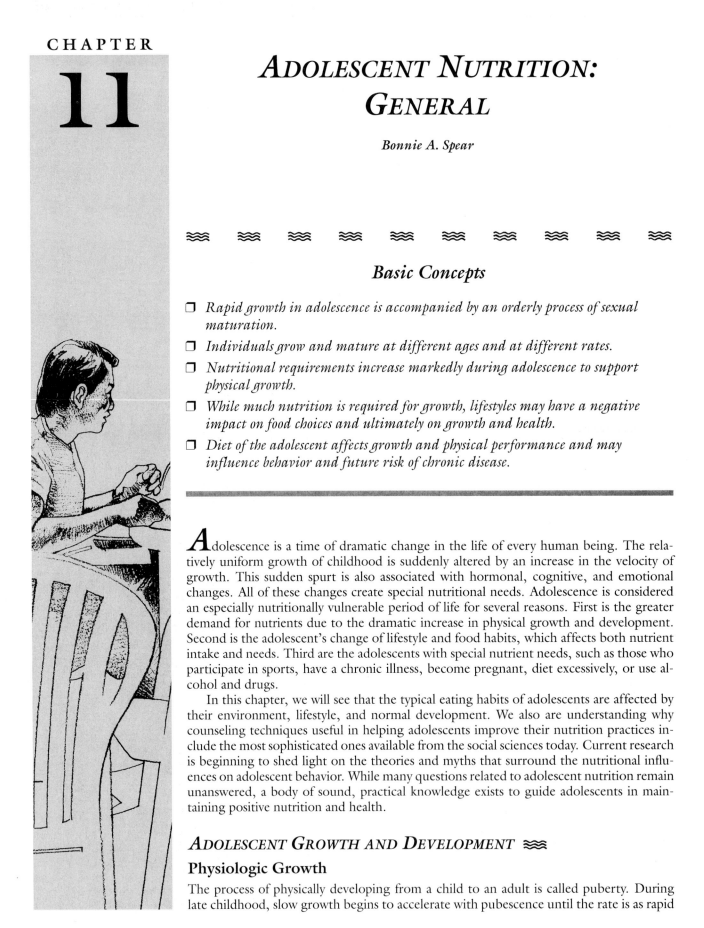

ADOLESCENT NUTRITION: GENERAL

Bonnie A. Spear

≋   ≋   ≋   ≋   ≋   ≋   ≋   ≋   ≋   ≋   ≋

Basic Concepts

❏ *Rapid growth in adolescence is accompanied by an orderly process of sexual maturation.*

❏ *Individuals grow and mature at different ages and at different rates.*

❏ *Nutritional requirements increase markedly during adolescence to support physical growth.*

❏ *While much nutrition is required for growth, lifestyles may have a negative impact on food choices and ultimately on growth and health.*

❏ *Diet of the adolescent affects growth and physical performance and may influence behavior and future risk of chronic disease.*

Adolescence is a time of dramatic change in the life of every human being. The relatively uniform growth of childhood is suddenly altered by an increase in the velocity of growth. This sudden spurt is also associated with hormonal, cognitive, and emotional changes. All of these changes create special nutritional needs. Adolescence is considered an especially nutritionally vulnerable period of life for several reasons. First is the greater demand for nutrients due to the dramatic increase in physical growth and development. Second is the adolescent's change of lifestyle and food habits, which affects both nutrient intake and needs. Third are the adolescents with special nutrient needs, such as those who participate in sports, have a chronic illness, become pregnant, diet excessively, or use alcohol and drugs.

In this chapter, we will see that the typical eating habits of adolescents are affected by their environment, lifestyle, and normal development. We also are understanding why counseling techniques useful in helping adolescents improve their nutrition practices include the most sophisticated ones available from the social sciences today. Current research is beginning to shed light on the theories and myths that surround the nutritional influences on adolescent behavior. While many questions related to adolescent nutrition remain unanswered, a body of sound, practical knowledge exists to guide adolescents in maintaining positive nutrition and health.

ADOLESCENT GROWTH AND DEVELOPMENT ≋

Physiologic Growth

The process of physically developing from a child to an adult is called puberty. During late childhood, slow growth begins to accelerate with pubescence until the rate is as rapid

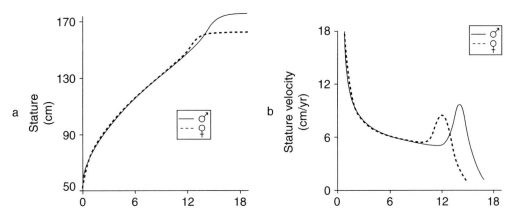

FIG. 11-1 (*a*) Growth in stature of typical boy (*solid line*) and girl (*dashed line*). (*b*) Growth velocities at different ages of typical boy (*solid line*) and girl (*dashed line*).

From Marshall, W.A. 1975. *Clin Endocrinol Metab* 4:4.

as that of early infancy. Although stature growth continues at an even pace until the growth spurt, adolescence is the only time following birth when the velocity of growth actually increases (fig. 11-1). Enormous variability exists in the timing of this change. Adolescents of a given chronologic age may vary widely in physiologic development. Due to this variability among individuals, age is a poor indicator of physiologic maturity and nutritional needs.

Because adolescents of the same age often differ markedly in size, it is impossible to use age alone in evaluating pubertal growth. An assessment of the degree of maturation of secondary sexual characteristics is useful not only in evaluating physical growth but also in detecting certain diseases and disorders associated with adolescence. Sexual maturity ratings (SMR), often called Tanner stages, are widely used to evaluate growth and developmental age during adolescence. These stages of growth correlate highly with other pubertal events.[1,2]

Sexual maturity ratings are based on the development of secondary sexual characteristics and are assigned on a scale of 1 (prepubertal) to 5 (adult). For boys, this scale is based on the progression of genital and pubic hair development; for girls, the development of breast and pubic hair. Figure 11-2 and table 11-1 describe each stage of development for boys and girls. Separate ratings should be established for each characteristic, because variations in the stage of maturity of each characteristic are not uncommon. Furthermore, although a mean value of the two ratings can be used as a general indicator of maturity, many physical changes that occur during puberty have greater correlation with one of the other ratings than with a mean value.

SMR 1, for all practical purposes, is an indicator of prepubertal development in both boys and girls; SMR 2 is the earliest visible signs of puberty. SMR 5 is generally considered to be evidence of adult growth, although height may continue to increase, and other physical changes may occur. Although great variability in growth is seen at any given chronologic age, growth proceeds in a sequential pattern, with only minor variations. In girls, the first signs of pubertal change is the development of breast buds. If this has not appeared by age thirteen, puberty is considered to be delayed, although this is likely to represent a normal variant rather than an endocrine abnormality. Peak height velocity in girls occurs early in the pubertal process, after pubic hair development reaches SMR 2, and menarche most often occurs after pubic hair and breast development reach SMR 4. Females manifest variability in age at onset and time required for completion of each stage of development. The first even to be noticed is breast budding at an average age of 10.6 years, with an age range of 9–13 years. Pubic hair usually develops later, but in one-third of all girls pubic hair appears before breast development. The average time elapsed from breast budding to breast stage 3 is one year. Average time elapsed before reaching adult breast development is four years.[3]

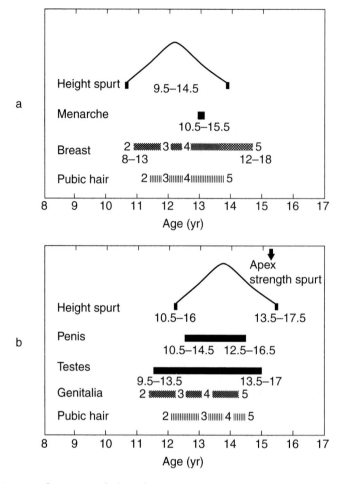

FIG. 11-2 Diagram of sequence of selected events at puberty in girls (*a*) and boys (*b*). *Cross-hatched and small vertical line bars with numbers* refer to developmental stages described in table 11-1.
From Marshall, W.A., and J.M. Tanner. 1970. *Arch Dis Child* 45:13.

In boys, the first sign of puberty is enlargement of the testes, but sometimes this is difficult to evaluate. If minimal enlargement of the genitals has not occurred by age 14 ½, puberty is considered to be delayed, although this, too, is likely to be of biological etiology. Peak height velocity in boys occurs after pubic hair development reaches SMR 3; often, genital development has reached SMR 4. Individual differences also occur in the rabidity with which an individual completes a sequence once it has started. Average boys have one year between genitalia stage 2 and genitalia stage 3 and three years between genitalia stage 2 and genitalia stage 5, but others may progress from genitalia stage 2 to stage 5 in two years.[3]

For health professionals who are not physicians or nurses, it is often difficult to assess secondary sexual characteristics, but many other physical changes correspond to each stage of development. For example, if a girl has already started her periods, she is probably at SMR 4 and has already completed most of her linear growth; therefore, her nutrient needs are beginning to decrease. However, it is important to note that girls who begin menstruation early (before age eleven) may have more linear growth after menarche than do girls who have later menarche. In boys, a faint mustache at the corners of the lip corresponds to SMR 3. This is the beginning of the peak height velocity, the time when he needs the peak in energy and nutrient intake.

Height attainment. During the pubertal process, teenagers attain approximately 15% of their final adult height and about 45% of maximal skeletal mass. Compared with girls, boys have a longer period of childhood growth before the adolescent growth spurt and a

TABLE 11-1   *Ratings of Sexual Maturation*

	Pubic Hair	Genitalia	Corresponding Changes
Boys			
Stage 1	None	None	Childhood
Stage 2	Small amount at outer edges of pubis, slight darkening	Beginning penile enlargement, testes begin to enlarge, scrotum reddened and changed in texture	Increased activity of sweat glands
Stage 3	Covers pubis	Penis longer, testes continue to enlarge, scrotum further enlarged	Voice begins to change, faint mustache/facial hair begins, axillary hair present, beginning of peak height velocity (PHV) (growth spurt 6–8 in)
Stage 4	Adult type, does not extend to the thighs	Penis wider and longer, scrotal skin darker	End of PHV, voice deepens, acne may be severe, facial hair increases, hair on legs becomes darker
Stage 5	Adult type, spreads to the thighs	Adult penis and testes	Able to grow full beard, muscle mass increases significantly
Girls			
Stage 1	None	None	Childhood
Stage 2	Small amount, downy on medial labia	Small breast bud	Increased activity of sweat glands, beginning of peak height velocity (PHV) (growth spurt 3–5 in)
Stage 3	Increased, darker, and curly	Larger but no separation of the nipple and the areola	End of PHV, beginning of acne, axillary hair present
Stage 4	More abundant, coarse texture	Increased size, areola and nipple form secondary mound	Acne may be severe, menarche begins
Stage 5	Adult, spreads to medial thighs	Adult distribution of breast tissue, continuous outline	Increase in fat and muscle mass

Adapted from Tanner, J.M. 1962. *Growth at adolescence,* 2d ed. Oxford: Blackwell Scientific Publications.

higher peak velocity (or maximum speed) in height growth, resulting in an average final height difference between males and females of 5.2 inches.[2] In females, stature growth ceases at a median of 4.8 years after the onset of menarche or at a median age of 17.3 years. In males, stature growth stops at a median age of 21.2 years; however, there is great variability. The total increment in height achieved after menarche varies inversely with age of menarche. Most females gain no more than 2 to 3 inches (5.1–7.6 cm) after the onset of menses. Girls who have early menses grow much more after menarche and for a longer period than do girls with later menarche. Excessive or less-than-normal growth can be detected by plotting height changes on the grids in appendices A and B.

Weight gain and body composition changes. The rate of weight gain during adolescence parallels that of the height spurt. In males, peak height velocity coincides with peak weight velocity. In contrast, peak weight velocity in females occurs six to nine months prior to height rate changes.[4] Weight gain during this period accounts for approximately 50% of the ideal adult weight.

For both males and females, elevated androgen levels have a growth-promoting effect. However, the female sex hormones, estrogen and progesterone, promote the deposition of proportionately more fat than muscle tissue in girls.[4] In the prepubertal period, the proportion of fat and muscle in males and females tends to be similar (body fat about 15%

and 19%, respectively), and lean body mass is about equal for both sexes. However, under the influence of testosterone and the anabolic adrenal androgens, boys gain proportionately more muscle mass than fat, experience increased linear growth to produce a heavier skeleton, and develop greater red blood cell mass than girls. Males have more lean body mass per unit height than females.[5] Lean body mass significantly increases in boys, with muscle mass doubling between the ages of ten and seventeen years. As adults, the normal percentage of body fat is about 23% for females and about 15% for males. This striking difference in adolescent growth between males and females influences nutritional needs. Because the adolescent male experiences greater gain in bone and lean tissue than the female does, he often requires more protein, iron, zinc, and calcium for development of these tissues. Another reason for the male's larger requirements for these nutrients is his greater rate of growth.

Measurement of growth. Knowing the relationship between the milestones of sexual development and physical growth enables the clinician to assess the progress of growth in an adolescent at a particular time and gives an indication of the extent of future growth. Thus, pubertal development can be monitored clinically by using weight and height charts and Tanner stages (sexual maturity ratings). For example, a sixteen-year-old female who has experienced her menarche and has progressed beyond stage 4 of breast development, but who is not as tall as her peers, would be considered to be close to her adult height. Excessive or less-than-normal growth can be detected by plotting height changes on the standard growth grids. In the preceding example, if the sixteen-year-old girl's height corresponds to the 25th percentile for her age, her physical maturation is considered to be normal. The major cause of short stature during adolescence is genetically late initiation of puberty, although conditions such as chronic disease and skeletal and chromosomal abnormalities also account for certain children being shorter than normal. Hormonal imbalances leading to abnormal growth are rare.

Weight can be plotted on a grid similar to that for height to determine whether an individual is keeping pace with peers or exceeding them in total weight at a particular age. For the first time, growth grids developed in 1998 allow assessment of weight-for-height-age using BMI. This will be described more in the assessment section later in this chapter.

Acne. Initiated by the influence of hormones on the sebaceous glands, acne is a normal characteristic of adolescent development. It occurs in varying degrees of severity in teenagers, mediated by factors such as stress and phase of the menstrual cycle. Traditionally, dietary factors have been blamed for the appearance of acne, but studies have shown no correlation between ingestion of foods and the appearance or degree of this condition.

Education about the physiologic basis for the development of acne supports teenagers in their efforts to control it. Effective medications include oral antibiotics, topical applications of benzoyl peroxide and tretinoin, and an oral synthetic retinoid 13-*cis*-retinoic acid (Accutane), a vitamin A derivative. Although very effective in treating acne, 13-*cis*-retinoic acid can cause an increase in serum triglycerides and total cholesterol that is reversed after the medication is discontinued. Adolescents taking Accutane should have their lipid levels checked before and during treatment and should start appropriate diet therapy, if necessary. Women should also avoid unprotected sexual activity, because Accutane is a teratogen and mutagen.[6]

Vitamin A is the most effective vitamin for treating acne, because it reduces the production of sebum (the white, fatty substance found in the body's pores). Vitamin A is the base for many of the topical acne products, as well as Accutane. It is important to remember that large amounts of vitamin A may be toxic. Additionally, vitamin E helps regulate the level of vitamin A. Laboratory evaluations have shown that animals deficient in vitamin E have difficulty in processing vitamin A; thus, adolescents should be encouraged to have diets adequate in vitamins A and E. Additionally, zinc may play a role in the development and treatment of acne; if so, zinc may be related to the free fatty acid production of the pilosebaceous follicle. Low levels of serum zinc have been found in those suffering most from acne, suggesting that a zinc deficiency may exacerbate the condition.[7]

TABLE 11-2 *Comparison of Erikson's and Piaget's Models for Emotional and Cognitive Development*

Age (Years)	Erikson (Emotional)	Piaget (Cognitive)
0–2	*Phase I:* Basic trust versus mistrust	*Sensorimotor period:* Learning through senses and manipulation
2–4	*Phase I:* Autonomy versus shame and doubt	*Preconceptual period:* Classification by a single feature (e.g., size); no concern for contradictions
4–8	*Phase III:* Initiative versus guilt	*Initiative thought period:* Intuitive classification (e.g., awareness of conservation of mass concept)
8–12	*Phase IV:* Industry versus inferiority	*Concrete operations period:* Logical thought development; learning to organize
12–20	*Phase V:* Ego identity versus role confusion	*Formal operations period:* Comprehension of abstract concepts; formation of "ideals"
20 onward	*Phase VI:* Intimacy versus isolation	———
Middle adulthood	*Phase VII:* Generativity versus stagnation	———
Late adulthood	*Phase VIII:* Integrity versus despair	———

Psychosocial Development

Span and scope of adolescence. *Adolescence* is the term applied to the period of maturation of both mind and body and therefore may be applied to humans before, after, and during puberty. Along with physical growth, emotional, social, and intellectual development are rapid during adolescence.[2] Milestones in psychologic development are shown in table 11-2. The ability to use abstract thinking, as opposed to the concrete thought patterns of childhood, enables the individual to accomplish these tasks. Planning ahead and connecting facts into integrated ideas becomes possible. With the accomplishment of the developmental "tasks of adolescence" as seen in fig. 11-3, the person is prepared for a role in adult society.

Implications for nutritional issues. Many of the tasks of adolescence relate to the nutritional health of the individual. For example, emotional maturity allows teenagers to develop their own value system. As a result, they can choose foods that will enhance their health rather than make their choices by responding to less healthful characteristics of foods, as they may have done in childhood. They may go through a time of experimentation while they are learning to make wise choices.

Body image. Developing an image of the physical self that includes an adult body is an intellectual and emotional task intertwined with nutritional issues. Adolescents often feel uncomfortable with rapidly changing bodies. At the same time, being very much affected by influences outside themselves, they want to be like their most perfect peers and the idols of their culture. Stereotypes in the mass media reinforce such images. Teenagers may wish certain body parts were larger and other parts were smaller. They may want to grow faster or slower. These feelings can lead them to try to change their bodies by manipulating their diets, an impulse that certain commercial interests are quick to exploit. Young women who have not developed a mature body image may unnecessarily restrict the amount of food they eat in response to weight gained with the development of secondary sexual characteristics. Hoping to achieve the muscular appearance of adult males, young men are tempted to use nutritional supplements. Phases of adolescent development are discussed in the box on p. 269.

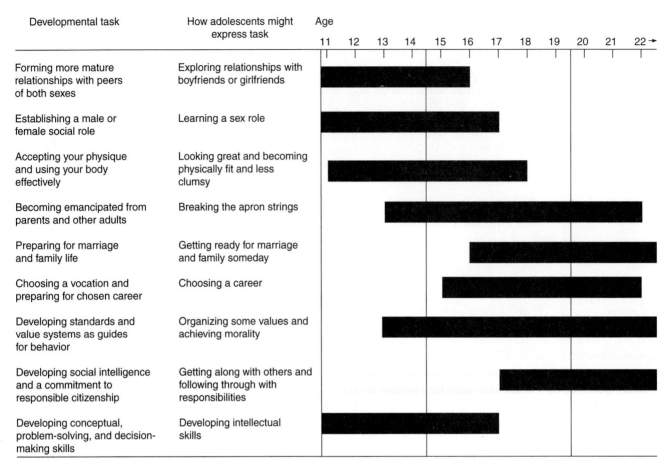

FIG. 11-3   Developmental tasks in adolescence.

Adapted from Thornburg, H. 1975. *Contemporary adolescence: Readings,* 2d ed. Monterey, CA: Brooks/Cole.

NUTRITIONAL REQUIREMENTS ≋

Growth as a Basis for Nutritional Requirements

Little specific experimental data exist on which to base the nutrient needs of adolescents. The Recommended Dietary Allowances (RDAs) for energy are based on median energy intakes of adolescents followed in longitudinal growth studies.[5] The RDAs for protein in this group are calculated from growth rate and body composition data, assuming protein utilization for growth is comparable with maintenance data in adults. As noted earlier, because of wide variability in growth rate, physical activity, metabolic rate, physiologic state, and adaptability, it is difficult to estimate specific nutrient requirements for adolescents. In addition, human studies involving youth are costly, and permission to use them as subjects is difficult to attain.

For practical reasons, the RDAs[5] for adolescents are categorized by chronologic age, rather than maturational development. Thus, practitioners should use RDAs with caution, particularly in individual assessments. For groups of teenagers, the RDAs can be used as general guidelines in evaluating the probability of populations at risk of consuming inadequate diets. However, in comparing an individual's intake with the RDA, one must remember that the RDAs include a safety factor; thus, individual intakes below the RDA do not automatically mean that the intakes are deficient or that the individual is not meeting his or her needs. An adolescent's nutritional status must be assessed on an individual basis, using information from clinical, biochemical, anthropometric, dietary, and psychosocial assessments.

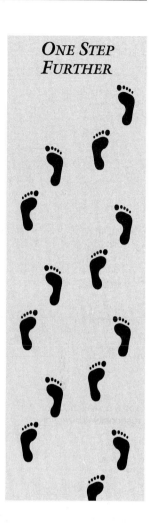

Phases of Adolescent Development

Early adolescence

Challenges parental authority and value system.

Holds a fascination with sexuality, although he or she has generally not yet entered into sexual relationships.

Compares him- or herself with others.

Relies greatly on peers for self-esteem.

Most comfortable with same-sex peer group.

Holds vague and unrealistic plan for career.

Deals with the "here and now" and has trouble with the future.

Middle adolescence

Continues to challenge parents' authority and shifts to peer group.

Attempts to become comfortable with his or her body and is concerned with looking more attractive.

Conforms with peers.

Begins heterosexual relationships.

Begins to develop career plans.

Challenges previously taught values and struggles with issues of morality.

Capacity and capability for abstracting increase.

Late adolescence

Separates him- or herself from family and identities; is not dependent on rebellion from parents.

Relies greater on own values while peers have become less important.

Prefers intimate, caring relationships.

Focuses on future planning for career.

Has a sense of perspective and is able to think through problems with alternatives.

Begins to develop a degree of financial independence.

Energy

The Recommended Dietary Allowances for energy for teenagers of various chronologic ages and for each sex are shown in table 11-3. As with other nutrients, the RDAs for energy do not include a safety factor for increased energy needs, such as illness, trauma, and stress, and are considered to be only average needs. Actual needs for adolescents vary with physical activity and stage of maturation.

Few studies have investigated the relationship between growth and caloric intake. On average, males tend to increase their caloric intake steadily to approximately 3,470 kcal per day at age sixteen years. From sixteen to nineteen years, the intake decreases to approximately 2,900 kcal per day. In females, the caloric intake increases to age twelve, with a peak calorie level of 2,550 per day, followed by a decline in calories to eighteen years, with intakes averaging 2,200 kcals/day. The caloric intake of girls at three stages of development (prepubescent, rapidly growing, and postpubescent) is related to stage of physiologic development, not to age. Wait[8] found that relating energy needs to height is the preferred index for determining calorie needs, and the use of kcal/cm is a rough predictor of energy needs. An estimated range for females eleven to eighteen years of age is 10–19 kcal/cm; for males eleven to eighteen years of age, 13–23 kcal/cm. Review table 11-3 for kcal/cm based on the RDAs.

Protein

Adolescents' protein needs, like those for energy, correlate more closely with the growth pattern than with chronologic age. Using the RDA for protein in relation to height is probably the most useful method of estimating need (review table 11-3). The daily protein recommendations for adolescents are approximately 0.3 g/cm height ranging from

TABLE 11-3 Recommended Energy and Protein Allowances

Age (Years)	kcal/day	kcal/kg	kcal/cm	Protein g/day	g/cm
Females					
11–14	2,200	47	14.0	46	0.29
15–18	2,200	40	13.5	44	0.26
19–24	2,200	38	13.4	46	0.28
Males					
11–14	2,500	55	16.0	45	0.28
15–18	3,000	45	17.0	59	0.33
19–24	2,900	40	16.4	58	0.33

Reprinted with permission from Recommended Dietary Allowances, 10th ed. © 1989 by the National Academy of Sciences. Published by National Academy Press, Washington, DC.

0.29 to 0.32 g/cm height for males and 0.27 to 0.29 g/cm height for females.[9] Average intakes of protein are well above the RDAs for any age group. There is little evidence to show that insufficient protein intakes occur in the adolescent population.[10] However, if energy intakes become insufficient for any reason, such as economic problems, chronic illness, or attempts to lose weight, dietary protein may be used to meet energy need and, thus, may be unavailable for synthesis of new tissue or for tissue repair. This may result in a reduction of growth rate and a decrease in lean body mass, despite an apparent adequate protein intake. Current dieting patterns of adolescent females that result in restricted caloric intakes represent potential health problems when protein sources are used to meet energy needs. Protein metabolism is particularly sensitive to caloric restriction in adolescents during their growth spurt.

Minerals

During adolescence, all mineral needs increase. Adolescents at the peak of their growth velocity require large quantities of nutrients. They have been shown to incorporate twice the amount of calcium, iron, zinc, magnesium, and nitrogen into their bodies during the years of the growth spurt, compared with that of other years. Dietary surveys have consistently shown that calcium and iron are marginal in adolescents' diets. These low intakes are often due to their popular food choices, including convenience foods, fast foods, and sugar-containing snacks.

Calcium. Due to accelerated muscular, skeletal, and endocrine development, calcium needs are greater during puberty and adolescence than in childhood or the adult years. At the peak of the growth spurt, the daily deposition of calcium can be twice that of the average during the adolescent period between ten and twenty years. In fact, 45% of the skeletal mass is added during adolescence.

The DRI for calcium is 1,300 mg for all adolescents.[11] Calcium requirements are expressed as adequate intakes (AIs). The AI is believed to cover the needs of all individuals in a group, but the lack of data or uncertainty in the data preclude the ability to specify the percentage of people covered by this intake. This is especially true for adolescents. The National Institutes of Health Consensus Development Conference Statement on Optimal Calcium Intake[12] recommended 1,200–1,500 mg calcium per day for adolescents eleven to twenty-four years. In its statement, the committee acknowledged that there appears to be a threshold level of dietary calcium that is necessary to allow growing adolescents to achieve their genetically predetermined peak bone mass. Dietary survey data indicate that adolescents, particularly females, are at greatest risk for inadequate calcium intake.[13] Calcium intake tends to decline among females from ten to seventeen years of age. Consumption surveys show an average intake for females to range from 780 to 820 mg per day. In males, the average intake is from 800 to 920 mg per day. The National Health and Nutrition Examination Survey (NHANES) has also shown a drop in dietary intakes of adolescents from NHANES II (1976–1980) to NHANES III (1988–1991):[14]

Age	Calcium Intakes	
	NHANES II	**NHANES III**
	(1976–1980)	(1988–1991)
6–11	1,209 (mg/day)	867 (mg/day)
12–15	854 (mg/day)	796 (mg/day)
16–19	725 (mg/day)	822 (mg/day)

Additionally, there is evidence to suggest that high soft drink consumption contributes to low calcium intake in this age group, because adolescents may be substituting soft drinks for milk. It is estimated that 14% of total caloric intakes in males and 15% of total caloric intakes in females can be attributed to soft drink consumption. Males average $2\frac{1}{2}$ oz servings of soft drinks per day but only $1\frac{1}{2}$ cups of milk per day, while females average $1\frac{3}{4}$ 12 oz servings of soft drinks but less than 1 cup of milk per day.[15] Pronounced bone loss in animals has been observed with excess phosphorus or insufficient calcium intakes. Teenagers may have low Ca:P ratios due to large consumption of high-phosphorus soft drinks, but additional research is needed to determine the effect of decreased intakes of milk in combination with increased intakes of soft drinks and processed foods high in phosphorus. Additionally, the caffeine increases the excretion of calcium in the urine. Since only 5% of soft drink consumption is caffeine free, caffeine can play a significant role in the bone mineralization in growing adolescents.

Iron. During adolescence, iron requirements are increased. Dallman[16] notes that in boys there is a sharp increase in the requirements for absorbed iron from approximately 1.0 to 2.5 mg/d. This increase reflects not only an expanding blood volume but also a rise in hemoglobin concentration, which occurs with sexual maturation in males. After the growth spurt and sexual maturation, there is a rapid decrease in growth and in the need for iron. Consequently, there is an opportunity to recover from an iron deficiency that might have developed during peak growth. In females, the growth spurt is not as great, but menstruation typically starts about one year after peak growth. The mean requirement for absorbed iron reaches a maximum of approximately 1.5 mg/d at peak growth but settles to a mean of approximately 1.3 mg/d because of the need to replace menstrual iron losses.

In girls on marginal iron intakes with increased losses, iron deficiency anemia may result from growth demands. Conversely, iron deficiency may limit growth during adolescence. Additionally, anemia in adolescence may also impair the immune response. A study of Indian children aged one to fourteen indicated that the cell-mediated immune response and the bactericidal capacity of leukocytes (in vitro methods) were significantly depressed in those with hemoglobin concentrations below 10 mg/d.[16]

Reports from dietary surveys indicate that the iron intakes of adolescents with normal dietary patterns were between 12.5 and 14.2 mg/d for females, compared with 13.6 to 18.0 mg/d for males.[17] The American diet contains an estimated 6 mg iron/1,000 kcal.[17] Adolescent females, who typically have lower caloric intakes than males, may have more difficulty in obtaining adequate levels of iron from their diets.

The National Health and Nutrition Examination Survey III (NHANES III) reported that iron deficiency was found in 14.2% of the fifteen- to eighteen-year-old females and 12.1% of the eleven- to fourteen-year-old males.[13] Iron deficiency is prevalent in adolescents of both sexes and in teens of all races and socioeconomic levels.[10]

Zinc. Zinc is known to be essential for growth and sexual maturation. Although plasma zinc levels decline during pubertal development, the retention of zinc increases significantly during the growth spurt. This increased utilization may lead to more efficient use of dietary sources, but limited intake of zinc-containing foods may affect physical growth as well as the development of secondary sexual characteristics. Additionally, there is limited research in the area, but there is some evidence that adolescents with low serum zinc levels may have increased problems with acne.

Although the roles of other minerals in the nutriture of adolescents have not been studied well, the importance of magnesium, iodine, phosphorus, copper, chromium, cobalt, and fluoride is well recognized. The possibility of interactions among these nutrients cannot be overlooked.

Vitamins. The need for vitamins is increased during adolescence. Due to the increase in energy demands, thiamin, riboflavin, and niacin are required in increased quantity for the release of energy from carbohydrates. With great tissue synthesis, there is an increased demand for vitamin B_6, folic acid, and vitamin B_{12}. There are also increased requirements for vitamin D (for rapid skeletal growth), and vitamins A, C, and E are needed for new cell growth. Although there are few reports of low serum vitamin C levels in teens, those who habitually avoid fruits and vegetables and those who smoke cigarettes may be at higher risk for deficiency. As with other nutrients, vitamin needs are most associated with the degree of maturity rather than chronologic age, due to the demands of growth. In most cases, these vitamins can be provided by a well-chosen diet, without vitamin supplements. Exceptions occur in adolescents who are dieting, have an eating disorder or chronic disease, or chronically make poor food choices.

EATING BEHAVIOR ≈

Typical Nutritional Patterns

Surveys of nutrient intake have shown that adolescents are likely to be obtaining less vitamin A, thiamin, iron, and calcium than recommended. They also ingest more fat, sugar, protein, and sodium than is currently thought to be optimum.[18,19]

While concern is often expressed over the habit of eating between meals, it has been shown that teenagers obtain substantial nourishment from foods eaten outside traditional meals. The choice of foods they make is of greater importance than the time or place of eating. Emphasis should be placed on fresh vegetables and fruits as well as whole-grain products to complement the foods high in energy value and protein that they commonly choose.[20]

Irregular Meals

The number of meals teenagers miss and eat away from home increases from early adolescence to late adolescence, reflecting the growing need for independence and time away from home. The evening meal appears to be the most regularly eaten meal of the day. Females are found to skip the evening meal, as well as breakfast and lunch, more often than males.

Breakfast is frequently neglected and is omitted more by teenagers and young adults under twenty-five years of age than by any other age group in the population. It is likely that females are more apt to miss breakfast than are males because of a pursuit of thinness and frequent attempts at dieting. Many teenage girls believe that they can control their weight by omitting breakfast or lunch. Young women who are dieting should be counseled that this approach is likely to accomplish just the opposite. By midmorning or lunchtime, they may be so hungry that they eat more than if they had had at least simple foods in the early morning.

Vegetarian Diets

Adolescents do, on occasion, take on special diets, such as vegetarian routines. This can mean anything from eliminating red meat to omitting all animal products, such as eggs, fish, poultry, dairy products, and even gelatin. Such diets can be healthful, if planned with care. A sample "vegan" (strict vegetarian) diet is provided in the box on p. 273.

Sample Menu of an Adequate Vegan Diet for a Thirteen-Year-Old

Breakfast
Orange, 1 medium
Oatmeal, 3/4 cup
Soymilk, 6 oz
Bread, whole-wheat, 1 slice
Jam, 2 tsp

Lunch
Tofu-miso soup with 1 tsp miso, 4 oz tofu
Sandwich of hummus (1 medium pita bread, 2 tsp hummus, $\frac{1}{2}$ cup spinach, 2 slices tomato)
Carrot juice, 6 oz
Figs, dried, 3

Dinner
Casserole of beans ($\frac{3}{4}$ cup brown rice, $\frac{1}{2}$ cup navy beans, 1 tsp safflower oil, 1 cup broccoli, $\frac{1}{2}$ cup yellow squash, $\frac{1}{4}$ cup onion)
Kale, cooked, $\frac{3}{4}$ cup

Snack
Watermelon, 1 slice
Strawberries, 1 cup
Gorp ($\frac{1}{4}$ cup almonds, $\frac{1}{2}$ oz pumpkin seeds, $\frac{1}{4}$ cup sunflower seeds, $\frac{1}{4}$ cup raisins)

Jacobs, C., and J. Dwyer. 1988. Vegetarian children: Appropriate and inappropriate diets. *Am J Clin Nutr* 48:811.

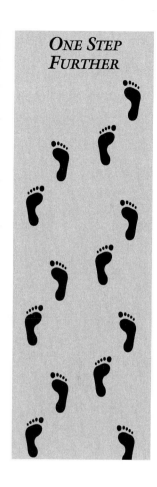

ONE STEP FURTHER

Factors Influencing Eating Behavior

By the time a person reaches adolescence, the influences on eating habits are numerous and the formation of those habits is extremely complex, as shown in fig. 11-4. The growing independence of adolescents, increased participation in social life, and a generally busy schedule of activities have a decided impact on what they eat. They are beginning to buy and prepare more food for themselves, and they often eat rapidly and away from home.

Advertising. While the basic foundation for eating habits is found in the family, the influences on eating behavior originating outside the home in modern America are great. By the time Americans become adolescents, they have been influenced by ten years of television food commercials and the eating habits portrayed in television programs. The average teenager will have watched over a million food commercials, the majority of which are for products with a high concentration of sweetness and fat.

Ease of obtaining ready-to-eat foods. The ease of obtaining food that is ready to eat also influences the eating habits of teenagers. Through vending machines, at movies and sporting events, and at fast-food outlets and convenience grocery stores food is available at numerous times throughout the day. During the time of their peak growth velocity, adolescents may need to eat often and in large amounts and are able to use foods with a high concentration of energy. However, they usually need to be more careful of amounts and frequency once growth has slowed.

Nutritional limitations of fast foods. The following factors appear to be the major nutritional limitations of fast-food meals:

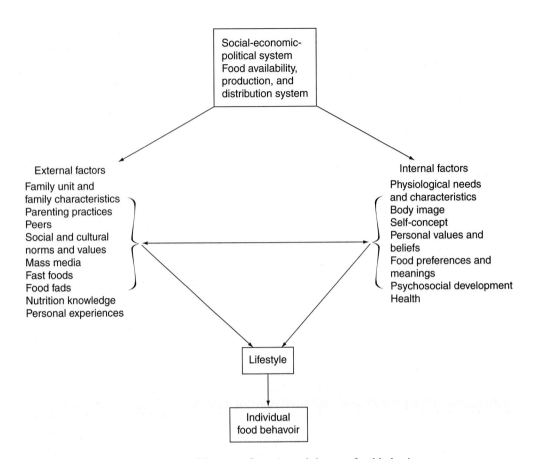

FIG. 11-4 Schematic diagram of factors influencing adolescent food behavior.

- *Calcium, riboflavin, vitamin A.* These essential nutrients are low unless milk or a milkshake is ordered. Extensive consumption of soft drinks contributes to low intakes of these nutrients, in addition to magnesium and vitamin C.[21]
- *Folate, fiber.* There are few sources of these key factors.
- *Fat.* The percent of energy from fat is high in many meal combinations.
- *Sodium.* The sodium content of fast-food meals is high.
- *Energy.* Common meal combinations are excessive in kilocalories when compared with the amounts of nutrients provided.

Although fast foods can contribute nutrients to the diet, they cannot completely meet the nutritional needs of teenagers. Both adolescents and health professionals should be aware that fast foods are acceptable nutritionally when they are consumed judiciously and as a part of a well-balanced diet.[20] When they become the mainstay of the diet, there is cause for concern.[22] A nutrient imbalance may not appear to be a problem until a number of years have gone by, unless a specific problem, such as a chronic disease, exists.

Through health and science education at school, adolescents appear to know what they should and should not eat.[23] However, overcoming barriers to act on that knowledge is the goal. Teens identify the biggest barrier as time. Teens perceive themselves as too busy to worry about food, nutrition, meal planning, and correct eating habits. Additionally, as shown in table 11-4, adolescents have mainly negative associations with healthy foods but positive associations with junk foods.[24] In order for adolescents to improve their eating habits, counseling must center on fitting proper nutrition into allowable time, must make selection of healthy foods easier, and must make it appealing to teens and their peers.

During the time of peak growth velocity, adolescents usually need to eat often and in large amounts. They are able to use foods with a high concentration of energy; however, they need to be more careful of amounts and frequency of eating when growth has slowed.

TABLE 11-4   Adolescents' Perceptions of "Junk" Food Versus "Healthy" Food

"Junk" Food	"Healthy" Food
Being with friends	Being with parents
Being away from home/parents	Staying home
Enjoyment/pleasure	Being concerned with weight and appearance
Being at the mall/store	Meals
Snacks	Self-Control
Not being in control, overeating, guilt, disgust	

Adapted and used by permission from Chapman, G., and H. Maclean. 1993. *JNE* 25:108.

Poor eating and overeating habits adopted during adolescence may ultimately contribute to a number of debilitating diseases.

Hypertension and Hyperlipidemia

Pediatric epidemiology programs have established that the major adult cardiovascular diseases, coronary-artery disease and essential hypertension, begin in childhood. Cardiovascular risk factors change during periods of growth and development, and there are ethnic (black-white) and male-female differences that relate to adult heart disease.[25] These risk factors have been shown to "track" over a fifteen-year period and are predictive of adult levels.[26] Cardiovascular risk factors also tend to cluster—for example, obesity correlates with higher blood pressure and with adverse serum lipoprotein changes. Adolescents with high blood cholesterol levels are also more likely to have elevated levels as adults. Attention should be paid to screening children and adolescents in families with a history of premature cardiovascular disease or parental hypercholesterolemia.[27] The screening criteria are as follows: 1) children and adolescents whose parents or grandparents, at age fifty-five years or less, were found to have coronary atherosclerosis through diagnostic coronary arteriography or who suffered a documented cardiovascular or cerebrovascular event or sudden cardiac death, 2) children and adolescents with a parent who has an elevated blood cholesterol, and 3) adolescents at high risk, such as adolescents who smoke or who are obese. The following is a guide to the risks of particular levels of blood lipids for ages two to nineteen years by sex:

	Total Cholesterol (mg/dl)	Risk	LDL-Cholesterol (mg/dl)	Risk
Males	175–1,990	Moderate	110–130	Moderate
	≥190	High	>130	High
Females	178–200	Moderate	115–140	Moderate
	≥200	High	>140	High

The nutritional recommendations of the National Cholesterol Education Program are appropriate for all children over the age of two years. Helping adolescents understand the importance of current lifestyle factors on later disease processes is a challenge but is not impossible. If an adolescent is hypertensive or there is a strong family history of hypertension, a diet controlled in sodium and total energy is a part of long-term nutritional care. The challenge is in making the information practical in the adolescent's hectic lifestyle, much of which revolves around consuming food that is high in fat, low in fiber and nutrients, and limited in variety. Promoting healthy lifestyle behaviors should include discussions of not only food choices but also the avoidance of smoking and alcohol use and increasing physical activity.

Dental Caries and Periodontal Disease

It is becoming apparent that the cause of dental caries is a complex process involving the interaction of several factors. The minerals of the tooth enamel are in constant equilibrium with the oral environment. It is necessary, therefore, to consider not only the presence of fermentable carbohydrates but also such factors as food solubility, mineral composition, and the buffering capacity of the oral environment. Adolescents' propensity to snack on refined carbohydrates is conducive to tooth decay. Since 80% of the average person's total incidence of dental lesions occur in the teenage years, this is the time to encourage habits built on choosing alternatives to sugar-containing foods.[28]

Gingivitis increases in prevalence during the teenage years, and **periodontal disease** often follows. Little is known about the role of nutrition in periodontal disease, although nutritional deficiency, widespread in underdeveloped countries with a high incidence of periodontal disease, has been implicated. Inadequate intake of these nutrients in the teenage years can have an adverse effect on the health of the gums in later life.

Gingivitis
(L *gingiva*, gum of the mouth) Inflammation of the gum tissue in the mouth surrounding the base of teeth.

Periodontal disease
(Gr *Peri*, around; L *dens, tooth*) General term for disease of tissues surrounding the tooth, affecting its integrity and stability and contributing to tooth loss.

Role of Parents

In order to encourage adolescents to form reasonable eating habits, parents should give their children increased responsibility and choice within the range of nourishing foods as they are growing up. By the time they are teenagers, they will need some freedom to use the kitchen. This is true for young men as well as for young women.

Substance Use and Abuse

Substance abuse in adolescence is a public health problem of major significance and concern. The substances most widely abused by adolescents are tobacco, smokeless tobacco, alcohol, marijuana, and cocaine. The strongest predictor of drug use by an adolescent is association with a peer group that uses drugs, although poor parenting and drug use by parents are also strong influences. Adolescents who are left alone for long periods of time are more likely to use drugs and to start using them earlier than are those who are with families or other positive supervised group activity more of the time. Over 90% of high school seniors have consumed alcohol; in one study one out of seven seniors admitted they had been inebriated once a week. While use of marijuana has declined during the past several decades, cocaine use has increased. While rates of tobacco use have remained stable since the early 1980s, the rate among females has increased, and the age of beginning use has declined for all teenagers. Smokeless tobacco, in the form of chewing tobacco and snuff, is typically used by male adolescents in rural areas and by young white male athletes, from 7% to 25% in populations studied. It has caused significant oral damage, including cancer, and thus is cyclical in its relationship to nutritional status.

Overall, about 10–15% of teenagers have had no experience with drugs and alcohol, 70–80% have experimented, 10–15% have definable problems, and somewhat less than 1% are chemically dependent, addicted. Cognitive, emotional, and social development is likely to be retarded in the last group.[29]

Impact on nutritional status. Two small studies have been published of nutritional status in drug- or alcohol-abusing teenagers: one study was of a racially mixed group and the other was of a Native American population.[30,31] Deficient *nutrient levels* were not found in blood samples from either group, and neither reported consuming less of the nutrients studied than they needed or than nonusing peers. However, in the study that reported food choices, those of the abusers were different from those of the controls in that most of the nutrients they consumed came from snack foods and meat products. Fruits, vegetables, and milk were left out of their usual dietary patterns. Thus, though the adolescents studied did not have deficiencies that were measured either biochemically or in reported consumption, the long-term effects of their characteristic dietary habits, coupled with exposure to alcohol, would account for the development of the nutritional disorders seen in adult abusers. Studying the nutritional status of eighteen- to twenty-five-year-old drug abusers would be useful in the exploration of the natural history of deficiency diseases among alcohol and drug abusers. In summary, it can be said that the effect of substance abuse on nutritional status of any individual depends on the substance, the amount, the duration and frequency of use, the prior health and nutritional status, the stage of physical growth, and the nutritional adequacy of the diet consumed.

Identification and referral. Since the incidence of greatest abuse is among eighteen- to twenty-five-year-old individuals, all health professionals need to be aware of the indicators of drug use, so that they can refer adolescents with a definable problem for treatment before they reach a more advanced stage of chemical dependency. These indicators include:

Rash	Dyspnea on exertion
Muscle weakness	Faintness
Vomiting	Hangover
Diarrhea	Blackouts
Stomach pain	Nervousness
Nausea	Depression
Indigestion	Tiredness
Bleeding gums	Insomnia
Sore tongue	Somnolence
Taste loss	Headache
Appetite loss	Seizures
Memory loss	

Nutritional assessment, intervention, and support are components of the comprehensive physical and psychologic rehabilitative process of adolescent substance abusers.

ASSESSMENT OF NUTRITIONAL STATUS ≋

Teenagers are in a fluctuating state of balance between supplying their bodies with needed nutrients and using up the nutrients. At any one time, this flow is the teenagers' nutritional status. (Assessment of nutritional status was described in chapter 2.) Modification for the adolescent requires use of the sexual maturity ratings and specific data base with which to compare height, weight, and weight-height proportion.

Assessment of Growth

Weight and height can be plotted on growth grids to determine whether an individual is maintaining his or her growth pattern (growth channel). The relationship between weight and height can be evaluated by using the NCHS BMI growth grids for adolescents up to nineteen years of age.

Use of body mass index ($BMI = kg/m^2$), which is highly correlated with body fatness, can also indicate weight status. An adolescent's BMI is calculated by dividing body weight (in kg) by the square of the adolescent's height (in meters). Consult a BMI table to determine the adolescent's weight status. BMIs below the 5th percentile should be explored. These adolescents should be assessed for organic diseases or eating disorders. Adolescents with BMIs ≥ 85th percentile and ≤ 95th percentile are at risk for overweight and should receive a nutritional assessment to determine health risk (see chapter 12 on obesity). Adolescents with BMIs ≥ 95th percentile for age and gender are overweight and should have an in-depth medical assessment.[32,33,34]

A skinfold evaluation yields a further degree of precision. For example, a low skinfold measurement in an individual above the 75th percentile weight-for-height indicates a state of being overweight but *not* overfat. An assessment of muscle and arm circumference can confirm the muscular composition. However, a skinfold at the 95th percentile or greater suggests obesity. (Measurement of skinfolds is further discussed in chapter 2.) Figure 11-5 provides a system for evaluating a teen's weight/fitness status.

Sexual Maturity Rating

The evaluation of sexual maturity is an essential factor in making a valid nutritional assessment of an adolescent in a normal clinical setting. By knowing the stage of sexual maturity of the adolescent (review fig. 11-2), it is possible to determine whether the full height has been reached or growth can still occur. Also, it is possible to determine whether the proportion of fat to muscle seen is that which the individual has developed as an adult or has obtained at one stage as a still-developing adolescent. Thus, if a young woman at stage 1 of sexual maturity is at the 90th percentile weight-for-height, she will continue to grow

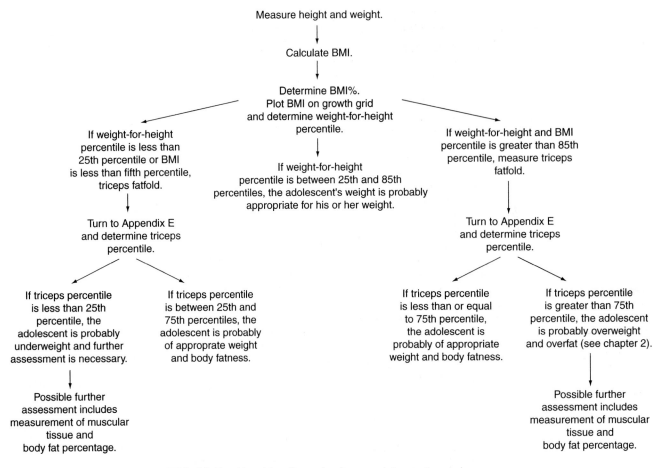

FIG. 11-5   Algorithm for evaluating an adolescent's weight.

in height and has a greater potential to stay within the bounds of normal body composition than has a female of the same age, the same weight-for-height, but who has experienced menarche and is at stage 4 of sexual maturity.

Nutrition Environment

The nutrition environment, the combination of factors that influence nutritional status, is an important consideration. Such factors as general medical history, socioeconomic status, medications, alcohol or tobacco use, family attitudes, and peer group food practices all contribute to the adolescent's food choices. Nutrition assessment includes the study of both the nutritional status and the nutrition environment of the individual adolescent. The methods described in Chapter 2 will be used to help the health professional understand the effect they have on the adolescent's eating habits. A probing interview by a sensitive nutritionist who has had experience communicating with adolescents will also be required to find out how an individual teenager feels about and manages food.

Nutritional Care Plan

Assessment of all factors in the environment that may influence nutriture is essential if appropriate action to meet needs is going to be initiated as a personal **nutritional care plan.** The extent to which the total nutrition environment is studied depends on the projected use of the nutrition assessment. For example, a great deal of detailed information reflecting nutritional status is needed for a thirteen-year-old male with Crohn's disease who is scheduled for a course of **parenteral nutrition.** Information about the

Nutritional care plan
The person-centered care plan, based on nutritional assessment data and evaluation, for individual nutritional care and education to promote health and prevent or treat disease.

Parenteral nutrition
(Gr *para,* beyond, beside; *enteron,* intestine) Nourishment received not through the gastrointestinal tract but, rather, by an alternate route, such as injection into a vein; intravenous feeding of elemental nutrients.

Teenagers and TV: How Do We Increase Physical Activity?

Teenagers from twelve to seventeen years of age watch television about twenty-one hours per week. This estimate does not include any additional hours spent watching videos or playing video or computer games. The sedentary habits of many teens are likely to be contributing to the rising prevalence of obesity in this age group. As many as 30% of teens are obese. The relationship between hours spent watching television and inappropriate body weight gain among adolescents is controversial. Television viewing may be substituting for other activities with a higher energy expenditure and that contribute to a positive energy balance. Watching television has been associated with a lowered resting metabolic rate, which may indirectly add to weight gain. Increased television viewing could lead to increased consumption of energy-dense snacks, raising the total energy intake while limiting energy expenditure in physical activity. All of these factors are likely to be involved. An important goal for nutrition and health educators working with teens should be making available to them physical activities that focus on fun and fitness. School health programs can help students develop exercise patterns that provide a foundation for lifelong fitness. After-school or leisure time programs can encourage participation in physical activities that teens enjoy and that are compatible with their lifestyle and social pattern.

Some suggestions for developing exercise programs for teens are:

- Focus on physical activities that you can do when you are alone or bored: bicycle riding, walking, skating, jogging, aerobic dancing, shooting baskets.
- Organize contests in which everyone can participate, regardless of their athletic ability: offer prizes for walking, skating, or riding a bicycle a certain distance (maybe fifty miles) or for walking or dancing for a certain number of hours (maybe twenty hours) over a certain number of weeks or months.
- Emphasize team activities in which everyone on the team is active: basketball, volleyball, soccer, racquetball.
- Promote participation rather than winning in team sports; give small prizes or recognition to everyone who plays, not only to the team that wins.
- Encourage the formation of small groups to encourage and support each other in exercise activities: "get fit with a friend."
- Favor exercise activities that do not require expensive uniforms or equipment and that carry a low risk of injury: walking, jogging, basketball, soccer, volleyball, aerobic dancing.

Gortmaker, S.L., W.H. Dietz, and L.W.Y. Cheung. 1990. Inactivity, diet, and the fattening of America. *J Am Diet Assoc* 90:1247.

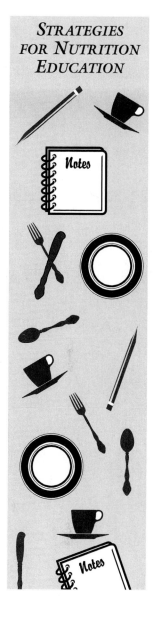

STRATEGIES FOR NUTRITION EDUCATION

nutrition environment would be less vital at this time. However, nutritional care planning for a newly diagnosed fifteen-year-old female with insulin-dependent diabetes mellitus (IDDM) would require both nutritional status evaluation and assessment of the nutrition environment. Without both components, the care plan cannot adequately address physiologic nutritional needs and the adolescent's ability to meet them.

NUTRITION FOR FITNESS AND SPORTS ≋

Young athletes are particularly vulnerable to nutrition misinformation and unsafe practices that promise enhanced performance. Pressures to achieve optimum performance encourages athletes to experiment with supplements and **ergogenic aids** in order to achieve the "competitive edge." Inappropriate use of supplements, unsafe weight loss practices, and inadequate fluid and nutrient intakes can adversely affect the adolescent's health and can limit ultimate growth.

Ergogenic aids
Supplements taken to increase performance or build muscles.

Fluids

Adequate fluids intake and prevention of dehydration are critical for young athletes. This is especially true for the younger adolescent. In fact, heat illness ranks second to head injury among noncardiac reported causes of death in secondary school athletes. Children and young adolescents, compared with adults, are at highest risk for becoming dehydrated and developing hyperthermia because:

- They have a lower sweating rate (absolute and per sweat gland), which potentially decreases their capacity to dissipate heat through evaporation of the sweat.
- They experience greater heat production in exercise and have less of an ability to transfer heat from the muscles to the skin.
- They have a greater body surface area, which can result in excessive heat gain in extreme heat and heat loss in the cold.
- They have a lower cardiac output, which reduces their capacity for heat transport from the core to the skin during strenuous exercise.
- They acclimatize to exercising in heat more gradually. A young adolescent may require five or six sessions to achieve the same degree of acclimatization acquired by an adult in two or three sessions in the same environment.[35]

It is not only the actual temperature but also the humidity that impact on an individual's ability to dissipate heat. The higher the humidity, the less sweat that will be evaporated from the skin, thereby decreasing the body's ability to cool itself and increasing the risk of heat-related illness.

There are certain adolescents that are at a higher risk for developing a heat illness due to certain diseases or medical conditions. Excessive fluid loss may occur in children and adolescents with bulimia, congenital heart disease, diabetes mellitus, gastroenteritis, fever, and obesity. Additionally, insufficient fluid intake may occur in persons with anorexia nervosa, cystic fibrosis, mental retardation, or kidney disease. Children who are obese experience heat illness more frequently because (1) only a small amount of heat is needed to increase the temperature of a large amount of fat mass, (2) fat mass has a lower water content than lean body mass and there is a higher amount of fluid lost in persons who have higher fat mass, and (3) obese children expend more effort than lean children in the same intensity of exercise and therefore increase their overall body temperature more quickly. These teens should be considered high-risk and should be watched more closely when they are physically active, but they should not be kept from participating in activities. If kept properly hydrated, these children's medical conditions can often be improved with a consistent physical activity program.[36] It is important to recognize the signs and symptoms of dehydration and what to do if these symptoms are present.[37] See the box on p. 281.

However, the key to treating heat illness is to prevent it. Nutrition professionals should take the lead in counseling athletes in prevention. The following should be done to prevent heat-related illness:

- Exercise during the coolest times of day (before 10:00 A.M. and after 6:00 P.M.).
- Gradually increase exercise in hot weather (intensify workouts over a two-week period).
- Schedule fluid breaks every fifteen to twenty minutes during any activity lasting longer than one hour.
- Avoid the use of excessive clothing or equipment. Mesh jerseys, lightweight shorts, and low-cut socks allow more sweat to evaporate than do sweat suits and heavy gear.
- Drink cold water (40–50° F) *before* and *after* exercise.
- Drink 4–8 oz of cold water every ten to fifteen minutes *during* activity.
- Weigh before and after exercise—replace each pound of weight loss with 16 oz (2 cups) of water.
- Eat a balanced diet and do not skip meals. The necessary salts, minerals, and vitamins can be obtained in a basic, healthy nutrition plan.

Although plain water is all that is needed and readily available, teens may be more likely to drink sufficient amounts of fluids if they are given flavored fluids. Although sports

Heat Illness Signs to Watch Out For

Heat cramps	Thirst Chills Clammy skin and throbbing heart Muscle pain and spasms Nausea	Drink 4–8 oz of cold water every 10–15 minutes. Move adolescent to shade and remove any excessive clothing.
Heat exhaustion	Reduced sweating Dizziness Headache Shortness of breath Weak, rapid pulse Lack of saliva Extreme fatigue	Stop exercise and move to a cool place. Take off wet clothes and place ice bag on head. Drink 16 oz (2 cups) for each pound of weight lost.
Heat stroke	Lack of sweat Lack of urine Dry, hot skin Swollen tongue Visual disturbances Hallucinations Fainting Rapid pulse Loss of consciousness Low blood pressure Unsteady gait Shock	*Call for emergency medical treatment.* Place ice bags on back of head. Remove wet clothing. If athlete is conscious, help take a cold shower.

ONE STEP FURTHER

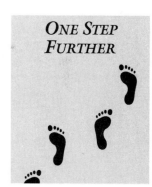

Hydration Guidelines for the Athlete

Before exercise	Drink 4–8 oz one to two hours before exercising and 4–6 oz ten to fifteen minutes before beginning activity.
During exercise	Drink at least 4–8 oz every 10–15 minutes.
After exercise	Drink at least 16 oz for every pound of weight lost. If a preexercise weight is not available, a minimum of 16 oz of fluids should be consumed.

ONE STEP FURTHER

drinks have not been shown to improve performance, some studies have shown that young athletes who drink sports drinks are more likely to consume more fluids than those who drink plain water.

Undiluted fruit juice and carbonated sodas should never be used during activity, because they typically contain too much carbohydrate and may cause stomach upset (cramps) and may delay the fluids getting into the blood. Caffeinated beverages should also be avoided, because they encourage increased fluid loss.

Carbohydrate

Carbohydrate is the most efficient fuel for athletic performance—especially intense aerobic and anaerobic activity. The energy from carbohydrate sources can be released within exercising muscles up to three times faster than can energy from fat. Therefore, carbohydrate is the preferred fuel for working muscles. The only problem is that the body can store

Glycogen
Principal carbohydrate reserve, which is primarily stored in the liver and muscles. It is readily converted into glucose.

only a limited amount of carbohydrate as **glycogen** (in the liver and muscles). When carbohydrate is burned for fuel during exercise, it must be replaced, or the athlete will have less and less energy when exercising.

Research has shown that athletes who have poor mental performance during competition and training eat a low-carbohydrate diet. These athletes have a lower level of concentration, have more periods of moodiness, and are more irritable, compared with athletes who eat a high-carbohydrate diet. This is because carbohydrates affect certain chemicals in the brain and control mood and mental sharpness.

A targeted diet for an active adolescent should be about 50–55% carbohydrate, 15–20% protein, and 25–30% fat. Most athletes find it more helpful in determining needs as amount needed per unit of body weight than as a percentage of total calories. The estimated carbohydrate intake is 3–5 g of carbohydrate per pound of body weight. For a 120-pound athlete, this ranges from 270 to 500 g of carbohydrate per day. Carbohydrates can come in the form of fluids, simple carbohydrates, or complex carbohydrates.[35]

Protein

Protein is an essential part of the adolescent athlete's diet. However, the key to protein's successful role in the athlete's diet is moderation. Protein doesn't need to take a special place in the diet—only 15–20% of calories should come from protein. There are many mythical and magical claims for the use of protein. The adolescent athlete is especially susceptible to promotional literature—anything to get "the competitive edge." It is important for the adolescent to understand that the only way to build muscles is to eat appropriate amounts of protein and to exercise, exercise, exercise.

As with carbohydrates, protein recommendations are made in terms of grams of protein per unit of body weight. For adolescents, the recommendation is to eat 0.6–0.9 g of protein per pound of body weight. Although these are overall recommendations, other factors may affect protein needs:

Carbohydrate intake. If the carbohydrate intake and energy levels are lower than needed, then the athlete may use protein for energy needs and not have protein available to build lean body mass.

Training level. Adolescents who are training at an elite level or at a very intense level may need to increase their protein intake, but protein intakes in adolescents should not exceed 1.0 g/lb.

Protein quality. As a rule, animal proteins are of higher biologic value than plant protein. If an athlete eats only plant protein, a higher intake of protein may be necessary.

Ergogenic Supplements

As previously mentioned, adolescents are vulnerable to nutrition misinformation and unsafe practices that promise improved performance, including "performance-enhancing" supplements. Supplements promising increased muscle mass, increased strength, and improved ability should be used with caution and in most cases avoided. Many of these supplements increase the risk for dehydration and have little impact on still developing muscle mass.

Research is lacking on the use of dietary supplements and other performance-enhancing aids by adolescent athletes. Unfortunately, many self-proclaimed "experts" and clever marketing strategies by companies are eager to convince athletes that their products improve athletic performance. These "experts" may claim that muscle fatigue and soreness are due to certain vitamin and muscle deficiencies. In reality, fatigue is probably secondary to insufficient calories, insufficient carbohydrate, or dehydration.[37] Supplements fall into three main categories, including protein/amino acids, vitamin/mineral supplements, and hormonal/enzymatic supplements.

Protein/amino acids. Supplements of protein or excessive protein intake can be dangerous. Ingestion of single amino acids or in combinations, such as arginine and lysine, may interfere with the absorption of certain essential amino acids. An additional concern is that substituting amino acid supplements for food may cause deficiencies of other nutrients such as iron, niacin, and thiamin, found in protein-rich foods. Amino acid supple-

TABLE 11-5 *Which Tastes Better?*

Amino Acids	Cheerios (1 oz) + Milk (1 c)	Amino Acid Supplement
Threonine	329 mg	24 mg
Isoleucine	588 mg	40 mg
Lysine	492 mg	135 mg
Methionine	171 mg	20 mg
Cysteine	144 mg	0 mg
Phenylalanine	425 mg	280 mg
Tyrosine	346 mg	8 mg
Valine	519 mg	38 mg
Arginine	465 mg	500 mg
Histidine	205 mg	0 mg

ments have not been shown to increase muscle mass or to burn body fat. High protein intakes require additional fluid for metabolism and excretion of waste products and may therefore make athletes more susceptible to dehydration. In most cases, food can provide more amino acids than can supplements, at a significantly lower cost. (Table 11-5 compares cereal and milk with an amino acid supplement marketed to adolescents.) Finally, no margin of safety is available for ingesting large doses of amino acids, and the long-term risks have not been identified.

Vitamin/mineral supplements. Individuals who consume marginal amounts of nutrients from food may benefit from supplementation with vitamins and minerals, but no scientific evidence supports the general use of supplements to improve athletic performance. For the child who is unable to incorporate certain foods into the diet, who is chronically ill, or who is restricting intake, a multivitamin and mineral supplement may be prudent to ensure adequate intake of micronutrients. However, there is no place in the diet of a healthy child for megadoses of vitamin or minerals. Unsupervised use of large amounts of vitamin and mineral supplements raises safety concerns.[35]

Hormonal/enzymatic supplements. This type of supplement gets the most advertising and promises the most improvement in athletic performance. The increase in marketing and advertising is due in part to the passage of the Dietary Supplement Health and Education Act (DSHEA) in 1994, which created a category of supplements called "dietary supplements." This category includes vitamins, minerals, amino acids, herbs, and other botanical preparations, which do not fall under Food and Drug Administration (FDA) approval. This has led to ergogenic aids' being classified on the market as foods.[38] Many of the claims advertised and written about supplements are not supported by published studies. In some instances, there is no scientific evidence to support claims; in other cases, research findings are extrapolated to inappropriate applications. There are hundreds of products marketed in this category. It would be impossible to cover all of these in this chapter, so just a few are reviewed.

Chromium picolinate. Serves as a cofactor in the action of insulin in lipid and carbohydrate metabolism. Claims for this product include an increase in muscle mass, a decrease in body fat, and an increase in energy. These claims are based on two poorly controlled and never published studies. Two well-controlled studies were conducted, in which athletes were given either chromium picolinate or placebo. In both cases, muscle mass and strength increased in both (due to increase in activity), but there was no difference between the two groups. In November 1996, the Federal Trade Commission (FTC) ordered three companies that manufactured chromium picolinate to stop making unsubstantiated weight loss and health claims.[38]

Creatine monohydrate. The supplement form of creatine. It is derived from the amino acids arginine, glycine, and methionine. The discovery that creatine (Cr) and phosphocreatine (PCr) content in human muscle can be increased by oral ingestion of

---

TABLE 11-6   *Position Paper: Creatine Supplements*

- Creatine supplementation may cause an electrolyte imbalance. More specifically, it may create a reversal in the muscle's calcium-phosphorus ratio. A disruption of the calcium-phosphorus ratio could potentially interfere with the muscle's contraction/relaxation mechanisms. As a result the muscle may contract/shorten when it's supposed to relax/stretch or vice versa. This may cause tetanic muscle cramping and muscle strains.
- Creatine supplementation research is preliminary and lacks valid longitudinal studies. Also lacking to date is research on the effects of creatine supplementation on combined strength training and conditioning/agility program.
- A team/individual success will be commercially marketed by the food supplement industry as evidence of product efficacy to immature and highly impressionable youth (their primary market). Such marketing hyperbole undermines the efforts of our organization to be responsible to our community youth and exploits the talents/efforts of our players.
- Current evidence suggests that creatine supplementation may be advantageous to a bodybuilder interested in "ornamental" muscle development [but] disadvantageous for football players interested in "functional" muscular development. As a result, the Tampa Bay Buccaneers do not endorse supplementation as a training adjunct to our players.

---

supplemental creatine has led to numerous research studies and the use of this product by millions of athletes. Research has shown increases in performance in athletes who already had low levels of muscle Cr and PCr (due to vegetarianism or poor intake). Other research studies have shown increases in body mass and increased performance resulting from the ingestion of Cr monohydrate; however, there is some evidence that significant portions of this weight gain are due to total body water, not just lean body mass. Other research studies have shown no difference in performance on single-effort sprint activity. Trainers working with athletes who use Cr monohydrate over prolonged periods have noticed increases in muscle cramping and muscle strains. They have also noticed an increased incidence of dehydration in athletes using the product. Additionally, there have been no research studies conducted on the long-term effects or the risks associated with ingestion by teenagers who are still developing lean body mass. The concerns over the safety of the product have led more than thirty-three professional athletic teams to disapprove of its use.[38] Table 11-6 shows excerpts from the Tampa Bay Buccaneers position on the use of creatine supplements.

Androstenedione. Very little was heard about androstenedione until the 1998 baseball season, when Mark McGwire was on the verge of breaking Roger Maris' home-run record and a bottle of Androstene-50 was seen on his locker shelf. This product's claim is that it automatically boosts testosterone and thereby increases muscle mass and strength. It is advertised as an alternative to anabolic steroid. There is much written about the dangers, especially to teenagers, of anabolic steroid. To date, there have been no controlled research studies conducted on Androstene-50. Since researchers have known about this product for more than fifty years, there appears to be little evidence to indicate that oral ingestion of androstenedione increases muscle mass. In fact, the initial results of one controlled study actually show a decrease in testosterone, not an increase.[39] However, there is major concern that even the slightest andrionic effect of taking this product may be extremely dangerous to still-growing athletes. These dangers include premature closure of the epiphyseal plates, limits on ultimate adult height, and alterations in mood.

Well-meaning but misinformed coaches and parents may encourage adolescents to take supplements in order in improve their performance, but providing teens with supplements can give them the wrong idea and may encourage poor eating habits that will affect their overall health. Additionally, they may erroneously associate improvement with the supplement, rather than with hard work and training. Parents, coaches, and health professionals must emphasize how many foods, as opposed to supplements, promote muscle growth and optimal performance.[35]

Preexercise Intake

The preexercise meal intake is important because it prevents the athlete from getting hungry during the event and provides carbohydrate to maintain optimal levels of blood glucose for exercise. Many athletes have "special" competition foods they are convinced they must eat for success; the preexercise meal is often ritualistic and psychologically important to the athlete. While allowing for individual preferences, the meal/snack should include foods that are high in carbohydrate, low to moderate in protein, and low in fat and fiber. High-fat foods, such as cheeseburgers, candy bars, and heavy meats, should be avoided, because the fat delays the stomach emptying time. Exercising on a full stomach may cause nausea and vomiting, which are dangerous in contact sports, such as football.

Current guidelines indicate that 1–4 g of carbohydrate/kg body weight should be consumed one to four hours before exercise. To prevent gastrointestinal distress, the carbohydrate content of the meal should be reduced close to the exercise period. For example, a meal of 4 g/kg carbohydrate could be eaten four hours before the event, while only 1 g/kg should be eaten one hour before the event.[35]

Postexercise Replacement

The time immediately after exercise is important for muscle recovery. Research has shown that the rate of muscle glycogen storage is increased for the first two to four hours postexercise. This suggests that delaying the carbohydrate intake for too long after exercise will reduce muscle glycogen storage and may impair recovery. It is recommended that 0.75 g carbohydrate be consumed within the first two hours postexercise. Because most athletes have difficulty in eating immediately after exercising, athletes should be encouraged to drink high-carbohydrate beverages immediately after exercise and then to eat high-carbohydrate foods within the next two hours.

Risk of Injury

Research on the development of **epiphyseal cartilage** in animals shows strength increases from birth with a decline in rate prior to sexual maturation and an actual decrease in strength during puberty. Studies indicate that the incidence of acute or sudden epiphyseal injuries in humans peaks during adolescence.

The growth spurt may also increase the susceptibility to overuse injury by causing an increase in muscle-tendon tightness about the joints and an accompanying loss of flexibility. Longitudinal growth occurs initially in the long bones of the extremities and in the spinal column, and the muscle-tendon units elongate in response to this change; this situation creates a temporary disparity between muscle-tendon and bone lengths. This suggests that, during periods of rapid growth, children have temporary "structural growth lags," which cause a somewhat heightened susceptibility to injury. Although problems do not ordinarily arise at normal levels of activity, frequent intense training or collision with other players may lead to injuries.

Some sports medicine physicians suggest that male athletes at SMR 3–4 should not be allowed to participate in wrestling or football. These individuals are in the period of fastest bone growth and may be at greatest risk of epiphyseal injury and ligament strains.

With respect to noncontact sports and individual events, coaches and parents should be sensitive to the possibility that periods of growth are accompanied by an increased risk of injury. For boys, this is SMR 3–4; for girls, SMR 2–3. Teens should have a reduced training load during this period. In fact, some elite dance teachers have been aware of this phenomenon and decrease the intensity of training for dancers during the growth spurts. Such an approach is no less applicable to young female gymnasts, who at high levels of competition may be training up to thirty hours each week.

Epiphyseal plate
Part of the long bones that develops differently from the shaft of the bone and is separated at first from the shaft by a layer of cartilage to allow for growth.

CASE STUDY

Susan, A Female Adolescent

Susan is a thirteen-year-old who has been referred to you by her family physician. Susan is on the cross-country team, but her mother is concerned that she is not eating right, and her doctor wants you to give her some nutritional advice. She tells you that her coach has told her she needed to lose weight so she could increase her time. Additionally, she states that she has become a vegetarian in order to eat a healthier diet. A physical exam by her physician shows that she is between Tanner stage 2 and 3 for development, she weighs 90 lb, and she is 62 inches tall.

Questions for analysis

1. List at least four questions you would include in your assessment session with this young person. Why would you include these questions?
2. What are the particular nutritional requirements for a teenage girl in Tanner stage 2–3?
3. What are the additional nutritional needs because Susan is an athlete?
4. How would you address the coach's concern about the need to lose weight?
5. How would you talk to Susan regarding the vegetarian diet?
6. What advice would you give this teen's parents?

NUTRITION COUNSELING FOR ADOLESCENTS ≋

Facilitating Change

Attempts to help adolescents improve their nutritional status must be approached with skill, especially because of their growing independence. Nutrition counselors must know adolescents' physical and psychologic development, lifestyles, and habits, as well as appropriate methods of communicating with them.

Strategies for change. Sophisticated strategies to add knowledge, alter attitudes, and change behavior must be used in any setting if the objective is to influence an adolescent's eating habits. Providing knowledge or teaching can be done in a variety of settings from the classroom to the hospital bedside. Altering attitudes is much more difficult and usually demands an individualized experience. Facilitating the adoption of new behavior is even more difficult and requires a lengthy period of time. The adolescent will have to feel positive about any plan before it can succeed. In fact, much effort must be directed toward encouraging the person to want to change before introducing steps to bring the change about.

Personalized counseling. Besides changes in attitude, the counselor must impart knowledge in an especially meaningful and individualized manner. Finally, behavior change can be approached in increments that are sufficiently realistic to ensure personal success. It is important to remember that it is not the attempt but the success that builds self-efficacy; therefore, nutrition counseling may need to start slowly and then gradually make goals more difficult.

Role of parents. Parents must be appropriately involved in the counseling process. They need help in being supportive, as opposed to being intrusive, as the adolescent makes changes. Both adolescents and their parents must be helped to see the importance of focusing on the process of making change rather than solely on the desired goal of self-care. A sure understanding of both the physical and social sciences, along with a liberal injection of art, are needed in nutrition counseling for adolescents and their parents. It is indeed a challenging field.

The Health Care Team

Adolescent health care is one of the most demanding of clinical problems. As such, it is best handled as a team effort. Any one professional will generally not possess the skills to meet all the client's needs. This does not mean that certain problems are the responsibility of any one profession to the exclusion of others. Each professional team member can support and reinforce the messages and guidance provided by other team members. Team conferences aid in the coordination of care and in team efficiency in meeting identified needs and in noting the client's progress in solving various problems. Nutritionists and other professionals who are in positions to influence program planning can help develop clinical teams for the care of adolescents.

Summary

Adolescence is a period of tremendous change. A major change is one of physical size, which can occur only if sufficient nutrition is available. For the most part, boys require larger amounts of nutrients than do girls. An exception to this generalization is the mineral iron, which requires regular replacement due to monthly menstrual loss. Most adolescents have a considerable amount of freedom when it comes to food choices and eating behavior. The quality of the teen's diet is determined not only by the foods available at home and at school but also by access to and resources for the purchase of fast foods and convenience snacks. Concerns about body weight may adversely affect nutritional status; motivation to prepare optimally for sports may have a positive effect. The degree to which eating behaviors in adolescence are carried forward into adult life may either positively or negatively influence health during the adult years.

Review Questions

1. Sequence the steps in sexual development in boys and girls.
2. Demonstrate how to assess the status of body fatness in an adolescent.
3. List screening criteria for a high risk of premature cardiovascular disease.
4. List the pros and cons of ergogenic aids.
5. List the criteria for determining nutritional needs for adolescents who are prepubertal and who are in the middle of their peak height velocity.
6. Describe adolescent cognitive development.
7. Identify ways to prevent heat illness in the physically active adolescent.

WEIGHT-RELATED CONCERNS AND DISORDERS AMONG ADOLESCENTS

Dianne Neumark-Sztainer
Jillian K. Moe

≋ ≋ ≋ ≋ ≋ ≋ ≋ ≋ ≋ ≋ ≋ ≋

Basic Concepts

❏ *The developmental changes associated with adolescence place these individuals (especially girls) at high risk for establishing behaviors which are aimed at changing their appearance to feel better about themselves.*

❏ *Disordered eating patterns (and sometimes purging practices) may have mild to severe consequences.*

❏ *A number of environmental circumstances contribute to the development and progression of weight-related problems.*

❏ *Comprehensive, multidisciplinary treatment programs have been formulated to address the more serious forms of eating disorders.*

❏ *Treatment goals for obese adolescents need to be based on appreciation of issues that are important in adolescent growth and development.*

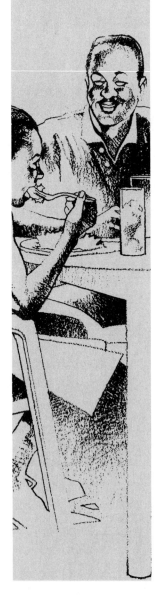

*I*n most parts of the world, getting enough food for growth, development, and maintenance of body weight is a major concern. However, in many industrialized societies, there are strong social pressures emphasizing thinness, an abundance of easily accessible food, and a limited need to be physically active in order to survive. These conditions have led to a proliferation of weight-related concerns and disorders associated with overweight and fears of being overweight. Weight-related concerns may or may not be accompanied by excessive body weight. They range from mild body dissatisfaction to life-threatening eating disorders, such as **anorexia nervosa.** Weight-related concerns and disorders are prevalent during adolescence and have potentially serious consequences for the young person's physical and psychosocial development.

The focus of this chapter is on weight-related concerns and disorders during adolescence. It begins with an explanation as to why weight-related conditions tend to be prevalent and are of particular concern during this period of the life cycle. The spectrum of weight-related disorders is presented, ranging from anorexia and **bulimia nervosa** to obesity, including anorexic/bulimic behaviors, unhealthy dieting, and **binge eating disorder.** A justification is provided for focusing on the entire spectrum, not only on the more severe conditions—in particular, when developing interventions for adolescents. Prevalences of each of the weight-related conditions on the spectrum are given in order to better understand the scope of the problem. Similarities in causal pathways leading to these conditions are described. More detailed descriptions of anorexia nervosa, bulimia nervosa, and obesity are provided, with some key points on etiology, potential consequences, assessment, and treatment. The chapter concludes with a discussion about the prevention of the entire spectrum of weight-related concerns and conditions.

More emphasis needs to be placed on the prevention, early identification, and proper treatment of these prevalent and serious conditions within homes, schools, clinics, fitness facilities, youth organizations, community centers, restaurants, and society at large. All members of society can contribute to the reduction of weight-related concerns and conditions among adolescents through counseling and educational work in clinics, schools, and other settings; through advocacy work with the media; and through personal conversations with children and adolescents regarding weight-related issues. The information in this chapter provides the basics for this work, while a partial list of resources for further information and outreach work is provided at the end of the chapter.

Why Focus on Adolescents? ≋

Although weight-related concerns and disorders occur throughout the life span, many appear to peak in prevalence and severity during adolescence. The changes occurring during adolescence place youth at increased risk for the development of weight-related concerns. These changes include physical and physiologic changes, such as rapid growth, sexual development, changes in body shape, and hormonal changes. Large psychologic and social changes also occur during adolescence that are related to one's search for a personal identity, a desire for more independence, moodiness, a preoccupation with body image and appearance, increased desire for social activities with friends, increased need and desire for contact with the opposite sex, and conflicting needs to belong to a group as well as to individualize.[1]

Physical/Physiological Changes

The rapid changes in growth and development during adolescence lead to increased nutritional needs. However, eating patterns may be less than ideal during this period, due to busy schedules of youth and their parents, increased opportunities and desire for eating outside of the home, and a low sense of urgency regarding health.[2] Therefore, many youth are at risk for inadequate intake of some nutrients, such as calcium, and excessive intake of others, such as fat.[2–4]

The rapid physical changes also place adolescents at high risk for body dissatisfaction. For example, since growth spurts among girls tend to begin at about eleven to twelve years of age and growth spurts among boys tend to begin about two years later, girls may feel uncomfortable being taller than boys and boys may feel uncomfortable being shorter than girls. Among girls, the widening of hips due to the widening of bones and normal fat accumulation may lead to a feeling of being "fat," particularly as many women seen in the media (movies, television, and magazines) have very slender hips. Changes in sexual organs, the growth of body hair, and increased sweating may affect feelings of insecurity and may lead the adolescent to feel as though he or she does not have control over his or her body. Some adolescents may try to gain control over these physical changes by controlling their food intake. The negative impact of these changes on body image is more likely to occur if reinforced by social norms. Conversely, if social norms tend to support these changes, they are more likely to lead to feelings of pride. It is noteworthy that many of the physical changes that occur among adolescent males, such as the widening of shoulder muscles, are viewed in a positive way, whereas normal changes that occur among adolescent girls, such as the widening of the hips, may be viewed less favorably. This may contribute to the large gender differences in prevalences of body dissatisfaction and eating disorders.

Psychologic and Social Changes

A central theme throughout adolescence is finding one's identity. One's developing physical identity may be strongly intertwined with one's overall identity during this phase of life. Therefore, adolescents who are dissatisfied with their bodies may be at increased risk for overall low self-esteem. Although research has not consistently shown that overweight

Anorexia nervosa
(Gr *anorektos,* without appetite; L *nervosa,* nervous or emotional disorder) Severe psychophysiologic eating disorder, usually seen in girls and young women, in which the person does not lack appetite but is psychologically unable to eat and refuses food, becoming extremely emaciated.

Bulimia nervosa
(L *bous,* ox; *limos,* hunger; *nervosa,* nervous or emotional condition) Psychophysiologic eating disorder, seen mainly in girls and young women, marked by alternate gorging on large amounts of food, followed by self-induced purging with vomiting, laxatives, or exercise; weight usually remains fairly stable and within a normal range.

Binge eating disorder
Condition characterized by binge eating with no subsequent attempt at purging, often leading to weight gain.

youth as a group have lower self-esteem than nonoverweight youth,[5,6] an unsupportive social environment may place an overweight adolescent at increased risk for poor self-esteem. This may lead to the use of unhealthy weight control behaviors in a desperate attempt to lose weight. For example, in a research study in which individual interviews were conducted with overweight adolescents, one girl discussed the painful impact of being mistreated by others on her self-esteem and on the self-esteem of overweight people in general:

I know there are a lot of people who are overweight, or think that they're overweight, they have very low self-esteem and stuff like that. And, I think that part of the reason is that because, I mean you're trying to build up your self esteem and yet they just keep knocking it down, knocking it down, knocking it down. . . . So, it's like the harder you struggle the farther, the farther that you fall behind. And then eventually you have no self-esteem and sometimes you break down. Sometimes you close yourself out of the world.[7]

Adolescents may be particularly sensitive to comments from others, such as parents, coaches, and health care providers regarding their changing body shape. Care needs to be taken to avoid making comments that may be construed as criticism and magnified by the adolescent. Moodiness is common during adolescence, due to hormonal changes and other life stresses, and mood changes may be accompanied by imbalances in eating behaviors and exaggerations in the way in which the body is perceived.

An increased need and desire for social contact with peers—and, in particular, with peers of the opposite sex—may cause adolescents to be overly concerned with their appearance. Adolescents may feel that they would be more socially desirable if they were more attractive or thinner and may go to extremes to reach this ideal. If attempts at weight loss are achieved and are met with support from significant persons in their environment, susceptible adolescents may continue to lose weight beyond that which is viewed as attractive by family and friends, and an eating disorder may develop with a force of its own. The need to belong to a peer group may also increase adolescents' susceptibility to social pressures to be thin or to otherwise have a body shape like others in the peer group.

In short, adolescence is a period of rapid physical and psychosocial changes that place youth at risk for increased weight-related concerns and conditions. The increased nutritional needs for growth and development during this period place adolescents who are severely restricting their food intake at risk for adverse short- and long-term health complications. Therefore, it is important to focus on weight-related concerns and conditions during this phase of the life cycle.

THE SPECTRUM OF WEIGHT-RELATED DISORDERS ≋

A strict definition of "eating disorders" includes only conditions such as anorexia nervosa, bulimia nervosa, and, more recently, binge eating disorder. Terms such as "weight-related disorders," "weight-related conditions," and "eating disturbances" may be used instead of the more formal term "eating disorder" in order to encompass a broader range of conditions. One way to view weight-related conditions is on a spectrum with obesity on one end, anorexia and bulimia nervosa at the other end, and a range of other weight-related disorders in the middle, such as anorexic/bulimic behaviors, unhealthy dieting, and binge eating disorder (fig. 12-1). This spectrum may be viewed as ranging from conditions as-

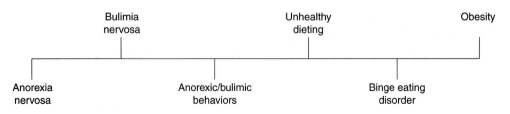

FIG. 12-1 The spectrum of weight-related behaviors.

sociated with being extremely underweight to conditions associated with being extremely overweight (fig. 12-2). This type of spectrum approach has its flaws; for example, anorexia nervosa is not the "opposite" of obesity, and persons engaging in unhealthy dieting behaviors are not necessarily in the middle of the spectrum in terms of their weight. However, a spectrum is very useful for understanding and teaching about weight-related disorders—in particular, when discussing issues of prevention and early detection among adolescents. The spectrum serves as a reminder that it is essential to direct our attention toward the milder conditions and not only to focus on the more dramatic conditions. While engagement in anorexic behaviors and unhealthy dieting may not be frequent or intense enough to meet the formal criteria for being defined as an eating disorder, these behaviors may negatively impact health and may lead to the development of more severe eating disorders. Furthermore, the spectrum approach also reminds practitioners to avoid focusing on only one condition, such as obesity, in prevention and treatment. The danger of focusing on only one condition is that it may inadvertently lead to an increase in other conditions, such as unhealthy dieting and anorexic and bulimic behaviors.

While it is important to be aware of the differences among the conditions, an awareness of their similarities may aid in understanding their etiology and the best ways to work toward treatment and prevention. The similarities among the conditions on the spectrum include body image and food intake concerns, albeit to different degrees for different persons and conditions. In addition, all of these conditions have a social component, which largely results from societal attitudes toward body shape and size. The psychologic component tends to differ greatly across these conditions, as well as within individuals with the same condition.

Prevalence of Weight-Related Conditions

It is important to be aware of the prevalence of weight-related conditions, to plan accordingly for interventions aimed at the prevention and treatment of a condition. Conditions that are prevalent among youth warrant interventions that can reach large numbers of youth, such as school-based interventions. Conditions that affect a small

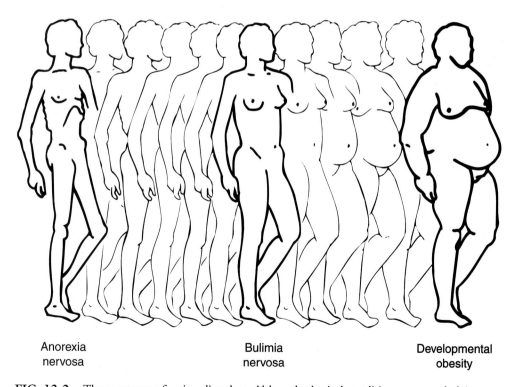

Anorexia nervosa   Bulimia nervosa   Developmental obesity

FIG. 12-2 The spectrum of eating disorders. Although physical conditions vary, underlying psychologic characteristics are held in common across the spectrum.

TABLE 12-1 *Estimated Prevalence and Brief Descriptions of Weight-Related Disorders*

Disorders	Prevalence Estimates	Brief Descriptions
Anorexia nervosa*	0.2–1.0% of adolescent females and young women	Condition characterized by self-starvation, weight loss, intense fear of weight gain, and strong body image distortion.
Bulimia nervosa*	1–3% of adolescent females and young women	Condition characterized by binge eating with subsequent purging by self-induced vomiting, laxative abuse, excessive exercise, and periods of fasting.
Anorexic/bulimic behaviors*	10–20% of adolescent females	Behaviors characteristic of anorexia nervosa and bulimia nervosa but not done frequently enough or with the degree of severity necessary to meet the formal diagnostic criteria for either condition.
Dieting behaviors	40–60% of adolescent females and 15% of adolescent males attempting to lose weight	Varies from healthy weight loss behaviors, such as eating less fat or more fruits and vegetables, to unhealthy behaviors, such as skipping meals or periods of starvation.
Binge eating disorder	2.6% of college-age youth	Condition characterized by binge eating, with no subsequent attempt at purging, often leading to weight gain.
Obesity	12% of adolescents using BMI >95th percentile, 22% of adolescents using BMI >85th percentile	Characterized by excess body tissue, measured as BMI above the 95th percentile for age; between the 85th and 95th percentiles for age is considered overweight or at risk for overweight.

*Prevalence rates of these behaviors are considerably lower among males than females.

percentage of the adolescent population, yet may have severe health implications, warrant more intensive individual or small-group interventions. Prevalence estimates and brief descriptions of each of the weight-related conditions shown on the spectrum are outlined in table 12-1. More detailed descriptions of obesity, anorexia nervosa and bulimia nervosa appear in later sections of this chapter, due to their severity and relatively high prevalence among adolescents.

Prevalence of Anorexia and Bulimia Nervosa

Anorexia nervosa is a serious condition characterized by self-starvation and an intense fear of being fat. Bulimia nervosa is an eating disorder characterized by the consumption of large amounts of food cycled with compensatory behaviors, such as self-induced vomiting, laxative use, and excessive food restrictions or exercise. Diagnostic criteria for anorexia and bulimia nervosa are shown in tables 12-2 and 12-3, respectively.[8] Among adolescent females and young women, estimates of anorexia nervosa range from 0.2% to 1.0%,[9,10] and reliable estimates of bulimia nervosa range from 1.0% to 3.0%.[11] In other words, it is estimated that out of 100 adolescent females or young women, 1–3 will develop a serious eating disorder. Anorexia and bulimia nervosa tend to be more prevalent among females than among males; about 9 out of 10 individuals with these conditions are female. Some of the factors that may contribute to the higher prevalence of these conditions among females than among males include stronger sociocultural pressures to be thin; changing societal expectations of women for which adequate role models are not always available; and increased vulnerability to sexual exploitation. In spite of the lower prevalence rates of eating disorders among males, it is important to note that they do occur, and their onset must be identified as early as possible in order to increase the likelihood of successful outcomes.

Prevalence of Anorexic/Bulimic Behaviors

Some adolescents engage in anorexic or bulimic behaviors, but with less frequency or intensity than required for a diagnosis of an eating disorder. Behaviors typically included in this category include self-induced vomiting, laxative use, use of diet pills, fasting or ex-

TABLE 12-2 **Diagnostic Criteria for Anorexia Nervosa**

Diagnostic Criteria for 307.1 Anorexia Nervosa

- Refusal to maintain body weight at or above a minimally normal weight for age and height, such as weight loss leading to maintenance of body weight less than 85% of that expected or failure to make expected weight gain during period of growth, leading to body weight less than 85% of that expected.
- Intense fear of gaining weight or becoming fat, even though underweight.
- Disturbance in the way in which one's body weight or shape is experienced, undue influence of body weight or shape on self-evaluation, or denial of the seriousness of the current low body weight.
- Amenorrhea in postmenarchal women—that is, the absence of at least three consecutive menstrual cycles (a woman is considered to have amenorrhea if her menstrual periods occur only following hormone (e.g., estrogen) administration.

Specify **type:**

Restricting type: during the episode of anorexia nervosa, the person has not regularly engaged in binge eating or purging behavior (i.e., self-induced vomiting or the misuse of laxatives, diuretics, or enemas).

Binge eating/purging type: during the episode of anorexia nervosa, the person has regularly engaged in binge eating or purging behavior (i.e., self-induced vomiting or the misuse of laxatives, diuretics, or enemas).

Reprinted with permission from *Diagnostic and Statistical Manual of Mental Disorders,* Fourth Edition. Copyright 1994 American Psychiatric Association.

TABLE 12-3 **Diagnostic Criteria for Bulimia Nervosa**

Diagnostic Criteria for 307.51 Bulimia Nervosa

A. Recurrent episodes of binge eating. An episode of binge eating is characterized by both of the following:
  - Eating, in a discrete period of time (e.g., within any two-hour period), an amount of food that is definitely larger than most people would eat during a similar period of time and under similar circumstances.
  - A sense of lack of control over eating during the episode (i.e., a feeling that one cannot stop eating or control what or how much one is eating).
B. Recurrent inappropriate compensatory behavior in order to prevent weight gain, such as self-induced vomiting; misuse of laxatives, diuretics, enemas, or other medications; fasting; or excessive exercise.
C. The binge eating and inappropriate compensatory behaviors both occur, on average, at least twice a week for three months.
D. Self-evaluation is unduly influenced by body shape and weight.
E. The disturbance does not occur exclusively during episodes of anorexia nervosa.

Specify **type:**

Purging type: during the current episode of bulimia nervosa, the person regularly engages in self-induced vomiting or the misuse of laxatives, diuretics, or enemas.

Nonpurging type: during the current episode of bulimia nervosa, the person has used other inappropriate compensatory behaviors, such as fasting or excessive exercise, but has not regularly engaged in self-induced vomiting or the misuse of laxatives, diuretics, or enemas.

Reprinted with permission from *Diagnostic and Statistical Manual of Mental Disorders,* Fourth Edition. Copyright 1994 American Psychiatric Association.

TABLE 12-4   *Diagnostic Criteria for Eating Disorder Not Otherwise Specified*

307.50 Eating Disorder Not Otherwise Specified

This category is for eating disorders that do not meet the criteria for any specific eating disorder. Examples include:

A. For females, all of the criteria for anorexia nervosa are met except the individual has regular menses.

B. All of the criteria for anorexia nervosa are met except that, despite significant weight loss, the individual's current weight is in the normal range.

C. All of the criteria for bulimia nervosa are met except that the binge eating and inappropriate compensatory mechanisms occur at a frequency of less than twice a week or for a duration of less than three months.

D. The regular use of inappropriate behavior by an individual of normal body weight after eating small amounts of food (e.g., self-induced vomiting after the consumption of two cookies).

E. Repeatedly chewing and spitting out, but not swallowing, large amounts of food.

F. Binge eating disorder: recurrent episodes of binge eating in the absence of the regular use of inappropriate compensatory behaviors characteristic of bulimia nervosa.

Reprinted with permission from *Diagnostic and Statistical Manual of Mental Disorders,* Fourth Edition. Washington, DC: Copyright 1994 American Psychiatric Association.

treme dieting, binge eating, and excessive exercise. Physical activity is generally viewed as a health-promoting behavior, yet excessive physical activity should be monitored, as it may be a sign of a weight-related disorder. Due to the importance of these behaviors, a formal category has been established for eating disorders that do not meet the criteria for any specific eating disorder.[8] This category is called Eating Disorder Not Otherwise Specified (EDNOS) (see table 12-4). Due to the heterogeneity of these behaviors, it is more difficult to estimate the prevalence of anorexic and bulimic behaviors. In a large population-based study of Minnesota adolescents in grades 7–12, 12% of the girls reported that they had made themselves vomit for weight control purposes at least once in their lives, and 2% reported having used laxatives or diuretics for weight control purposes. Rates were lower among boys: 6% reported vomiting and less than 1% reported laxative or diuretic use.[12] Binge eating (eating large amounts during a short period of time and feeling out of control while eating) was reported by 30% of the girls and 13% of the boys.[12] From a review of the literature, Fischer et al. estimated that as many as 10–50% of adolescent girls have participated in occasional self-induced vomiting or binge eating and up to 20% have scored in the abnormal range on standardized tests of eating attitudes and behaviors.[13] Based on a review of the more reliable research findings, it seems reasonable to estimate that 10–20% of adolescents have engaged in anorexic or bulimic behaviors.

Prevalence of Dieting Behaviors

Dieting behaviors are consistently reported by a high percentage of the adolescent population, particularly by girls. Based on their review of the literature, Fischer et al. concluded that as many as 50–60% of adolescent girls consider themselves overweight and have attempted to diet.[13] In a national survey of high school youth, 44% of the female students and 15% of the male students reported that they were trying to lose weight. An additional 26% of the female students and 15% of the male students reported that they were trying to keep from gaining weight.[14] However, estimates tend to vary across studies, in accordance with how dieting is assessed. Furthermore, adolescents may interpret the term *dieting* differently when asked if they have dieted. For some youth, *dieting* refers to healthful eating behaviors, such as eating less fat or more fruits and vegetables, while for others *dieting* means skipping meals or "starvation."[15] Dieting behaviors among youth are of concern, in that they are often used by youth who are not overweight. Furthermore, unhealthful dieting behaviors in which meals are skipped, energy intake is severely restricted,

TABLE 12-5 *Research Criteria for Binge Eating Disorder*

Recurrent episodes of binge eating. An episode of binge eating is characterized by both of the following:
- Eating, in a discrete period of time (e.g., within any two-hour period), an amount of food that is definitely larger than most people would eat in a similar period of time under similar circumstances.
- A sense of lack of control over eating during the episode (i.e., a feeling that one cannot stop eating or control what or how much one is eating).

The binge eating episodes are associated with three (or more) of the following:
- Eating much more rapidly than normal.
- Eating until feeling uncomfortably full.
- Eating large amounts of food when not feeling physically hungry.
- Eating alone because of being embarrassed by how much one is eating.
- Feeling disgusted with oneself, depressed, or very guilty after overeating.
- Marked distress regarding binge eating.
- Binge eating that occurs, on average, at least two days a week for six months.

Note: The method of determining frequency differs from that used for bulimia nervosa; future research should address whether the preferred method of setting a frequency threshold is counting the number of days on which binges occur or counting the number of episodes of binge eating. The binge eating is not associated with the regular use of inappropriate compensatory behaviors (e.g., purging, fasting, excessive exercise) and does not occur exclusively during the course of anorexia nervosa or bulimia nervosa.

Reprinted with permission from *Diagnostic and Statistical Manual of Mental Disorders,* Fourth Edition. Copyright 1994 American Psychiatric Association.

or food groups are lacking are common. Dieting behaviors have been found to be associated with inadequate intakes of essential nutrients, such as calcium.[16–18] Furthermore, dieting behaviors leading adolescents to experience hunger or cravings for specific foods may place them at risk for binge eating episodes. Dieting among adolescents should not be viewed as a normative and acceptable behavior.

Prevalence of Binge Eating Disorder

Binge eating disorder (BED) has recently been proposed as a distinct diagnostic entity and is now listed in the appendix of the *Diagnostic and Statistical Manual of Mental Disorders,* fourth edition *(DSM-IV)* (table 12-5). BED is defined by recurrent episodes of binge eating at least two days a week for at least six months. BED differs from bulimia nervosa in that binge eating is not followed by compensatory behaviors, such as self-induced vomiting.[8,19]

BED is more prevalent among overweight clinical populations (30%) than among community samples (5% of females and 3% of males).[19] Although studies on adolescents have assessed the prevalence of binge eating, few studies have assessed prevalence rates of BED. In a college student sample, the rate of BED was 2.6%. In contrast to other weight-related conditions, significant differences were not found between male and female students.[8,19]

Prevalence of Obesity

Obesity is defined as the presence of excess body tissue. Overweight is the excess amount of body weight that includes muscle, bone, fat, and water. Due to difficulties in distinguishing between the two, these terms are often used interchangeably. Body mass index (BMI) is most commonly used for obesity assessment among youth. BMI is a weight-stature index (weight in kilograms/height in meters^2) and therefore takes both weight and height into account in the assessment of obesity. In assessing the presence of obesity and in determining prevalence rates of obesity, comparisons are often made to population norms derived from the first National Health and Nutrition Examination (NHANESI), which was a large national study done between the years 1976 and 1980.[20,21] According to Himes and Dietz, adolescents with BMI values above the 95th percentile of population norms are defined as overweight, and adolescents between the 85th and 95th percentiles are considered "at risk for overweight."[22] However, it should be noted that including only youth above the 95th percentile is a rather conservative measure of obesity.

Prevalence rates of obesity among adolescents have increased significantly in the United States.[23–25] Data from NHANES show that, in 1976–1980, 5.7% of adolescents (aged twelve to seventeen years) were overweight (BMI >95th percentile). The prevalence of overweight increased to 12% of adolescents in 1988–1994 using the same cut-off point. Therefore, the prevalence of overweight doubled among adolescents during a period of less than two decades. Using a less conservative measure of overweight (BMI >85th percentile), 21.7% of adolescent males and 21.4% of adolescent females in the United States are defined as overweight (or at risk for overweight, according to Himes and Dietz).[22,24]

Patterns of Distribution in the Population

Anorexia nervosa appears to be far more prevalent in industrialized societies, in which there is an abundance of food and in which being attractive is linked to being thin, especially for females. Historically anorexia nervosa has been viewed as an upper-class condition, with higher prevalence rates among youth from higher socioeconomic backgrounds. However, the social class effect seems to have weakened in recent years.[26,27] This may be due to spreading of social norms emphasizing thinness and success across all social classes.

In examining rates of anorexia nervosa over time and by sociodemographic characteristics, data may be biased by differences in referrals for treatment. If clinical data are used in establishing prevalences of conditions, only persons who have sought out treatment are counted. Individuals with more financial resources and a higher awareness of the symptoms of anorexia nervosa may be more likely to seek out treatment. Some research has focused on population-based samples of youth in order to avoid this clinical bias. Within population-based studies, it is more difficult to determine whether someone has an eating disorder, but it is easier to examine trends across socioeconomic status and ethnicity.

Population-based research has found that girls with higher socioeconomic backgrounds are more likely to diet than are girls with lower socioeconomic backgrounds, but they are also less likely to report vomiting, the use of laxatives, and binge eating.[12,28] Ethnic differences are also apparent. For example, higher rates of body satisfaction, lower perceptions of overweight, and less dieting have been found among African American girls, as compared with Caucasian girls.[12]

The prevalence of obesity also differs across socioeconomic status and ethnicity in the United States, with a higher prevalence among persons from lower socioeconomic levels and minority status. For example, 30% of African American adolescent girls are at risk for overweight (BMI >85th percentile), as compared with 22% of Caucasian girls.[24,25]

High-Risk Subgroups of the Adolescent Population

It has been noted that weight-related concerns and conditions tend to peak during adolescence. Furthermore, these conditions are more likely to have detrimental consequences during this period than during adulthood, due to the physical and psychosocial development that occurs during adolescence. There are subgroups of the adolescent population that appear to be at particular risk for weight-related conditions and for potential adverse effects. Four groups are particularly worthy of mention, in that health care providers, educators, and parents might not suspect weight-related conditions among these youth.

The first group includes athletes—in particular, those participating in sports in which the body tends to be exposed or in which there is a need to maintain a particular body shape, size, or weight.[29–33] Boys participating in sports such as wrestling may undergo extreme measures to "make weight" that can be fatal, while other boys may suffer from distorted body images and want to be larger.[34] In spite of the evidence that dancers and gymnasts may be at increased risk for unhealthy dieting and anorexic and bulimic behaviors, and that this may severely interfere with their ability to perform, pressure may still be placed on these young athletes to restrict their energy intake. Disordered eating can have serious health effects, resulting in amenorrhea due to low body fat and hormonal changes and osteoporosis due to calcium loss. Termed the female athlete triad, disordered eating, amenorrhea, and osteoporosis can have serious and long-lasting effects on young athletes.[35,36]

A second group that may be at increased risk for weight-related conditions included youth following a vegetarian diet. Vegetarians are about twice as likely as nonvegetarian youth to engage in frequent dieting, four times as likely to engage in intentional vomiting, and eight times as likely to use laxatives.[37] Thus, although a vegetarian diet may have numerous benefits, adolescent vegetarians should be monitored for eating behaviors and body image attitudes.

The third group worthy of mention is youth with chronic illness. Youth with a range of chronic illnesses are at increased risk for engaging in excessive dieting and anorexic/bulimic behaviors.[38,39] The potential adverse effects of engaging in these behaviors are particularly large for youth with conditions such as diabetes mellitus. In spite of an increased awareness of health-related issues, desires for increased control and a need to be like other teenagers may contribute to the onset of weight-related conditions among youth with chronic illness.

Finally, youth who have experienced either sexual or physical abuse may be at increased risk for a range of weight-related conditions.[40-44] Therefore, questions about past abuse experiences should be included in the clinical assessment of youth, and, for youth reporting abuse, further screening should address weight-related conditions.

ETIOLOGY OF WEIGHT-RELATED CONCERNS AND CONDITIONS ≋

Although each weight-related condition has specific factors contributing to its etiology, a number of general principles apply across conditions. The main similarity is that all of the weight-related conditions have a complex etiology involving interactions between multiple factors—namely, a range of psychologic, biologic, familial, sociocultural, environmental, and behavioral factors. Furthermore, these factors interact with each other on the causal pathway to weight-related conditions. Therefore, obesity is not caused only by behavioral factors, such as a lack of physical activity, but by a range of factors, including drive for thinness, biologic disposition to obesity, lack of opportunities for physical activity in one's neighborhood, familial eating patterns, and eating and physical activity behaviors. Environmental factors, such as a lack of safe physical fitness facilities within the vicinity of one's home, influence an adolescent's level of physical activity, and, if there is a biologic disposition toward obesity, an adolescent's risk of gaining weight and becoming obese increases. Anorexia nervosa is not caused only by sociocultural norms emphasizing thinness but also by the interaction of these social norms with other factors, such as difficult familial relationships, low self-esteem, and dieting behaviors. Furthermore, once the dieting begins, its likelihood of continuing depends on factors in the social environment, such as familial and societal norms supporting weight loss, and personal factors, such as body image and self-esteem.

In the prevention and treatment of weight-related conditions, it is essential to be aware of the wide range of factors contributing to the onset of a condition. Although an intervention may not address all of these factors, an awareness of their impact is essential to developing an intervention plan and setting reasonable outcome expectations. Although all of the weight-related conditions have multicausality, for each individual various factors' contributions to the onset and continuation of a weight-related condition may differ in strength. For example, for some overweight youth, biologic factors may be the main contributors, while, for others, eating patterns may be a stronger factor. Therefore, although it is important to recognize the multicausality of these conditions, it is also important to recognize individual differences in developing an intervention plan.

An etiologic model showing the pathway leading to the onset of a weight-related condition, whether it is obesity or anorexia nervosa, is shown in figure 12-3. This is a simplified model of complex phenomena. While the contribution of specific risk factors may vary somewhat for different weight-related conditions, and from individual to individual, these

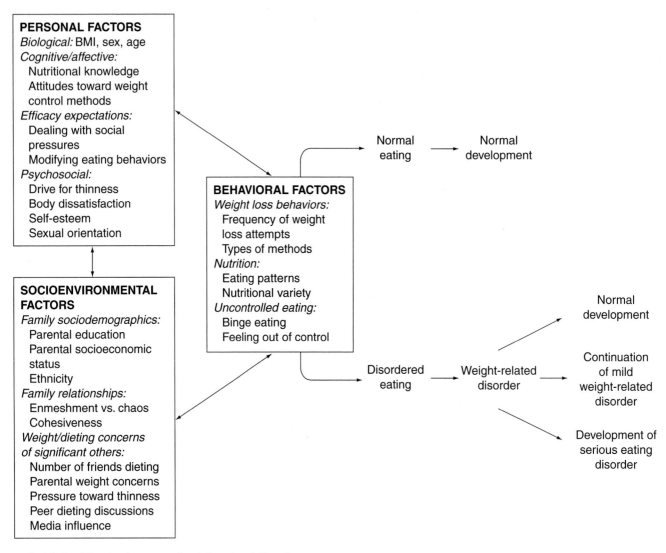

FIG. 12-3   The development of weight-related disorders.

Adapted from Neumark-Sztainer, D., Butler, R., and Palti, H. Personal and socioenvironmental predictors of disordered eating among females. *Journal of Nutrition Education.* 1996; 28:195–201.

factors can be organized into similar broad domains. The model incorporates a number of principles from social cognitive theory:[45,46] socioenvironmental, personal, and behavioral factors are shown to interact with each other and together influence health behaviors and outcomes.[47] Personal factors contributing to the onset of weight-related disorders include developmental, cognitive/affective, and psychologic factors. Socioenvironmental factors include sociocultural norms, familial factors, peer norms and behaviors, and food availability. Behavioral factors include eating behaviors, dieting and other weight management behaviors, physical activity levels, coping behaviors, and behavioral skills.[48] The result of these joint factors may be the onset of disordered eating behaviors, such as self-induced vomiting or binge eating. Over time, these behaviors may disappear, continue, or develop into more serious weight-related conditions, such as bulimia nervosa or obesity.

Through a recognition of the multicausality of weight-related conditions, similarities in causal factors and their patterns of interactions across conditions, and condition-specific and individual-specific causal factors, practitioners are better equipped to develop more effective interventions aimed at the prevention and treatment of weight-related conditions among youth.

The Extremes of the Spectrum: A Closer Look ≋

Anorexia nervosa and bulimia nervosa are at one end of the spectrum, while obesity is at the other. Many of the principles discussed in the following sections on anorexia and bulimia nervosa may be applied to understanding the other conditions on the spectrum—anorexic and bulimic behaviors, unhealthy dieting, and binge eating disorder—although to different degrees.

Anorexia Nervosa

Anorexia nervosa is the most severe condition on the spectrum of weight-related conditions, in terms of its impact on morbidity and mortality. It is characterized by self-starvation and an intense fear of being fat. The effects of anorexia nervosa on body weight are clearly seen in figure 12-4. It is a disease that has attracted the attention of professionals and laypersons due to the irony of its nature—self-starvation among an abundance of food. The condition defies the basic principles of survival, which have always been aimed at gathering enough food to avoid hunger. The name of this disease is somewhat of a misnomer, since loss of appetite (anorexia) is rare. Rather, there is a need to feel that one can control one's food intake in spite of extreme hunger.

A new condition? Although in the past few decades accounts of anorexia nervosa in the medical literature have been much more common than before, there are early descriptions in the scientific literature of adolescents who seem to have had anorexia nervosa. For example, in 1694 Morton vividly described a case of "nervous consumption," which is now referred to as anorexia nervosa:

Mr. Duke's daughter in St. Mary Axe, in the year 1684, and the Eighteenth year of her Age, in the month of July fell into a total suppression of her Monthly Courses from a multitude of Cares and Passions of her Mind but without any Symptom of the Green-Sickness following upon it. From which time her Appetite began to abate, and her Digestion to be bad; her Flesh also began to be flaccid and loose. . . . She wholly neglected care of her self for two full Years. . . . I do not remember that I did ever in all my Practice see one, that was conversant with the Living so much wasted with the greatest degree of a Consumption, (like a Skeleton clad only in skin) yet there was no fever. . . . Only her appetite was diminished. . . . She was after three months taken with a Fainting Fit and dyed.[49]

It is unclear whether the increased accounts of anorexia nervosa in the medical literature are due to an increase in the actual number of cases or to an increased recognition of the condition among individuals with anorexia nervosa, family members of these individuals, and health care providers. There are a number of indications that the incidence of anorexia nervosa has increased over time, particularly the milder forms of this condition.[10,26]

Description. The essential features of anorexia nervosa are refusal to maintain body weight over a minimal normal weight for age and height; intense fear of gaining weight or becoming fat, even though underweight; a distorted body image; and amenorrhea (in females). (Review the diagnostic criteria in table 12-2).

Usually, weight loss is accomplished primarily through a reduction in total food intake. Individuals may begin by excluding foods from their diets that they perceive as high-calorie food, but most eventually progress to a very restricted diet, limited to only a few foods. Additional methods of weight loss include purging and increased or excessive exercise. Weight loss is usually viewed as an impressive achievement and a sign of extraordinary self-discipline, while weight gain is perceived as an unacceptable failure of self-control. Although some individuals with anorexia nervosa may acknowledge being thin, they typically deny the serious medical implications of their malnourished state. The experience and significance of body weight and shape are distorted among individuals with anorexia nervosa. Some individuals feel globally overweight, while others realize that they are thin but are still concerned that certain parts of their bodies are "too fat." The self-esteem of individuals with anorexia nervosa is highly dependent on their body shape and size. Usually, amenorrhea follows weight loss, but it is not unusual for amenorrhea to appear before noticeable weight loss has occurred.[8]

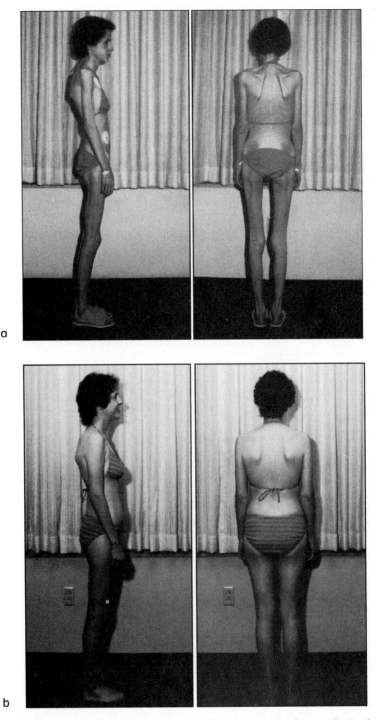

FIG. 12-4 (*a*) Anorexic woman before treatment. (*b*) Same patient after *gradual* refeeding, nutritional management, and psychologic therapy.

Courtesy Sycamore Hospital, a division of Kettering Medical Center, Dayton, Ohio.

TABLE 12-6   *Common Signs and Symptoms of Anorexia Nervosa*

- Wearing loose, baggy, heavy clothes to hide thinness.
- Excessive weight loss in relatively short time period.
- Loss of menstrual cycle.
- Dry, cold skin.
- Lanugo: Very fine hair on arms, legs, back, face, or chest.
- Insomnia and hyperactivity.
- Distorted body image.
- Extreme, excessive, and rigid exercise routines.
- Extreme fear of gaining any weight.

There are two types of anorexia nervosa: restricting and binge eating/purging. In the restricting type, the individual does not regularly engage in binge eating or purging behaviors; in the other, there are regular episodes of binge eating and purging behaviors. In both types, however, there is a refusal to maintain a minimally normal body weight.

The mean age at onset of anorexia nervosa is seventeen years of age. However, some data suggest that the incidence of anorexia nervosa tends to have a bimodal peak at ages fourteen and eighteen years. The onset of this condition is often associated with a stressful life event, such as leaving home for college or experiencing changes in familial relationships.[8] Recovery rates are estimated at 40–50% for individuals with anorexia nervosa.[50]

The adolescent with anorexia nervosa is often brought to professional attention by family members after marked weight loss, or failure to make expected weight gains, has occurred. By the time the individual is profoundly underweight, other signs of the disease may be present, such as hypothermia, bradycardia, hypotension, edema, lanugo (soft hair on the body), and a variety of metabolic changes. Unfortunately, denial of the condition by the adolescent or the family is common and can delay the diagnosis and treatment, resulting in a poorer prognosis. Early recognition of possible signs of anorexia nervosa and seeking out of professional help is likely to decrease significantly the time and intensity of treatment and improve chances for a successful recovery. Some of the key symptoms of anorexia nervosa are listed in table 12-6.

Consequences. The most dire consequence of anorexia nervosa is death. An estimated 10–15% of patients with anorexia nervosa die from their disease, although difficulties arise in assessing mortality rates.[51] Karen Carpenter, a well-known singer, and Christy Henrich, a world-class gymnast, died of complications of anorexia nervosa. Reasons for fatality from anorexia include a weakened immune system due to undernutrition, gastric ruptures, cardiac arrhythmias, heart failure, and suicide.

Other medical complications that are not necessarily fatal but that can lead to permanent physical and neurologic damage include the side effects of laxative use—such as dehydration, abdominal cramping, muscle cramps, and electrolyte imbalances, which affect neurologic functioning. Also, the regular use of diet pills may lead to insomnia, mood changes, irritability, and when taken in extremely large doses, psychosis.[52] Cessation of the menstrual cycle also is one part of the diagnostic criteria for anorexia nervosa and is partly due to loss of body fat and weight, but is also due to hormone irregularity due to stress, malnutrition, and psychologic factors. Many patients with anorexia complain of being cold, generally thought to be due to diminished functioning of the hypothalamic-pituitary system in the brain and low levels of body fat accompanying extreme weight loss.[50]

Psychologic complications common in anorexia nervosa include distorted body image, depression, and social isolation.[18,50,53] Moodiness, anxiety, irritability, intolerance of others, low self-esteem, hopelessness, rigidity, and ritualistic habits are also common.[53] There are also severe consequences for the family of an adolescent with anorexia nervosa, due to the pain caused by watching one's child or sibling whither away and the daily impact of this illness on regular family rituals, such as eating meals.

Etiology. There is no single cause for anorexia nervosa; rather, a range of biologic, psychologic, familial, and sociocultural factors contribute to the development of the disease.[54,55] Questions exist as to the relative contribution of each of these factors to the onset of anorexia nervosa, and research continues to elucidate causal pathways.

Biologic factors include gender, heritability, and neurotransmitter abnormalities. Gender is a strong predisposing factor in the development of eating disorders. Studies indicate that men and women perceive and respond to hunger in different ways,[56] and dieting changes brain serotonin in women but not men.[57] Studies with twins indicate that eating disorders may run in families. In studies of identical twins, nine out of sixteen identical twins of patients with anorexia had anorexia as well, while only one out of fourteen fraternal twins of patients with anorexia also had the disease.[58,59] Differences in neurotransmitter concentrations—namely serotonin and norepinephrine—have been documented in patients with anorexia nervosa.[60,61] However, hormone, neurotransmitter, appetite, mood, and menstruation abnormalities may all be present in patients with anorexia, thus making it difficult to establish cause and effect relationships between anorexia nervosa and neurotransmitters.[62]

Psychologic factors contributing to the onset of anorexia nervosa include poor body image, a strong drive for thinness, and low self-esteem. Adolescents with anorexia nervosa are likely to be perfectionists and high achievers yet may suffer from low self-esteem. Feeling an intense need for mastery over their lives, adolescents with anorexia nervosa may feel in control only of their weight and food intake.[63,64] Bruch describes anorexia nervosa as related to deficits in the sense of self and development of autonomy.[65] These deficits may be related to family dynamics or relationships within the family. Minuchin[66] discusses **emeshed,** overprotective family systems that do not allow for individual development of appropriate roles, which may foster the development of anorexia nervosa as a coping mechanism for adolescents. However, there are large differences between individual and familial characteristics of youth with anorexia nervosa, and care should be taken in making assumptions about either.

Emeshed
Intertwined, as in family relationships that capture and diminish individual autonomy or self-regard.

Sociocultural factors may contribute significantly to the onset of anorexia nervosa and other weight-related conditions. In many industrialized societies, culture puts extreme pressure on women to be thin, causing widespread body dissatisfaction and leading to unhealthy dieting, which can lead to the development of an eating disorder among vulnerable youth. The average woman in the United States is about 5 ft 4 in and weighs 145 lb, while the average model is 5 ft 10 in and weighs 110 lb, 20–25% less than the average woman. To set up the average model as the ideal for the average woman creates an unhealthy standard for women and girls. Through the images and messages in advertising and the media, society makes unrealistic demands on women and men in terms of what bodies should look like. Adolescents are faced with these continual media influences, which contribute to the diet and thinness obsession prevalent in society; as a result, adolescents can have an unrealistic image of what they should look like.[8,67]

Assessment. Prior to developing a treatment plan, a thorough assessment is needed to determine the presence of anorexia nervosa, the type of anorexia, and the severity of the condition. In addition, a thorough assessment of the factors contributing to anorexia nervosa is necessary. Youth who do not meet the full diagnostic criteria for an eating disorder, yet are displaying some of the symptoms, should receive nutritional and psychologic treatment as needed and should be closely monitored to prevent the advancement of symptoms to an eating disorder diagnosis.

Reiff and Reiff suggest gathering information on a range of factors, including family history; exercise history; sports involvement; diet history; sources of nutritional information used by the person; beliefs about food, hunger, and weight; food fears; history of food or weight-related conditions of self, family, or friends; and expectations from nutrition therapy.[68] They also suggest using the "Are You Dying to Be Thin?" questionnaire shown in table 12-7. Although this questionnaire was not designed to be a diagnostic tool, it may be helpful in determining whether there is a tendency toward anorexia nervosa or other eating disorders.

Treatment. Because the severity of anorexia nervosa varies from patient to patient, each patient has individual treatment needs. In general, a multidimensional approach is recommended that focuses on weight restoration and cessation of weight reduction behaviors, improvement in eating behaviors and nutritional status, and improvement in psychologic and emotional state.[69,70]

TABLE 12-7   Dying to Be Thin Questionnaire

Due to an increase in publicity and public awareness, anorexia nervosa (key symptom: extreme weight loss due to self-starvation accompanied by an intense fear of being fat or gaining weight) and bulimia nervosa (key symptom: binge eating—eating what the individual considers to be too much food in a way that feels out of control—followed by purging) are becoming more and more openly acknowledged.

The following questionnaire will tell you whether or not you think or behave in a way that indicates that you have tendencies toward anorexia nervosa or bulimia nervosa.

Directions: Answer the questions below honestly. Respond as you are now, not the way you used to be or the way you would like to be. Write the number of your answer in the space at the left. Do not leave any questions blank unless instructed to do so.

_____   1.   I have eating habits that are different from those of my family and friends.
      1] Often   2] Sometimes   3] Rarely   4] Never

_____   2.   I find myself panicking if I cannot exercise as I planned because I am afraid I will gain weight if I don't.
      1] Often   2] Sometimes   3] Rarely   4] Never

_____   3.   My friends tell me I am thin, but I don't believe them because I feel fat.
      1] Often   2] Sometimes   3] Rarely   4] Never

_____   4.   *(Females only)* My menstrual period has stopped or become irregular due to no known medical reasons.
      1] True   2] False

_____   5.   I have become obsessed with food to the point that I cannot go through a day without worrying about what I will or will not eat.
      1] Almost always   2] Sometimes   3] Rarely   4] Never

_____   6.   I have lost more than 15% of what is considered a healthy weight for my height (e.g., female, 5'4" tall, healthy weight = 122 lbs., lost 20 lbs.) and currently weigh that weight or less.
      1] True   2] False

_____   7.   I would panic if I got on the scale tomorrow and found out I had gained two pounds.
      1] Almost always   2] Sometimes   3] Rarely   4] Never

_____   8.   I find that I prefer to eat alone or when I am sure no one will see me, thus make excuses so I can eat less and less with friends and family.
      1] Often   2] Sometimes   3] Rarely   4] Never

_____   9.   I find myself going on uncontrollable eating binges during which I consume large amounts of food to the point that I feel sick and make myself vomit.
      1] Never   2] Less than 1 time per week   3] 1–6 times per week   4] 1 or more times per day

_____   10.   *(NOTE: Answer only if your answer to #9 is "1," otherwise leave blank.)* I find myself compulsively eating more than I want to while feeling out of control and/or unaware of what I am doing.
      1] Never   2] Less than 1 time per week   3] 1–6 times per week   4] 1 or more times per day

_____   11.   I use laxatives or diuretics as a means of weight control.
      1] Never   2] Rarely   3] Sometimes   4] On a regular basis

_____   12.   I find myself playing games with food (e.g., cutting it up into tiny pieces, hiding food so people will think I ate it, chewing it and spitting it out without swallowing it, keeping hidden stashes of food) and/or telling myself certain foods are bad.
      1] Often   2] Sometimes   3] Rarely   4] Never

_____   13.   People around me have become very interested in what I eat and I find myself getting angry at them for pushing me to eat more.
      1] Often   2] Sometimes   3] Rarely   4] Never

_____   14.   I have felt more depressed and irritable recently than I used to and/or have been spending an increasing amount of time alone.
      1] True   2] False

_____   15.   I keep a lot of my fears about food and eating to myself because I am afraid no one would understand.
      1] Often   2] Sometimes   3] Rarely   4] Never

TABLE 12-7—Cont'd.

_____   16.   I enjoy making gourmet and/or high calorie meals for others as long as I don't have to eat any myself.
       1] Often   2] Sometimes   3] Rarely   4] Never

_____   17.   The most powerful fear in my life is the fear of gaining weight or becoming fat.
       1] Often   2] Sometimes   3] Rarely   4] Never

_____   18.   I exercise a lot (more than 4 times per week and/or more than 4 hours per week) as a means of weight control.
       1] True   2] False

_____   19.   I find myself totally absorbed when reading books or magazines about dieting, exercising and calorie counting to
       the point that I spend hours studying them.
       1.] Often   2.] Sometimes   3.] Rarely   4.] Never

_____   20.   I tend to be a perfectionist and am not satisfied with myself unless I do things perfectly.
       1.] Almost always   2.] Sometimes   3.] Rarely   4.] Never

_____   21.   I go through long periods of time without eating (fasting) or eating very little as a means of weight control.
       1.] Often   2.] Sometimes   3.] Rarely   4.] Never

_____   22.   It is important to me to try to be thinner than all of my friends.
       1.] Almost always   2.] Sometimes   3.] Rarely   4.] Never

Scoring
Step 1: Add scores together. **Total is** _____.

Step 2: Compare your score with the table below.

38 or less—Strong tendencies toward anorexia nervosa.

  39–50—Strong tendencies toward bulimia nervosa.

  50–60—Weight conscious. May or may not have tendencies toward an eating disorder. Not likely to have anorexia or bulimia
       nervosa. May have tendencies toward compulsive eating or obesity.

 Over 60—Extremely unlikely to have anorexia or bulimia nervosa; however, scoring over 60 does not rule out tendencies to-
       ward compulsive eating or obesity.

If you score below 50, it would be wise for you to (1) seek more information about anorexia nervosa and bulimia nervosa and
       (2) contact a counselor, pastor, teacher, or physician in order to find out if you have an eating disorder and, if you do, talk
       about what kind of assistance would be best for you.
If you scored between 50 and 60, it would be a good idea for you to talk to a counselor, pastor, teacher, or physician in order to
       find out if you have an eating disorder and, if you do, how to get some help.
If you score over 60, but have questions and concerns about the way you eat and/or your weight, it would be a good idea for you to talk
       to a counselor, pastor, teacher, or physician in order to determine if you have an eating disorder and, if you do, how to get some help.
NOTE! Eating disorders are potentially life-threatening disorders which can be overcome with the proper information, support,
       and counseling. The earlier you seek help, the better, although it is never too late to start on the road to recovery.

Immediate inpatient medical care may be necessary for medical stabilization if the person is at a dangerously low weight or is experiencing life-threatening electrolyte imbalances or cardiac abnormalities. Inpatient treatment on a medical service may be followed by an inpatient stay on a psychiatric service or at a residential treatment facility for more in-depth treatment of the eating disorder.

The treatment team generally consists of a medical doctor, psychiatrist, psychologist, dietitian, and nurse. In addition, the team may include a recreational or art therapist, social worker, dentist, and schoolteacher. The adolescent with the eating disorder and family members (in particular, parents) should also be viewed as part of the treatment team. The roles of each of the members on the treatment team at one inpatient program are shown in table 12-8. The team works together with the patient to attain an appropriate, individualized approach for recovery.

*TABLE 12-8　Roles of Team Members, Patients, and Families
in the Treatment of Eating Disorders*

Physician: Completes medical evaluation, oversees general medical care of patient.

Nursing staff: Develops and maintains treatment schedule with team, provides emotional and conflict resolution support to patient, monitors patient compliance with treatment program.

Psychologist: Individual, group, and/or family therapist, helps patient reassess and improve body image and coping skills.

Psychiatrist: May also function as therapist, manages medications.

Nutritionist/dietitian: Helps patient increase knowledge and confidence in choosing foods and making meal plans as part of nutrition therapy, helps patient discern emotional ties to eating.

Social worker: Works as community liaison between school and patient, may also be a family or group therapist in either inpatient or outpatient treatment.

Activities therapist: May include occupational therapist, physical therapist, and music or art therapist; addresses the patient's life-skill or physical needs or other therapy needs.

Schoolteacher: Serves as a link to patient's reintroduction into school setting if necessary, can promote eating disorder prevention education in schools.

Parent(s)/family: Support patient's treatment plan in manner recommended by treatment team; integral to treatment approach via family therapy, family education, or support for the patient.

Patient: Is an active member of the team, needs to be receptive to treatment in order for these approaches to be successful and recovery to begin.

Adapted from Kreipe, R. E., and M. Uphoff. 1992. Treatment and outcome of adolescents with anorexia nervosa. *Adolescent Medicine: State of the Art Reviews* 3(3):519–540.

Common components of treatment include regular individual, group, and family therapy, nutritional therapy through regular meetings with a registered dietitian, and specific therapy activities aimed at improving body image, socialization, and self-esteem. Some research shows that eating disorder clients can benefit greatly from group therapy.[50] Often, patients with anorexia express an overwhelming aloneness with regard to their eating disorder and gain immeasurable support from hearing others with similar feelings. However, for anorexia nervosa, there is often the fear that youth will "learn each other's" tricks in group work, and competition may occur. Family therapy can also be very useful in identifying issues related to onset of the anorexia and in assisting the family in developing new patterns of relating to one another, and it is usually recommended for working with adolescents with eating disorders. Family therapists can help the family explore and modify ingrained, emeshed family patterns and improve their communication with each other.[70]

In addition, medication can be used to treat anorexia and is part of the American Psychiatric Association guidelines,[70] but not all patients respond to or even accept a recommendation to begin medication.[62,71] The most widely used and researched medications for eating disorders are the antidepressants. Other groups of drugs have been used with less success, including antipsychotics, lithium carbonate, and appetite stimulants.[70,71] Estrogen replacement therapy may also be used to reduce the risk of osteoporosis due to calcium loss in some patients with severe chronic amenorrhea.[72]

Other conditions may be seen in patients with anorexia, with depression the most common diagnosis. The evaluation of depressive symptoms needs to be done by a qualified professional and may contribute to the decision to use medications in treatment. Other common diagnoses include mood disorders, chemical dependency, obsessive-compulsive disorder, and some personality disorders. Patients diagnosed with anorexia and any of these other disorders require treatment plans that appropriately address recovery from both diagnoses.[71]

Research suggests that the combination of group therapy, nutritional counseling, psychotherapy, and possibly medication provides the most beneficial treatment approach to facilitate recovery for the client.[69,71] However, relapse often accompanies the recovery process; thus, treatment of anorexia nervosa involves a long-term approach and a strong commitment by the patient and the treatment team.

Nutritional Goals of Treatment. Abnormal nutritional status and dietary patterns are the key components of anorexia nervosa and other weight-related conditions that need

CASE STUDY

Sarah: A Compulsive Female Athlete

Your ninth-grade sister, Sarah, is the star basketball player on the junior varsity team and is known for her speed and agility on the court. Preseason practice has just started, and her coach has told her he is considering moving her to the varsity team if she "proves herself" in practice and games the first half of the season. She begins to run for thirty minutes after practice every night to work on her speed and endurance, and you can hear her doing calisthenics late at night in her room. Her runs get longer and longer, and she starts to skip eating dinner with the family, with the excuse that she has homework. She has become irritable with your parents, and the two of you have started fighting every day about trivial things. You begin to notice that her clothes look baggy, and she looks tired and worn. When she brings home her nearly straight-*A* report card at the end of the term, she bursts into tears over the one *A–* she received and says she needs to work a lot harder. She stays in her room, doing homework, all weekend, leaving only for her nightly run, which now lasts about ninety minutes. One day, two months into basketball season, her best friend, Jessie, tells you she is worried about Sarah because she never eats and she has lost weight.

Questions for analysis
1. What symptoms is Sarah displaying that suggest she may have an eating disorder?
2. What can you and Jessie do to help Sarah? Who would you talk to about your concerns?
3. Who else do you think should be involved?

to be addressed in treatment. The role of the dietitian or other nutrition counselor is crucial. Patience and empathy need to be combined with firmness in working with an adolescent with anorexia nervosa or other eating disorder. Time needs to be taken to develop a relationship of trust. In order to be most effective, the nutrition counselor should have some knowledge of behavioral strategies, adolescent health, psychology, and eating disorders, as well as solid training in nutrition. Rock and Curran-Celentano have outlined the goals and strategies of nutritional care for patients with anorexia nervosa (see table 12-9).[73] They state that nutrition education tools that are used with patients with anorexia nervosa are usually based on a food group or exchange system. The goal is to teach a new approach to food choices, emphasizing nutrient density or other health-promoting qualities, rather than to prescribe a rigid diet. Working with a food plan in the outpatient setting, the dietitian can guide patients toward increased quality and quantity of the diet. Formerly forbidden foods can be introduced gradually. Empathetic guidance of a nutrition counselor provides reassurance to the adolescent, who is usually terrified of excessive and uncontrollable weight gain.[73]

Bulimia Nervosa

The term *bulimia nervosa* comes from the ancient *Latin* words "bulim os," which translates to "ox hunger."[74] As previously mentioned, bulimia nervosa is an eating disorder characterized by the consumption of large amounts of food with subsequent purging by self-induced vomiting, laxative or diuretic abuse, enemas, and/or obsessive exercising. Whereas anorexia nervosa is characterized by severe weight loss, in bulimia nervosa there may be weight maintenance or extreme weight fluctuations due to alternating binges and fasts. In some individuals, there is overlap between anorexia and bulimia nervosa.

Description. The essential features of bulimia nervosa are recurrent episodes of binge eating (rapid consumption of a large amount of food in a discrete period of time); a feel-

TABLE 12-9   *Goals and Strategies of Nutritional Care*
for Patients with Anorexia Nervosa

1. Increased energy intake to promote weight restoration, initially 800–1200 kcal/day, with a gradual increase to achieve the goal weight gain (e.g., 0.5 to 1.0 kg/wk).
2. Specific meal plan and dietary guidelines to promote normalization of intake, including limitations on foods that patients may refuse to eat and accommodation of patient preferences that permit nutritional adequacy and weight gain.
3. A new approach to food choices, based on nutrient contributions and other qualities, rather than energy content.
4. Formerly forbidden foods introduced with reassurance and sensitivity to a fear of uncontrollable eating and weight gain.
5. Adequate dietary calcium to permit improved bone mineralization as weight is restored and hormonal abnormalities are corrected.
6. Low-dose daily multiple vitamins with minerals, especially if patients are chronically ill.
7. Avoidance of strategies to reduce energy intake and manage hunger (such as overuse of caffeine-containing beverages, chewing gum, and modified food products) or promote energy expenditure (such as excessive exercise).

From Rock, C. L., and J. Curran-Celentano. 1996. Nutritional management of eating disorders. *The Psychiatric Clinics of North America* 19(4):701–713.

TABLE 12-10   *Common Signs and Symptoms of Bulimia Nervosa*

- Eating in secret.
- Disappearance into bathroom for long periods of time to induce vomiting.
- Bingeing and purging from once a week to five times a day.
- Abuse of alcohol or drugs.
- Possible weight fluctuations.
- Extreme fear of gaining even a small amount of weight.
- Distorted body image.
- Dry skin and dry brittle hair.
- Swollen salivary glands under the jaw and along sides of face from bingeing and purging.
- Depression, guilt, fear, and mood swings.
- Fatigue and cold sweats from rapid changes in blood sugar levels.

ing of lack of control over eating behavior during the binge; self-induced vomiting, use of laxatives or diuretics, strict dieting or fasting, or vigorous exercise in order to prevent weight gain; and persistent overconcern with body shape and weight.

Many individuals with bulimia nervosa keep their eating disorder a secret and maintain normal or above normal body weight. Because of their secretive bingeing and purging habits and general absence of severe weight loss, people with bulimia nervosa can often successfully hide their eating disorder for years.[8,75] People with bulimia nervosa can be overweight, underweight, or of average weight for their height and body frame. Bulimia nervosa may be preceded by a history of dieting or restrictive eating, which are thought to contribute to the binge-purge cycle. Some common signs and symptoms of bulimia nervosa are listed in table 12-10.

The onset of bulimia nervosa is generally at a later age than that of anorexia nervosa. The average age of onset is seventeen to twenty-five years, but, because of the secrecy of the disorder, many patients do not seek treatment for years.[76] Recovery rates are quite high, with recovery estimates of 50–60%.[50]

Females with bulimia nervosa tend to come from families in which there is chaos or conflict.[76] Low self-esteem, depression, and lack of self-control over their lives contribute to the development of the disorder.[76] The characteristic binge/purge cycle of bulimia nervosa is used to avoid pain, problems, and anxiety. Patients often describe a feeling of "emptiness," defined as emotional hunger by psychologists, which the patient translates into a type of physical hunger.[77] The binge/purge is a method to meet these hunger needs, but not gain weight from the extra calories. After the binge and purge, the patient feels angry, disappointed, and disgusted and renews her commitment to restrict her food intake and stop bingeing. This semistarvation period and the related hunger is a setup for the binge portion of the cycle, and it occurs again.[64] Unlike patients with anorexia, those with bulimia usually recognize that they have a problem and are more likely to seek help for their eating disorder on their own.[62]

Consequences. Mortality for bulimia nervosa appears to be lower than for anorexia nervosa. Based on a review of the existing literature, Woodside has estimated that approximately 5% of patients die of their disease, usually due to heart failure resulting from electrolyte abnormality or to suicide.[50]

Common medical complications of bulimia nervosa include electrolyte imbalance leading to irregular heartbeat, heart failure and kidney damage; dehydration, constipation, and intestinal atrophy from laxative dependency; throat damage, esophageal tears, and broken blood vessels in the eyes from vomiting; dental problems, including erosion of tooth enamel, sensitivity to heat and cold, and shortening of the teeth; and irregular menstruation.[50,62,64,76]

Bulimia nervosa may also lead to a number of psychosocial consequences. The need for secrecy about bingeing and purging may lead to lying and may interfere with personal and work relationships. Stealing may be necessary in order to obtain enough money to purchase large quantities of food, especially among adolescents who do not have an income. In addition, the consumption of large amounts of food may lead other family members to not have enough food or to be angry because their food was consumed. Binge-purge cycles may be accompanied by depression, mood swings, and feelings of low self-control, low self-worth, and emptiness.

Etiology. The causes of bulimia nervosa are similar to those of anorexia nervosa and encompass a similar range of biologic, psychosocial, and sociocultural factors. In twin studies with identical twins, if one twin had bulimia, the chance that the other twin did also was 23%, which is eight times higher than in the general population.[78] Differences in neurotransmitter concentrations have also been documented in patients with bulimia—namely, low serotonin concentrations and alterations in the hormones that regulate hunger.[60,61] Again, it is difficult to establish cause and effect between bulimia and chemical alterations in the body.

Psychologic issues of low self-esteem, depression, and anxiety, as well as conflict within the family, have all been implicated in the development of bulimia nervosa. Also characteristic of patients with bulimia is a higher than normal level of substance abuse, particularly alcohol abuse. Studies have shown up to a third of women with bulimia also have alcohol and drug problems, with the eating disorder the primary disorder in most cases.[79]

The sociocultural factors contributing to the development of bulimia are similar to those implicated in anorexia nervosa. Society's message for women to be thin and meet the media ideal of beauty often goes hand in hand with food and alcohol advertising. Adolescents faced with these messages may resort to bulimia as a way to be able to eat in a culture with an abundant and reliable food supply yet still strive to meet society's ideal body image.[8]

Treatment. As with anorexia nervosa, each patient with bulimia nervosa has individual treatment needs, but the primary components of treatment are stabilization of binge/purge behaviors, nutritional rehabilitation, therapy as necessary, and often medication. Because patients with bulimia have chaotic eating patterns and often lose their ability to discern hunger and fullness, a structured meal plan is necessary to reintroduce them to a more normal eating pattern.[50] Treatment goals should also include working with the

CASE STUDY

Melissa: A Mother's Concern

You are a nutritionist working in a family practice clinic. One of your appointments today is with a nineteen-year-old girl named Melissa, who is home on summer break from college. Her mother called you a few weeks ago, saying that Melissa recently told her she has been vomiting after meals and after eating a great deal at other times, all during the school year. She also said her resident hall advisor and her roommate are very concerned about her. Her mother said that, when Melissa was home over winter break, she saw an empty laxative box in the trash in Melissa's room but thought nothing of it at the time. She also said that Melissa has always been just the right weight for her height, but now she looks too thin. Melissa has agreed to come in to see you today, but she is very quiet when you first start talking to her.

Questions for analysis
1. Given the limited information you have, how would you address the situation with Melissa, and what questions would you ask her?
2. What nutritional advice would you give her?
3. What would you tell her mother when she asks you what she can do to help Melissa?

patient to identify high-risk situations, the times that are typically considered binge times, or situations that elicit anxiety and distress, which typically lead to a binge.[76,77] New coping mechanisms must be learned in order to deal successfully with these situations and avoid binge/purge behaviors.

Psychotherapy treatment should focus on educating and assisting the patient to understand her feelings and the connections between her eating patterns and her emotions. Learning to express needs and feelings in an assertive manner will decrease her need to cover emotions with food. Cognitive-behavioral therapy can help restructure poor, unrealistic body image thoughts, low self-esteem, powerlessness, depression, and other negative thoughts.[77] Group and family therapy can be very useful in this restructuring and can educate family members as to how they can help the patient, either through support or by changing their own actions and comments.[50]

Use of medication has been shown to be effective in treatment of bulimia nervosa. Use of fluoxetine (Prozac) at a dose of 60 mg/day has been shown to decrease binge behaviors by 67% and purge behaviors by 56%.[77,80] Other medications, similar to those that have been used with anorexia patients, have been used in the treatment of bulimia but have not been shown to have significant effects;[50,77] thus, fluoxetine is the most commonly used medication in the treatment of bulimia.

Nutritional Goals of Treatment. As with anorexia nervosa, empathetic and knowledgeable guidance is the basis for effective nutrition counseling in bulimia nervosa.[73] Meal planning to establish regular eating and discouraging dieting are part of the first stage of an intervention program, in addition to teaching about body weight regulation, the adverse effects of dieting, and the physical consequences of bulimic behaviors.[81] The most essential element in the program may be helping the patient establish a pattern of regular eating, such as three planned meals and two or three planned snacks per day.[81] The basic principles and goals of nutritional care for patients with bulimia nervosa have been outlined by Rock and Curran-Celentano and are shown in table 12-11. An important benefit of providing sessions devoted to nutrition in the overall treatment program is that these sessions can function as the arena for discussion about food, so that psychotherapy can be devoted

TABLE 12-11   *The Basic Principles and Goals of Nutritional Care for Patients with Bulimia Nervosa*

1. Regular pattern of nutritionally balanced planned meals and snacks.
2. Adequate but not excessive levels of energy intake, with the goal of weight maintenance.
3. Adequate dietary fat and fiber intake, with the goal of promoting meal satiety.
4. Avoidance of dieting behavior, excessive exercise, and associated strategies, such as overuse of caffeine-containing beverages and modified products.
5. Inclusion of formerly forbidden foods in the diet, with the goal of minimizing food avoidances, using behavioral strategies.
6. Dietary recordkeeping and review to assess progress and plan strategies.
7. Stimulus control strategies, with the goal of controlling exposures and high-risk situations.
8. Weighing at scheduled intervals only.

From Rock, C. L., and J. Curran-Celentano. 1996. Nutritional management of eating disorders. *The Psychiat. Clin. No. Amer.* 19(4):701–713.

to psychologic issues. The emphasis in a cognitive-behavioral therapy program is on the regularity of eating, rather than the composition of the meals and snacks, and many patients benefit from detailed assistance in meal planning.[73] Components rated as helpful by individuals with bulimia nervosa at twelve to fifteen months' follow-up after treatment included being encouraged to eat a balanced diet, eating regular meals, and avoiding binge foods.[82]

Obesity

Obesity is not regarded as an eating disorder, since it does not necessarily have a psychologic component that has contributed to its etiology. Although for some individuals psychologic distress may contribute to its onset, behavioral factors (eating and physical activity) and a biologic predisposition toward obesity are generally viewed as much stronger predictors of obesity. As previously discussed, obesity has increased considerably in prevalence over the past two decades in the United States and is viewed as a major public health concern.

Description. As previously mentioned, obesity is the presence of excess body tissue, and overweight is the excess amount of body weight, but these terms are often used interchangeably. BMI (weight in kilograms/height in meters^2) is often used in assessing overweight, since it takes height into account in determining whether one is overweight and to what degree.

Consequences. The potential consequences associated with obesity result from both the condition itself and society's reaction to obesity. Health risks of obesity include hypertension, insulin resistance diabetes mellitus, and cardiovascular disease.[83] Research has shown that obesity in childhood and adolescence is associated with the development of risk factors for cardiovascular disease[84] and with increased morbidity and mortality after a fifty-year follow-up period, independent of adult body weight.[85] The economic costs associated with the physical consequences of obesity are high and have been found to range from 2.0% to 5.5% of total health care costs in a number of countries.[86–89] This high cost suggests the importance of strategies aimed at the prevention of obesity.

In addition to the higher risk for these physical consequences, overweight youth are at risk for a number of psychosocial consequences, largely due to social norms regarding weight-related issues. Weight-related stigmatization of overweight individuals has been documented for different age and gender groups in a variety of settings. Overweight adolescents may be particularly vulnerable to weight-related stigmatization due to the strong emphasis on appearance during adolescence. Fifty overweight adolescent girls were interviewed, and all but two of them described situations in which, due to their weight, they had been mistreated by family members, other children, employers, or strangers.[90] In a study of more than 30,000 adolescents, overweight youth were at greater risk than nonoverweight youth for weight-related concerns and disordered eating behaviors.[6] The potential psychosocial consequences of obesity may be strongly influenced by social norms for thinness within the adolescent's family, peer group, and larger society. Potential consequences include poor body image, low self-esteem, and social isolation. Research has found mixed results regarding associations between overweight status and global self-esteem, probably due to the heterogeneity of this group.[5] Therefore, some overweight adolescents experience more negative psychosocial consequences than others.

Etiology. Multiple factors contribute to the onset of obesity among children and adolescents. A child who has a biologic disposition toward obesity, lives in a society in which high-fat and high-calorie foods are readily accessible and the need to be physically active is minimal, and has grown up in a family in which energy-dense food is served and being physically active is not the norm, is at increased risk for obesity. A review of the scientific literature suggests that there has been a shift in beliefs about key etiological factors over the past two decades. More emphasis is currently being placed on the interaction between genetic dispositions toward obesity and environmental factors that provide more opportunities for overeating and underexercising, and less emphasis is being placed on the psychologic factors that place one at greater risk of overweight and obesity.

Sedentary lifestyles are believed to be a large contributor to the increase in the prevalence of obesity. Societal changes, such as increased technology, have played a large role in leading to more sedentary lifestyles. As previously noted, the prevalence of obesity is higher among individuals from lower socioeconomic backgrounds and minority groups. Adolescents and children living in neighborhoods in which it is unsafe to play outside or otherwise be active or in which fitness facilities are not accessible are less likely to be physically active. Youth from families or cultural backgrounds in which it is not encouraged or acceptable to be physically active are at increased risk for obesity. In addition, youth from low socioeconomic backgrounds or from families in which parents work long hours may be more likely to eat fast food, which tends to have a high energy and fat content.

Treatment. The aims of obesity treatment include weight loss or maintenance (in relation to changes in height), improved nutritional intake, increased physical activity, and increased self-acceptance. If the success of treatment is determined by all of these outcomes, and not only changes in degree of overweight, both health care providers and patients are more likely to perceive their efforts as successful. The aims for weight control and self-acceptance do not seem contradictory, as it is important for the overweight adolescent to have an overall positive self-image and to accept the fact that he or she may never be thin, only thinner or healthier.

Himes and Dietz have recommended that adolescents with a BMI ≥95th percentile for age and gender should be considered overweight and should have an in-depth medical assessment to determine underlying diagnoses (see fig. 12-5).[22] They have further recommended that youth with BMIs ≥85th percentile but <95th percentile should be considered at risk for overweight and should have a second-level screen. The second-level screen includes five areas that indicate additional health risk: 1) family history of premature heart disease, obesity, hypertension, or diabetes mellitus; 2) high blood pressure; 3) high total cholesterol (>200 mg/dl); 4) large increment in BMI; an increase over the previous year of two BMI points; and 5) concern about current weight by the adolescent. If any of these second-level items are positive, the adolescent should be followed up or referred for further in-depth medical assessment. If the second level of screening is negative, youth should receive preventive counseling. Issues to be discussed include nutrition guidance, with a focus on healthy weight control, strategies to increase physical activity levels, body image issues, weight-related stigmatization, and sources of social support.[91]

Overweight adolescents were asked for their recommendations for school-based programs for overweight youth. Their top ten recommendations are listed in table 12-12. Many of the principles are applicable to individual and group counseling within the clinical setting. The notion of receiving support is clearly very important to overweight

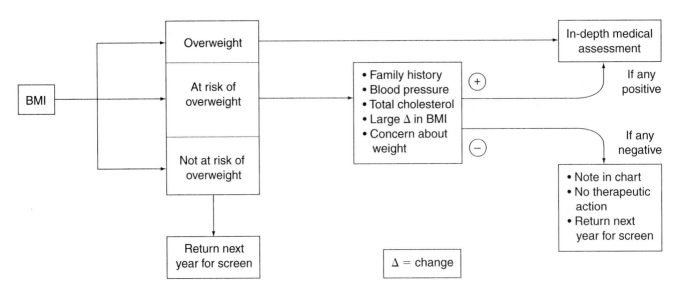

Fig. 12-5   Schematic representation of recommended overweight screening in adolescence.
Am J Clin Nutr American Society for Clinical Nutrition.

***TABLE 12-12   Ten Main Recommendations from Overweight Youth
for School-Based Weight Control Programs***

1. Have a leader who understands the difficulties faced by overweight teens. Try to have a leader or co-leader who is or has been overweight.
2. Provide a supportive, caring, and accepting environment for the participants.
3. Have discussions on nonweight-related issues aimed at helping the participants feel better about themselves. Relate to the participants as teens, not only as *overweight* teens.
4. Make the program fun! Avoid sitting around too much and have lots of physical activity.
5. Offer out-of-classroom and out-of-school activities, such as walking in the park, going to the YMCA as a group, playing softball, going to jazzercise classes, shopping together, and having healthy picnics.
6. Include activities aimed at increasing nutritional knowledge and skills, including food tasting, food preparation, and identification of low-cost foods.
7. Be sensitive to the social stigma associated with being overweight in program recruitment and planning.
8. Try to reduce "technical" barriers to participation by offering the program at a convenient time, at low or no cost, and by providing transportation if necessary.
9. In program evaluation, assess improvements in self-perceptions, eating and exercise skills and behaviors, and perceived social support from the group, in addition to weight loss and maintenance.
10. Involve youth in all stages of planning prior to program implementation and throughout the program.

Neumark-Sztainer D., Story M. Recommendations from overweight youth regarding school-based weight control programs. *Journal of School Health.* Vol. 67, No. 10, p. 428–433. December 1997. Reprinted with permission. American School Health Association, Kent, Ohio.

CASE STUDY

Jake: A Boy Worried About His Weight

Jake is a fourteen-year-old boy who comes to see you in the school clinic with a referral from his doctor for weight loss. He is currently over the 95th percentile weight-for-height, and he says he would like to lose some weight so kids in school won't tease him anymore. In talking with him, you learn that in his free time he likes to play computer games and watch movies with his family. He lives near the school and goes home for lunch every day, which usually consists of a large helping of leftovers from dinner the night before and a couple of glasses of soda. He tells you his mother is trying to lose weight, too, and she is starting to buy "a lot of that low-fat stuff" for his family.

Questions for analysis
1. What ideas do you have for nutritional goals that would help Jake lose weight?
2. What approaches to increasing physical activity might work for Jake?
3. What other issues do you think are important to address?

youth and needs to be addressed. Furthermore, in light of the high degree of weight-related stigmatization to which overweight youth are exposed, it seems important to work with overweight youth in recognizing and dealing with this mistreatment. Interventions should include components for the family and other significant others, in order to provide them with the tools for supporting the overweight adolescent in both weight control and self-acceptance.

Nutritional goals of treatment. The nutritional goals of treatment for obesity are to 1) balance energy intake and expenditure in order to allow for a moderate weight loss or decrease in weight gain in proportion to height gain; 2) avoid the use of unhealthy weight control behaviors; 3) ensure an adequate nutritional intake, with particular attention to such nutrients as calcium; and 4) develop healthy eating patterns that can be continued on a long-term basis. Realistic modifications in weight should be encouraged in order to avoid frustration and ensure an adequate intake to meet the adolescent's nutritional needs. Overweight youth are at risk for unhealthy weight control behaviors; therefore, special attention needs to be directed toward the monitoring and prevention of these behaviors. Unhealthy weight control methods should be discouraged, and some youth will need to learn to accept their larger body size as normal for them. "Dieting" should be avoided, as it tends to be viewed as a temporary behavior, whereas increased emphasis should be placed on the development of life-long healthy eating and physical activity patterns. Recommended changes include having regular meals, increasing consumption of fruits and vegetables, avoiding foods high in fat and sugar, and increasing physical activity. Adolescents need to be involved in the development of an eating plan that suits their lifestyle. It is often helpful for them to record their food intake over a number of days in order to identify areas for change.

THE PREVENTION OF WEIGHT-RELATED DISORDERS ≋

A number of factors point to the need for activities aimed at the prevention of weight-related disorders. These factors include the high prevalence of weight-related disorders, potential severe consequences associated with weight-related disorders, high costs of treatment, and difficulties encountered in bringing about full recovery. A meaningful decrease in the prevalence of weight-related concerns and disorders is not likely to be brought on by better treatment facilities but, rather, by better prevention activities. Over the past decade, increased attention has been directed toward the importance of prevention.[92–97]

Primary and Secondary Prevention

Primary prevention is needed for children and adolescents who do not yet exhibit weight-related concerns or symptoms of disorders. Due to the high prevalence of dieting and body dissatisfaction among youth, it seems logical to aim interventions at the population-at-large. In addition, more intensive activities aimed at the secondary prevention of weight-related disorders are needed for high-risk youth. High-risk youth include those who have an overweight parent, those who express extreme weight concerns, those from difficult family backgrounds, or those who are engaging in unhealthy weight control behaviors. Both primary and secondary prevention are critical in decreasing the prevalence of weight-related concerns and disorders.

Factors to Be Addressed

Factors to be addressed in interventions aimed at the prevention of weight-related disorders include those that play an etiologic role in the development of eating disturbances, that are amenable to change, and that are suitable for addressing within the designated setting. As discussed previously, weight-related disorders are multifactorial, and developmental, cognitive, genetic, psychologic, behavioral, familial, and sociocultural factors contribute to their etiology. More sensitive issues may be addressed within the clinical setting, such as familial and psychologic concerns, while the school setting may be a more suitable place for addressing less sensitive topics, such as sociocultural influences on body image, and for identifying youth who should be referred for further screening and counseling.

Settings for Prevention

Activities aimed at the prevention of weight-related disorders among adolescents need to occur in various settings if they are to be effective. These settings include homes, health care settings, schools, and other community organizations. In addition, broader societal activities are needed to modify social norms, images seen in the media, and advertisements for unhealthy weight control products.

Home. Within the home, parents need to strive to teach their children about healthy eating and physical activity without encouraging excessive weight concerns and dieting behaviors. This is challenging within a society that makes it easy for youth to eat unhealthy food, be sedentary, and be concerned about their body shape. Parents should avoid dieting and negative comments about their own bodies and should try to role-model positive body image attitudes, positive eating behaviors, and physical activity. Whenever possible, family meals should be encouraged, as they offer the opportunity for healthy eating and communication. Parents also need to provide enough structure and encouragement for their children without placing too many restrictions on them or too much pressure to succeed. Finally, parents need to help their children feel good about themselves, regardless of their weight or appearance. Parenting an adolescent presents numerous challenges, and opportunities for learning and support in a non-judgmental atmosphere are essential.

Health care settings. Within health care settings, adolescents should be screened routinely for weight concerns, dieting behaviors, and weight-related disorders. Individual and group sessions for high-risk youth and their families should be provided. Health care providers should work together with schools and other community groups in order to provide a system in which youth can be identified in the early stages of a weight-related disorder, can be referred for help as needed, and can receive follow-up care.

Schools. Schools appear to be suitable settings for prevention efforts, due to their large, captive audience of youth, the natural learning environment, and their opportunities for peer interactions. However, classroom interventions have met with limited success,[98,99] suggesting the importance of a more comprehensive school-based approach.[100] The sug-

TABLE 12-13   *Suggested Components of a Comprehensive School-Based Program*
for Preventing Weight-Related Disorders

Staff training	Examination of their own body image and eating behaviors, knowledge about weight-related disorders, and skills for working with youth and program implementation.
Classroom interventions for the general student body	Modula specifically aimed at preventing weight-related concerns and disorders; options for approaches include 1) feminist approach, 2) weight control and nutrition, and 3) promotion of life skills, such as self-esteem and assertiveness.
Integration of relevant material into existing curricula	Relevant information integrated into existing classes, such as science, art, history, health, and physical education.
Smaller and more intensive activities for high-risk students	Small-group work or individual counseling for overweight students or students with excessive weight preoccupation and unhealthy dieting behaviors.
Referral system within school and between school and community	Training of school staff to be alert to warning signs; referral mechanism to ensure that students don't get overlooked and those in need get help.
Opportunities for healthy eating at school	Options for attractive nutrient-dense and low-fat foods at affordable prices in cafeteria, vending machines, and school events.
Modifications in physical education and sport activities	Increased time being active in physical education classes; involvement of more students in after-school sports; increased sensitivity to needs of overweight youth in physical education classes.
Outreach activities to the community	By students, staff, and parents (e.g., contact with local media).

Adapted from Neumark-Sztainer, D. 1996. School-based programs for preventing eating disturbances. *J. School Health* 66:64–71.

gested components of a comprehensive school-based program are outlined in table 12-13. Suggested approaches toward working with students include a feminist approach, a focus on weight control and nutrition, and a broader focus on overall life skills, such as assertiveness, self-esteem, and communication. For example, a feminist approach might focus on sociocultural norms overemphasizing thinness, increased openness to gender equality, and increased acceptance of a wider range of acceptable body weights. Care needs to be taken to avoid glamorizing eating disorders, increasing curiosity levels about anorexic and bulimic behaviors, and overemphasizing the importance of weight control, in order to avoid an inadvertent increase in weight-related disorders. Staff training should include increasing awareness of their own body image attitudes and eating behaviors, knowledge about the spectrum of weight-related disorders, and skills for working with youth.[100]

Society. If weight-related disorders are to be prevented, changes at the broader, societal level are needed. Substantial resources need to be devoted to meaningful prevention interventions. Broader types of images need to be portrayed in the media. The public needs advocates in letting companies know that certain advertisements, such as those in which extremely thin body shapes or unhealthy foods are promoted, are not acceptable. Huge strides have been made in decreasing the acceptability of racial discrimination and the discrimination of persons with disabilities in the United States; similar efforts are needed to decrease the acceptability of size discrimination and to promote a wider acceptance of different body shapes and sizes.

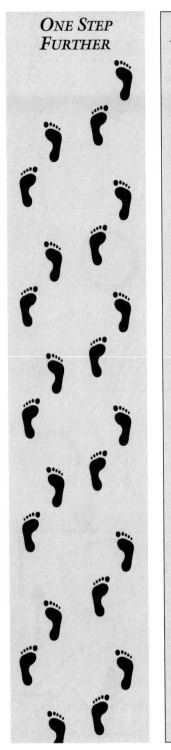

ONE STEP FURTHER

Resources for More Information About Eating Disorders

Books

Eating Disorders and Obesity: A Comprehensive Handbook. Kelly D. Brownell and Christopher G. Fairburn (eds.). New York: Guilford, 1995.

Handbook of Assessment Methods for Eating Behaviors and Weight-Related Problems: Measures, Theory, and Research. David B. Allison. Thousand Oaks, CA: Sage, 1995.

Handbook of Eating Disorders: Theory, Treatment, and Research. George Szmukler, Chris Dare, and Janet Treasure (eds.). New York: John Wiley & Sons, 1995.

Organizations

Academy for Eating Disorders (AED)
c/o Division of Adolescent Medicine
Montefiore Medical School
111 East 210th St.
Bronx, NY 10467
(718) 920-6781

American Anorexia/Bulimia Association
293 Central Park West, Suite IR
New York, NY 10024
(212) 501-8351

Anorexia Nervosa and Related Eating Disorders, Inc.
P.O. Box 5102
Eugene, OR 97405
(541) 344-1144

Eating Disorders Awareness & Prevention, Inc.
603 Steward St., Suite 803
Seattle, WA 98101
(206) 382-3587
Fax (206) 382-4793
http://members.aol.com/edapinc/home.html

Harvard Eating Disorders Center
356 Boylston St.
Boston, MA 02116
(617) 236-7766, Voice-mail ext.: 100
(888) 236-1188, Voice-mail ext.: 100
(617) 236-2068 fax
info@hedc.org
http://www.hedc.org/

International Association of Eating Disorders Professionals (IAEDP)
123 NW 13th St. #206
Boca Raton, FL 32901
(407) 338-6494

National Association of Anorexia Nervosa and Associated Disorders (ANAD)
Box 7
Highland Park, IL 60035
Hotline: (847) 831-3438
Fax: (847) 433-4632
E-mail: anad20@aol.com
http://members.aol.com/anad20/

National Center for Nutrition and Dietetics of the American Dietetic Association (ADA)
216 West Jackson Boulevard
Chicago, IL 60606-6995
(312) 899-0040
Nutrition hot line: (800) 366-1655

National Eating Disorders Organization
6655 South Yale Ave.
Tulsa, OK 74136
http://www.laureate.com/nedointro.html

Overeaters Anonymous (OA) Headquarters
World Services Office
P.O. Box 440-0
Rio Rancho, NM 87174-4020
(505) 891-2664

The National Eating Disorders Information Center
CW-134, 200 Elizabeth St.
Toronto, Ontario, M5G 2C4
Canada
(416) 340-4156

Summary

Weight-related concerns and disorders are prevalent among adolescents and may be associated with severe physical and psychosocial consequences. Weight-related concerns and disorders are best viewed on a spectrum, ranging from anorexia and bulimia nervosa to obesity and including anorexic/bulimic behaviors, unhealthy dieting, and binge eating disorder. All of these disorders have a complex etiology involving interactions among psychologic, biologic, familial, sociocultural, environmental, and behavioral factors. Factors relevant for the adolescent with a weight-related disorder need to be identified and addressed in treatment. The complex nature of weight-related disorders suggests that a multidisciplinary treatment approach is desirable. The nutritional component is key in treatment and should be addressed by a dietitian trained in behavioral strategies, adolescent health, psychology, and eating disorders. The high prevalence of weight-related disorders, their severe consequences, and the high costs and difficulties of treatment point to a need for more interventions aimed at prevention by a range of people in many settings.

Review Questions

1. What are some of the advantages of using a spectrum approach to learning about weight-related concerns and disorders?
2. Why are adolescents at risk for weight-related concerns and disorders?
3. What are some of the signs and symptoms of anorexia nervosa? bulimia nervosa?
4. What are the nutritional goals of treatment for anorexia nervosa? bulimia nervosa? obesity?
5. What factors contribute to the onset of weight-related concerns and disorders among adolescents?
6. How would you assess which of the factors in #5 is relevant to an adolescent prior to treating him or her for a weight-related disorder?
7. How would you address the factors in #5 in prevention interventions?
8. In your opinion, is it possible to simultaneously prevent two or more of the weight-related disorders shown on the spectrum (e.g., anorexia nervosa *and* obesity)? Justify your answer.

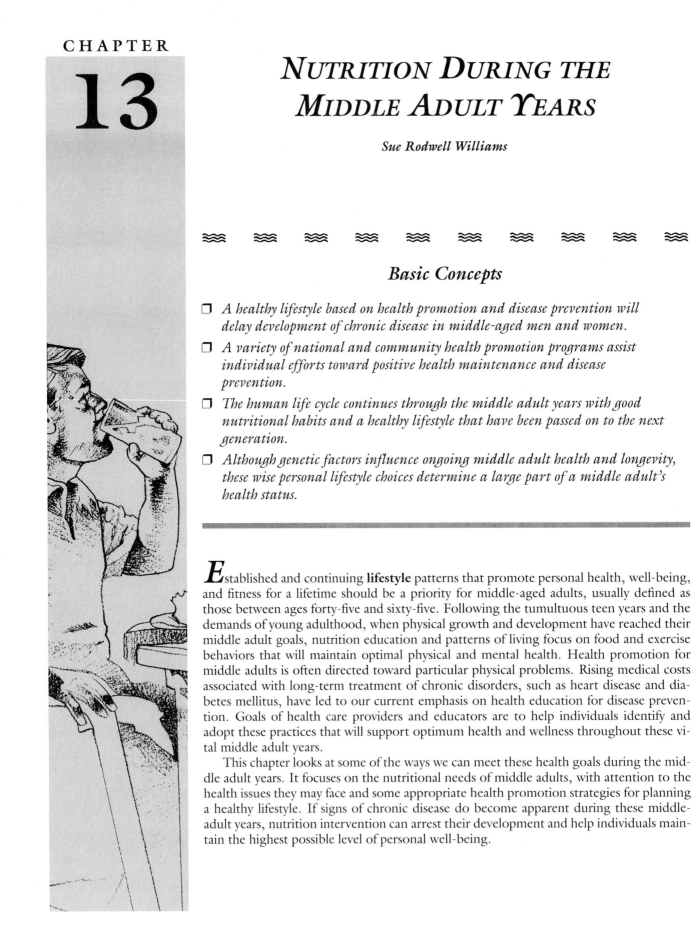

NUTRITION DURING THE MIDDLE ADULT YEARS

Sue Rodwell Williams

≋ ≋ ≋ ≋ ≋ ≋ ≋ ≋ ≋ ≋

Basic Concepts

❏ *A healthy lifestyle based on health promotion and disease prevention will delay development of chronic disease in middle-aged men and women.*

❏ *A variety of national and community health promotion programs assist individual efforts toward positive health maintenance and disease prevention.*

❏ *The human life cycle continues through the middle adult years with good nutritional habits and a healthy lifestyle that have been passed on to the next generation.*

❏ *Although genetic factors influence ongoing middle adult health and longevity, these wise personal lifestyle choices determine a large part of a middle adult's health status.*

*E*stablished and continuing **lifestyle** patterns that promote personal health, well-being, and fitness for a lifetime should be a priority for middle-aged adults, usually defined as those between ages forty-five and sixty-five. Following the tumultuous teen years and the demands of young adulthood, when physical growth and development have reached their middle adult goals, nutrition education and patterns of living focus on food and exercise behaviors that will maintain optimal physical and mental health. Health promotion for middle adults is often directed toward particular physical problems. Rising medical costs associated with long-term treatment of chronic disorders, such as heart disease and diabetes mellitus, have led to our current emphasis on health education for disease prevention. Goals of health care providers and educators are to help individuals identify and adopt these practices that will support optimum health and wellness throughout these vital middle adult years.

This chapter looks at some of the ways we can meet these health goals during the middle adult years. It focuses on the nutritional needs of middle adults, with attention to the health issues they may face and some appropriate health promotion strategies for planning a healthy lifestyle. If signs of chronic disease do become apparent during these middle-adult years, nutrition intervention can arrest their development and help individuals maintain the highest possible level of personal well-being.

MIDDLE ADULT HEALTH, WELLNESS, AND LIFESTYLE ≋

Concept of Wellness

Health and *wellness* are words that cannot be used interchangeably. *Health* is most simply defined as the absence of disease, although the World Health Organization has expanded this definition to include complete physical, mental, and social well-being, not merely the absence of disease or dysfunction. The concept of wellness carries this state of being one step further. It seeks to develop the maximal potential of individuals within their own environments. This implies a balance between activities and goals: work versus leisure, personal needs versus the expectations and goals of others, and lifestyle choices versus health risks. Wellness is a positive dynamic state as a person strives toward a higher level of function.

Wellness represents a continuum from high-level wellness and optimum health to low-level wellness, illness, and death. Various body functions differ in their level of wellness from time to time. As one system or function improves, another may deteriorate. However, an area of strength may compensate for an area of weakness or stress. For example, excellent physical health may help a middle adult cope with the severe emotional stress that occurs with the death of a family member, job loss, dissatisfaction with a job, or disapproval of the peer group.

Lifestyle
Unique pattern of living—which, depending on its form, can be negative or positive in its health results.

Approaches to Health and Well-Being

Every day individuals are bombarded with messages that encourage actions to improve their health. However, people approach personal health decisions in many different ways, and these approaches may differ at different stages in the life cycle. A healthy child may see little need for appropriate health behavior, whereas an overweight middle-aged man with above normal serum lipid levels may be concerned about his risk of heart disease and may consider changing his lifestyle to modify predisposing factors. In general, people use one of three approaches to health care: traditional, preventive, or wellness.

Traditional approach. The **traditional approach** to health leads to change only when the symptoms of illness or disease already exist, and the individual seeks out a physician to diagnose and cure the condition. This is the pattern usually followed for acute illnesses that develop suddenly and are cured with specific drugs or treatment. Because major chronic problems, such as heart disease or cancer, develop over a period of years, long before overt signs become apparent, this approach is of little value for lifelong positive health.

Traditional approach
Approach to health that provides directions for dealing with a diagnosed problem.

Preventive approach. The **preventive approach** to health, especially at middle adulthood, focuses on identifying risk factors that increase a person's chances of developing a particular health problem and on making behavior choices that will prevent or minimize such risks. Preventive measures include screening programs to detect the development of a problem while it is still asymptomatic, thus allowing early intervention.

Preventive approach
Approach to health that seeks to identify and reduce risk factors for disease.

Wellness approach. The **wellness approach** emphasizes positive lifestyle choices that enhance physical and mental well-being. On this basis, people may choose to consume more vegetables and whole-grain cereals and fewer foods high in fat, salt, or sugar. The wellness approach begun early in life, and especially continued into middle adulthood, allows the development of full personal potential while retarding the onset of degenerative changes and chronic disease.

Wellness approach
Approach to health that promotes positive planning of a healthy lifestyle for physical and mental well-being.

Determinants of Health Status

Good or poor health is usually determined by five factors: heredity, environment, health outlook, health care, and lifestyle. The first of these factors, heredity, is beyond the individual's control, but the remaining four factors can, at least to some extent, be modified by the middle adult who wishes to achieve better health.

Environment. Our environment has two dimensions: the physical environment and the social environment. The *physical environment* encompasses both the near environment and the extended surrounding area. Middle adults and their families living in poor housing with ineffective plumbing and no refrigerator are highly susceptible to infection and disease. Poor air and water quality or contaminated food also influences health status. The *social environment* can be friendly or hostile. A middle adult may have family or friends for emotional support or be essentially alone. The environment may be fast-paced, with high expectations for performance, or may have low expectations and few demands.

Health outlook. The health outlook of middle adults relates to personal perceptions of one's own health and well-being, although perception and reality may not necessarily agree. Generally, people who think of their health as excellent or good have a longer life expectancy than those who always consider their health as fair or poor. Often, self-rating of health is a stronger predictor of life expectancy than actual physical status based on a medical examination. Positive personal feelings about one's health usually reflect a similar attitude toward life in general that supports positive adjustment and adaptation.

Health care. Middle-aged adults may or may not have personal control of needed health care. People in lower socioeconomic groups do not always have access to the same level or quality of medical care as those in higher-income groups. Poor reading skills, limited education, or a language barrier may hinder an individual who is attempting to carry out instructions from a health professional about a change in health habits or steps in the treatment of disease. Health care also includes wise self-care, such as seeking medical care when symptoms so indicate, following directions when using medications (including over-the-counter drugs), and exercising regularly.

Lifestyle. The term *lifestyle* refers to a person's unique pattern of living. These patterns reflect our values and beliefs. They involve what, how much, and when an individual chooses to eat, whether or not an individual exercises regularly, and whether an individual uses addictive drugs. Use of time is a lifestyle choice. One middle adult, for example, may spend leisure time watching television and consuming large amounts of alcohol and snack foods high in sodium and fat. Another person of similar age may spend leisure time practicing tennis or may choose to walk rather than drive to a nearby store. A middle adult may relieve stress in harmful ways by overeating, smoking, or abusing alcohol. For another, appropriate outlets involving exercise, counseling, or relaxation techniques may be the choice.

Actually, health and wellness throughout adulthood are to a great extent the result of lifestyle choices. In general, when we consider what determines health status, we find that much of this influence is under our personal control. Diet, exercise, smoking habits, use of addictive substances, and stress management all contribute to this total. For middle adults exhibiting early signs of chronic disease, or for those at risk because of genetic background, adoption of positive health behaviors can slow or interrupt the degenerative disease process.

Health Promotion

Definitions. The current increased focus of public attention on health promotion began with the benchmark 1979 publication of *Healthy People: The Surgeon General's Report on Health Promotion and Disease Prevention*.[1] This report was of special interest in middle adult health care. The goal was to help adults maintain and enhance their well-being by making use of preventive health services and lifestyle modification strategies. While lifestyle changes are a major component of health promotion, health strategies also include educational, economic, and environmental adjustments that support behavior conducive to good health. For example, a middle adult with poor reading skills attempting to select a diet lower in saturated fat and cholesterol may need help understanding food labels or could benefit from meal planning materials that emphasize pictures. Health promotion requires a combination of intervention strategies to bring about behavioral change.

Models for behavioral change. Health and nutrition educators are learning more about the social and psychologic factors that influence behavioral change. For example, by understanding how middle adults choose to alter their behavior, programs can be developed to encourage positive change. Three models of behavior change illustrate this process: the health belief model, the locus of control model, and the concept of self-efficacy.

Health belief model. The health belief model was developed to explain how a person who does not have a disease chooses to change behavior and alter risk factors to prevent future development of this disease.[2] This model suggests that the decision for action is based on three factors: 1) the individual's perception of vulnerability to the disease, 2) the seriousness of the disease, and 3) the degree of difficulty in implementing the lifestyle changes required. For example, a middle adult woman of forty-five whose mother is now confined to a wheelchair as a result of osteoporosis and bone fractures (see p. 347–49) may begin to exercise regularly and select calcium-rich foods.

Locus of control model. People perceive the world and their ability to control events occurring around them in different ways. Some individuals perceive the day-to-day events in their lives as being under their (internal) control. They assume responsibility for their life choices and the physiologic and psychologic components of their well-being. For example, middle adults with an internal **locus of control** tend to be more successful in weight management, as they assume responsibility for the body weight.[3,4] Other individuals, with an external locus of control, consider their health status to be the result of outside forces beyond their control and, thus, take less responsibility for their lifestyle behaviors. Such middle adults may view their elevated blood pressure as caused by a genetic sensitivity to sodium and decide that reducing sodium intake will not be effective in reducing their risk. Some persons consider all life happenings to be a matter of chance, with no particular basis of control. It may be difficult to motivate these individuals to alter lifestyle behavior to improve well-being.

Locus of control
(L *locus*, place, site) Perceived control center over one's life.

Concept of self-efficacy. The concept of self-efficacy, especially in the middle adult years, relates to an individual's belief that he or she will be able to make and maintain the health-related changes desired. This feeling of empowerment is based on the facts or skills provided to the individual that support behavioral change. Nutritionists, registered dietitians, and other health team members who become involved in health promotion must learn to recognize clients' beliefs and attitudes relating to behavioral change and must develop programs and skills to meet their needs.

Health Care Reform

The primary goal of health and nutrition education is the optimum health status of individuals in all population groups. This public health approach, designed to assure each member of society appropriate access to health assessment and intervention, is receiving increased attention within the framework of proposals for ongoing health care reform. A major concern is the fact that many Americans have very limited access to health care. Although most people receive health insurance coverage as a fringe benefit through their employer, many people who work for small companies or are self-employed do not have health insurance. Nearly 37 million people in the United States have no health insurance, and about one-fourth of these are children.[5] As a result, health care services are less available to them. Because they must pay directly for all services, they often postpone seeking care, with the result that their condition worsens. Uninsured persons also have less access to preventive health services, such as nutrition counseling to facilitate weight loss and a possible reduction in elevated blood pressure levels.

A second concern with the current health care delivery system is its emphasis on treating existing medical problems, with limited attention to health promotion strategies. As a result, Americans are not nearly as healthy as they could be. At the same time, over the past decade, health care costs have been increasing rapidly, by more than 10% per year, considerably faster than personal income.[5] The high cost of technologic improvements in medical care, such as open heart surgery and kidney transplantation, has partly contributed to these rising costs. Programs that address prevention of diseases, including breast cancer, heart disease, and stroke, will not only decrease long-term health care costs but also contribute to an increased level of wellness and quality of life. A nutritious and prudent diet, combined with regular physical activity, is the cornerstone for public health intervention.

COMPONENTS OF A PRUDENT, HEALTHY LIFESTYLE ≋

Recommendations to Americans relating dietary fat to heart disease began to appear in the late 1950s and remain essentially the same today after forty years of continuing study.[6] Coronary heart disease has a multiple risk factor profile, including premature coronary disease in middle adults under sixty years of age.[7] Two research conclusions have now been

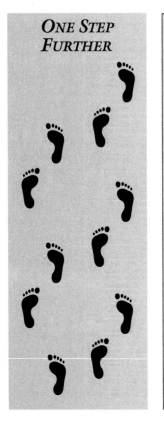

ONE STEP FURTHER

Recommendations for Healthy Eating

- Reduce total fat to 30% or less of total kilocalories, saturated fat to less than 10% of total kilocalories, and cholesterol to less than 300 mg per day; polyunsaturated fatty acids should not exceed 10% of total kilocalories.
- Each day eat five or more servings of fruits and vegetables, especially dark green and deep yellow vegetables and citrus fruits; eat six or more servings from breads, cereals, or legumes.
- Maintain protein intake at a moderate level, not more than two times the RDA.
- Balance energy intake and physical activity to maintain appropriate weight; avoid diets that are either excessive or severely restricted in kilocalories.
- Limit alcohol consumption to less than 1 oz per day (the equivalent of two 12 oz cans of beer, two 3.5 oz glasses of wine, or two average cocktails).
- Limit daily intake of salt (sodium chloride) to 6 g or less, including salt added in cooking or at the table and that found in highly processed foods or pickled items.
- Maintain adequate calcium intake with servings of low-fat and nonfat dairy products and dark green vegetables; use of calcium supplements by healthy people to raise intake above the RDA is not justified.
- Avoid taking dietary supplements that contain any nutrient in amounts above the RDA.
- Maintain an optimal intake of fluoride, particularly during the years of tooth formation and growth.

Modified from Committee on Diet and Health, Food and Nutrition Board. 1989. *Diet and health: Implications for reducing chronic disease risk.* Washington, DC: National Academy Press.

established: 1) risk factors include high blood cholesterol, diabetes, overweight, and cigarette smoking and 2) the overall risk for cardiovascular disease and all-cause mortality increases substantially with each additional risk factor.[8]

Health promotion activities for middle adults should focus on the lifestyle behaviors known to influence long-term health. These behaviors include dietary patterns, exercise patterns, ability to manage stress, and addictive behaviors related to smoking and alcohol use.[9]

Dietary Recommendations

Absolute proof of a relationship is especially difficult to establish when evaluating a multifaceted issue such as diet and associated health risks. When developing dietary recommendations, policy makers must always balance the potential benefits of the recommended dietary pattern against the possible adverse effects. Another consideration when developing dietary recommendations is the practicality of the diet for implementation by the public. For example, the production of leaner animal products may be as important as public education in lowering dietary fat levels.

In 1989, an expert panel was commissioned by the Food and Nutrition Board of the National Research Council to develop dietary recommendations that would assist people in reducing their risk of chronic disease.[10] These early recommendations, designed for use by nutritionists, government policy makers, and the public, remain essentially the same today. They are outlined in the box on p. 322.

These recommended nutrient and energy guides are based on their relation to established chronic disease risks.

Fats. Diets high in saturated fat and cholesterol are associated with increased incidence of atherosclerosis and coronary heart disease. Also, high-fat diets contribute to the development of obesity and increase cancer risk. One issue related to reducing dietary fat centers on the fact that red meat, an important source of bioavailable iron and zinc, and dairy foods, important sources of calcium and riboflavin, can be high in total fat, saturated fat, and cholesterol.

Fats and cholesterol can be limited by using moderate amounts of lean meat, poultry without skin, fish, and low-fat or nonfat dairy products without sacrificing intakes of other important nutrients. Total fat and saturated fat can be reduced further by using polyunsaturated vegetable oils and margarines, as well as fewer fried foods. Research findings suggest that regular consumption of coldwater fish such as herring and mackerel, high in omega-3 polyunsaturated fatty acids, may be beneficial to health; however, ingesting fish oil capsules is not recommended.[11] It also appears that monounsaturated fats, such as oleic acid, present in nuts, canola oil, and olive oil have a favorable effect on serum lipoprotein patterns and might be a prudent substitute in part for polyunsaturated fatty acids. Trans-fatty acids produced in the processing of polyunsaturated fats, although present at very low levels, are believed to increase atherosclerotic damage to the arterial wall.

Complex carbohydrates. The energy value (kilocalories) lost from the diet when fat is reduced can be replaced by eating more vegetables, fruits, grains, and legumes. Plant foods rich in complex carbohydrates and fiber reduce chronic disease risk in several ways. First, a diet high in plant foods is likely to be low or moderate in fat. Also, the soluble fiber found in plant foods independently lowers blood lipid levels and thereby lowers cardiovascular disease risk. Fruits and vegetables are good sources of potassium, which seems to play a role in moderating blood pressure levels in some people and thereby may reduce the risk of stroke. **Carotenoids** present in dark green and deep yellow fruits and vegetables offer some protection against some forms of cancer. Dark green, leafy vegetables and citrus fruits, particularly oranges, are rich in folacin, a vitamin of special importance to young women planning a pregnancy. Finally, the insoluble fiber component of plant foods assists in maintaining proper function of the large bowel and lower gastrointestinal tract and decreases risk of colon cancer.

Protein. Protein intakes among most age groups in the United States are usually well in excess of the recommended amounts.[12] Protein intakes greater than two times the Recommended Dietary Allowance (RDA) are associated with increased incidence of certain cancers and coronary heart disease, mainly as a result of the high levels of saturated fat and cholesterol usually associated with diets high in animal protein. High protein intakes could lead to increased urinary loss of calcium and increased risk of osteoporosis. It has been suggested that long-term consumption of excessive levels of dietary protein might contribute to degenerative changes in renal function; however, this effect has not been demonstrated in human subjects.

Energy. Continuing trends among middle adults include decreased energy intakes, decreased physical activity, and increased body fat as defined by body mass index (BMI).[13] Physical activity even at moderate levels allows an energy intake sufficient to obtain recommended levels of important vitamins and minerals, to assist in maintaining reasonable weight for height, and to improve fitness. Excess body weight increases risk of premature coronary heart disease, hypertension, noninsulin-dependent diabetes mellitus (NIDDM), and gallbladder disease. Weight loss decreases that risk, even if desirable weight is not attained. A loss of even 10 lb of body weight can lower blood pressure and serum lipid levels and can improve glucose tolerance.[11] Excessive alcohol consumption, which adds kilocalories that provide few other nutrients, not only undermines energy balance but also increases risk of heart disease, liver disease, high blood pressure, some forms of cancer, and nutrient deficiencies.

A diet low to moderate in fat supports energy balance. A daily menu in which fat provides no more than 30% of total energy contains reduced kilocalories, as compared with a similar menu comprised of high fat foods. In one program, women who substituted reduced-fat foods for the food items they normally consumed lost 2.4 kg over a twelve-week period, although reduced energy intake was not a goal of the program.[14] Moreover, in contrast to carbohydrate, dietary fat requires less metabolic energy for conversion to storage in adipose tissue. Thus, energy balance may be related to the proportion of energy consumed from fat independent of the total energy content of the diet.

Minerals. Intakes of salt (sodium chloride) above 6 g per day (2,400 mg/day) are associated with elevated blood pressure in genetically sensitive individuals.[10] However, it is not possible at this time to identify those individuals. The recommended level of intake

Carotenoids
Any of a group of red and yellow pigments chemically similar to and including the carotene found in dark green and yellow vegetables and fruits.

(2,400 mg sodium or less) is likely to prevent the development of high blood pressure in sensitive individuals and is not deficient for the general population. Foods that are pickled or prepared in brine should be used sparingly.

Calcium is receiving increased attention, based on the reports associating low calcium intake in middle adults with elevated blood pressure and increased risk of bone fracture. At the same time, there is no strong evidence that calcium intakes above the recommended amount carry any benefit.

A recent study in Finland found increased risk of myocardial infarction among men with high-normal body iron stores.[15] This study has not been duplicated by other researchers but does suggest that frequent consumption of food products highly fortified with iron may not be prudent for middle-aged men.

Supplements. Protein, vitamin, and mineral supplements in excess of the RDA have not been shown to be beneficial, and excessive intakes of vitamins B_6, A, and D and iron have been shown to be harmful, leading to toxicity or inappropriate interactions with other nutrients.[10] Amino acid supplements proposed to enhance development of lean body mass and fitness can be dangerous to health if amino acid imbalances are created. The long-term health risks and benefits related to supplementation have yet to be identified.

Exercise and Physical Fitness

Positive effects of exercise. Regular physical exercise during the middle adult years, when maturing middle adults tend to become less active, contributes to health and fitness in many ways. Some of these benefits include improved energy balance, body composition, cardiac efficiency, and serum lipid levels.

Energy balance. One of the most obvious health benefits of exercise for the middle adult is its role in energy balance and weight management. Increasing energy expenditure with exercise allows a higher energy intake in food, increasing the likelihood of obtaining adequate amounts of all important nutrients without inappropriate weight gain. An indirect effect of exercise is increased glucose uptake and utilization by muscle cells in the trained versus the untrained individual. Increased uptake of glucose by muscle can help prevent the development of NIDDM or can lower serum glucose levels in middle adults who have this disease.

Body composition. Physical exercise strengthens middle adult muscle fibers and helps prevent age-related loss of lean body mass and increase in body fat. Exercise strengthens bone by stimulating bone formation and preventing bone loss. Regular physical stress on the bone through exercise that increases the gravity pull of body weight on bone, as occurs in walking, jogging, dancing, and bicycling, can prevent or retard the onset of osteoporosis, a common bone disorder among middle-aged and older men and women.

Cardiovascular efficiency. Regular exercise increases the middle-aged person's ability to do physical work with increased cardiovascular efficiency and decreased recovery time. Maximal oxygen consumption increases, while heart rate and blood pressure levels decrease both during exercise and at rest. Improved condition of the heart as a pump and reduced fat deposition in the arterial wall contribute to the maintenance of appropriate blood pressure levels in those exercising regularly. Blood pressure levels increase with age among those with sedentary lifestyles.[16]

Serum lipid levels. Physical activity retards middle-age degenerative changes through its effect on serum lipid levels. Daily exercise increases serum levels of high-density lipoproteins (HDLs), which help protect against coronary-artery disease by removing cholesterol molecules from the blood before they can enter the arterial wall. At the same time, physical activity assists a low-saturated-fat, low-cholesterol diet to significantly lower low-density lipoproteins (LDLs), which carry cholesterol to the cells and increase cardiovascular risk.

Exercise and disease risk. Physically fit middle adults have a lower risk of premature death from all causes, as compared with their less-fit peers. In a study of more than 10,000 male Harvard College alumni aged forty-five to eighty-four, mortality rates from coronary heart disease and all other causes were 23% lower in those who had begun a moderately vigorous sports program.[17] Those benefited most who expended about 2,000 kcal per week in exercise; however, walking at least nine miles per week or climbing at least twenty flights of stairs per week also reduced risk. This suggests that such simple changes in lifestyle as taking the stairs rather than the elevator or parking the car at a greater distance from a store entrance can improve the level of fitness and general health. A brisk walk of thirty minutes per day, an exercise level within the physical ability of most middle adults, can result in a moderate level of fitness.

The duration and resulting energy expenditure of exercise may be more important than the intensity. Regular exercise reduces the incidence of coronary heart disease and death, even among those with elevated serum cholesterol and blood pressure levels and increased BMI. In fact, in a Norwegian study of mortality risk of coronary death among healthy middle-aged men, the risk was about half in men with a high level of fitness, despite the presence of other risk factors, as compared with those less fit.[18] Regular exercise may be most critical for individuals who already suffer from several negative risk factors.

Development of an exercise program. A sedentary individual, regardless of age, should undergo a physical examination before embarking on a strenuous exercise program. This is especially important for middle adults, an age period when heart disease frequently begins to occur. Both men and women should pay attention to body signals, as recent research indicates that middle adult women with ischemia are at the same increased risk for cardiovascular disease as men with ischemia.[19] Ischemia is a deficiency of blood in a part of the body due to constriction or obstruction of a blood vessel, especially deficiency of blood supply to the heart muscle. The appearance of pain suggests that it is time to slow down or stop. To prevent muscular or skeletal injury, or a cardiovascular incident, the progression in both duration and intensity of exercise must be gradual. Cardiovascular exercise requires an increase in heart rate to 70% of maximum (pulse: 220 minus age), continued for at least twenty minutes. However, this level may need to be achieved over a period of time. For a person with cardiovascular problems, heart rate must be monitored carefully.

An individual may be motivated to initiate an exercise program to improve or maintain health, but long-term adherence is more likely if the person enjoys the activity and has family support. Activities of great intensity that are perceived to require great exertion or carry risk of injury are less likely to be begun or continued. Walking is an ideal activity, contributing to energy expenditure and cardiorespiratory fitness, while providing a transition to more vigorous exercise if desired. Characteristics of exercise programs that promote continuing participation include:

- No need for specialized facilities or equipment.
- Limited discomfort.
- Potential for incorporation in the daily routine.
- Opportunity for social interaction.

Health professionals need to give particular attention to the transitions in lifestyle often associated with a decline in physical activity. These include the transition from high school or college to a work situation, a change in residence, or recovery from an illness or injury. Suggestions for exercise activities are given in table 13-1.

Stress Management

Stress is a physiologic or psychologic reaction to a life event. The event may be starting a new job, moving to a different city, getting married, or experiencing the death of a family member. The stress response is the same, whether initiated by a positive or negative event. Stress can result in adverse physiologic symptoms, including 1) gastrointestinal distress—for example, nausea, vomiting, or diarrhea; 2) irregular sleep patterns; 3) increased muscle tension, with resulting headache or backache; and 4) cardiovascular responses, resulting in constriction of blood vessels and rapid pulse.

Everyone experiences one or more of the symptoms of stress occasionally, but the danger lies in the long-term consequences of continuing, unalleviated stress. Continued gastric upset and inappropriate secretion of stomach acid can lead to peptic ulcers and associated stomach problems. Heart disease is accelerated by high blood pressure that occurs over time as a stress response. Psychologic distress can have a detrimental effect on food intake. This can result in patterns of overeating or binge eating, leading to inappropriate weight gain or, at the other extreme, anorexia or bulimia nervosa, now increasing among young adults.

Stress
Sum of biologic reactions to adverse stimuli—physical, mental, emotional, and internal or external—that disturb the state of homeostasis and sense of well-being.

TABLE 13-1　*Energy Cost of Various Physical Activities**

Activity	kcal/kg/hr
Aerobic dancing	8.9
Bicycling (moderate speed)	2.5
Bicycling (racing)	7.6
Golf	3.9
Rowing in race	16.0
Running	7.0
Skating	3.5
Skiing (cross-country)	5.9
Swimming (2 mph)	7.9
Tennis	5.3
Walking (3 mph)	2.0
Walking (4 mph)	3.4

*Does not include basal metabolism

Because poorly managed stress is a threat to both physical and mental health and occupational safety and productivity, cognitive and behavioral approaches have been developed for stress reduction. Group and individual counseling help people improve their understanding and attitudes, develop constructive coping mechanisms, and learn positive approaches to problem solving. Behavioral approaches include reduction in use of alcohol, caffeine, or nicotine, along with increased exercise, rest, and relaxation.

ADDICTIVE BEHAVIORS HARMING HEALTH ≈

Addiction

(L *addictio,* a giving over, surrender) State of being enslaved to an undesirable practice that is physically or psychologically habit-forming to the extent that its cessation causes severe trauma.

Some personal habits can become **addictions** and harm health. Each year, two of these addictive behaviors, cigarette smoking and alcohol abuse, continue to disrupt lives and families, harm health, and cause death.

A third form of addictive behavior, eating disorders, poses difficult problems, often rooted in the adolescent years (see chapter 11 and centered on misuse of food.)

Cigarette Smoking

Incidence. Cigarette smoking is considered the greatest single preventable cause of illness and premature death in the United States.[20] A current U.S. Department of Health and Human Services report examining underlying causes of death indicates that, although heart disease and cancer are listed as the nation's leading killers, tobacco use is the largest underlying culprit, followed by poor diet.[21] A major concern of health professionals is the prevalence of cigarette smoking among teenagers and young adults. By the age of sixteen, 21% of teenagers have begun to smoke. Most adult smokers had started to smoke by age twenty.[22]

Cigarette use differs according to ethnic and socioeconomic group. More black men than white men smoke, and more black women than white women smoke, probably contributing to the higher incidence of heart disease, hypertension, and stroke in the black population.[23] Middle adults who did not complete high school are more likely to smoke than are their better educated peers.[22]

Health problems. Cigarette smoking is a major risk factor for many chronic conditions, accounting for 87% of lung cancer deaths, 21% of coronary heart disease deaths, and 18% of stroke deaths.[20] Cigarette use accelerates the development of atherosclerotic lesions, leading to the estimate that more than 40% of deaths from coronary heart disease occurring among men and women less than sixty-five years of age are attributable to smoking.[20] Smoking exacerbates the risk associated with alcohol use, high blood pressure, and diabetes mellitus.

Mortality risk for both sexes increases with the number of cigarettes smoked and is higher for those who began smoking at a younger age. By middle age, a person smoking two packs of cigarettes a day has a life expectancy eight to nine years shorter than a non-smoker of similar age.[20] Until recently, prevalence of lung cancer was lower among women, as relatively fewer women were smoking. Lung cancer has now passed breast cancer as the leading cause of death in women.[23]

Smokers who quit smoking experience both immediate and long-term benefits. Risk of coronary artery disease is reduced within the first few years. Risk of lung cancer drops substantially in five to nine years but still remains two times that of the lifelong smoker after twenty years of smoking cessation.[20] Although further deterioration of the lungs is arrested, smokers with obstructed air passages cannot anticipate major improvement, despite cessation of smoking.

Treatment programs. A positive result of smoking cessation programs has been the overall decline in adult smokers over the past twenty-five years from 40% to 27% of the population.[20] In fact, nearly half of all living adults who ever smoked have quit. Smoking cessation programs have focused on behavior modification techniques and coping strategies to assist with the physiologic, psychologic, and social factors related to nicotine addiction. Fear of unwanted weight gain may deter some people from joining a smoking cessation program. Contrary to common belief, average weight gain was found to be only 2.8 kg (6 lb) in men and 3.8 kg (8 lb) in women.[24] Major weight gain of 13 kg (28 lb) or more occurred in only 10% of the men and 13% of the women. Black persons, those under the age of fifty-five, and those who smoked at least fifteen cigarettes a day were more likely to gain weight. Attention to weight control is usually included in such health education programs.

Alcohol Abuse

Incidence. In the United States, alcohol consumption peaks in young adulthood and continues at a relatively high level among middle-aged adults. About 80% of the men in this age group are currently drinkers and 13% are heavy drinkers, consuming fourteen or more drinks per week, assuming 0.5 oz of ethanol per drink.[23] About 50–60% of middle adult women drink, but only 3% drink heavily. Fewer black and Hispanic men and women are currently drinkers, as compared with white men and women. Among Native Americans, the rate of alcohol abuse remains high. The U.S. Indian Health Service (IHS) has identified alcoholism as the most significant health problem of American Indians and Alaska Natives.[21]

Health problems. Inappropriate use of alcohol has a negative effect on nutritional status and enhances risk of chronic disease. Alcohol has a toxic effect on the gastrointestinal tract and reduces the absorption of many nutrients, including vitamins B_6 and B_{12}, folate, and zinc. Alcohol further contributes to malnutrition by adding kilocalories (7 kcal/g) to the diet that provide no protein or essential vitamins or minerals. This problem of nutrient density is evident in the diets of some middle adults for whom alcohol kilocalories replace about one-third of the nonalcohol food kilocalories. Although this practice is intended to avoid weight gain, it further decreases intakes of iron and calcium, nutrients already low in their diets.

Continuing alcohol abuse contributes to deteriorating health through its association with elevated serum LDL-cholesterol and triglyceride levels, hypertension, and liver disease. Although it was believed that liver damage resulted from a lack of food and nutrients rather than from the direct toxic effect of alcohol itself, studies have found the development of liver abnormalities in well-nourished alcohol abusers. Regular use of alcohol increases risk of stroke and cancer of the oral cavity and esophagus. Depletion of liver stores of vitamin A is a consequence of alcohol abuse and may contribute to the relationship observed between alcohol consumption and cancer of the liver, breast, and pancreas.

The paradox of alcohol consumption lies in its effect on serum levels of HDL-cholesterol, the so-called good cholesterol. Increased levels of HDL-cholesterol are associated with low to moderate drinking, often defined as no more than two drinks per day. This is likely the basis for the epidemiologic findings that coronary artery disease risk is lower in persons consuming these low to moderate levels of alcohol. At the same time, the potentially devastating effects of excessive alcohol intake on health and overall mortality preclude any recommendation that individuals increase their alcohol intake or start to drink if they do not already.

Screening tests. The cost of alcoholism is high, in both lives lost and the financial burden of care. The United States' combined lifetime prevalence of addiction and dependence ranges from 11% to 16%, with hospitalized medical patients showing even greater numbers of 15% to 60%, depending on the population studied. For example, in one year alone—1990—more than 65,000 Americans lost their lives because of alcohol abuse, 22,000 of them on the highways.[25, 26] The National Center for Health Statistics indicates that the financial burden of alcohol abuse continues at a high level, reaching about $150 billion in 1995 (up from $128 billion in 1986)—more than the total cost of cardiovascular disease.[26] Thus, screening tests to identify early signs of alcohol abuse before it becomes lethal are crucial medical tools. Two basic types of tests are used, questionnaires and biochemical tests.

Questionnaires. An example of a commonly used screening tool is the *CAGE* questionnaire included as part of a history-taking interview. It can be used to help detect a suspected alcoholic, whether he or she is in denial or not.[26,27] Its name is an **acronym** that indicates its focus: *c*utting down, *a*nnoyance by criticism, *g*uilt feelings, and *e*ye-openers. It is short, easy to use, and relatively nonintimidating. Nonalcoholics are eliminated from alcohol abusers, who answer three of the four questions in the affirmative:

- *C* Have you ever felt you should *c*ut down on your drinking?
- *A* Have people *a*nnoyed you by criticizing your drinking?
- *G* Have you ever felt bad or *g*uilty about drinking?
- *E* Have you ever taken a drink first thing in the morning to get rid of a hangover or to steady your nerves (*e*ye-opener)?

Biochemical tests. Because alcohol abuse affects many body systems and metabolites, a single marker does not provide an effective screening tool. Screening test strategies involve combinations of tests, which can be arranged in parallel, in series, or both, according to the kind of computer analysis needed. A combination of tests is interchangeably called a *battery, panel,* or *profile* of tests, such as the classic clinical test battery in the standard automated *sequential multiple analyzer* (SMA-6, SMA-12).[26,27]

The SMA-6 is essentially a panel of renal tests; the SMA-12 can include renal tests, electrolyte tests, and commonly used clinical chemistry tests. For example, a battery of tests used to screen for alcohol abuse may include tests for standard hematologic values, liver enzymes, and serum lipid concentrations.[26]

Treatment programs. Alcohol addiction programs have two phases—initial detoxification treatment and maintenance of behavior change.[28] At times, physicians may prescribe disulfiram (Antabuse) to help alcoholics abstain from drinking. This drug does not cure alcoholism; it interferes with the normal metabolic breakdown in the liver of **acetaldehyde,** the highly toxic initial substance ordinarily produced from alcohol metabolism. Powerful reactions to the buildup of unmetabolized acetaldehyde toxicity occur when the person drinks even small amounts of alcohol. These serious and highly unpleasant toxic reactions can include throbbing headache, flushing, breathlessness, nausea, thirst, palpitations, dizziness, and fainting. Fear of such events may deter the alcohol abuser from drinking even small amounts of alcohol, but it does not solve the underlying problem of addiction.

By its nature, a chemical dependency such as alcoholism has biologic, psychologic, and social components that require a health care team approach to meet comprehensive needs and to solve problems.[29]

- *Biologic component.* Chronic alcohol (drug) poisoning causes brain and liver dysfunction.
- *Psychologic component.* Progressive brain dysfunction creates personality disorganization—the "addictive personality."
- *Social component.* Secondary relationship problems interfere with functioning and support systems at home, on the job, and with friends.

Experienced leaders in the field of addictive behavior indicate that, in terms of maintaining the behavioral change, all paths lead to the difficult job of relapse prevention.[28] This self-control task requires training in stress-coping skills and lifestyle changes. Such training helps addicted persons deal with guilt and self-blame by recognizing that their addictive behavior has certain negative consequences and that these behaviors can be

Acronym

(Gr *acros,* topmost, foremost; *-onym,* word, name) Word or name formed from the initial letters or groups of letters of words in a set series.

Acetaldehyde

Chemical compound, intermediate metabolic product in the breakdown of alcohol by liver enzymes.

changed.[28] In the team approach to the health care of people with alcohol abuse problems, an experienced registered dietitian with special training in rehabilitative care is needed to provide comprehensive nutrition care,[25,29,30] including:

- Initial and ongoing nutritional assessment.
- Nutritional management of meals and supplements that help addicted individuals develop normal eating patterns.
- Nutrition education and counseling that help addicted individuals develop an eating plan to support stable recovery.

HEALTH PROMOTION AND CHRONIC DISEASE ≋

Within this century, nutrition research has shifted from the identification of nutrients and deficiency symptoms to the study of the effect of diet and lifestyle on the diseases of civilization, such as heart disease and cancer. An abundant food supply along with a decrease in physical activity made possible by modern technology have contributed to the widespread prevalence of chronic diseases, especially during the middle adult years. Chronic diseases, in contrast to acute conditions, are lifelong and can only be managed, not cured. The long-term health care costs associated with these diseases have led policy makers and health professionals to identify risk factors associated with these conditions and to develop public education approaches that support risk reduction.

Atherosclerotic Heart Disease

Prevalence and impact. The major cause of death in the United States and other Western societies is disease of the heart and blood vessels, accounting for nearly half of all deaths. Nearly 18% of these deaths occur in middle adult persons under sixty-five years of age.[22] Risk is low in early adulthood but increases rapidly with age. Although mortality rates from cardiovascular disease have declined by one-fourth over the past two decades as a result of better medical care following a heart attack, therapeutic intervention such as development of drugs to lower serum lipids and blood pressure, and changes in diet and exercise patterns, improvement has not been equal across ethnic groups. Black men are twice as likely to die of a stroke and black women have higher death rates from heart disease, as compared with the general population.[13]

Development of atherosclerosis. Atherosclerosis, a pathologic series of events occurring in the coronary arteries supplying blood to the heart muscle and the cerebral arteries supplying blood to the brain, actually begins in childhood. Lipid deposits appearing as fatty streaks in children may regress or progress to form fibrous plaques of accumulated fat and debris. Ulceration or hemorrhage into the plaque, causing swelling, can occlude the lumen of the artery, resulting in tissue breakdown as blood supply is interrupted. Arterial injury in the coronary arteries results in coronary heart disease. This most commonly occurs in middle age and carries equal risk of myocardial infarction, or heart attack, for both men and women.[19] Occlusion or hemorrhage in a cerebral artery usually occurs ten to twenty years later, resulting in a stroke, with possible paralysis or loss of speech, vision, hearing, or memory. Elevated serum total cholesterol or LDL-cholesterol levels and high blood pressure levels increase the severity of atherosclerosis, although high blood pressure is more closely associated with problems in the cerebral arteries.

Risk factors and coronary heart disease. Genetic, dietary, and lifestyle factors, as described in table 13-2 influence the development of atherosclerosis and heart disease. Intervention strategies have been directed toward diet- or drug-induced reductions in LDL-cholesterol levels, smoking cessation, weight loss, limited use of alcohol, and increases in physical activity.

High intakes of dietary cholesterol and saturated fatty acids lead to increased LDL-cholesterol levels, whereas polyunsaturated fatty acids when substituted for saturated fats lower both HDL- and LDL-cholesterol concentrations. Monounsaturated fatty acids appear to decrease LDL-cholesterol levels without lowering HDL-cholesterol levels. Soluble fiber, commonly found in oat bran and starchy vegetables, also appears to lower serum LDL-cholesterol levels. Physical activity increases HDL-cholesterol levels, as does

TABLE 13-2   *Factors Contributing to Cardiovascular Disease Risk*

Personal Characteristics (No Control)	Lifestyle Behaviors (Intervene and Change)	Background Conditions (Screen and Treat)
Sex	Stress/ability to cope	Hypertension
Age	Cigarette smoking	Diabetes mellitus
Family history	Alcohol abuse	Hyperlipidemia (especially
	Sedentary lifestyle	hypercholesterolemia)
	Obesity	
	Food habits	
	Excess fat	
	Excess salt	
	Excess sugar	
	Excess kilocalories	
	Low fiber	

moderate use of alcohol. The effect of the omega-3 polyunsaturated fatty acids on serum LDL-cholesterol levels is uncertain, although these fatty acids do interfere with the formation of unwanted blood clots in the coronary arteries.

Intervention trials for coronary heart disease. Several large-scale diet-heart trials have been conducted with middle-aged hypercholesterolemic men to evaluate strategies for reducing mortality from coronary heart disease. Interventions to reduce serum cholesterol levels have included diets low in fat and saturated fat and lipid-lowering drugs. A general finding has been that reduction in coronary risk is directly proportional to the decrease in serum cholesterol levels. Over the short term, a 1% decrease in serum cholesterol levels results in a 2% decrease in coronary risk; over the long term, a 1% decrease in serum cholesterol levels may result in as much as a 3% decrease in coronary risk. Other nutrients now receiving attention regarding a possible role in cardiovascular risk are vitamins C and E and beta carotene.[31] Men and women who consumed vitamin E supplements containing 10 to 100 times the RDA over several years had decreased risk; however, further research is needed to determine the safety and effectiveness of long-term consumption of vitamin E before this can be recommended to the general public.

A study in San Francisco evaluated the influence of lifestyle changes without surgical or drug intervention on atherosclerotic damage.[32] After one year, a measurable decrease in fatty plaques in the coronary arteries was observed in men and women who exercised regularly, stopped smoking, and followed a vegetarian diet with less than 10% of energy coming from fat. Such a diet could be deficient in essential fatty acids, vitamin B_{12}, zinc, and iron and should not be followed without close medical supervision. However, this study provided evidence that lifestyle changes over a long-term period not only retard but may actually reverse coronary-artery disease. A diet less restrictive in fat, combined with other positive lifestyle changes may also lead to significant reduction in coronary risk.

Hypertension

Hypertension, or sustained elevated arterial blood pressure, increases risk of stroke, coronary heart disease, and kidney damage. Obesity is associated with elevated blood pressure levels, which decrease during periods of active weight loss. It appears that regular exercise can prevent the usual age-related increase in blood pressure levels and can lead to a decrease in elevated levels.[16]

Risk reduction and hypertension. Dietary factors associated with hypertension are alcohol, calcium, and various electrolytes, including sodium and potassium. Excessive ingestion of alcohol, more than 1 oz of alcohol each day, can raise blood pressure.[16] The effect of nutrients on hypertension is less well understood. Epidemiologic data suggest that habitual intake of more than 6 g salt, or 2,400 mg sodium, per day increases the risk of hypertension in salt-sensitive individuals.[16] Dietary calcium has been associated with high blood pressure in some but not all U.S. surveys. On the other hand, a liberal potassium intake (from food sources) may protect against developing hypertension and play an ameliorative role in those with blood pressures above normal. Epid data also suggest that when dietary intakes of fruits and vegetables were increased by middle-aged people with hypertension, 38% of them were able to reduce their antihypertensive medication, and their blood pressure remained well controlled.[33]

Individual response. The impact of sodium restriction or calcium or potassium supplementation on blood pressure levels is a highly individual response. Clinical trials resulting in no significant change in mean blood pressure among all participants have produced striking decreases in blood pressure levels in particular individuals. Diets limited in sodium but generous in food sources of potassium and calcium may be of general benefit. Reductions in dietary sodium should be strongly encouraged for black Americans, among whom salt sensitivity and hypertension are highly prevalent.[16] Potassium supplementation with potassium chloride, unless medically supervised, is not recommended and is especially dangerous for those using potassium-sparing diuretics or with compromised kidney function.

Overweight and Obesity

Incidence of overweight. In the United States, 32% of white and black men; 32% and 49% of white and black women, respectively; and 40% and 48% of Mexican American men and women, respectively, are overweight, and these numbers are increasing.[34] Between 1976 and 1991, the prevalence of overweight increased 8% among adults, and mean body weight increased 3.6 kg. Americans in all social and ethnic groups are attempting to lose weight, but most gain it back. The diets chosen are often low in protein, vitamins, and minerals, as well as kcalories, and lead to nutrient depletion. Very-low-calorie diets (VLCD) containing 500–800 kcal have been used in medical clinics to bring about rapid weight loss; however, such diets are dangerous when unsupervised. Moreover, extremely low-energy diets do not help the dieter develop new eating patterns; consequently, when the dieter discontinues and resumes the usual eating pattern, he or she is likely to regain the weight. This can establish a cycle of weight gain, weight loss, and weight gain, which over a period of years can be more detrimental to health than the initial overweight. An approach to weight loss that includes an increase in energy expenditure in the form of physical activity along with a reasonable decrease in energy intake is more effective than either strategy alone (see the box on p. 332).

Obesity and disease risk. Obesity is an independent risk factor for cardiovascular disease, as well as a contributor to the development of elevated blood pressure and serum cholesterol levels. Obesity promotes degenerative **osteoarthritis** and bone-joint disease, reducing flexibility and hindering mobility. In a fifteen-year follow-up of 698 older women, those considered to be overweight (BMI >27) when first measured were twice as likely to become disabled and unable to carry groceries or perform housekeeping chores as those who had been normal weight.[35] Because physical exercise is difficult, the obese individual is more likely to be sedentary, which sustains the obesity and further contributes to degenerative changes.[36] Obesity is a significant factor in the development of noninsulin-dependent diabetes mellitus (NIDDM), as enlarged fat cells resist the action of insulin.

The influence of obesity and overweight on mortality risk is controversial. Life insurance statistics indicate that individuals greatly above or below average weight are more likely to die at younger ages. In early reports, underweight persons had an even greater mortality rate than overweight persons. This led to the assertion by some health professionals that being slightly overweight might actually be protective, particularly in the presence of severe illness or disease. Long-term follow-up of participants in the Framingham Heart Study revealed that high mortality among the underweight men was related to cigarette smoking.[37] Eighty percent of the underweight middle-aged men were cigarette smokers, as compared with only 55% of the overweight men.

The age when an individual becomes obese also influences mortality from cardiovascular disease. Middle adults who become obese before age fifty-five have a higher risk of

Osteoarthritis
(Gr *osteon* + *arthron*, joint; *-itis*, inflammation) A form of arthritis in which joints undergo degenerative changes, resulting in stiffness, pain, and swelling; arthritis in the hip, knee, or spine can result in some degree of disability.

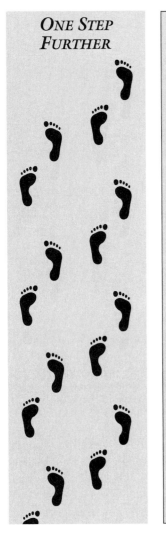

ONE STEP FURTHER

Weight Reduction: The High Cost of False Hope

At any given time, 65 million Americans are trying to lose weight. It is estimated that they spend at least $51 billion a year on weight loss products and services. The weight loss industry has continued to market new diets, formulas, and gimmicks to those who are desperate to shed unwanted pounds. Unfortunately, many of these efforts end in failure, and the obese dieter is again left in despair or worse. At present, the weight loss industry is largely unregulated, and advertisements present a false hope of success. Very-low-calorie diets may be a threat to health when followed without medical supervision. Even hospital-based programs with appropriate nutrition counseling and social support may impose unrealistic weight goals on individuals who have never achieved ideal weight, despite a lifetime of effort.

A more successful and appropriate approach is weight management without dieting. This nondieting approach involves five steps:
1. Provide counselor and peer support. Many overweight individuals are socially isolated, and dieting failure reinforces these feelings. Group interaction with peers who have similar problems provides acceptance and understanding.
2. Develop normal eating patterns. Chronic dieters often restrict intake by skipping meals or fasting. Encourage eating of three meals each day, even though energy intake may increase.
3. Increase exercise gradually. Exercise will burn calories and allow more flexibility in food choices. Walking is an appropriate activity. Begin with short sessions (five minutes, if necessary) to avoid pain or stiffness.
4. Reduce dietary fat gradually. Over time, help the dieter reduce current fat intake to 20–30% of kilocalories. High-fat diets are more likely to lead to weight gain than are low-fat diets.
5. Accept the body weight achieved through appropriate diet and exercise. A lower body weight that does not approach ideal weight still contributes to functional benefits in blood pressure, serum lipid, and serum glucose levels.

A weight loss of even 10% sustained for a lifetime will be of greater benefit than extensive weight lost that is promptly regained.

Begley, C.E. 1991. Government should strengthen regulation in the weight loss industry. *J Am Diet Assoc* 91:1255.

Foreyt, J.P., and G.K. Goodrick. 1993. Weight management without dieting. *Nutr Today* 28(2):4.

mortality than those who become obese after age fifty-five. Regardless of body weight at age twenty-five, excess weight gain during the middle adult years increases cardiovascular risk, whereas voluntary weight loss among those who are overweight can reduce their risk. Men appear to be more sensitive than women to the detrimental effects of weight gain and overweight. The location of body fat also influences risk. Men with thick layers of body fat in the abdominal region have higher risk of coronary artery disease and death than those with similar amounts of fat about their hips. In fact, the site of accumulated fat, abdominal area versus the hips, may explain in part the increased mortality risk of men versus women with similar BMIs. Even mild overweight can be detrimental to the maintenance of good health. A weight loss of 10 to 15 pounds can bring about a significant drop in elevated blood pressure and reduction in serum LDL-cholesterol levels.[38]

Cancer

Cancer development. Cancer is the second leading cause of death in the United States. One researcher suggests that one-third of all cancers are diet-related.[10] Dietary fat, fiber, the antioxidant vitamins A, C, and E, and the vitamin A precursor, beta carotene, have been evaluated as to their influence on cancer risk. Dietary components may interact at various stages in cancer development. They may also influence the development of cancer in particular organs or tissues.

Three stages of abnormal cell growth transform a normal cell into cancerous tissue:
1. *Initiation.* An irreversible genetic alteration in a normal cell is brought about by a carcinogen, which makes the cell capable of uncontrolled growth.
2. *Promotion.* The abnormal cell is stimulated to grow and produce a cancer.
3. *Progression.* The tumor cells invade healthy tissues and spread throughout the body.

Linoleic acid has been shown to interact at all stages to promote carcinogenesis. In contrast, naturally occurring compounds present in the cruciferous vegetables, (such as broccoli, cauliflower, and brussels sprouts), block both the initiation and promotion of cancer development in the cell. Dietary antioxidants may destroy **free radicals,** which can initiate carcinogenesis, or actually reverse the process after it has begun.

Diet and cancer. Dietary fat, particularly saturated fat, has been implicated in the development of breast, prostate, and colon cancer, although findings differ according to where and how the studies were performed. For example, fat intakes per person are higher in countries with generally higher rates of breast cancer. However, studies that have examined the fat intakes of large groups of women in relation to their subsequent development of breast cancer have found no direct relationship. Incidence of breast cancer is higher among obese women. Possibly, the high-energy density of foods containing a high proportion of fat contribute to development of obesity and thereby influences cancer risk. Epidemiologic studies have related high intakes of red meat to increased incidence of colon cancer.[39]

Nutrition has a wellness role in maintaining health and preventing illness, especially in relation to cancer. This role is evident in the American Cancer Society's new dietary guidelines:[40]
1. Choose most of the foods you eat from plant sources; eat a variety of fruits, vegetables, and grains.
2. Limit your intake of high-fat foods, particularly from animal sources.
3. Be physically active; achieve and maintain a healthy weight.
4. Limit consumption of alcoholic beverages, if you drink at all.[40]

These guidelines are displayed in the now familiar Food Guide Pyramid, emphasizing national and state "5 a Day for Better Health" programs, which encourage Americans to eat five or more servings of fruits and vegetables every day.[41] This emphasis stems from certain compounds found in plants, thus called phytochemicals ("plant chemicals"), which ongoing research indicates have promising effects in the chemoprevention of cancer.[42,43] As indicated, these compounds include food nutrients—vitamin A and its analogues, vitamin C, and vitamin E—as well as nonnutritive substances, such as indoles, isothiocyanates, dithiolthiones, and organosulfur.[42] The American Dietetic Association is working with the government and the food industry to ensure that the public has accurate scientific information in this emerging field.[44]

The strongest evidence associating a dietary component with reduced cancer risk exists for fiber and cancer of the colon. It has been proposed that colon cancer risk would decrease by 31% if daily fiber intake were to increase by 13 g (the amount of fiber in one apple and 1/2 cup of cooked legumes).[45] The protective effect of fiber against colorectal cancer may relate to its bulk, which dilutes the bile acids that are present. Fiber also hastens the passage of the food bolus through the digestive tract, thereby shortening the time during which ingested carcinogens are in contact with the intestinal wall. Finally, diets high in fiber may be low in dietary constituents, such as fat, that promote carcinogenesis.

Diabetes Mellitus

Diabetes mellitus is a metabolic disorder characterized by high blood glucose levels and abnormal carbohydrate utilization caused by inappropriate levels of insulin. Insulin-dependent diabetes mellitus (IDDM) results from destruction of the beta cells of the pancreas. Because no insulin is secreted by the pancreas, insulin must be supplied by injection, or death will result. Destruction of the beta cells is believed to occur through an autoimmune reaction of genetic origin. Age of onset is usually in childhood. However, depending on the individual self-care management under medical supervision, at middle adult years chronic disease usually seen in older persons may already have developed.

Free radical
An unstable, high-energy cell molecule with an unpaired electron that causes oxidation reactions in unsaturated fatty acids and may act as a carcinogen.

CASE STUDY

The Patient with Cancer

Kate is a thirty-five-year-old mother of three young children. She was admitted to the hospital three weeks ago with multiple enterocutaneous fistulas. She weighed 52 kg (116 lb) on admission and is 165 cm (5 ft 6 in) tall. Kate had undergone a hysterectomy four months before admission, following a recurrence of cervical cancer. During the chemotherapy that followed for seven months, she had regular bouts with nausea and anorexia. Surgery was performed again. Her fistulas continued to drain for two weeks postoperatively, during which she tolerated clear liquids only. An intravenous drip of 10% glucose and 45% normal saline was ordered to supplement fluids and kcalories. This week, she developed peritonitis and has had a fever of 39° C (102° F) for the past twenty-four hours. Her weight has dropped to 41 kg (90 lb); drainage from the fistulas has become odorous. Kate was placed in isolation today and was advised by her physician that he intended to start her on total parenteral nutrition (TPN) and to take some more tests to determine her progress.

Questions for analysis

1. What types of nutritional assessment procedures would be used by the TPN team for planning Kate's nutrition therapy? Explain the purpose of each.
2. Account for Kate's increased energy and protein needs.
3. Why did Kate develop nausea and anorexia during chemotherapy? What are the implications of this for recovery? Outline a TPN team plan for evaluating and controlling nausea and vomiting in patients undergoing chemotherapy.
4. What personal concerns would you expect Kate to have? What resources may help her obtain the personal and physical support she probably needs?

Noninsulin-dependent diabetes mellitus (NIDDM), formerly referred to as adult-onset diabetes, usually occurs in middle adults after age forty and is generally associated with obesity. It is more likely caused by secretion of an inappropriate form of insulin or resistance of oversize adipose cells to the action of insulin, rather than a deficiency of insulin. Treatment usually involves weight reduction and dietary intervention. The dietary pattern most commonly prescribed in the past was high in carbohydrates (50–60% of kcalories) and low in fat (less than or equal to 30% of kcalories). Ongoing studies have indicated that a moderating of this nutrient ratio may be beneficial in controlling serum glucose and lipid levels in some patients with NIDDM. Recent guidelines indicate that fat intake may increase up to 40% if monounsaturated fat is emphasized (20% of total kcalories).[46] Regular exercise is important, and, if necessary, oral hypoglycemic drugs are prescribed. Atherosclerotic coronary disease is a frequent complication of this disorder; thus, diets high in soluble fiber and low in cholesterol and saturated fat are advisable. Maintaining appropriate weight for height and avoiding alcohol intake are important preventive measures for lowering risk.

NUTRITION AND HEALTH PROMOTION PROGRAMS 〰

National Cholesterol Education Program. The National Cholesterol Education Program (NCEP) sponsored by the National Heart, Lung, and Blood Institute was begun in 1985 in response to the published findings from large-scale intervention studies that reducing elevated blood cholesterol levels reduces the rate of heart attacks and associated mortality. Revised guidelines released in 1993 have added standards for serum HDL-cholesterol levels to be used in evaluation and treatment.[11] The NCEP encourages a team approach with physicians, dietitians, nurses, and pharmacologists in developing intervention strategies and materials to educate health professionals, patients, and the public. The guidelines presented in table 13-3 emphasize dietary intervention as a primary treatment

TABLE 13-3 *Classification of Blood Cholesterol Levels and Recommended Follow-Up for Persons with No Evidence of Coronary Heart Disease (CHD)*

Total Blood Cholesterol	HDL-Cholesterol	Recommended Actions
<200 mg/dl (desirable)	≥35 mg/dl	Provide general guidelines for diet, physical activity, and risk reduction.
	<35 mg/dl	Do fasting lipoprotein analysis (total, HDL-, and LDL-cholesterol). Recommendation based on LDL-cholesterol results (see below).
200–239 mg/dl (borderline high) ≥240 mg/dl	≥35 mg/dl and fewer than two risk factors*	Provide information on dietary modification, physical activity, and risk-factor reduction. Reevaluate in one to two years.
	<35 mg/dl or 2 or more risk factors*	Do fasting lipoprotein analysis (total, HDL-, and LDL-cholesterol). Recommendation based on LDL-cholesterol results (see below).
		Do fasting lipoprotein analysis (total, HDL-, and LDL-cholesterol).
		Recommendation based on LDL-cholesterol levels:
		LDL-cholesterol <130 mg/dl (desirable) Provide general guidelines for diet, physical activity, and risk reduction. Reevaluate within five years.
		LDL-cholesterol 130–159 mg/dl (borderline high-risk); fewer than two risk factors.* Provide information on Step I diet (fat ≤ 30% total kcal; saturated fat 8–10% total kcal). Encourage physical activity. Reevaluate annually.
		LDL-cholesterol 130–159 mg/dl (borderline high-risk); two or more risk factors *or*
		LDL-cholesterol ≥160 mg/dl (high-risk) Initiate intensive diet therapy. Evaluate for other CHD risk factors.*

From U.S. Department of Health and Human Services. 1993. *Second report of the expert panel on the detection, evaluation, and treatment of high blood cholesterol in adults,* NIH pub. no. 93-3095. Washington, DC: U.S. Government Printing Office.
*Positive risk factors:
  Age: male ≥45 year
  female ≥ 55 years or early menopause without estrogen replacement
  Family history of premature coronary artery disease
  Cigarette smoking
  Hypertension
  Diabetes mellitus
  HDL-cholesterol <35 mg/dl

and present a rational approach applicable to persons of different ages and health statuses. Use of drugs to lower serum cholesterol levels is reserved for persons with the following:
- Known coronary heart disease.
- Risk factors in addition to elevated serum cholesterol.
- Serum cholesterol levels that remain high despite dietary intervention.

Because diagnosis of high blood cholesterol depends on the accuracy of a blood test, standardized procedures for cholesterol testing have been established. The NCEP has defined intervention strategies for children and adolescents whose blood cholesterol levels or family history places them at risk. Findings from national surveys conducted between 1960 and 1991

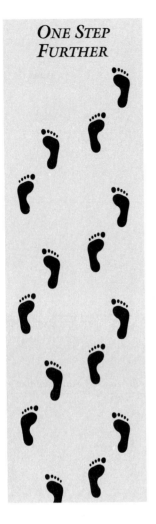

ONE STEP FURTHER

National Health Promotion and Disease Prevention Objectives

Since its beginning, the U.S. Public Health Service has had responsibility for disease prevention and has developed programs for the eradication of nutritional deficiency diseases, such as pellagra, and the control of infectious diseases. In the late 1970s, Congress directed this agency to establish national goals for health promotion and disease prevention, publicized nationwide as the 1990 Health Objectives for the Nation. The goals included improved health status, improved health services, improved public awareness of personal health strategies, and improved health and nutrition monitoring. By 1985, there was significant progress toward meeting many of the 1990 objectives, with major reductions in illness and death among specific groups of infants, children, and adults.

Based on this success, regional hearings were organized to allow professional organizations, community health groups, and state and local governments to provide input toward the development of new national health objectives for the 1990s, targeted for the year 2000. With the findings of these regional hearings, the U.S. Department of Health and Human Services, Public Health Services issued the new goals in 1990: *Healthy People 2000: National Health Promotion and Disease Prevention Objectives**

The target areas are:

- *Health promotion.* Behavioral lifestyle factors that influence health and well-being, including the use of tobacco, alcohol, and drugs; nutrition, physical fitness, and mental health.
- *Health protection.* Health problems related to the physical and social environment, including violence and abusive behavior, air quality, waste disposal, and occupational safety and health.
- *Preventive health services.* Preventive services directed toward specific health problems, such as sexually transmitted disease, adolescent pregnancy, heart disease and other chronic conditions, maternal and infant health problems, and human immunodeficiency virus (HIV).

---

*United States Department of Health and Human Services. 1991. Healthy people 2000: National health promotion and disease prevention objectives, DHHS pub. no. (PHS) 91-50212. Washington, DC: U.S. Government Printing Office.

indicate that mean serum cholesterol levels in adults ages twenty to seventy-four years have declined from 221 to 206 mg/dl.[47] More than 50% of this decrease has occurred since 1976.

Dietary counseling and drug intervention requiring professional supervision usually take place in a physician's office or health care facility, but public education to promote preventive dietary changes and to encourage screening of those at high risk must target the community. The overall goal is to provide practical dietary information "wherever people eat." Major supermarkets can distribute heart healthy recipes, provide shelf markers noting the cholesterol and sodium contents of important foods, and serve as sites for blood cholesterol screening. Restaurants need to offer menu items carrying a heart healthy logo. School and worksite cafeterias may sponsor contests featuring menu items low in cholesterol and saturated fat. The NCEP has developed sample menus using foods from the traditional American diet, as well as items common to Mexican American, Asian American, and vegetarian diets to assist people in making appropriate food choices (table 13-4).[11] Support from community businesses, local health care agencies, and volunteers can make these programs possible. A multifaceted community-based program sponsored by the state department of public health in South Carolina resulted in an 8.9% decrease in the use of animal fats by black and white adults.[48] Thirty-percent of those interviewed also reported looking at restaurant nutrition information when making their selections. Such programs encourage participation in screening and follow-up counseling.

Community Sites for Health Promotion

The popular emphasis on health and wellness has led community groups in schools, hospitals, and local government agencies to become involved in health promotion. In the private

TABLE 13-4 *Heart Healthy Sample Menus for Various Food Patterns*

Traditional American Cuisine	Mexican American Cuisine	Asian American Cuisine	Lacto Ovo Vegetarian Cuisine
Breakfast			
Bagel, plain	Cantaloupe	Banana	Orange
Margarine	Farina prepared with skim	Whole-wheat bread	Pancakes made with 1% milk
Jelly	milk*	Margarine	and egg whites*
Cereal, shredded wheat	White bread	Orange juice	Pancake syrup
Banana	Margarine	Milk, skim	Margarine
Milk, skim	Jelly		Milk, 1%
Orange juice	Orange juice		Coffee
Coffee	Hot cocoa prepared with skim		
Milk, skim	milk		
Lunch			
Minestrone soup, canned,	Beef enchilada	Beef noodle soup, canned,	Vegetable soup, canned, low-
low-sodium	Tortilla, corn	low-sodium	sodium
Roast beef sandwich	Lean roast beef*	Chinese noodle and beef salad*	Bagel
Whole-wheat bread	Vegetable oil	Sirloin steak	Processed American cheese,
Lean roast beef,	Cheddar cheese, low-fat and	Peanut oil	low-fat and low-sodium
unseasoned*	low-sodium	Soy sauce, low-sodium	Spinach salad
American cheese, low-fat	Onion	Carrots	Spinach
and low-sodium	Tomato	Squash	Mushrooms
Lettuce	Lettuce	Onion	Olive oil dressing, regular-
Tomato	Chili peppers	Chinese noodles, soft type	calorie*
Margarine	Refried beans prepared with	Steamed white rice*	Apple
Apple	vegetable oil*	Apple	Iced tea
Water	Carrots	Tea, unsweetened	
	Celery		
	Milk, skim		
Dinner			
Flounder*	Chicken taco	Pork stirfry with vegetables	Omelette*
Vegetable oil	Tortilla, corn	Pork cutlet*	Egg whites
Baked potato*	Chicken breast without skin*	Peanut oil	Green pepper
Margarine	Vegetable oil	Soy sauce, low-sodium	Onion
Green beans seasoned with	Cheddar cheese, low-fat	Broccoli	Mozzarella cheese made
margarine*	and low-sodium	Carrots	from part skin milk
Carrots seasoned with mar-	Guacamole	Mushrooms	Vegetable oil
garine*	Salsa	Steamed white rice*	Brown rice seasoned with
White dinner roll*	Corn, seasoned with	Milk, skim	margarine*
Margarine	margarine*	Tea, unsweetened	Carrots, seasoned with mar-
Frozen yogurt	Spanish rice prepared with		garine*
Iced tea, unsweetened	margarine*		Whole-wheat bread
	Banana		Margarine
	Coffee		Fig bar cookies
	Milk, skim		Tea
			Honey
Snack			
Popcorn*	Popcorn	Wonton soup prepared with	Corn flake cereal
Margarine	Margarine	low-sodium broth	Milk, 1%
		Tea, unsweetened	

From U.S. Department of Health and Human Services. 1993. *Second report of the expert panel on detection, evaluation and treatment of high blood cholesterol in adults,* NIH Pub. no. 93-3095. Washington, DC: U.S. Government Printing Office.
*No salt is added in recipe preparation or as seasoning. All margarine is low-sodium.

sector, health maintenance organizations (HMOs), businesses, and health clubs are providing health education and screening programs for their members and employees.

Hospital-Based Community Programs

The increasing number of hospitals becoming involved in health promotion is reflective of their changing role from institutions providing care for the sick to those providing a continuum of health care, including education for disease prevention, monitoring, and follow-up care when the patient returns home. Hospital programs include community screening programs to identify those at major risk for chronic disease and educational programs describing lifestyle patterns that reduce risk. Programs may involve blood pressure and cholesterol screening and education, nutritional assessment and nutrition counseling, and weight management with support groups for long-term weight loss.

Some hospitals are marketing health promotion services to local employers. These services include employee assistance programs offering counseling and treatment for such problems as alcohol and drug dependency, occupational health services for monitoring the safety of the work environment or treating work-related illness or injury, and wellness programs emphasizing improvement of lifestyle habits.

Health Maintenance Organizations

General organization. Health maintenance organizations, which are based on a concept first developed in the early 1900s, currently operate under federal law regulating their practice that was enacted in the 1960s. They present the option of prepaid medical care, usually by group medical practices. Subscribers pay a set fee per individual or family and in turn are guaranteed all health services required, including visits to physicians and other health care professionals, hospital care, and related services. HMOs negotiate fees with hospitals, pharmacies, and specialty practice consultants.

As providers of health care services, HMOs have both advantages and disadvantages. From the consumer's point of view, HMOs provide an opportunity to control one's own health care costs, as all services required are provided for the set fee. Such a system effectively insulates an individual or a family against the financial devastation that can result from a catastrophic illness or injury. Also, HMOs have a financial incentive to encourage preventive health care. The traditional fee-for-service system rewards providers for treating illness. One disadvantage of the HMO is that individuals may not be able to choose their care provider but, rather, must accept the provider under contract to the HMO. Also, any arrangement that does not provide a fee per unit of service may result in a provider's limiting services in an effort to control costs.

Health promotion activities. HMOs have taken a leadership role in health promotion activities, often in response to member requests. Seminars and ongoing classes are offered on such topics as diet and weight control, smoking cessation, stress management, and physical fitness. Some provide health education libraries; professional counselors, including nutritionists and registered dietitians; extensive printed material from public sources; handouts authored in-house; lists of recommended books; or newsletters. Many HMO members consider health education to be an important component of their membership services.

Worksite Wellness Programs

Goals. Worksite wellness programs have expanded rapidly in recent years. Now 81% of worksites offer at least one health promotion activity. Companies with more than fifty employees are most likely to sponsor health promotion programs.[49] The incentive for establishing such programs has come at least in part from escalating medical care and insurance costs. Employers have sought to identify causes of this rise and to intervene appropriately.

Health screening programs evaluating blood pressure and serum cholesterol levels or promoting smoking cessation, nutrition and weight management, physical fitness, and stress management are the most commonly offered. Nutrition programs have been reported to be the most effective wellness programs, improving health in 59.6% of participants. In one study, stress-management training improved productivity and outlook in 46.5% of the workers.[49]

Evaluation. Results from many programs indicate that not only do employees lose excess weight, stop smoking, or lower their blood pressure or serum cholesterol levels but this reduction in risk continues after the formal program has been completed. The success of worksite programs is attributed to the systematic monitoring that provides employees with information about their condition and offers continued support. A worksite program focusing on dietary changes in middle-aged men reported a mean decrease in serum cholesterol levels from 238 mg/dl to 210 mg/dl that was sustained over a period of one year.[50]

Employer-assisted alterations in the environment that support health promotion are also important to the success of a program. Establishing a smoke-free workplace, eliminating cigarette machines, and ensuring low-fat, nutritious food options in the employee cafeteria or vending machines are important when developing a strategy for program evaluation.

Cost-effectiveness. Decreasing health risk factors does reduce illness and subsequent health costs, although not immediately. In fact, health care costs may rise during the first six months following health risk screening when medical intervention needs become apparent. After this initial rise, however, costs decline and this trend continues. In a comparison of worksite wellness participants and nonparticipants from the same company, health care costs over a one-year period were one-third lower for those receiving health education. Other companies have reported that physically fit employees had 3.5 fewer sick days each year.[50] Worksite programs offer vast potential for education and intervention in all aspects of health risk.

Health Clubs

Increasing media attention to physical fitness and weight control has fostered the rapid expansion of for-profit health clubs that offer a variety of services for a comprehensive membership fee. Aerobic exercise and use of physical conditioning equipment are the most common activities, although fitness evaluations and development of personal exercise programs may also be provided. Facilities may include a swimming pool, a tennis court, or racquetball courts. Nutrition and diet counseling is often available. Unfortunately, in some situations, the individuals providing dietary evaluations or instruction are not professional nutritionists or registered dietitians.

Health Fairs

More than 2 million people visit health fairs each year. These health fairs are sponsored by service organizations, hospitals, home health agencies, and professional health-related associations. They take place in shopping malls, parking lots, community centers, and parks. They feature displays, posters, hand-out materials, and screening tests for common disorders. Staffed by both professional and lay volunteers, health fairs have as their major purpose health education, and sponsors make an effort to attract both the general population and targeted groups.

Because health fairs are unregulated, little is known about the numbers of persons reached or the screening procedures attempted. An organization that offers assistance to health fair sponsors estimates that more than 1.5 million measurements of height and weight and more than 20 million blood chemistry tests are performed each year at health fairs. Screening tests to detect health problems may be offered as an incentive to attract participants.

Be Cautious About Health Fair Tests

The criteria for health fair tests and the degree of follow-up within such screening programs concern health professionals. False alarms for the well participants as well as false reassurance for the person at risk are an issue in situations in which test conditions and the sheer number of tests performed contribute to error. Despite these limitations, blood cholesterol screening does appear to motivate individuals to seek professional care when indicated. In one community, 74% of those with identified elevated blood cholesterol levels sought help, resulting in a 4.5% decrease in blood cholesterol levels over the next year.* Health fairs serve an important role in drawing attention to healthy lifestyle choices and in emphasizing personal responsibility for one's own health.

---

*Maiman, L.A. Et al. 1994. Public cholesterol screening in the previously diagnosed, misuse of resources or beneficial function. *Am J Prev Med* 10:20.

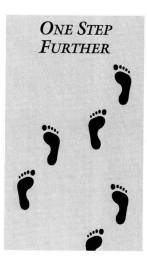

ONE STEP FURTHER

MIDDLE ADULT STAGE OF THE LIFE CYCLE ≋

The world over, a healthy beginning for each child depends on the degree to which young and middle adults, especially women, have the opportunity and support to nourish their own state of healthy maturity.[50] A healthy adult maturity depends on physiologic, cultural, and psychosocial strengths born of individual and societal health values that produce healthy lifestyles.

Adult Homeostasis

After the turbulent physical growth and sexual development of adolescence under the control of growth and sex hormones, the human body's growth pattern levels off into a state of adult **homeostasis.** The word was first used by Boston physiologist Walter Cannon (1871–1945) to describe what he called the "wisdom of the body." In a state of gene regulation and feedback, the "body's wisdom" maintains an internal dynamic equilibrium and stability within the ebb and flow of its parts through a balancing system of homeostatic mechanisms. Physically, then, the adult body has grown up, has attained its full genetic size and strength, and has leveled off in a stable state of tissue maintenance and function. In the two decades of middle adult years, ages forty-five to sixty-five, the human body levels off in a state of tissue maintenance and function.

This dynamic balance between body parts and functions is life-sustaining. All body constituents are in a constant state of flux, although some tissues are more actively engaged than others. This concept of dynamic equilibrium can be seen in carbohydrate and fat metabolism, but it is especially striking in protein metabolism. The adult body's state of metabolic stability results from a balance between the rates of tissue protein breakdown and resynthesis. In earlier growth years, the tissue protein synthesis rate is higher, so that the necessary new tissues can be formed. In later adult years, as in the aging process in the elderly, the rate of tissue protein breakdown gradually exceeds that of synthesis, and the older adult body slowly declines.

Body Composition

Body composition of the maturing middle adult is maintained within a rather wide range of individual variance according to sex, weight, and age (see chapter 2). The most metabolically active tissue is the lean body mass compartment. It requires the greatest amount of energy and is larger in men than in women, accounting for 30–65% of the total body weight. The lean body mass is larger in middle adults who continue to be physically active and consume a low-fat diet. As in previous adult years, the fat compartment is larger in women than in men and may vary in average-weight adults from about 14–30% of total body weight. In overweight middle adults, too prevalent a situation among Americans due to a relatively sedentary lifestyle and a rich diet, the fat compartment is larger. It is smaller in persons who continue to exercise regularly and eat less fat. In general, as middle adults grow older and become less physically active, the lean body mass decreases and the relative fat tissue increases. The water compartment of average-weight middle adults accounts for about 20% of total body weight. It is larger in thin or less fat persons and smaller in fat persons. The mineral compartment, the smallest part of middle adult body composition, accounts for only about 5–6% of body weight, most of it in the skeleton.

Physiologic Maturity

The middle adult reached physiologic maturity in the young adult years and now continues tissue growth only on a healthy maintenance basis. There is full development of body functions, including sexual **maturation** and reproductive capacity. This reproductive capacity continues for a number of years in middle-aged men; however, a women's childbearing years end with her menopause at about age fifty.[52] During middle and older adulthood, there is a gradual cell loss and reduced cell metabolism, with a gradual reduction in the performance capacity of most organ systems. Individuals vary widely in the rate and

Homeostasis

(Gr *homoios,* same, unchanging; *stasis,* stability) State of the body's internal physiologic balance through constant feedback and adjustment, the operation of homeostatic mechanisms that maintain a dynamic equilibrium within the body in relation to its external environment.

Maturation

(L *maturus,* mature) Process or stage of attaining one's full physical, psychosocial, and mental development. Individual genetic potential guides physical and mental development, which in turn bears the imprint of environmental, psychosocial, and cultural influences.

order at which these changes occur. In general, the age-related decline in lean body mass accelerates in later life.

Psychosocial Maturity

Psychosocial development continues in individual and changing patterns throughout adulthood with its unique potentials and fulfillments. Throughout the human life cycle, food not only meets nutritional requirements for physical growth and tissue maintenance but also relates intimately to personal psychosocial development. Over the past thirty-five years, Erikson's classic structure of human development in relation to society and culture has greatly influenced our view of the human life cycle.[53] In this pattern, the three adult stages—young, middle, and older—of the human life cycle complete the whole and give meaning to human development.

In the years of middle adulthood, the psychosocial problem people face is generativity versus self-absorption. The middle adult's older children have grown and have gone to make their own lives. For some, these are the years of the "empty nest." For others, these years are an opportunity for expanding personal growth—"it's my turn now." There is a coming to terms with what life is all about and great opportunity of finding expression for stored learning in passing on life's teachings. To the degree that these inner struggles are not won, there is increasing self-absorption, a turning-in on oneself, and a withering rather than a regenerating spirit of life.

BASIC NUTRIENT NEEDS ≈

Physiologic Gender Differences

With adolescent and young adult growth and development behind them, middle adults experience a leveling off of physiologic needs. Profound body changes have occurred in earlier growth years.

Adult males arrive at this middle point of their lives with completed muscle mass development and long bone growth. He is usually the larger of the two middle adult forms. Middle adult women generally have developed increased amounts of subcutaneous fat deposit during prior pregnancies, particularly in the abdominal area. This pelvic girdle of fat is often a source of anxiety to many figure-conscious middle adult women.

With such profound physical body changes and individual differences, largely revolving around sexual development and decline, as well as mature adult roles and responsibilities in a complex society, it is small wonder that many psychosocial tensions result in middle adulthood.

Middle Adult Dietary Recommendations

The physiologic differences between the sexes account for differing energy and nutrient recommendations for middle adult men and women. The comparative dietary needs of middle adults, in relation to surrounding younger and older adult groups, are shown in table 13-5.[54]

Energy (kilocalories). The larger male body size and muscle mass in middle adults accounts for the greater need for energy, especially since the lean body mass is the most metabolically active tissue in the body composition. In adults, the resting energy expenditure (REE) per unit of total body weight, a measure of metabolic rate, differs by approximately 10% between the sexes. The remainder of energy need, which is much smaller than that for metabolic needs, is for physical activities. In the past, due to occupational differences, men and women often had markedly different energy expenditures, but their occupational activity requirements now are quite similar. Note that these recommended height-weight reference figures are actual medians for the U.S. population of the designated age, as reported by the National Health and Nutrition Examination Survey II (NHANES II) and are not meant to imply ideal height-to-weight ratios. Additional kilocalories are required to support pregnancy and lactation.

TABLE 13-5 *Age and Sex Comparisons of Recommended Dietary Allowances (1989) for Adults*

Age (Years) or Condition	Sex	Weight*		Height*		Energy†	Protein	Major Minerals		
		kg	lb	cm	in	kcal	g	Calcium (mg)	Phosphorus (mg)	Magnesium (mg)
Young adults, 19–24	F	58	128	164	65	2,200	46	1200	1,200	300
	M	72	160	177	70	2,900	58	1200	1,200	300
Middle adults, 25–50	F	63	138	163	64	2,200	50	800	800	280
	M	79	174	176	70	2,900	63	800	800	350
Older adults, 51+	F	65	143	160	63	1,900	50	800	800	280
	M	77	170	173	68	2,300	63	800	800	350
Pregnancy						+300	60	1,200	1,200	320
Lactation						+500	65	1,200	1,200	355
						+500	62	1,200	1,200	340

RE: retinol equivalents (see full RDAs); α-TE: alpha-tocopherol equivalents (see full RDAs); NE: niacin equivalent (see full RDAs)
*Medians of U.S. population survey figures (NHANES II); does not imply ideal height-weight ratios
†Light to moderate activity

Protein. The adult protein allowances are based on a daily protein intake of approximately 0.75 to 0.80 g/kg of body weight for both sexes and all three age groups. An additional allowance of 10 g/day of protein throughout pregnancy and 15 g/day during lactation is indicated.

Minerals. Adult allowances are sufficient if provided on a continuing basis by a well-balanced diet. Two minerals need emphasis: calcium and iron. The allowance for calcium has been increased from 800 to 1,200 mg/day for young adults to ensure peak skeletal bone mass, which is attained roughly by age thirty-five.[54,55] In comparison, the middle adult allowance remains at 800 mg/day, although some increase may be needed for post-menopausal middle adult women, who should have an increased intake to prevent calcium loss from bone and the development of osteoporosis (p. 347–49).[55] Poor middle adult diets may also be deficient in iron, which is needed to prevent iron deficiency anemia. During the reproductive years, women require more iron intake to prevent deficiency due to menstrual blood loss, so their iron allowance is 15 mg/day; for men, it is 10 mg/day. Iron recommendations during pregnancy are 30 mg/day, which is difficult to attain by diet, so a supplement is usually needed.[55] No increase is needed during lactation.

Vitamins. Intake of the middle adult vitamin allowances is usually met by ordinary, well-balanced diets. The problem in some cases may stem from inadequate normal intake rather than from an increased need. A well-selected, mixed diet usually supplies all the vitamins in normally needed quantities. There may be increased therapeutic needs in illness, which should be evaluated on an individual basis.

Dietary pattern. The publication *Nutrition and Your Health: Dietary Guidelines for Americans,* currently issued in its newly developed joint fourth edition by the U.S. Departments of Agriculture and of Health and Human Services, provides a good basic guide for choosing a diet to promote health.[56,57] Other general food guides are discussed in chapter 1.

MIDDLE ADULT WOMEN'S NUTRITION AND HEALTH ISSUES ≈

Pregnancy and Lactation

Primordial follicle
(L *follis,* a leather bag) Primitive ovarian follicle formed during fetal life; a sac- or pouch-like cavity; a small secretory sac or gland. A mature ovarian follicle is an ovum surrounded by specialized epithelial cells.

The normal female reproductive years extend about five years into the early middle adult period, with menopause usually occurring around age fifty to fifty-five. At this end of the woman's reproductive capacity, only a few **primordial follicles** remain in the ovaries, and these last few follicles shortly degenerate.[58] During a middle adult woman's final years of her reproductive period, she will probably continue her contraceptive program of previ-

TABLE 13-5   *Age and Sex Comparisons of Recommended Dietary Allowances (1989) for Adults—Cont'd.*

Trace Elements				Fat-Soluble Vitamins					Water Soluble Vitamins					
Iron (mg)	Zinc (mg)	Iodine (μg)	Selenium (μg)	A (μg RE)	D (μg)	E (mg α-TE)	K (μg)	C (mg)	Thiamin (mg)	Riboflavin (mg)	Niacin (mg NE)	B₆ (mg)	Folate (μg)	B₁₂ (μg)
15	12	150	50	800	10	8	60	60	1.1	1.3	15	1,5	180	2.0
10	15	150	70	1,000	10	10	70	60	1.5	1.7	19	2.0	200	2.0
15	12	150	55	800	5	8	65	60	1.1	1.3	15	1.6	180	2.0
10	15	150	70	1,000	5	10	80	60	1.5	1.7	19	2.0	200	2.0
10	12	150	55	800	5	8	65	60	1.0	1.2	13	1.6	180	2.0
10	15	150	70	1,000	5	10	80	60	1.2	1.4	15	2.0	200	2.0
30	15	175	65	800	10	10	65	70	1.5	1.6	17	2.2	400	2.2
15	19	200	75	1,300	10	12	65	95	1.6	1.8	20	2.1	280	2.6
15	16	200	75	1,200	10	11	65	90	1.6	1.7	20	2.1	260	2.6

ous adult years. Most commonly, this method is oral contraceptive agents—the "pill"—which is based on hormonal suppression of fertility by preventing ovulation but allowing menstruation to occur, or she may have chosen, together with her physician and attending trained professionals, to use Norplant, the most recently developed (1990) method of contraception.[59,60] In this long-term, reversible system, the contraceptive drug levonorgestrel is implanted by a medical specialist and prevents pregnancy for up to five years. The implant can be medically removed at any time during that period. The drug used apparently prevents pregnancy by preventing ovulation.

Nutrition and Pregnancy Planning

Ideally, every pregnancy should be planned. However, for many reasons this is not always the case. However, if pregnancy occurs during this last five-year period of fertility in the middle adult woman's experience, she will want to plan a healthy lifestyle, including both positive nutritional support and physical fitness. A helpful daily food guide for women that covers the reproductive years, developed by the California Department of Health Services, is given in table 13-6.

Menopause

There is a progressive decline in estrogen secretion toward the end of a woman's reproductive life. When she is approximately fifty years of age, her sexual cycles become irregular and ovulation fails to occur in many of them. This period during which the cycles cease altogether and the female sex hormones diminish rapidly is called menopause. The cause of menopause is the "burning out" of the ovaries. Few primordial follicles remain, and production of estrogen by the ovaries decreases as the number of primary follicles approaches zero and the final ones involute and disappear. For most middle adult women, this menopausal period is a normal physiologic process with no marked physical or psychologic symptoms. Approximately 15% of women, however, experience a variety of symptoms, such as "hot flashes" with extreme flushing of the skin, sensations of **dyspnea**, irritability, fatigue, anxiety, and in a few cases occasional psychotic states.[58] In such cases, estrogen therapy may be indicated.

Dyspnea
(Gr *dysnia*, difficult breathing)
Difficult or labored breathing.

Middle Adult Women and Weight

The health problem of obesity, defined as an excessive accumulation of body fat, has been regarded traditionally as the result of overeating. However, studies of twins have indicated that there is a strong genetic component to body fat accumulation and its distribution.[61,62] Men and women differ genetically in their respective sex chromosomes. Men carry an XY combination pair of X (female) and Y (male) chromosomes, whereas women carry a complete XX combination. Cell division of the male XY chromosomes produces

TABLE 13-6 *Daily Food Guide for Women*

Food Groups	One Serving Equals	Recommended Minimum Servings		
		Nonpregnant		Pregnant/ Lactating
		11–24 Years	25+ Years	
Protein foods Provide protein, iron, zinc, and B-vitamins for growth of muscles, bone, blood, and nerves; vegetable protein provides fiber to prevent constipation	**Animal protein:** 1 oz cooked chicken or turkey 1 oz cooked lean beef, lamb, or pork 1 oz or ¼ cup fish or other seafood 1 egg 2 fish sticks or hot dogs 2 slices luncheon meat **Vegetable protein** ½ cup cooked dry beans, lentils, or split peas 3 oz tofu 1 oz or ¼ cup peanuts, pumpkin, or sunflower seeds 1½ oz or ⅓ cup other nuts 2 tsp peanut butter	5 A half-serving of vegetable protein daily	5	7 One serving of vegetable protein daily
Milk products Provide protein and calcium to build strong bones, teeth, healthy nerves and muscles, and to promote normal blood clotting	8 oz milk 8 oz yogurt 1 cup milk shake 1½ cups cream soup (made with milk) 1½ oz or ⅓ cup grated cheese such as cheddar, Monterey, mozzarella, or Swiss) 1½–2 slices presliced American cheese 4 tbsp parmesan cheese 2 cups cottage cheese 1 cup pudding 1 cup custard or flan 1½ cups ice milk, ice cream, or frozen yogurt	3	2	3
Breads, cereals, grains Provide carbohydrates and B-vitamins for energy and healthy nerves; also provide iron for healthy blood; whole grains provide fiber to prevent constipation	1 slice bread 1 dinner roll ½ bun or bagel ½ English muffin or pita 1 small tortilla ¾ cup dry cereal ½ cup granola ½ cup cooked cereal ½ cup rice ½ cup noodles or spaghetti ¼ cup wheat germ 1 4 in pancake or waffle 1 small muffin 8 medium crackers 4 graham cracker squares 3 cups popcorn	7 Four servings of whole-grain products daily	6	7

Food group	Serving sizes		
Vitamin C–rich fruits and vegetables Provide vitamin C to prevent infection and to promote healing and iron absorption; also provide fiber to prevent constipation	6 oz orange, grapefruit, or fruit juice enriched with vitamin C; 6 oz tomato juice or vegetable juice cocktail; 1 orange, kiwi, mango; $1/2$ grapefruit, cantaloupe; $1/2$ cup papaya; 2 tangerines	$1/2$ cup strawberries; $1/2$ cup cooked or 1 cup raw cabbage; $1/2$ cup broccoli, brussels sprouts, or cauliflower; $1/2$ cup snow peas, sweet peppers, or tomato puree; 2 tomatoes	1 1 1
Vitamin A–rich fruits and vegetables Provide beta-carotene and vitamin A to prevent infection and to promote wound healing and night vision; also provide fiber to prevent constipation	6 oz apricot nectar or vegetable juice cocktail; 3 raw or $1/4$ cup dried apricots; $1/4$ cantaloupe or mango; 1 small or $1/2$ cup sliced carrots; 2 tomatoes	$1/2$ cup cooked or 1 cup raw spinach; $1/2$ cup cooked greens (beet, chard, collards, dandelion, kale, mustard); $1/2$ cup pumpkin, sweet potato, winter squash, or yams	1 1
Other fruits and vegetables Provide carbohydrates for energy and fiber to prevent constipation	6 oz fruit juice (if not listed above); 1 medium or $1/2$ cup sliced fruit (apple, banana, peach, pear); $1/2$ cup berries (other than strawberries); $1/2$ cup cherries or grapes; $1/2$ cup pineapple; $1/2$ cup watermelon	$1/4$ cup dried fruit; $1/2$ cup sliced vegetable (asparagus, beets, green beans, celery, corn, eggplant, mushrooms, onion, peas, potato, summer squash, zucchini); $1/2$ artichoke; 1 cup lettuce	3 3 3
Unsaturated fats Provide vitamin E to protect tissue	$1/8$ medium avocado; 1 tsp margarine; 1 tsp mayonnaise; 1 tsp vegetable oil	2 tsp salad dressing (mayonnaise-based); 1 tbsp salad dressing (oil-based)	3 3 3

Adapted from California Department of Health Services, Maternal and Child Health. 1990. *Nutrition during pregnancy and postpartum period: A manual for health care professionals.* Sacramento: CDHS.
NOTE: *The Daily Food Guide for Women may not provide all the calories you require. The best way to increase your intake is to include more than the minimum number of servings recommended.*

the final mature sperm cells, half male (Y) sperm and half female (X) sperm. The sex of the offspring depends on which of these two types of sperm fertilizes the ovum. Thus, it should not be surprising that women may differ from men in the prevalence of obesity, its time of onset, and their responses to treatment. This genetic factor in obesity helps explain the "yo-yo" pattern of dieting that compounds the weight problem for many women, as a successful diet will reduce body weight and fat stores but cannot change individual genetic makeup.

Once a person has expressed this genetic predisposition to gain weight, and for women this occurs most often in the early adult years, the obesity tends to develop increasingly in the middle adult years. The obesity is likely to recur unless major changes that promote health and fitness and a healthy lifestyle are made in lifetime habits and environmental factors.[63] Thus, regular exercise and physical activity needs to be a part of that healthy lifestyle. Although the effects of exercise on weight loss may be minimal in the short term, long-term follow-up studies of both men and women show that those who make regular exercise a part of their long-term lifestyle have dramatically better success at keeping weight off with improved food habits based on moderation and variety.[62]

These study results should encourage middle-aged adult women whose health concerns include regional body fat distribution, especially abdominal body fat, with its association with potential development of chronic disease risks for cardiovascular problems, hypertension, and diabetes. In women, body fat is usually localized in the hips and thighs (*gynoid,* or lower body fat distribution). In middle adult men, body fat is usually localized in the abdominal region (*android,* or upper body fat distribution). However, this sex-related distribution pattern can vary among individual men and women. In both sexes, abdominal body fat tends to increase with age, but, with the reduction of the female sex hormones at menopause, postmenopausal women experience an acceleration of this upper body fat accumulation.

Coronary Heart Disease

Gender differences. Through earlier adult years, a large gender gap exists between men and women in the incidence of cardiovascular disease, with men at much greater risk, developing the view of heart disease as a "man's disease." However, the gap closes rapidly with menopause, and heart disease is the leading cause of death for American women aged fifty years and older, accounting for a large number of the nearly 500,000 deaths of men and women annually. Very few women develop cardiovascular disease before menopause, due to the protective effect of the female sex hormone estrogen. Thus, women develop coronary heart disease at the same rate as men, but six to ten years later. Current research indicates that women with ischemia, deficiency of blood supply to the heart muscle due to functional constriction or obstruction of blood vessels serving this vital tissue, are at the same increased risk for cardiovascular disease mortality as men.[19]

Risk factors. Postmenopausal middle adult women face the same risk factors for cardiovascular disease as do men (review table 13-2). They are just as vulnerable to the blood lipid factors, especially elevated cholesterol and the LDLs carrying cholesterol to the cells, that are now recognized as major risk factors in the development of coronary heart disease. A high level of LDL is an independent risk factor in both men and women, but a high serum triglyceride level is an independent risk factor only in women. Women with diabetes and those who are overweight and hypertensive are at higher risk, and those who smoke compound it much further. The devastating effects of smoking leading to peripheral vascular disease and coronary heart disease are now experienced by women as well as men. Thus, the coronary heart disease risk profile of a woman can be assessed by a few simple indicators: serum cholesterol, blood pressure, serum glucose, weight, and smoking status. The positive approach of planning a healthy lifestyle, as described earlier, will reduce these risk factors and increase general fitness and well-being.

Noninsulin-Dependent Diabetes Mellitus (NIDDM)

Gender differences. NIDDM, the onset of which occurs in adulthood, is closely related in predisposing risk factors for women described for cardiovascular disease. It occurs mainly in postmenopausal middle adult women aged forty-five to sixty and has a greater impact on women than on men, sometimes requiring insulin during the initial treatment period to counteract its degree of impaired glucose tolerance. The reasons for this differing gender impact are not entirely clear. It would seem from current studies that obesity (especially an upper body or abdominal pattern of distribution) and elevated serum lipids (especially triglycerides), combined with a low HDL value and the postmenopausal woman's lack of estrogen, help set the stage for impaired glucose tolerance in middle adult women.[63,64]

Dietary recommendations. The current standard of dietary guidelines for diabetes management of the American Diabetes Association and the American Dietetic Association, which generally follow guidelines of the American Heart Association's "prudent" diet, provide the present basis for individual care of diabetes. Some interesting initial data from recent NIDDM studies, however, document plasma glucose and lipid response to diets that vary from these current standards in the relative amount and type of dietary carbohydrate and fat. Studies have shown a persistent elevation of serum triglycerides, an independent heart disease risk factor for women, with the usual high-carbohydrate/ low-fat ratio of the standard diet guides. Improvement in serum lipid levels has occurred with moderation of dietary fat to include more use of monounsaturated fat. For treatment of middle adults with NIDDM, it would appear that an adjustment of the nutrient ratios may achieve better control of serum glucose and lipids: 1) carbohydrate lowered from a high of 60% to 45–50% of total kilocalories, mostly complex in form, with little, if any, sucrose; 2) fat moderated from 30% to 35% to 40% of total kilocalories, with the small increase in monounsaturated fat; and 3) protein kilocalories remaining the same at 15–20%. Researchers and practitioners agree, however, that any general population guideline must always be applied with reasonable common sense to individuals.

Breast Cancer

Breast cancer is a significant health issue for women. At some time during their lives, mostly in middle adult years, one out of ten American women will develop breast cancer, a rate that has not changed despite current advances in treatment. Diagnosis of breast cancers at earlier stages is achieved through widespread screening. However, researchers agree that only prevention efforts will decrease cancer incidence and prolong survival, because most women with breast cancer do not have a family history or any of the other known risk factors, which include fibrocystic disease, **nulliparity,** or first pregnancy after age thirty. Thus, prevention strategies need to be applied to all women. There is an increasing consensus that obesity and the high-fat American diet are primary risk factors and that weight reduction and maintenance on a low-fat, high-fiber diet provide a valuable and practical strategy for breast cancer prevention. Such long-term maintenance goals require planning for a lifetime of healthy lifestyle.

For some years, a vast body of **epidemiologic** evidence has supported this association of increased dietary fat and subsequent increase in incidence of breast cancer in populations migrating to the United States, but controlled studies to rule out other confounding factors from the analysis are needed. Current studies are examining nutritional, hormonal, and physiologic data in conjunction with dietary and lifestyle change that will clarify these effects for breast cancer prevention.

Osteoporosis

Bone growth and maintenance. The health problem of osteoporosis in women's later adult years has its roots in earlier growth, development, and maintenance of skeletal bone mass. Thus, it provides an excellent example of the importance of the life cycle preventive approach of planning for a healthy lifestyle. Skeletal homeostasis is a sophisticated response to the alternating pattern of the three basic factors involved in building and maintaining bone mass: nutritional state, physical activity, and hormonal status.[53] There is also a strong genetic role in the development of bone mass in women by the age of about twenty-five, independent of calcium and other nutrients, but dietary factors, physical activity, and hormonal factors constantly modulate the genetically predetermined quantity, size, and shape of bone.

Nulliparity
(L *nullus,* none; *parere,* to bring forth, produce) Reproductive status of a woman who has never given birth to a viable child.

Epidemiology
(Gr *epidemios,* prevalent; *-ology,* study) Study of factor determining the frequency and distribution of diseases in population groups.

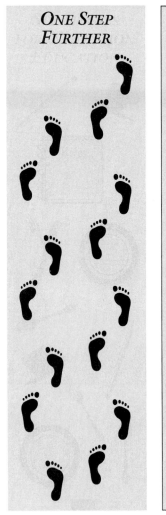

ONE STEP FURTHER

Further Reading

Greene, G.W., and S.R. Rossi. 1998. Stages of change for reducing dietary fat intake over 18 months. *J Am Diet Assoc* 98:529.

Sikand, G. et al. 1998. Medical nutrition therapy lowers serum cholesterol and saves medication costs in men with hypercholesterolemia. *J Am Diet Assoc* 98(8):889.

These authors describe the beneficial effects of reducing dietary fat and cholesterol in middle adults, in both long-term costs of cholesterol-lowering drug use and improved health.

Jordan, V.C. 1998. Designer estrogens. *Scientific American* 279:60.

This article describes how new drugs, so-called designer estrogens, are helping women with health problems during and after menopause in middle adult women.

Kritchevsky, D. 1998. History of recommendations to the public about dietary fat. *J Nutr* 128:449S.

This very interesting article by a pioneer in research and community involvement to develop guidelines for reducing total fat and cholesterol in the American diet describes his experiences and indicates that the general health picture related to coronary heart disease keeps improving.

Polsinelli, M.L. et al. 1998. Plasma carotenoids as biomarkers of fruit and vegetable servings in women. *J Am Diet Assoc* 98(2):194.

Steinmetz, K.A. and J.D. Potter. 1996. Vegetables, fruit, and cancer prevention: A review. *J Am Diet Assoc* 96(10):1027.

These two very helpful articles review the various substances in certain fruits and vegetables that help protect against cancer. Steinmetz and Potter provide a useful review of many of these substances and their mechanisms of action.

Tepper, B.J., and R.M. Nayga. 1998. Awareness of the link between bone disease and calcium intake is associated with higher dietary calcium intake in women aged 50 years and older: Results of the 1991 CSFII-DHKS. *J Am Diet Assoc* 98(2):196.

This brief report centers on the relation of calcium intake and bone disease in middle adult women around menopause, average age sixty-seven, who were subjects in the larger research programs Continuing Survey of Food Intake of Individuals (CSFII) and its companion instrument, the Diet and Health Knowledge Survey (DHKS). Women who were aware of the link between calcium intake and bone disease consumed 76 mg more calcium per day than did women who were unaware of this relationship.

Trabecular

(L *trabes,* a little beam) Small bones in the ends of long bones at joints such as wrist, vertebrae, and hips.

Life cycle bone development. Childhood bone growth is gradual in concert with the child's overall body growth and development, but with puberty a rapid growth period begins. During the healthy adolescent growth spurt of young girls after menarche, under the added stimulus of estrogen secretion of the developing ovaries, large quantities of calcium, between 150 and 350 mg/day, are retained by the skeleton.[53] Calcium absorption efficiency is high during this three- to five-year period, but dietary calcium must also be sufficient to sustain this high retention rate. Peak adult bone mass is reached by about thirty-five years of age, although cortical bone tissue, the hard outer layer, may reach its full mass during the early adult decade of the twenties. The smaller **trabecular** bone tissue completes its development later, at age thirty-five or afterward. These trabecular bones, which are found in the ends of the long arm bones at the wrists, the vertebrae, and the proximal femurs at the hips, are most susceptible to fractures, beginning at menopause. Men may sustain fractures at these same sites, but their fracture rates are very much lower than female rates, largely due to the man's greater bone mass and shorter life span.[53] During the decade before menopause, which now occurs in most North American women in the United States and Canada in their early fifties, bone mass begins to decrease at a very low rate, and level of calcium intake appears to have no major effect on the status of this bone mass. At menopause, the rate of estrogen secretion drops sharply and gradually ceases, a physiologic event that has major impact on the turnover of bone in nearly all women, making them more vulnerable to osteoporosis. If such signs do develop, estrogen replacement therapy may be needed. Continuing an appropriate level of regular exercise during older adult years also helps maintain the bone mass attained in the premenopausal years.

Dietary recommendations. Since the current RDA for calcium for young adults aged nineteen through twenty-four has been raised to 1,200 mg/day, matching the already established allowance for adolescent girls, the increased demand for calcium to meet rapid bone growth during this period should be ample for skeletal bone mass needs. The RDA for calcium for women twenty-five to fifty is set at 800 mg/day, which is sufficient for active women. After menopause, however, rather than the continued 800 mg/day, the calcium intake probably needs to be increased to 1,000 mg/day.[53] Additional calcium supplementation cannot overcome the negative calcium balance that follows the loss of ovarian estrogens. Studies of premenopausal and postmenopausal women suggest that a threshold of calcium intake must be met at the different life cycle stages in order to enhance absorption and retention of calcium, independent of other factors. In short, women who practice good nutrition as a healthy lifetime habit, including not only adequate amounts of calcium but also other bone-building nutrients, such as protein, phosphorus, and vitamin D, can develop optimal bone mass during adolescence and young adult years and can maintain that bone mass at a higher level during their postmenopausal years. Planning for a healthy lifestyle is the middle adult woman's health-promotion, disease-prevention approach to osteoporosis, as well as the other health issues of women discussed.

Summary

Middle adult health and wellness for both men and women depend on a healthy lifestyle throughout this vital period of life. Although genetic factors play a role in determining level of health, lifestyle choices are the major determinant of well-being and the onset and severity of chronic diseases that begin to appear in middle age. Components of a healthy lifestyle include a sound diet, with attention to risk factors associated with excess fat, cholesterol, sodium, and body weight; regular physical exercise; stress management; smoking cessation; and avoidance of alcohol abuse. Addictive behaviors related to cigarette smoking and alcohol abuse harm health and require special treatment programs. Chronic diseases of the cardiovascular system, hypertension, diabetes mellitus, and cancer have all been related to one or more of these lifestyle behaviors. A number of health programs have been developed at the national and community levels to heighten public awareness and encourage appropriate behavioral change. These public and professional activities include hospital-based community programs, health maintenance organization (HMO) programs, worksite wellness programs, health clubs, community screening programs, and health fairs.

A comparison of the nutrient energy needs of middle adult men and women reflects their gender differences in body composition and size, as well as in physiologic function. Women encounter gender-based health issues in their middle adult years, including weight concerns and health problems such as heart disease, diabetes, breast cancer, and osteoporosis.

Review Questions

1. Describe various approaches to middle adult health promotion. Which do you think has the greatest application to current health issues? Why?
2. List and discuss five components of a healthy lifestyle. How does each influence risk of the major chronic diseases? Develop a healthful one-day food plan for a middle adult of your choice, indicating daily activities that would influence the meal pattern or food selection.
3. Describe three addictive behaviors that harm middle adult health. In each case, outline an appropriate treatment program, with special attention to nutritional needs.
4. During the middle adult years, how do women's nutritional needs differ from those of men? Account for each gender difference.
5. Describe the gender differences in bone mass growth and development over the life cycle that create a greater risk for middle adult women of developing osteoporosis.
6. Critique the need for "menopausal nutritional products."

NUTRITION AND THE AGING ADULT

Eleanor D. Schlenker

≋ ≋ ≋ ≋ ≋ ≋ ≋ ≋ ≋ ≋ ≋

Basic Concepts

❑ *People sixty years of age and older—the fastest growing segment of the population—sometimes need nutritional support services to maintain healthy independent living.*

❑ *In most individuals, aging brings about a gradual decline in normal physiologic functions.*

❑ *Energy needs decrease with age, but protein, vitamin, and mineral needs do not decrease and may even increase, making nutrient density important in meal planning.*

❑ *Vitamins and minerals are the nutrients most likely to be lacking in an older person's diet; they also are most adversely affected by multiple medications, both over-the-counter and prescription drugs.*

❑ *Numerous social, physiologic, and economic factors influence food and nutrient intake in older people.*

❑ *Many of the physiologic changes and chronic diseases associated with aging may be prevented or postponed by a healthy lifestyle that includes an appropriate diet, continued physical activity, and not smoking.*

*T*he number of older people in our society and around the world is increasing rapidly. One in eight Americans is age sixty-five or older. By the year 2030, it will be one in five.[1] The fastest growing segment within the older population is the eighty-five and older group. These shifts in population have far-reaching implications for our society, from public policy regarding health care costs and the need for health care reform to increasing efforts by food manufacturers to develop preprepared products that are attractive to older consumers. This increase in the number of older people presents both a challenge and a responsibility to the health professional. Food and nutrition programs that promote continuing physical and mental well-being in healthy older people will become increasingly important. Specialized nutrition services designed to maintain the highest possible level of independence and functional capacity in older people with declining health must be developed.

In this chapter, we will look at the changing nutrient needs of the aging population. We will explore the environmental, personal, and health factors that influence their nutrient needs and physical well-being. We will seek effective intervention strategies, keeping in mind the individual differences, resources, and needs of each older person.

GROWTH AND DIVERSITY IN THE OLDER POPULATION ≋

Population Trends

In the United States, age sixty-five—the typical age of retirement—is often used as a benchmark to characterize the older population, but **chronologic age** is a poor measure of physical health, mental alertness, or zest for life. Also, individuals continue to change as they age, so that sixty-five-year-olds differ markedly from ninety-year-olds. To evaluate these differences and recognize when they occur, United States census reports group older people into three age categories.

- Those age sixty-five to seventy-four are the young-old.
- Those age seventy-five to eighty-four are the aged.
- Those age eighty-five and older are the oldest-old.[2]

As the over-sixty-five group increases in number, it also will increase in diversity. Men and women age eighty-five and over are more likely to have serious health problems and depend on others for grocery shopping or meal preparation, whereas the young-old may still be employed. At younger ages, the numbers of men and women are about equal, but at older ages women outnumber men. Today the older population is predominantly white, but African American, Native American, Asian American, and Hispanic elderly will make up an increasing proportion of the over-sixty-five segment as **life expectancy** continues to rise in those groups.[2]

Changes in Life Expectancy

Basis for the changes. Although life expectancy has increased at all ages since 1900, the most dramatic increase has occurred in infancy and childhood. For men, life expectancy at birth has increased from forty-eight years to seventy-two years since 1900; for women, life expectancy has increased from fifty-one to seventy-nine years.[2] However, life expectancy at age sixty-five has increased only four years in men and seven years in women over this time period, despite improvements in medical care and the control of infectious disease. This suggests that the growth of the older population does not reflect an increase in the maximum life span but, instead, indicates the extended life span of those who in the past would have died in infancy or childhood.

Influencing factors. Gains in life expectancy have not been equal across all population groups. Women can expect to live longer than men do, and white persons can expect to live longer than black persons can. Increased smoking among women may reduce their life expectancy in future years, as death rates from lung cancer continue to climb and now exceed death rates from breast cancer. Level of education and income influences both self-care and accessibility to health care services, and low education and income levels contribute to the lower life expectancy of black Americans.

Causes of death. The leading causes of death in the United States are heart disease, cancer, and **cerebral hemorrhage** (stroke).[2] All three causes are related to degenerative changes associated with aging and personal lifestyle. In contrast, the leading cause of death in 1900 was infectious diseases, such as pneumonia, now controlled with antibiotic drugs. A healthy lifestyle that includes an appropriate diet, limited amounts of or no alcohol, no smoking, and regular exercise will delay the onset of chronic disease and will improve the health status of the expanding aging population.

Socioeconomic Characteristics of the Aging Population

At one time, old age was associated with poor health, illness, and dependency. This view led to the assumption that most older people live in nursing homes. In fact, 95% of people over age sixty-four live in the community with their spouses, other family members or friends, or alone; only 5% live in long-term care facilities.[2] The differences in life expectancy within the older population contribute to differences in living arrangements. Most older men are married and live with their wives. In contrast, half of all older women

Chronologic age
Age of an individual based on the number of years lived.

Life expectancy
Average remaining years a person of a given age, sex, and race can expect to live, based on statistical population averages.

Cerebral hemorrhage
Rupture of an artery in the brain; also referred to as cerebrovascular accident or stroke.

are widows, and many live alone. Widowed white women tend to maintain individual households, whereas widowed Hispanic and African American women are more likely to live with other family members.[2]

Older women, older people living alone, and people age eighty-five and over are more likely to have low incomes and poor diets. Usually, couples have a more adequate income than single individuals, and they have more money to spend on food. Black and Hispanic elderly people are more likely than white elderly people to have incomes below the **poverty line.** Government programs such as food stamps or **congregate meals** can help those with limited money for groceries.

Poverty line
Minimum income required to provide the basic necessities of food, clothing, and shelter for an individual or a family as determined by a U.S. government agency.

Congregate meals
Group meals for older adults served in a social setting in the community and funded by Title III-C of the Older Americans Act.

PHYSIOLOGIC CHANGES IN AGING ≋

How and Why Do Physiologic Changes Occur?

Definition of the aging process. Numerous theories have been developed to explain the degenerative biologic and physiologic changes that begin about age thirty. In fact, no single theory or cause can explain the mechanisms that lead to changes as people age, just as no single theory can explain the development of a particular disease, such as cancer. The pattern and sequence of aging changes are always the same, but the rate at which these changes occur differs significantly from one person to another. Both genetic and environmental factors influence the rate of aging. Individuals with long-lived parents are more likely to survive beyond age seventy. Environmental factors, such as exposure to toxic chemicals or level of nutrition, influence the rate of physiologic aging and the length of life in experimental animals. In a later section, we will examine the benefits of an appropriate diet and exercise pattern on the physical health and life span of men and women.

Effects of the aging process. Aging changes occurring in body cells and tissues influence the nutritional health and physical well-being of older people. Among the cell types that continue to divide throughout life, such as skin cells, the rate of division slows with advancing age. Highly differentiated cells in the brain, muscles, and kidneys do not continue to divide throughout life but do undergo functional changes with time, and some cells die. As a result, organ systems become less efficient as fewer cells and less effective cells remain to carry on normal function.

Age-related changes in physiologic function were evaluated in the men participating in the Baltimore Longitudinal Study of Aging (BLSA).[3] This study has been ongoing for more than thirty years, and each man returns every two years for reevaluation. This makes it possible for researchers to observe not only what changes occur but also when they occur, and to compare men of different ages. The loss of function in important organ systems that occurred in these men between ages thirty and eighty is presented in figure 14-1. Notice that the amount of loss was influenced by the degree of coordination required among organ systems. Nerve conduction velocity, which involves only one organ system, exhibited less change than resting cardiac output, which requires both neural and muscular input. As a system becomes more complex, impairment becomes more obvious. An older person may walk with comparative ease on a level surface but find it difficult to climb stairs. Nevertheless, many older people get along quite well on a day-to-day basis.

Changes in Physiologic Function

Several organ systems are particularly important to the study of nutrition in older people. Loss of cognitive function or the ability to self-feed can lead to weight loss and poor nutritional status in the elderly. The cardiovascular and renal systems are fundamental to the delivery of nutrients to all tissues in the body and the removal of waste products. Changes in the gastrointestinal tract influence the availability and absorption of nutrients. In the following section, we will review some of the aging changes occurring in these organ systems.

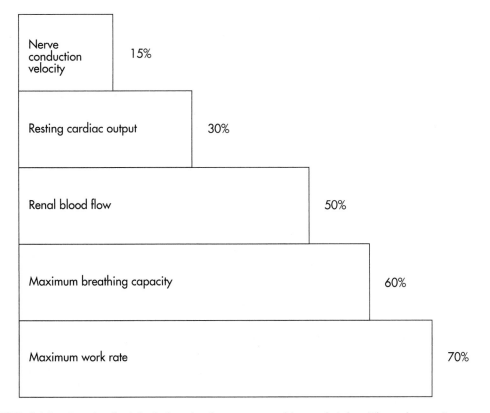

FIG. 14-1   Loss in physiologic function between ages thirty and eighty. These changes in physiologic function were observed in men participating in the BLSA.

Data from Shock, N.W., et al. 1984. *Normal human aging: The Baltimore Longitudinal Study of Aging*, NIH Pub No 84-2450. Washington, DC: U.S. Government Printing Office.

Brain and neural control.   Both structural and biochemical changes contribute to alterations in brain function in older people. There is general agreement that brain cells are lost with advancing age, although it appears that remaining cells establish new connections with each other to continue the transmission of nerve impulses and preserve a high level of cognitive function. Decreased blood flow to the brain as a result of atherosclerotic vascular changes contributes to a decline in cerebral function. Biochemical alterations in the aging brain sometimes lead to decreased synthesis of **neurotransmitters** (e.g., dopamine, serotonin, and acetylcholine) required for the conduction of nerve impulses. **Parkinson's disease,** a disorder occurring among older people that results in muscle rigidity, tremors, and shuffling gait, is believed to relate to the altered metabolism of dopamine.

Loss of brain cells, changes in the physical arrangement of brain cells, or reduced blood flow is associated with progressive and irreversible **dementia.** A particular type of dementia, **senile dementia of the Alzheimer type (SDAT),** results in rapid deterioration of cognitive function and the capacity for self-care. Patients forget how to use eating utensils and may lose the ability to swallow. Examination of tissues obtained from SDAT patients at autopsy has revealed above-normal levels of aluminum; however, there is no convincing evidence that the use of aluminum cooking utensils leads to the development of SDAT.

Cardiovascular system.   Age-related changes in the heart and circulatory system involve both structure and function. The work load of the heart increases because of the increased resistance to blood flow caused by atherosclerotic deposition and the loss of elasticity of the major arteries. At the same time, the heart's pumping action is diminished as the heart muscle loses strength. Consequently, less blood is pumped with each

Neurotransmitters
(Gr *neuron*, nerve; L *trans*, through, across; *missio*, a sending) Chemical substances, including compounds such as serotonin and acetylcholine, hormones, and several amino acids, that function as essential chemical messengers for sending or inhibiting nerve impulses across the synapses of connecting nerve cells.

Parkinson's disease
Neurological disorder described by English physician James Parkinson (1755–1824) and characterized by tremors, muscular rigidity, and abnormally decreased motor function and mobility; appears to relate to decreased synthesis of dopamine, a neurotransmitter.

Dementia
(L *de* + *mens*, mind) Progressive organic mental disorder causing changes in personality, disorientation, deterioration in intellectual function, and loss of memory and judgment; dementia caused by drug overdose, electrolyte or fluid imbalance, or insulin shock is reversed on treatment; dementia caused by injury or degenerative changes in brain tissue is not reversible.

Senile dementia of the Alzheimer type (SDAT)
Type of senile dementia first described by German physician Alois Alzheimer (1864–1915); causes progressive, irreversible degenerative changes in the brain, resulting in loss of neuromuscular function and mental capacity.

Cardiac output
Total amount of blood pumped by the heart per minute (average amount is 5 L).

Glomerular filtration rate
Measure of the amount of blood filtered by each kidney nephron per unit of time (ml/min).

Atrophic gastritis
Chronic inflammation of the stomach, causing damage to the mucosal lining and reduced secretion of hydrochloric acid and sometimes intrinsic factor; loss of intrinsic factor and the inability to absorb vitamin B_{12} leads to pernicious anemia.

heartbeat (**cardiac output**), and the flow of blood through the coronary arteries that supply nutrients to the heart muscle itself is decreased. Because of these changes, the aged heart is less able to adjust to physiologic stress and inappropriate exercise.

Changes in cardiovascular function contribute to the age-related rise in blood pressure observed in both sexes. Hypertension is a significant medical and nutritional problem among older people. Older African Americans are more likely to have hypertension than older white or Mexican American elderly. In the Third National Health and Nutrition Examination Survey (NHANES III), 72% of the African American elderly had elevated blood pressures, as compared with 53% of the white elderly and 55% of the Mexican American elderly.[4] Effective management of hypertension can involve weight loss, some degree of sodium restriction, regular exercise, and reduced alcohol intake.

Renal system. Kidney function changes in most people as they age because of a loss of cells and a 30% decrease in blood flow to the kidneys.[3] Because the **glomerular filtration rate** is slowed, it takes longer to remove drug metabolites or metabolic waste products from the blood. Thus, excessive protein intakes resulting in high blood urea nitrogen levels or megadoses of water-soluble vitamins should be avoided. The aging kidney is less able to concentrate urine, so a liberal fluid intake is essential.

Water balance. Fluid regulation and water balance are important matters in older people. Dehydration leads to seriously elevated blood sodium and potassium levels and is an ever-present danger in bed-bound elderly people with low fluid intake. Water balance is also a problem in relatively healthy elderly people. A study measuring fluid intake in younger and older people reported that the older subjects had a diminished sense of thirst.[5] After six hours of fluid deprivation, not only did the older people have less feeling of thirst, but they also drank less water than was needed for fluid replacement once water became available. This problem with water intake is compounded by the fact that the older kidney is less able to conserve water and reduce the amount of water lost as urine. Therefore, records of fluid intake become very important in the care of debilitated older people with limited access to water.

Gastrointestinal function. There is little evidence to support the idea that advancing age results in dysfunction of the stomach, small intestine, and colon.[6] However, gastrointestinal discomforts, including nausea, heartburn, and constipation, increase in frequency. Such discomforts often relate to feelings of anxiety, side effects of drugs, or poor eating and bowel habits. Gastrointestinal distress does not necessarily indicate nutrient malabsorption.[6] People with no discomfort may absorb nutrients poorly, whereas others with persistent distress may absorb nutrients normally.

Digestive enzymes must be present in sufficient amounts to support the breakdown of food into the nutrient form that is absorbed. For the most part, a lack of digestive enzymes does not impair absorption in healthy older people. Because digestive enzymes are normally secreted at levels substantially above what is required, even reduced levels are usually sufficient to break down the protein, fat, and carbohydrate consumed. One alteration in digestive function that does occur is reduced secretion of hydrochloric acid caused by a chronic inflammation of the lining of the stomach known as **atrophic gastritis.** In a group of community-living Boston elderly,[7] 40% of those above age eighty had atrophic gastritis. This alteration in the normal acid environment of the stomach can interfere with the absorption of iron, calcium, and vitamin B_{12}. Low levels of the enzyme lactase have been associated with lactose intolerance and reduced intakes of dairy foods by some older people. Age-related changes in the absorption of particular vitamins and minerals will be discussed in later sections.

NUTRITION AND THE LIFE SPAN ≋

Since antiquity, people have been searching for potions to preserve health and prolong life. Ponce de Leon came to the New World seeking the "fountain of youth." Francis Bacon, who lived from 1591 to 1626, recommended the scientific evaluation of the relationship between diet and longevity. Unfortunately, Bacon's recommendations for research are only beginning to receive attention.

Animal Studies

Researchers have evaluated the influence of diet on aging and the length of life in experimental animals. A general finding is that animals given diets restricted in kilocalories yet adequate in protein, vitamins, and minerals live 40% longer than animals given unlimited access to food.[8] More important, however, degenerative changes associated with the aging process, such as increases in plasma cholesterol levels and decreases in immune function, are delayed in the restricted animals. Also, the incidence of chronic diseases, such as renal disease, cardiac disease, and cancer, are lower for the restricted animals. Through these studies, researchers may learn more about the mechanisms that control the aging process and the way that nutrition influences these mechanisms.

Human Studies

Limited information now exists regarding the influence of lifelong dietary habits on health and longevity. Following an individual over time—in a **longitudinal study**—is necessary to evaluate the influence of diet and lifestyle on physiologic aging and the appearance of chronic disease. Recent studies have looked at nutrition and health habits in older people in the United States and elsewhere and have related these findings to long-term health and well-being. We will review several examples of these studies.

California study. An ongoing study that began with 7,000 adults living in Alameda, California,[9] examined the influence of the following health practices—adequate sleep, regular meals (including breakfast), desirable body weight, not smoking, limited or no use of alcohol, and regular physical activity—on life expectancy and physical health. Not only did the men and women with better health practices have a longer life expectancy than those with poorer health practices, but they also were in better physical health. The people who were following six or seven health practices were only half as likely to be disabled in later life as those who followed three or fewer health practices. These patterns continued to age seventy and beyond. The findings from the Alameda Health Study suggest that nutrition education and intervention activities can benefit those who are already old.

Georgia centenarian study. This study evaluated the food patterns of elderly people in Georgia, including twenty-two centenarians.[10] Researchers reported that only 5% of the centenarians had to avoid any particular foods because of gastrointestinal distress; however, 37% had trouble biting or chewing certain foods. Their mean energy intake was 1,581 kcal, and 42% came from fat. It is interesting to note that all of these people had stable body weights throughout adulthood, despite their high fat intakes. Continued observation of this group will provide insight as to the dietary needs and preferences of individuals in extreme old age.

Mediterranean countries. Recent attention has been given to the regions of Crete, Greece, and southern Italy, where the rates of stroke and heart disease have been among the lowest in the world. The traditional Mediterranean diet is a plant-based diet with a high ratio of monounsaturated to saturated fat; liberal intakes of legumes, cereal foods, fruits, and vegetables; and low to moderate intakes of meat and dairy products. In recent years, however, the use of red meat and animal fats has increased nearly sixfold, and intake of beans has fallen by 80%.[11] Among 182 older Greek villagers followed over a five-year period,[11] the death rate was only 26% in the group that continued to follow the traditional diet but rose to 45% in those who increased their intakes of total fat and saturated fat and reduced their intake of plant foods. The Five a Day public health initiative to increase the use of fruits and vegetables in the United States supports the benefits of the Mediterranean diet.

Body weight studies. In younger age groups, the greater the deviation from average or recommended weight for a person of a given age, height, and sex, the greater the risk of death. Recent research conducted with more than 11,500 nurses[12] and with male Harvard alumni[13] indicated that, for middle-aged individuals, a body mass index (BMI) below the desirable range carries benefits for health and reduces mortality. However, the association between overweight, chronic disease, and mortality at older ages is less clear. A complicating factor when evaluating the influence of body weight on length of life in older people is the very high mortality among those who are severely underweight. An important consideration is the basis for the underweight. In other words, was the person always

Longitudinal study
Study of persons or populations that occurs over a long period of time and measures the effects of specific factors on the aging process and incidence and course of disease.

lean and active, is the person underweight because he or she smokes, or has the person lost weight as a result of declining health or disease? It appears that people who are lean and active at age fifty, and neither gain nor lose weight thereafter, have the lowest cardiovascular risk.[14] Individuals at heavier weights could benefit from increased exercise to assist in modest weight reduction. However, a recent review of nearly 5,000 people age sixty-five and older[14] found that weight loss after age fifty exceeding 10% of body weight is associated with increased frailty, physical disability, and poor health status.

English studies of early nutrition. Records from several English communities[15] have made it possible to evaluate the health status of middle-aged men and women based on their weight at birth. It appears that babies having a low birth weight as a result of poor growth in utero rather than premature birth are at increased risk as adults. This relationship between low birth weight and heightened risk of hypertension, noninsulin-dependent diabetes, and coronary heart disease is not related to smoking, obesity, or social class. A lack of nutrients during fetal development leads to permanent alterations in cholesterol metabolism and insulin patterns that contribute to increased risk. This finding emphasizes the need for optimum diets in pregnancy.

NUTRIENT REQUIREMENTS OF OLDER PEOPLE ≈

Recommended Dietary Allowances

The Recommended Dietary Allowances (RDAs)[16] for older people remain controversial. Because few studies have examined the nutrient requirements of elderly people, the RDAs for people over age fifty have been extrapolated from those for younger adults. Various issues relating to older people influence nutrient requirements and are described in the following sections.

Heterogeneity of older adults. For all but four nutrients, the Dietary Reference Intakes are the same for younger adults, ages thirty-one to fifty and older adults age fifty-one and over (see table 14-1). These recommendations do not address the fact that people fifty to sixty years old have different needs than even healthy adults eighty to ninety years old. For some nutrients, recent recommendations have established categories for individuals ages fifty-one to seventy and ages seventy-one and over.[17] Even within these age categories, older people differ greatly, as aging changes occur at different rates in different people.

Physiologic changes. Aging brings about changes in the relative proportions of body muscle and fat and organ system function. Changes in gastric secretions influence di-

TABLE 14-1 *Differences in Dietary Reference Intakes Between Younger and Older Adults*

Age/Gender	Iron (mg)	Vitamin B$_6$ (mg)	Calcium (mg)	Vitamin D (μg)
Women				
31 to 50 years	15	1.3	1,000	5
51 to 70 years	10	1.5	1,200	10
71 years and over	10	1.5	1,200	15
Men				
31 to 50 years	10	1.3	1,000	5
51 to 70 years	10	1.7	1,200	10
71 years and over	10	1.7	1,200	15

Adapted from Food and Nutrition Board. 1998. *Dietary Reference Intakes: Recommended levels for individual intake.* Washington, DC: National Academy of Sciences.

gestion and absorption and may increase the need for certain nutrients. Estrogen withdrawal following menopause alters calcium absorption rates and bone metabolism. Reduced ability of the renal system to excrete waste contraindicates excessive use of nutrient supplements.

Disease interactions. Chronic diseases influence nutrient requirements as a result of the disease itself and the side effects of the drugs prescribed in treatment. **Diuretics** used to treat hypertension can deplete the body of potassium, vitamin B_6, folate, and zinc. One researcher[18] has advocated the development of formulas based on disease complications and prescription drug use to establish nutritional risk and recommended intakes in older persons.

The current recommendations for adults ages fifty and under and fifty-one and older differ for iron, calcium, vitamin D, and vitamin B_6 (review table 14-1).[17,19] The iron allowance drops from 15 mg to 10 mg for women over age fifty as menstruation and the associated iron loss come to an end. Physiologic changes related to increased need for calcium, vitamin D, and vitamin B_6 will be discussed in a later section.

Energy Requirements

Energy needs decrease with age in most people based on changes in the resting energy expenditure (REE) and physical activity. In an older sedentary adult, the REE makes up 60–75% of the total energy expenditure (TEE).[20] Physical activity plays a major role in maintaining energy balance in the older person, and the kilocalories expended vary according to individual activity patterns.

Resting energy expenditure (REE). Sex, age, body size, thyroid status, and body composition influence the REE, but the major influence is the amount of lean body mass. Women at all ages have lower resting energy needs per unit of body height and weight than men, because they have a higher proportion of body fat and a lower proportion of lean body mass. On the average, REE decreases about 24% in men and 15% in women between the ages of twenty and sixty as lean body mass is lost and body fat accrues.[20] Data from the Baltimore Longitudinal Study of Aging (BLSA)(see p. 353) indicate that the REE continues to decline beyond age sixty as the loss of muscle continues.[20] Decreases in the REE in later life generally are not related to impaired thyroid function.

Physical activity. Regular exercise and physical training are being recommended for older adults in relation to energy expenditure, cardiovascular fitness, and preservation of muscle. Among the men in the BLSA,[21] energy expended in physical activity declined most sharply at younger ages rather than older ages. Daily energy expenditure decreased by 40 kcal between ages thirty-five and forty-four, 17 kcal between ages fifty-five and sixty-four, and 24 kcal between ages seventy-five and eighty-four. The decrease in energy expenditure in middle age no doubt contributes to the weight gain that often occurs over that period. Endurance training, such as walking several hours each week, leads to a measurable decrease in body fat, an improved abdominal-hip ratio, and decreased cardiovascular risk.

Strength training appears to be very beneficial for older adults. Not only does strength training increase energy expenditure by as much as 15%,[22] but it also prevents the loss of both muscle mass and muscle strength. These losses are associated with falls and **functional disability** in older adults. Strength training has been shown to restore lost muscle by increasing the size of existing muscle fibers. A strength training program with elderly people up to the age of ninety-six resulted in a 9% increase in leg muscle area and improved the ability of these individuals to walk without help.[22]

Recommended energy intakes. This RDA groups all people over the age of fifty, based on the idea that a continuing decrease in energy expenditure is neither inevitable nor desirable (table 14-2).[16] Current research, however, suggests that the current recommended energy intake may not be appropriate, particularly in men. A recent study conducted at the Human Nutrition Research Center in Boston[23] evaluated the TEE of fifteen healthy older men with an average age of sixty-nine and a body weight of 79 kg. The current RDA underestimated the energy requirement of these older men by 390 kcal. The men expended more energy carrying out routine physical tasks related to daily living

Diuretics
(Gr *diouretikos,* promoting urine) Drugs that decrease the reabsorption of water in the renal tubule and increase the loss of water through the urine; some types of diuretics induce loss of body sodium and potassium along with water; often used to treat hypertension.

Strength training
Type of training that involves generating muscle force against a resistance, as occurs in lifting or lowering weights; can help prevent loss of muscle mass or help restore muscle that has been lost.

Functional disability
Disability that interferes with activities of daily living, such as bathing, dressing, shopping, preparing meals, and eating.

TABLE 14-2   *Recommended Energy Intakes for Persons over Age Fifty*

	Women	Men
Body weight (kg)*	65	77
Body height (cm)*	160	173
Kcal/kg body weight	30	30
Kcal/day	1,900	2,300
Range of intake (variation of 20%)	1,520–2,280	1,840–2,760

Modified from Food and Nutrition Board, National Research Council. 1989. *Recommended Dietary Allowances.* 10th ed. Washington, DC: National Academy Press.
*Body weight and height are the median values of the U.S. population of this age as reported in NHANES II; the use of these values as reference values does not imply that the height-to-weight ratios are ideal.

than was assumed. Moving about seems to require more effort in older people with reduced muscle coordination. In contrast, a similar study carried out with ten healthy elderly women[24] with an average age of seventy-four and a body weight of 59 kg indicated that the current RDA is an appropriate estimate of energy expenditure in older women. However, the women studied were five years older than the men and may have been less physically active. Age and sex may influence energy metabolism differently in men than in women.

Problems with low energy intake. Many older people have energy intakes well below the recommended amounts. In NHANES III[25] **mean** energy intakes were 2,110 kcal/day and 1,578 kcal/day, respectively, for the men and women sixty to sixty-nine years of age. For the men and women ages eighty and older, energy intakes dropped to 1,776 kcal/day and 1,329 kcal/day, respectively. Black and Hispanic elderly people had lower energy intakes than their white counterparts in all age categories. Energy intake strongly influences intakes of vitamins and minerals. Among 691 older people in Boston,[26] those with energy intakes below recommended levels were more likely to consume inadequate amounts of vitamin B_6, folate, calcium, and zinc.

Protein Requirement

Protein needs of adults. Even well-nourished adults appear to lose body protein as a function of age. Total body nitrogen decreases from 1,320 g in the average young adult to 1,070 g in the average older adult.[27] Skeletal muscle contributes the major portion of the protein that is lost, with lesser amounts coming from vital organs, such as the heart or liver. Muscle mass makes up 45% of body weight in the young adult but only 27% of body weight beyond age seventy.

The change in body nitrogen content over adulthood has led to various interpretations of the protein requirement of older people. A decrease in skeletal muscle and organ mass could reduce the need for protein and amino acids for maintenance of remaining tissues. On the other hand, an inadequate intake of nitrogen could be responsible for the observed loss in body nitrogen. Recent work[22] suggests that a lack of physical activity in middle and older age contributes to the loss of body muscle, although inadequate levels of dietary protein would add to this loss.

Evaluation of protein requirements. The method used to evaluate protein requirements in older adults is the nitrogen balance method. Nitrogen balance studies determine the amount of protein that must be consumed to replace **obligatory nitrogen losses.** Obligatory nitrogen losses include cells lost from the skin, hair, and gastrointestinal tract, along with the nitrogen-containing products of protein metabolism. The balance method measures the ability of older individuals to effectively use the protein they are eating.

A recent study evaluating nitrogen balance in twelve older people ranging in age from fifty-six to eighty years[28] indicated that the current RDA for protein (0.8 g/kg body weight) may not be adequate to achieve optimum protein status in older people (see fig. 14-2). The

Mean
Mathematical term for the average of a group of numbers.

Obligatory nitrogen losses
Lowest levels of nitrogen excretion that can be reached by an individual despite all body conservation mechanisms.

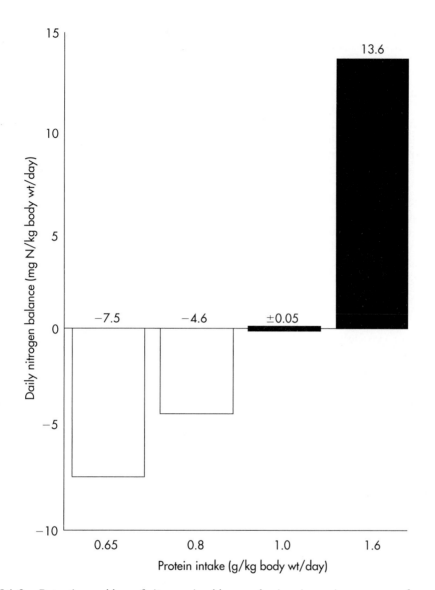

FIG. 14-2 Retention and loss of nitrogen in older people given increasing amounts of egg protein. The level of protein required for nitrogen balance has been calculated to be 1.0 g per kg of body weight.

From Campbell, W.W., et al. 1994. Increased protein requirements in elderly people: New data and retrospective assessments, *Am J Clin Nutr* 60:501; Uauv, R., N.S. Scrimshaw, and V.R. Young. 1978. Human protein requirements: Nitrogen balance response to graded levels of egg protein in elderly men and women. *Am J Clin Nutr* 31:779.

group given 0.8 g/kg body weight were in **negative nitrogen balance** (depleting their body stores) over the study period. In contrast, those given 1.6 g/kg body weight (two times the current RDA) were storing protein. The researchers[28] concluded that older people require 1.0 g/kg body weight to remain in nitrogen balance. If this is true, the current RDA for protein, even good-quality protein, is not adequate to assure positive protein status in many older adults.

Factors influencing protein requirements. Various conditions common to older people influence protein requirements. Low-grade infections, such as infections of the urinary tract and inflammation caused by osteoarthritis, result in a loss of body protein stores

Negative nitrogen balance
Situation in which the amount of nitrogen consumed is not sufficient to replace the amount of nitrogen lost through all excretory routes, resulting in a net loss of body nitrogen.

Corticosteroid hormones
(L *corticix*, bark, shell) Steroid hormones produced in the outer region (cortex) of the adrenal glands in response to stimulus by the adrenocorticotropic hormone (ACTH) from the pituitary gland or a synthetic derivative. These compounds affect carbohydrate, fat, and protein metabolism and include glucocorticoids, which act on glucose metabolism, and mineralcorticoids, which act on electrolyte (Na+) concentration and fluid-electrolyte balance.

as a result of the release and action of the **corticosteroid hormones.** Sufficient kilocalories are needed to allow the efficient use of dietary protein for tissue growth and repair. When kilocalories are limited, protein may be used for energy. The inability of some older people to maintain nitrogen balance on what would seem to be adequate levels of protein may relate to the energy content of their diet. The recommended energy intake of people over age fifty is 30 kcal/kg body weight;[16] however, dietary surveys[26] of healthy elderly people indicate that intakes are as low as 22 to 25 kcal/kg body weight. Older people participating in weight training need a protein intake of at least 1.0 g/kg body weight.[22]

Protein-energy malnutrition (PEM). Older people with debilitating diseases, such as congestive heart failure, often have low nutrient reserves and are particularly vulnerable to overt malnutrition. However, it appears that the protein status of apparently healthy older individuals can show significant change with short periods of inadequate intake. After only nine weeks on a low-protein diet (0.45 g/kg body weight), previously well-nourished older women demonstrated losses in lean body mass, muscle strength, and immune response.[29] PEM can be difficult to identify in an aged population, because assessment standards specific to older people have not been developed. Also, chronic diseases can bring about physiologic changes that interfere with nutritional evaluation. Fluid retention associated with cardiac failure can mask a loss in body weight.

Protein intake. Protein intake is adequate in many older Americans, but limited money for food or poor oral status, which makes chewing difficult, can lower intake. Both men and women ages eighty and older consume less protein than their counterparts ages sixty to sixty-nine.[25] African American and Mexican American elderly consume less protein than white elderly of the same age and sex. About half of all African American and Mexican American men over age sixty-nine eat less than the current RDA for protein, whereas most white men of that age consume at least the current RDA. Most white and black women ages eighty and over do not meet the RDA for protein. At greatest risk are those who are consuming inadequate levels of both protein and energy.

VITAMIN REQUIREMENTS OF OLDER PEOPLE ≈

Fat-Soluble Vitamins

Vitamin A. Age does not increase the requirement for vitamin A or reduce its absorption. In fact, vitamin A might be more easily absorbed by older people than younger people. Low serum vitamin A levels usually related to low intake and respond to dietary improvement; however, questions have been raised about the safety of long-term use of concentrated vitamin A supplements by the elderly. Healthy older people in Boston who took vitamin A supplements containing over 10,000 IU (about two times the RDA) for at least five years had elevated levels of vitamin A and certain enzymes associated with possible liver damage.[30] Dietary intakes of vitamin A are related to race and ethnic background. NHANES III[25] reported that about half of the white elderly met the RDA for vitamin A. In contrast, nearly half of the African American and Mexican American elderly consumed *less than* 60% of the RDA. Dietary intake can be influenced by income, since dark green and deep yellow vegetables high in beta-carotene (provitamin A) tend to be expensive, particularly in the winter months.

Vitamin E. Recent reports are associating high intakes of vitamin E with enhanced immune function in older people[31] and improved cognitive status in patients with SDAT.[32] However, further study is required before intakes in excess of the RDA can be recommended. Currently, dietary intakes of vitamin E fall below the RDA for many older people. In white men and women above age sixty, the **median** vitamin E intake is about 75% of the RDA.[25] African American and Mexican American elderly have a median intake of only 50% of the RDA. On the other hand, many older people routinely consume vitamin E supplements at levels 50 to 100 times the RDA. At this time, there is no reported evidence of toxicity resulting from megadoses of vitamin E; however, long-term intakes without medical supervision is unwise.

Vitamin D. The vitamin D status of older people is less than optimal. Dietary sources make only a limited contribution to the vitamin D requirement. In North America and

Median
Middle value in a series of numbers, so that half of the numbers are below the median and half of the numbers are above.

Europe, the average vitamin D intake is about 2.5 ug[33] (the former RDA was 5 ug[16]). Serum vitamin D levels are lower in winter, emphasizing the importance of sunlight in meeting body needs; however, age-related changes in the skin reduce the older person's ability to synthesize vitamin D. Appropriate levels of either dietary vitamin D or sun exposure offer some protection against loss of bone and possible bone fractures in elderly people when calcium is also consumed at recommended levels. Lack of vitamin D decreases calcium absorption and subsequently increases serum parathyroid hormone (PTH), causing a mobilization of calcium from the bone. In one study, older women who raised their vitamin D intake to 700 IU per day[34] suppressed this rise in PTH, which occurs in winter months when sunlight exposure is minimal. Homebound elderly with little or no exposure to sunlight are especially likely to be deficient in vitamin D. Based on current evidence showing the importance of vitamin D to bone health, the Food and Nutrition Board has set a new adequate intake[17] of 10 ug (400 IU) for men and women ages fifty-one to seventy years and 15 ug (600 IU) for men and women over age seventy who have limited exposure to sunlight.

Both fluid and nonfat dry milk are rich in calcium and fortified with vitamin D. Older adults having a cup of milk at each meal and one at bedtime will meet their suggested intakes for both calcium and vitamin D. (One quart of milk supplies about 1,200 mg calcium and 400 IU vitamin D.) In light of the known toxicity of vitamin D and the deleterious effect on bone of toxic doses, supplement levels higher than the current adequate intakes should be avoided.

Water-Soluble Vitamins

Thiamin, riboflavin, and niacin. Thiamin, riboflavin, and niacin act as coenzymes in energy metabolism. Thus, their RDAs are based on energy intake. Although energy intake tends to decrease in advanced age, continued intake of these vitamins at the levels recommended for younger adults assists in maintaining optimum enzyme levels. In a study of older Irish women[35] found to be deficient in thiamin, those given a thiamin supplement that raised red blood cell enzymes to normal levels had improved appetite, as compared with those given a **placebo.** Riboflavin requirements appear to increase when older people participate in physical training; however, this may relate to increased kilocalories. Poor thiamin status usually relates to low dietary intake or to excessive alcohol consumption.

Placebo
Inactive substance, such as water or sugar, used in nutritional studies to compare the effects of an inactive substance (control substance) with the effects of the test nutrient or compound.

Vitamin C. Ascorbic acid metabolism in older men differs from that of older women; older men have lower plasma ascorbic acid levels on intakes equal to or higher than those of older women. Older men require 150 mg/day to reach a plasma level of 1.0 mg/dl, whereas older women reach a plasma concentration of 1.0 mg/dl on intakes of 75 to 80 mg/day.[36] This difference likely relates to the higher proportion of lean body mass in men. Optimum intakes of vitamin C and other nutrients with antioxidant functions appear to reduce the risk of cataracts in older people.[37]

Vitamin B_6. Vitamin B_6 (pyridoxine) is a problem nutrient for many older people. Not only are intakes below recommended levels, but also many common prescription drugs interfere with its absorption. Vitamin B_6 is becoming increasingly important in respect to its role in preventing elevated blood homocysteine levels believed to contribute to coronary-artery disease and stroke. The current RDA for those above age fifty is 1.7 mg for men and 1.5 mg for women.[17] These RDAs remain controversial, as recent work with Boston elderly indicated that the actual requirement is about 1.9 mg.[19] This discrepancy between the actual requirement and the current RDA is especially critical for women, whose requirement far exceeds their recommended intake. It has been determined that 2.0 mg/day is required to maintain serum homocysteine levels in the normal range.[19]

Decreased use of meat, poultry, and fish because of chewing problems or financial constraints lowers vitamin B_6 intake. Frail elderly people with low energy intake may not be able to meet their requirement through food alone and may need a supplement. Bananas, potatoes, and other vegetables are also good sources of this vitamin.

Folate. Folate deficiency in older people is associated with poor dietary intake, low secretion of gastric acid, use of prescription drugs that interfere with folate absorption, and alcoholism. However, deficiency is seldom seen in healthy older people, despite intakes

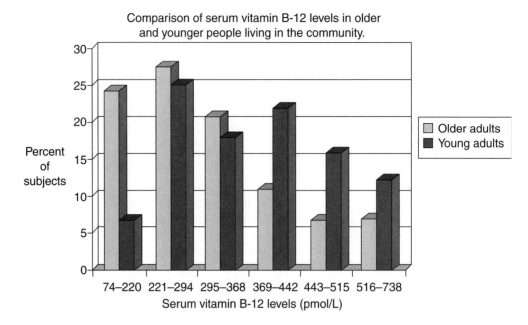

Comparison of serum vitamin B-12 levels in older
and younger people living in the community.

Serum vitamin B-12 levels (pmol/L)

FIG. 14-3 Comparison of serum vitamin B_{12} levels in older and younger people living in the community. The majority of the older people (ages sixty-five to ninety-nine) had serum vitamin levels at the lower end of the distribution; more of the younger people (ages twenty-two to sixty-three) had serum vitamin levels at the middle and upper end of the distribution.

Modified from Lindenbaum, J., et al. 1994. Prevalence of cobalamin deficiency in the Framingham elderly population. *Am J Clin Nutr* 60:2.

Achlorhydria

(L *a-*, negative; *chlorhydria*, hydrochloric acid) Absence or reduced amounts of hydrochloric acid in the gastric secretions resulting from changes in the cells lining the stomach.

well below the recommended level. New information associating low serum folate levels with high plasma homocysteine levels and increased risk of chronic disease has raised questions regarding the amount required to prevent deficiency versus the amount required for optimum health. Folate intakes reaching 400 ug/day, the current RDA for people age fifty-one and over,[17] seem to be sufficient to prevent a rise in plasma homocysteine; however, among financially advantaged elderly in Boston, 75% of the men and 90% of the women did not meet this level of intake on food alone.[19] African American, Mexican American, and low-income elderly who eat fairly low amounts of citrus fruits and fresh dark green vegetables are at particular risk of low intake. Folate fortification of flour may assist older people in raising their dietary levels.

Vitamin B_{12}. The absorption of vitamin B_{12} is a complicated process in people of all ages and requires intrinsic factor, a protein secreted by the gastric mucosa. Lack of intrinsic factor leads to vitamin B_{12} deficiency and, over time, changes in the brain and spinal cord, with deterioration of mental function, changes in personality, and loss of physical coordination. Sufficient amounts of gastric acid also are required to release food-bound vitamin B_{12} and make it available for absorption. In older people with **achlorhydria,** both intrinsic factor and gastric acid levels are lowered, and vitamin B_{12} absorption is impaired.

A recent survey of 548 surviving members of the Framingham Heart Study[38] found that serum cobalamin (vitamin B_{12}) levels decrease with age, even in healthy elderly people (see fig. 14-3). Low serum cobalamin levels were found in 40% of the elderly group (ages sixty-five to ninety-nine), as compared with 18% of the younger group (ages twenty-two to sixty-three). Moreover, 12% of the older group had elevated serum methylmalonic acid. Vitamin B_{12} is a required coenzyme for the conversion of methylmalonic acid to other compounds. The researchers concluded that many older people are metabolically deficient in vitamin B_{12}.

MINERAL REQUIREMENTS OF OLDER PEOPLE ≈

Iron

Most healthy older people maintain adequate iron status on intakes approximating the RDA. Daily iron losses in the form of desquamated cells from the skin and gastrointestinal tract are estimated to be less than 1.0 mg/day in older men and nonmenstruating women. This loss can be replaced with an intake of 10 mg/day. Pathologic conditions, such as peptic ulcers, undiagnosed cancer, or excessive aspirin use leading to continual blood loss through the gastrointestinal tract, can significantly deplete iron reserves. Low gastric acid levels can impair iron absorption, although poor absorption is less likely the cause of low iron stores than is chronic blood loss. Several factors were found to affect iron stores in 634 community-living elderly people[39] who were free of diseases causing iron loss. Intakes of heme iron, iron supplements, vitamin C, and alcohol were positively related to iron stores, but increased intakes of coffee resulted in lower iron stores.

Older men and women with low energy intakes often have low iron intakes. Fortified cereals can be a good source of iron, although older people need to be cautioned to avoid multiple daily servings of cereal foods fortified at a level of 15 mg of iron/serving, intended to meet the iron requirement of the menstruating female.

Calcium

Metabolism. Serum calcium levels must be maintained within very narrow limits to ensure normal function of the heart and nervous system. A decrease in serum calcium triggers the release of parathyroid hormone, (PTH) which restores serum calcium by 1) releasing calcium from the bone (**resorption**), 2) increasing calcium absorption in the intestines, and 3) increasing calcium reabsorption in the kidney. Prior to menopause, estrogen balances the action of PTH by making bone less sensitive to PTH and resorption. After estrogen withdrawal at menopause, bone becomes increasingly sensitive to PTH, and calcium mobilization accelerates. As bone resorption continues raising serum calcium, less PTH is released, lowering calcium absorption in the intestines. Thus, calcium losses increase while net absorption decreases. Estrogen also supports bone health by stimulating the conversion of vitamin D to **calcitriol,** the active metabolite necessary for calcium absorption.

Requirement. The calcium intake required to prevent calcium loss in postmenopausal women and older men has received careful study. The Food and Nutrition Board established an adequate intake of 1,200 mg for both men and women over age fifty (review table 14-1),[17] although a recent Consensus Panel on Optimal Calcium Intakes[40] recommended 1,500 mg for men and women age sixty-five and older. Researchers have demonstrated that calcium intakes of 1,000 to 1,500 mg/day can actually increase bone density in postmenopausal women.[34,41] Current intakes of all older ethnic and racial groups surveyed in NHANES III[25] fell below the goal of 1,200 mg. Mexican American women and African American men and women had the lowest intakes (median intakes between 400 and 500 mg). This indicates that half had intakes below 500 mg. Milks low in fat provide both calcium and vitamin D and are not excessive in kilocalories.

Chromium

Chromium is important in metabolism, since it facilitates the interaction of insulin with its receptor site on the cell membrane. Chromium intake and absorption are relatively low in all age groups. Healthy older Canadians on self-selected diets[42] had daily chromium intakes ranging from 21 ug to 274 ug, with a mean intake of 96 ug. Those with the highest intakes were drinking large quantities of tea, reported to be a good source. The current recommendation for an Estimated Safe and Adequate Daily Dietary Intake is 50 ug to 200 ug.[16] An American diet containing 1,600 kcal was found to supply only 25 ug of chromium; an energy intake of 2,300 kcal provided 33 ug.[16] In light of the low energy intakes of many older people, it is likely that chromium intake falls well below the recommended minimum in a considerable segment of this population.

Resorption
(L *resorbere,* to swallow again) Process by which bone is lost; the mineral crystals are dissolved, and the protein matrix is broken down and removed; cells responsible for bone resorption are the osteoclasts.

Calcitriol
Activated hormone form of vitamin D ($1,25(OH)_2D_3$); 1,25,dihydroxycholecalciferol; the two steps in the activation process take place in the liver and the kidney.

ONE STEP FURTHER

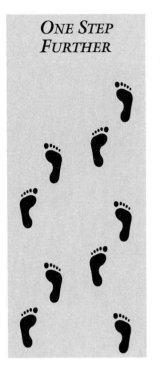

Food Guide Pyramid for Persons Fifty Plus

As people grow older, their food and nutritional needs change. It is important that older individuals and the health professionals who advise them have access to accurate and appropriate information about the foods required for disease prevention and continued good health. To meet this need, the American Dietetic Association joined with other health experts to develop the Food Guide Pyramid for Persons 50 Plus. This guide emphasizes nutrient density, convenience, and the need for fluids (see fig. 14-4). Although energy requirements often decline by as much as 25% over adulthood, the need for vitamins and minerals does not, so older people must be encouraged to choose foods that are good sources of the micronutrients. As people age, foods that are both easy to obtain and easy to prepare are important in meal planning. Because older people have a decreased sensitivity to thirst or may limit their fluid intake if incontinence is a problem, fluid requirements should be an important part of any nutrition education program for this age group.

The Food Guide Pyramid for Persons 50 Plus and other nutrition education materials designed for older people are available on the web site of the American Dietetic Association at *www.eatright.org*. Other sources of nutrition and health information for older people can be found on web sites maintained by the National Institute on Aging at: *http://www.nih.gov/nia/health/health.htm*, the Administration on Aging at *http://www.aoa.dhhs.gov*, and the Department of Health and Human Services at *http://www.healthfinder.gov/justforyou/seniors.htm*.

Zinc

Dietary zinc levels are influenced by total energy intake, total money spent for food, and food selection. Older men with energy intakes of 1,800 kcal consume about 10.6 mg of zinc (RDA = 15 mg). Older women consuming 1,300 kcal take in only 7.2 mg zinc, or 60% of their RDA.[43] In the average American diet, about 40% of the zinc is provided by meat, fish, and poultry, relatively expensive items in the food budget. The most common food source is beef. A diet based on dairy products and highly processed breads and cereals is low in zinc. A recent evaluation of menus served in adult boarding homes for elderly people[44] found that 60% provided less than two-thirds of the RDA for zinc. One population at particular risk for zinc deficiency is older vegetarians, whose primary dietary sources of zinc are low in bioavailability. Foods high in phytate reduce total zinc absorption. Zinc is important for taste sensation, wound healing, and the immune response. Each of these functions is altered in certain older people; however, zinc supplementation does not reverse these changes in people with adequate zinc status.[43] Optimum zinc intake is particularly important for healing **decubitus ulcers** and for recovery from surgery.

Decubitus ulcer
Bedsore caused by prolonged pressure on the skin and tissues covering a bony area; occurs in elderly people who are confined to bed or immobilized.

Fluid Intake

Water is supplied to the body through food, liquids, and water of oxidation. In younger people, the thirst mechanism ensures adequate fluid intake, but diminished sensitivity to dehydration and reduced sensation of thirst greatly lowers spontaneous fluid intake in older people (see p. 354). A frail individual who cannot drink without help is particularly vulnerable to low fluid intake and acute dehydration, and elderly people subject to incontinence may make a conscious effort to restrict fluids to avoid embarrassment. Patients given high protein supplements will become dehydrated if fluids are limited. Unless diagnosed with cardiac or renal complications, older people should drink a minimum of eight glasses of fluid each day.[5]

NUTRITIONAL AND CHRONIC DISORDERS IN THE AGED ≋

Carbohydrate Metabolism and Glucose Tolerance

Blood glucose levels. The ability to metabolize a given amount of glucose deteriorates with age. In younger people, abnormal glucose tolerance is associated with the develop-

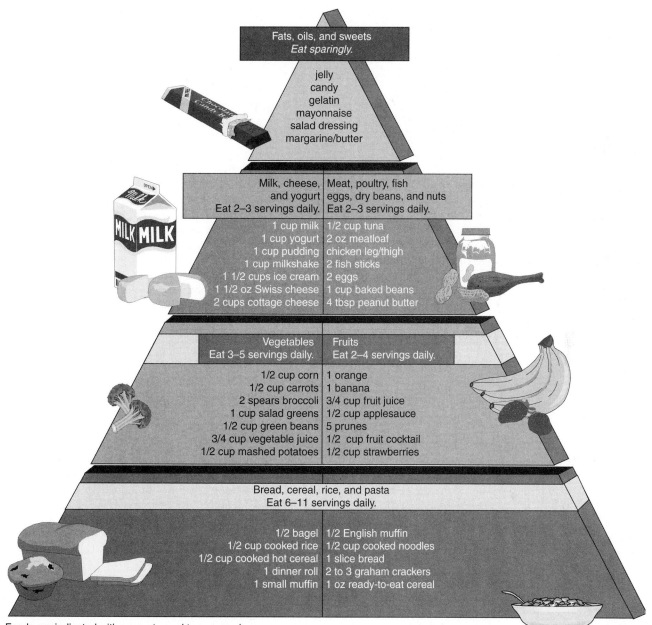

Foods are indicated with amount equal to one serving.

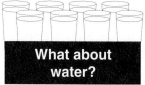

What about water? Adults need six to eight 8-ounce cups of water or liquid a day. Sources of liquid, in addition to water, are fruit and vegetable juices and milk. Caffeine-free coffees and teas and herbal teas are also good sources.

FIG. 14-4   Food guide pyramid for persons fifty plus.

The Food Guide Pyramid for Persons Fifty Plus, based on the USDA Food Guide Pyramid, was reprinted with permission of the American Dietetic Association and the American Dietetic Association Foundation, 216 W. Jackson Blvd, Chicago, IL 60606-6995, 1998.

ment of diabetes mellitus. In older individuals, the separation between disease-related changes and normal aging is less clear. Fasting blood glucose levels are not higher in older people; however, after a meal high in carbohydrates, blood glucose levels take longer to return to fasting levels in older people, as compared with younger people. The age-related increase in body fat and decrease in body muscle may contribute to this change in glucose utilization, as excessive fatness contributes to impaired glucose tolerance in all age groups. Physical activity promotes energy metabolism in skeletal muscle and the uptake of glucose for fuel; conversely, bed rest or a sedentary lifestyle reduces glucose movement into skeletal muscle and thereby could slow the fall of **postprandial** blood glucose levels to fasting levels.

Postprandial
Following a meal.

Physiologic aspects. At this time, it is not understood why glucose tolerance changes in even healthy older people. Except for those with diagnosed diabetes, older people secrete a sufficient amount of insulin from the pancreas to facilitate the movement of glucose into both fat cells and skeletal muscle. In fact, older people sometimes have higher insulin levels than younger people, although in older people fat cells may be enlarged and less sensitive to the action of insulin. Among 743 healthy men and women in the BLSA,[45] increases in abdominal fat and reductions in physical activity accounted for the differences in glucose tolerance between the young participants, ages seventeen to thirty-nine, and the middle-aged participants, ages forty to fifty-nine, but they did not account for the further decline in glucose tolerance in the oldest participants, ages sixty to ninety-two. Losing even 10 pounds and initiating regular physical activity can reduce elevated insulin levels and decrease one's risk of developing diabetes.

Bone Disorders in the Aging Adult

Loss of bone. Loss of bone in middle and old age has been observed in prehistoric skeletons from the year 2000 B.C. Osteoporosis (porous bone) is the clinical syndrome associated with a decrease in bone mineral and bone matrix and changes in the structure of remaining bone, causing increased fragility and risk of fracture. This condition results in bone pain, spinal deformity, and physical disability. At about age thirty, women begin to lose bone and, over their adult lives, lose as much as 35% of their **cortical bone** and 50% of their **trabecular bone;** men lose only about two-thirds as much.[46] Bone is lost from the spine, hip, and femur. All people lose bone as they age, but not all develop osteoporosis. The incidence of spontaneous hip fractures is such that, by age ninety, one in three women and one in six men will have a fracture.[46] The resulting immobility usually changes one's lifestyle. For example, an older woman may be forced to give up her home and enter a long-term care facility after breaking her hip. Osteoporosis also results in deformities of the spine, such as **kyphosis,** with accompanying pain.

Cortical bone
(Gr *corticis,* bark, shell) Long bone of the body extremities with a heavy, circular layer of bone surrounding the inner bone marrow.

Trabecular bone
(L *trabs,* a little beam) Small meshwork of bone at the end of the long bones; also the bone forming the connecting network between the vertebrae.

Kyphosis
(Gr *kyphos,* hunchbacked) Abnormal outward curvature of the upper back, resulting from age-related bone loss from the vertebrae; can cause extreme back pain.

Osteoporosis versus osteomalacia. Osteoporosis is the most common bone disease in older people. Bone mass is drastically reduced, but there is no change in the chemical ratio of mineral to protein matrix. Once thought to be relatively inactive, bone is now recognized to be an active tissue that undergoes constant remodeling throughout life. While old bone is being broken down at one location by osteoclasts, the cells that dissolve bone mineral and matrix, new bone is being formed at another location by osteoblasts, the cells that synthesize the protein matrix and accumulate the bone mineral to form new bone. With aging, this process becomes uncoupled, and bone is resorbed at a faster rate than it can be replaced. Impaired calcium absorption contributes to this imbalance.

Osteomalacia (adult rickets) is caused by a vitamin D deficiency and low absorption of calcium. Bone density decreases because of low mineral deposition in the available protein matrix. Vitamin D problems can relate to 1) low vitamin D intake and no exposure to sunlight, 2) malabsorption of dietary vitamin D, or 3) liver or renal disease, which interferes with the conversion of vitamin D to calcitriol. Osteoporosis and osteomalacia are compared in figure 14-5.

Factors influencing bone health. Many factors affect bone loss (see the box on p. 367). The most obvious predisposing factor is being female. The bone mass remaining at older ages is influenced by the amount of bone laid down during periods of

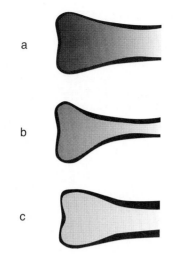

FIG. 14-5 Normal bone, osteoporosis, and osteomalacia. (*a*) Normal bone. (*b*) Osteoporosis, in which there is a reduced amount of bone of normal composition. (*c*) Osteomalacia, in which the amount of bone is normal but the composition is abnormal with reduced mineral density.

CHARACTERISTICS ASSOCIATED WITH LOWER BONE MASS

Genetic
Female
White or Asian race
Family history of bone disease
Extremely short or tall stature

Physiologic or Hormonal
Hyperparathyroidism
Hyperthyroidism
Diabetes mellitus
Premature menopause
Leanness

Environmental
Low calcium intake
Low exposure to sunlight
Low physical activity
Use of alcohol
Smoking

growth in childhood and adolescence. Men have greater bone mass than women at all ages and lose bone less rapidly. Black people have more bone than white people and are generally believed to be less likely to develop osteoporosis, although a recent study[47] indicated that blood metabolites produced by the breakdown of bone were elevated in black elderly nursing home patients. Lifestyle choices, including physical activity and use of cigarettes or alcohol, affect bone mass, and hormonal imbalances accelerate bone loss.

Prevention of osteoporosis. Promoting bone formation and preventing bone loss must begin with adolescent girls and continue with women of all ages. Regular physical exercise promotes bone health as the pull of gravity and body weight exerted on the bone preserve bone tissue. On the other hand, weightlessness, as occurs in space flight, or prolonged bed rest leads to rapid loss of bone mineral and matrix. Older people who exercise infrequently experience a higher rate of bone loss than do those who exercise several times a week. Weight training not only preserves bone mass but also may help restore bone in older individuals.

Raising calcium intake to recommended levels and assuring an adequate supply of vitamin D will slow bone loss. Hormone replacement therapy (HRT) reduces the activity of

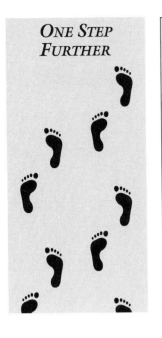

Use of Calcium Supplements

Media attention to the risks of bone fractures has led to mass marketing of calcium supplements. Although selection of high-calcium foods with high bioavailability should be a first priority in nutrition counseling, some older people will not consume dairy products because of lactose intolerance or cultural food preferences. Recommendations when choosing calcium supplements should include the following:

- Bioavailability of the calcium—calcium carbonate, lactate, gluconate, or citrate malate (used to fortify orange juice) are all reasonably well absorbed if consumed with a meal.
- Cost—which form or brand will provide the most calcium per tablet at the lowest cost?
- Safety—supplements containing bone meal or derived from other natural sources often contain lead, mercury, arsenic, or aluminum; if using products with vitamin D added, avoid total vitamin D intakes exceeding 600 IU (15 ug) per day.
- Level of calcium per tablet—tablets containing above 500 mg each stimulate the secretion of gastric acid and can result in gastrointestinal discomfort or **constipation.***

*Levenson, D.I., and R.S. Bockman. 1994. A review of calcium preparations. *Nutr Rev* S2(7):221.

---

the osteoclasts and has been shown to slow bone loss; however, questions remain regarding the long-term effect of estrogen replacement on the risk of breast and endometrial cancer. New drugs have been developed that decrease bone resorption or stimulate bone formation. Biphosphonate compounds, such as alendronate, inhibit osteoclast activity and bone resorption. Calcitonin derived from fish inhibits bone resorption and stimulates bone formation. Although new treatments are available, they are costly and involve close medical supervision, and they may be more effective on a short-term, rather than a long-term, basis. Preventing bone loss through appropriate lifestyle patterns is still urgent for all men and women.

Nutritional Anemia

Anemia

(Gr *a-*, negative; *haima*, blood) Blood condition marked by a decrease in number of circulating red blood cells, decrease in amount of hemoglobin in the red blood cells, or both.

Anemia brings about a decrease in the oxygen-carrying capacity of the blood. The subsequent oxygen deficit in the tissues causes an increased heart rate, shortness of breath, and weakness. Unfortunately, these symptoms are often thought of as typical of older people and go unnoticed as anemia develops.

Iron deficiency anemia. The most common anemia in older people is iron deficiency anemia. Blood loss through the gastrointestinal tract is a frequent and critical cause of iron deficiency in elderly people (see p. 363). Healthy older people have hemoglobin levels similar to healthy younger people, but several trends are apparent. In men, hemoglobin levels tend to be higher at younger ages, whereas women have lower hemoglobin levels during the childbearing years, but their iron status improves when menstruation ceases. Aged black people, particularly women, are more likely to have hemoglobin levels below 12 g/dl. People in their eighties or nineties have lower hemoglobin levels than people in their sixties or seventies.[48] Erythropoiesis is less efficient in advanced age because of changes in the bone marrow where new red blood cells are formed. Protein-energy malnutrition (PEM) depresses red blood cell production. Treating iron deficiency anemia requires careful evaluation. Giving supplemental iron to people who, in fact, have an anemia caused by vitamin B_{12} deficiency has serious consequences, as the progressive neural damage will continue. Self-medication with iron supplements is dangerous and can lead to **hemochromatosis** and liver damage.

Hemochromatosis

(Gr *haima*, blood; *chroma*, color) Disorder of iron metabolism characterized by excessive iron deposits in the tissues, especially the liver; results from iron overload caused by prolonged or inappropriate use of high-iron supplements.

Chronic low-grade infection associated with fever, inflammation, or renal disease interferes with hemoglobin synthesis. This produces an anemia characterized by a reduced

---

CASE STUDY

Bone Health in an Elderly African American

Mr. Perkins is an African American man who is eighty-nine years old and in fairly good health. He likes all kinds of meat and eats most fruits and vegetables. He doesn't like milk and has seldom drunk milk since his childhood. He spends most of his time in the house, watching television or talking on the telephone to his children and grandchildren, who live nearby. He has smoked all of his life but has recently tried to quit. Last week, an elderly neighbor down the street fell and broke his hip and had to go to live with his daughter until he is able to resume his daily activities. Mr. Perkins has been rather upset about this and is worried that it might happen to him.

Questions for analysis
1. Does Mr. Perkins have any risk factors for osteoporosis? If so, what are they?
2. What are some dietary changes you could suggest to decrease his risk of bone fracture?
3. What are some lifestyle changes that might decrease his risk of bone fracture?

---

number of red blood cells normal in size and hemoglobin content. This type of anemia, sometimes referred to as the **anemia of chronic disease,** is highly resistant to treatment.[49]
Megaloblastic anemia. A **megaloblastic anemia** arising from a lack of intrinsic factor or poor absorption of vitamin B_{12} requires immediate medical intervention in the older adult. A current medical dilemma is differentiating between such an anemia occurring as a result of atrophic gastritis (see p. 363) and a true pernicious anemia associated with a total loss of ability to produce intrinsic factor. Pernicious anemia was so named because of its persistent downward course to death. The implications of the age-related decline in blood vitamin B_{12} levels observed in the elderly population are poorly understood. If vitamin B_{12} is poorly absorbed and body stores are being depleted, blood levels can be expected to decline; however, many older people with blood levels below normal, observed over time, do not develop anemia. Conversely, older patients with normal blood vitamin levels and no indication of anemia can have neurologic and behavioral changes that in some instances improve with vitamin B_{12} supplementation.[49] Increasing numbers of older people are being given intramuscular injections of vitamin B_{12} as a preventive measure.

DRUGS AND NUTRITIONAL CONSIDERATIONS IN THE AGING ADULT 〰

Drug Use in Older Adults

Older people make up about 12% of the general population, yet they use about 35% of all prescription drugs.[50] This is not surprising, because many chronic diseases prevalent among older people are managed with prescription drugs. Hypertension, heart disease, and diabetes mellitus are the most commonly diagnosed medical conditions in the elderly. Physicians have more than 10,000 drugs to choose from in the diagnosis and treatment of disease, and this fact, coupled with the widespread assumption that there is a pill for every problem, makes the older population vulnerable to high drug use. Over two-thirds of older people take at least one drug daily, and many with multiple health problems take six or more.[50]

Older people are especially at risk of adverse nutritional effects from both prescription and over-the-counter (OTC) drugs. Nutritional status already may be jeopardized by less

Anemia of chronic disease
Anemia that occurs in elderly people that have chronic low-grade infections, inflammation, or kidney or liver disease; these conditions interfere with the release of iron needed for the production of hemoglobin, resulting in low numbers of red blood cells that contain normal levels of hemoglobin; this differs from iron deficiency anemia in that the body has adequate stores of iron; however, it cannot be released for making red blood cells.

Megaloblastic anemia
(Gr *mega,* great size; *blastos,* embryo, germ) Anemia caused by faulty production of red blood cells, resulting in abnormally large, immature cells; occurs as a result of folate or vitamin B_{12} deficiency.

than optimal nutrient intake, and long-term drug therapy has the potential for gradual depletion of existing nutrient reserves. The growing trend toward polypharmacy, or the use of multiple drugs at the same time, compounds the nutritional effects. Moreover, most drugs are tested on younger individuals, who have different rates of drug absorption, metabolism, and excretion, based on differences in body composition and renal function. These concerns point to the need for a greater emphasis on lifestyle interventions, rather than on drug therapy alone.

Mechanisms of Drug-Nutrient Interactions

Interference with normal processes. Drugs can interfere with nutrients at the point of ingestion, absorption, utilization, or excretion. Food intake may decrease because of drugs that depress appetite or cause nausea or vomiting. Interference with the secretion of digestive enzymes, alterations in pH, or increases in transit time brought about by particular drugs prevents the digestion of foods to the nutrient forms required for absorption. Competition for binding sites on the intestinal mucosa reduces nutrient absorption. Some drugs prevent the conversion of a vitamin into its active form, thereby negating its metabolic function. Other drugs form insoluble complexes with nutrients and prevent their absorption. In general, vitamins and minerals are most affected.

Depletion of nutrient reserves. Nutrient depletion is most likely to occur with a drug that inhibits absorption or with a drug taken for an extended period of time. A drug that acts as a vitamin **antagonist** or affects a nutrient, such as folate, that participates in a variety of biochemical reactions impairs metabolic function. For example, prescription drugs may contribute to low folate levels, which lead to elevated blood homocysteine and enhanced risk of disease (see p. 361-62). Finally, nutritional effects are most serious in those with poor nutritional status to begin with. Those with marginal nutrient reserves who consume multiple drugs over periods of years are at greatest risk.

Antagonist
(Gr *antagonisma,* struggle)
Agent that has a conflicting or an inhibiting action on another substance, often a vitamin.

Nutritional Aspects of Drugs

Effects of prescription drugs. The drugs prescribed most frequently for older adults are 1) diuretics, antihypertensives, and cardiac drugs; 2) drugs that affect the central nervous system, such as tranquilizers or drugs to prevent seizures; 3) drugs to manage diabetes mellitus; and 4) analgesics to control pain of osteoarthritis or other conditions.[50] Digoxin, a cardiac stimulant used to treat cardiac failure, causes anorexia and nausea, and these patients often exhibit significant weight loss and weakness. Diuretics that promote the excretion of water and sodium also promote the loss of potassium. Medicines used to control convulsions and seizures increase the need for vitamin D.[51] Common prescription and OTC drugs and their nutritional implications are described in table 14-3.

Effects of over-the-counter drugs. Because OTC drugs are easily obtained and commonly used, they are often perceived to be without risk. Patients may not report their use of these drugs to a physician, creating the possibility of a dangerous interaction with a prescription drug. Also, dosage may be increased above that recommended if the desired effect is not achieved.

The most common OTC drug is aspirin (acetylsalicylic acid), used to control arthritis, headache, and muscle pain. Prolonged use can induce iron deficiency anemia through irritation of the gastrointestinal tract and subsequent blood loss. Many elderly people also use gastrointestinal drugs. Continuous use of laxatives to relieve constipation can deplete body sodium and potassium and can lead to chronic diarrhea. Sodium bicarbonate and other antacids raise the gastric pH, inactivating thiamin and hindering the absorption of iron, calcium, and folate. Increasing use of common antacids containing calcium as supplements exacerbate this problem. Aluminum hydroxide–containing antacids bind phosphate and are known to cause phosphate depletion and accelerate bone loss. Unfortunately, some older people assume that all antacids contain calcium and may actually be hindering rather than helping their bone status.

TABLE 14-3 *Drugs Commonly Used by Older Adults and Their Nutritional Implications*

Drugs	Reasons for Use	Nutritional Implications
Prescription		
Anticonvulsant	Prevents or reduces the severity of seizures related to epilepsy or other condition	Can lead to folate deficiency; may interfere with bone mineralization by inactivating vitamin D and halting synthesis of vitamin K–dependent bone proteins
Antidepressant	Alters mood; relieves depression and increases feeling of well-being	Can lead to riboflavin deficiency; causes gastric irritation, constipation, dry mouth
Antihypertensive	Acts on central nervous system to lower blood pressure	Can lead to anorexia, disordered taste, vitamin B_6 deficiency
Cardiac stimulant	Increases the strength of the heart as a pump	Can lead to anorexia, nausea, weight loss, low potassium levels
Diuretic	Increases water loss via the urine to lower blood pressure	Causes loss of sodium, potassium, magnesium, and calcium; may cause irritation of the stomach and loss of appetite
Lipid-lowering drug	Increases excretion of bile acids to lower serum cholesterol levels	Can lead to deficiencies of vitamins A, D, E, K, B_{12}, and folate; can deplete iron
Tranquilizer	Alters mood; reduces anxiety and anxiousness	Can lead to riboflavin deficiency; causes constipation; decreases saliva, causing sore mouth and gums
Analgesic (NSAID)*	Reduces inflammation and relieves pain	Increases occurrence of gastric and duodenal ulcers; can cause sodium and fluid retention
Over-the-counter		
Analgesic	Relieves pain	Can cause gastric distress and iron deficiency based on blood loss from the gastrointestinal tract; can lower folate and ascorbic acid levels; some are high in sodium
Antacid	Neutralizes gastric acid; relieves gastric distress	Can cause constipation; depresses vitamin A absorption; inactivates thiamin; long-term use of aluminum-containing types deplete phosphorus; long-term use of magnesium-containing types increase risk of magnesium toxicity if kidneys are impaired
Antidiarrhea drug	Prevents or relieves diarrhea	Can cause nausea, vomiting, abdominal discomfort, constipation
Laxative	Prevents or relieves constipation	Abuse can deplete potassium and sodium, cause general malabsorption, dehydration; frequent use may result in laxative dependence

*Nonsteroidal antiinflammatory drug

Use and Abuse of Vitamin and Mineral Supplements

Many elderly people regularly use vitamin and mineral supplements. In a Wisconsin study of 2,152 middle-aged and older adults,[52] 44% of those age sixty-five and over took supplements, but only 34% of those below age sixty-five did. However, the supplements chosen do not always provide the nutrients that are in shortest supply. Although calcium intake is frequently low relative to recommended levels, calcium supplements were chosen by less than half of the Wisconsin supplement users. Supplement users who are concerned about health and nutrition often have higher nutrient intakes from food than do nonsupplement users.

Increasing attention to the possible benefits of megadoses of particular vitamins and minerals could increase supplement abuse among older people, with the potential for serious physical and nutritional consequences. One report of elderly women[53] identified individuals taking up to 25,000 IU of vitamin D, 3 g of calcium, and 400 mg of iron on a daily basis. Excessive intakes of calcium can interfere with the absorption of zinc and other trace minerals and can induce nutrient deficiency. Although the symptoms associated with vitamins A and D toxicities have been identified, symptoms related to excesses of other micronutrients are less well defined. Young women taking megadoses of vitamin B_6 reportedly have developed neurological problems and lost muscular control.[54] It is less likely that this toxicity syndrome would have been identified in elderly women, in whom such symptoms might be considered age-related. Inappropriate levels of folate can mask a vitamin B_{12} deficiency and thus should be avoided. Unfortunately, older people sometimes associate vitamin and mineral supplements with improved physical well-being and the prevention of health problems. Nutrition education should include advice for the prudent use of supplements. It is best to choose supplements containing no more than 100% of the recommended level, unless taken under a doctor's supervision.

Addictive Behaviors in the Older Adult

Alcohol or drug dependency in the elderly may go undetected. Dementia and depression occurring as a result of alcohol or drug dependence also are associated with medical conditions and changes in neurologic status; thus, the health professional may overlook the true cause. When substance abuse is identified, appropriate interventions include counseling, support groups, and substance-free structured environments.

Use of alcohol. Estimates of the prevalence of drinking problems among the elderly vary greatly from less than 5% to over 60%, depending on the population.[55] Physical and emotional distress, loneliness, and bereavement all contribute to increased use of alcohol. Among 991 older people in Boston,[26] 43% of the men and 28% of the women consumed alcohol at least once over the three-day record period, but use decreased with age. As people grow older, their tolerance to alcohol decreases, and adverse side effects increase, even in alcoholics. Alcohol interacts with drugs and medical conditions to worsen the negative effects. High alcohol intake puts the cardiac patient on digitalis at risk of toxicity. The alcohol abuser with insulin-dependent diabetes mellitus may develop dangerously low blood glucose levels. The risk of nutrient deficiency arising from long-term use of prescription or OTC drugs is markedly increased by excessive drinking.

Abuse of drugs. The use of illicit drugs is relatively uncommon in the elderly, although this problem will grow as younger users move into older age categories. However, the abuse of prescribed medications is becoming more prevalent as sedatives, **psychotropic** drugs, and analgesics are used to treat a greater variety of conditions. Caregivers may overmedicate individuals to make them docile and easier to control. Older people at home using mood-altering drugs to relieve depression or anxiety may consume increasing amounts as tolerance to the drug develops. Social withdrawal and the inability to perform household tasks may be the consequence of inappropriate drug use. Combining alcohol and psychotropic medications is especially dangerous, leading to delirium, muscle weakness, and serious medical complications.

Psychotropic
(Gr *psyche, trepein,* to turn) To exert an effect on the mind, altering behavior, mental activity, or emotional experience.

FOOD SELECTION IN OLDER PEOPLE ≈

Changes in Lifelong Food Patterns

Changes in lifestyle. In the older adult, food choices reflect lifelong attitudes and habits molded by the changing environment. To better understand the influence of lifestyle, health, and economic status on the food choices of older people, review the examples given in table 14-4. These factors act both individually and in combination with each other. The older woman who has taken pride in "cooking from scratch" may have to rely on preprepared items or home-delivered meals if her worsening arthritis makes working in the kitchen difficult. For older people on a fixed pension, rising costs of prescription drugs or other health care expenditures will reduce the money available for food. Changes in living situation or income contribute to poor nutrient intake in some older people, but not for all. The stereotype of the old person who eats only tea and toast is not substantiated by survey data from the United States or Europe. Helping older people solve their food problems involves seeking alternatives as their physical health or resources change and things have to be done differently.

Decreased energy intake and nutrient density. As people age, they consume less food. According to NHANES III,[25] energy intake in the men decreased 1,249 kcal over the adult years, from 3,025 kcal at ages twenty to twenty-nine, to 1,776 kcal at ages eighty and over. Among the women, energy intake decreased by 628 kcal, from 1,957 kcal to 1,329 kcal. Older people may compensate for their lower energy intakes by choosing foods more carefully, as indicated by the fact that vitamin A intake actually increased between ages twenty and eighty, from 1,026 RE to 1,207 RE among the men and from 786 RE to 1,083 RE among the women. Unfortunately, this pattern does not hold true for all nutrients. Zinc intakes decreased by 20–30% over this time period.[55] If older people decrease their energy intakes by consuming less of all foods, rather than selectively reducing their use of items lower in **nutrient density,** the overall quality of the diet suffers.

Changes in food availability. Changes in food preservation and food processing have multiplied the food items now available to the consumer. Frozen orange juice and frozen entrees designed for reheating in a microwave oven were unheard of when people now age sixty-five were young adults. The adoption of these new foods by older adults suggests that nutritious foods not formerly a part of the diet may be accepted if introduced in a positive way.

Nutrient density
Protein, vitamin, or mineral content of a food expressed in relation to its energy, or caloric, content.

Psychosocial Factors and Food Selection

Eating alone. Throughout life, eating is a social activity. Loss of spouse or friends means a loss of eating companions for the older person, who may now have to eat alone. Some

TABLE 14-4 *Influences on Food Choices of Older People*

Psychologic Factors	Physiologic Factors	Socioeconomic Factors
Social activity	Appetite	Age
Self-esteem	Sense of taste	Gender
Nutrition knowledge	Sense of smell	Income
Perceived health benefit	Dental status	Cooking facilities
Loneliness	Prescribed diets	Daily schedule
Bereavement	Chronic disease	Retirement/leisure time
Symbolism of food	Food intolerance	Education
Mental awareness	Health status	Distance to food store
Food likes/dislikes	Physical disability	Availability of transportation
Food beliefs	Physical exercise	Availability of familiar foods
	Use of drugs (prescribed and over-the-counter)	
	Vision level	

older people are content living and eating alone and may have done so most of their lives, whereas others are very lonely and dependent. Depression or the need for attention may be expressed as a food problem and may lead to significant weight loss.

Retirement. Retirement brings a change in lifestyle for both single adults and couples. For couples, both are at home and can participate in meal planning and preparation. For one group of retired couples, not only did the husbands participate in food-related decisions, but their participation had nutritional implications.[56] The greater the husband's involvement in meal planning and food purchasing, the better the diet. Nutrition education programs are often directed toward women, but leaders should make an effort to involve men. Men may be less bored with food activities and more receptive, and they can strongly influence food decisions in the retired family.

Physiologic Influences on Food Selection

Sensor changes. Most older people living in the community describe their appetite as good to excellent,[1] but anorexia is a side effect of many prescription drugs. Taste and smell influence the selection and enjoyment of food, and sensitivity to the four basic tastes—sweet, sour, salty, and bitter—seems to change with age. Dentures, poor oral hygiene, and certain prescription drugs contribute to unpleasant or disordered taste. When flavor enhancers, which are intense flavor mixtures, were added to foods served in a retirement home,[57] the residents ate more portions of protein foods, and their intakes of protein, thiamin, and zinc increased. The tendency of older people to add large amounts of salt to their food may be an attempt to strengthen flavor when taste is altered. Certain prescription drugs interfere with the flow of saliva, resulting in **xerostomia,** or dry mouth, causing problems with both swallowing and taste.

Dental problems. Periodontal disease, gingivitis, and tooth loss alter food choices in older people, particularly in those who are **edentulous.** Low-income older people may be prevented from seeking professional services for the preparation or repair of dentures. In a study of outpatients attending a medical clinic, loss of teeth and gum disease were strongly associated with involuntary weight loss. Dairy foods, eggs, ground meat, and well-cooked chicken and fish provide high-quality protein for those with chewing problems or mouth pain. Fruit juice, fresh fruit that is peeled and chopped, and steamed vegetables are good sources of vitamins A and C and folate.

Physical health. Older adults with poor vision or impaired mobility find it difficult to shop for groceries or prepare meals. Moving about the kitchen requires intense effort for a person who must grasp a cane or walker. Poor eyesight precludes reading nutrition labels or package directions. Peeling vegetables or fruit is painful or even impossible for someone whose hands are crippled with arthritis. These problems increase dependence on preprepared items that can be high in sodium and fat and low in vitamins and trace minerals. Nutrition education should assist older people in making healthful choices from the preprepared foods available.

Special diets. Existing health problems sometimes necessitate a prescribed diet limited in energy, fat, sodium, or cholesterol. Diets also may be self-prescribed, such as diets to alleviate arthritis that were obtained from a friend or salesperson. Elderly people need to be apprised of the dangers of following a "diabetic," low-fat, or weight loss regimen that is not appropriate for them.

Living Arrangements and Food Selection

Cooking facilities. Older people living in their own homes usually have a working stove, oven, and refrigerator. Those who live in rented rooms with no kitchen privileges are forced to eat in restaurants or elsewhere. They may heat foods on a hotplate or use a heating coil to heat water for soup or beverages. A small toaster oven or a microwave oven is a good investment for a person cooking for only one or two. The added advantage of a microwave oven is that it shuts off automatically.

Xerostomia
(Gr *xeros,* dry; *stoma,* mouth) Dryness of the mouth from lack of normal salivary secretions; can be caused by aging changes or certain drugs.

Periodontal disease
(Gr *peri,* around; *odove,* tooth) Inflammation and breakdown of tissues and ligaments that surround the tooth and hold it in place; periodontal disease is often the cause of tooth loss in older people.

Gingivitis
(L *gingiva,* gum; Gr *it is,* inflammation) Red, swollen and bleeding gums; can result from accumulation of plaque on the teeth or vitamin deficiency; sometimes occurs with diabetes mellitus; can result in gum pain when eating.

Edentulous
(L *e,* without; *dens,* tooth) Absence of natural teeth.

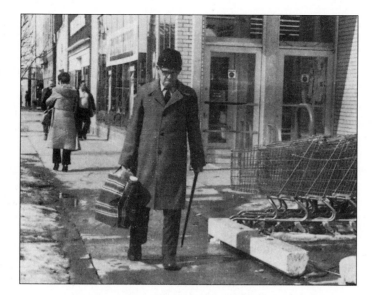

FIG. 14-6   Carrying groceries home from the store is a difficult task for older people.

Food shopping. Access to a grocery store is a problem for some older adults. In suburban or rural areas, stores can be at a distance, requiring either a car or a ride. In the city, an older person may have to ride a bus or walk to the store (fig. 14-6). During winter months, ice and snow create added difficulties for someone who must carry bundles home. For inner-city elderly, the nearest store is often a convenience store with high prices and limited selection, since downtown supermarkets are closing because of poor profit margins. Grocery delivery and shopping services are valuable programs for volunteer community agencies.

Household size. It is true that older people who live and eat alone are not always motivated to prepare adequate meals for themselves; however, personal characteristics, such as sex, age, income level, and health status, also pertain. Davis and co-workers[58] evaluated household size and dietary quality in 4,400 older adults who participated in a national study of the U.S. Department of Agriculture. In the women over age sixty-four, living alone did not increase the likelihood of a poor diet; in fact, 21% of the married women had poor diets, but only 17% of the single women did. The situation was completely reversed among the older men. One-fourth of the single men over age seventy-four had poor diets, compared with only 9% of the married men. Older men may find it difficult to prepare their own meals, as this was not expected of them as young adults. Another important finding was that total energy intake was the overriding factor in overall quality of the diet. The older people with diets lower in nutrients did not make poorer food choices; they just consumed less food (table 14-5). Those with poorer diets also spent less money for food and were more likely to be in poor health. Older people living alone may skip meals if they are sick and have no one to help with food preparation. **Congregate** (see p. 378) or home-delivered meals can increase total food intake in those with poor health or limited money for food.

Income Level and Food Selection

The income of older people has increased measurably in recent years; however, not all groups have shared equally in these gains.[59] Single elderly women and older African American, Mexican American, and Asian American men and women are more likely to be poor. Older households must spend a greater proportion of their income on food than younger households (20% versus 12%).[60] In a study of people age seventy and over who lived independently,[61] lack of money for food along with eating fewer than two meals a day and eating few fruits and vegetables were the strongest predictors of inadequate diets. Income does not influence all nutrients in the same way. In a U.S. government

Congregate meals
Group meals for older adults served in a social setting in the community and funded by Title III-C of the Older Americans Act.

TABLE 14-5   *Factors Affecting Dietary Quality in Older People*

	Men		Women	
	High-Quality Diet	Poor-Quality Diet	High-Quality Diet	Poor-Quality Diet
Energy intake (kcal)	2,136	1,222	1,593	934
Money spent for food per week	$19.42	$16.09	$19.02	$15.70
Participants in poor health	29%	51%	32%	45%

Modified from Davis, M.A. et al. 1990. Living arrangements and dietary quality of older US adults. *J Am Diet Assoc* 90:1667.

survey,[25] the lower-income elderly met the RDA for protein, suggesting that selecting good protein sources was a priority. In contrast, those with lower incomes consumed only 65–67% of the RDA for zinc and only 81–84% of the RDA for vitamin B_6. Older people with higher incomes were more likely to meet the RDA for both zinc and vitamin B_6. The elderly spend less money on food away from home than do younger groups; however, McDonald's estimates that 30% of their customers are above age sixty.[59]

Food stamps are available to older people meeting specific income guidelines. Unfortunately, only 22% of income-eligible older people use food stamps.[62] Older citizens may not know about the program, may lack transportation to the appropriate office to enroll, or may not apply because of pride.

Food Selection in Diverse Population Groups

As the older population is growing in size, it also is becoming more diverse. This means that nutritionists need to be familiar with the foods common to various cultures and ethnic groups. It is important to understand and respect the traditional food patterns of older people and to seek appropriate choices within these patterns that will support health.

African American elderly. Food records collected in NHANES III[25] revealed that older African American adults have lower intakes of energy, protein, and several important vitamins and minerals than do older white adults (see table 14-6). Traditionally, African American men and women above age sixty had higher intakes of vitamin A than white men and women of this age, because older African American families ate more servings of dark green and deep yellow vegetables, such as cooked greens and sweet potatoes, which are high in carotenes. Of major concern is the low intake of calcium among African American elderly, which increases their risk of osteoporosis. African American women above age seventy consume the least amount of food among African American women. This could relate to economic status, since 47% of elderly African American women have incomes below the poverty line.[59]

Mexican American elderly. Among elderly Mexican American women in Texas,[63] preferences for traditional ethnic foods exerted a greater influence on food choices than did income. Foods eaten frequently were flour tortillas, legumes, poultry, eggs, and organ meats. They cooked with saturated fats and had high intakes of sugar. Dairy foods, deep yellow fruits, and dark green vegetables were seldom used. Nutrient intakes obtained from a national sample of elderly Mexican Americans[25] reflected their selection of good protein sources, such as poultry, but their need to increase servings of foods rich in zinc. Older Mexican Americans should be encouraged to choose more foods high in vitamin A or carotenes, and Mexican American women need to increase their intake of calcium (review table 14-6).

Asian American elderly. Asian American elderly have a lower incidence of heart disease and diabetes mellitus than white and black elderly. However, a recent dietary study of 169 Chinese elderly, 90 Korean elderly, and 50 Japanese elderly residing in a senior apartment complex[64] found some serious nutrient deficiencies. Over half of the Chinese and Korean women were consuming less than two-thirds of the RDA for calcium.

TABLE 14-6   *Median Nutrient Intakes of Older Men and Women*
Ages Sixty to Sixty-Nine, by Race and Ethnic Group

	White		African American		Mexican American	
	Men	Women	Men	Women	Men	Women
Energy (kcal)	1,932.0	1,510.0	1,630.0	1,405.0	1,805.0	1,306.0
Protein (g)	79.0	60.0	67.0	51.0	74.0	53.0
Fat (g)	71.0	55.0	59.0	45.0	62.0	44.0
Vitamin A (μg RE)	914.0	816.0	551.0	431.0	613.0	435.0
Vitamin C (mg)	82.0	89.0	58.0	86.0	79.0	64.0
Folate (ug)	302.0	229.0	218.0	174.0	268.0	173.0
Vitamin B_6 (mg)	1.8	1.4	1.3	1.2	1.5	1.1
Calcium (mg)	734.0	660.0	480.0	399.0	810.0	494.0
Iron (mg)	14.7	10.7	10.6	9.3	13.5	8.7
Zinc (mg)	11.5	7.7	8.8	6.9	8.7	6.8

Data from Life Sciences Research Office, Federation of American Societies for Experimental Biology. 1995. *Third report on nutrition monitoring in the United States, Vol. I and II.* Washington, DC: U.S. Government Printing Office.

Energy intake was low, and vitamins A and C and riboflavin were also problem nutrients for the Chinese and Korean women. All of the men and the Japanese women had better diets. These elderly Asian Americans had not adopted American foods; instead, they continued to prefer their ethnic foods. Ethnic elderly may find it difficult to obtain their traditional foods at local food markets, and, if available, they may be higher in cost.

Food Selection Patterns and Nutrition Intervention

Food frequency patterns of older people[65,66] indicate that they consume bread and ready-to-eat cereals (both enriched and whole grain) regularly. Eggs and luncheon meats are the most common foods from the meat or protein group. Orange juice, bananas, lettuce, and potatoes are the fruits and vegetables included most regularly in meal planning. Milk is used frequently but in relatively low amounts, possibly as a whitener in coffee or tea. Missing from the diet is a dark green vegetable as a source of vitamin A precursors and an additional source of folate. Orange juice adds ascorbic acid, some folate, and some potassium to the diet, and bananas supply both potassium and vitamin B_6. Increased use of milk or other dairy foods is needed, and whole grain products should be encouraged. Alternatives to luncheon meats, often high in fat and sodium and low in zinc, iron, and other nutrients, should be explored.

Nutrition Screening Initiative

An urgent task for the nutrition professional is the identification of elderly people who have a less than optimum nutrient intake. When these individuals are identified, nutrition intervention can prevent any further nutrient-related deterioration in health. The Nutrition Screening Initiative is a national effort to seek out older people at risk. A panel of nutrition and medical experts developed and field tested a checklist of factors that are related to food intake and nutritional status in older people (fig. 14-7).[67] Older adults with a score of 6 or higher have a greater risk of low nutrient intake and chronic disease than those with lower scores. They should be referred to a nutrition professional for help with diet planning and information about nutrition and food support programs (see the following sections). The Determine Your Nutritional Health Checklist can be administered wherever older people are found and is a good starting point for discussing nutrition and health. The checklist should be completed at least once yearly to identify any new problems.

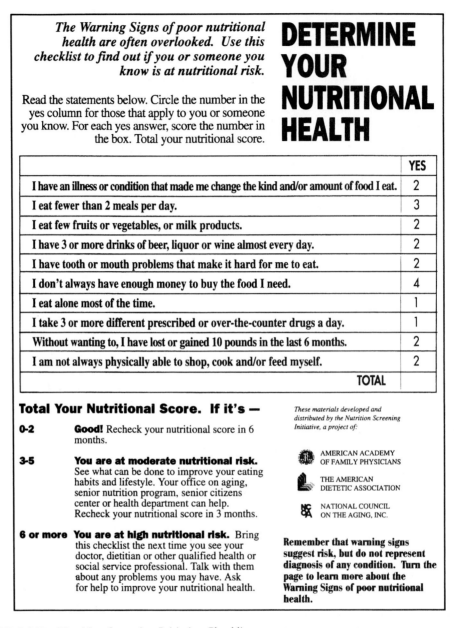

The Warning Signs of poor nutritional health are often overlooked. Use this checklist to find out if you or someone you know is at nutritional risk.

Read the statements below. Circle the number in the yes column for those that apply to you or someone you know. For each yes answer, score the number in the box. Total your nutritional score.

DETERMINE YOUR NUTRITIONAL HEALTH

	YES
I have an illness or condition that made me change the kind and/or amount of food I eat.	2
I eat fewer than 2 meals per day.	3
I eat few fruits or vegetables, or milk products.	2
I have 3 or more drinks of beer, liquor or wine almost every day.	2
I have tooth or mouth problems that make it hard for me to eat.	2
I don't always have enough money to buy the food I need.	4
I eat alone most of the time.	1
I take 3 or more different prescribed or over-the-counter drugs a day.	1
Without wanting to, I have lost or gained 10 pounds in the last 6 months.	2
I am not always physically able to shop, cook and/or feed myself.	2
	TOTAL

Total Your Nutritional Score. If it's —

0-2   **Good!** Recheck your nutritional score in 6 months.

3-5   **You are at moderate nutritional risk.** See what can be done to improve your eating habits and lifestyle. Your office on aging, senior nutrition program, senior citizens center or health department can help. Recheck your nutritional score in 3 months.

6 or more   **You are at high nutritional risk.** Bring this checklist the next time you see your doctor, dietitian or other qualified health or social service professional. Talk with them about any problems you may have. Ask for help to improve your nutritional health.

These materials developed and distributed by the Nutrition Screening Initiative, a project of:

AMERICAN ACADEMY OF FAMILY PHYSICIANS

THE AMERICAN DIETETIC ASSOCIATION

NATIONAL COUNCIL ON THE AGING, INC.

Remember that warning signs suggest risk, but do not represent diagnosis of any condition. Turn the page to learn more about the Warning Signs of poor nutritional health.

FIG. 14-7   Nutrition Screening Initiative Checklist.

Reprinted with permission by the Nutrition Screening Initiative, a project of the American Academy of Family Physicians, the American Dietetic Association and the National Council on the Aging, Inc., and funded in part by a grant from Ross Products Division, Abbott Laboratories.

NUTRITION AND FOOD PROGRAMS FOR OLDER PEOPLE ≈

Nutrition and the Continuum of Care

Older people differ in their general health, functional ability, mental capacity, and outlook on life. Thus, a full range of health, nutrition, social, and personal care services or, in other words, a continuum of care must be in place to support independent living and personal well-being at the highest possible level. A combination of services may provide long-term care in an institutional setting or in the person's home. Nutritional support services provided by family members, neighbors, and community agencies allow older people with some limitation of activity to continue to live independently. Support services may take the form of a ride to the grocery store or delivery of meals by a community

> **Innovative Approaches to Food Delivery**
>
> As the number of homebound elderly continues to escalate, the cost of daily meal delivery is becoming increasingly burdensome. Meal delivery in rural areas is especially costly and presents the added problem of maintaining foods at appropriate temperatures over an extended delivery time. One alternative to daily delivery of hot meals is weekly delivery of several frozen meals. This also allows recipients to choose what they want to eat on a particular day and at what time. For the homebound elderly who are able to move about within their homes, groceries can supplement either frozen or hot meals. Canned, dehydrated, freeze-dried, or other shelf-stable foods can provide a food reserve for weekends or other nondelivery days. Analysis of the relative cost-effectiveness and cost-benefit of alternative food delivery systems should be a priority as nutrition professionals seek to provide community-based long-term care for increasing numbers of aging adults.

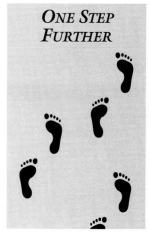

ONE STEP FURTHER

agency. Congregate meals that provide both a nutritious meal and an opportunity to socialize with others help maintain health and well-being in the relatively fit older adult.

National Nutrition Program for the Elderly (Title III-C)

Basic authorization. The Older Americans Act of 1965, as amended, is the major legislation providing programs for people age sixty and over. When established in 1972, the nutrition program was directed toward elderly people who might not eat adequately because they 1) could not afford to do so, 2) lacked the skills to select and prepare nourishing meals, 3) had limited mobility, which hindered shopping and cooking, and 4) felt rejected and lonely and lacked incentive to cook and eat alone.

Congregate and home-delivered meals. The congregate meal program, funded under the Older Americans Act is intended to make meals available at little or no cost in a social environment. Meal sites are in community centers, municipal buildings, public housing, senior citizens centers, and churches. Meals are served Monday through Friday in urban locations but on fewer days in rural locations. Important criteria in selecting a location are accessibility and familiarity to older people in the community. See the case study on p. 378, which describes a potential client for a congregate meal program in an urban community.

Since the congregate meal program was initiated, the older population has changed in both age and health status. There are more people age seventy-five and over, and these individuals are more likely to be frail, chronically ill, and homebound. To meet this emerging need, amendments to the Older Americans Act have authorized increasing funding for home-delivered meals. Mid 1990s statistics[68] report that 127 million meals were served to 2.3 million people at congregate sites and more than 113 million meals were served to 877,000 elderly in their homes. About 2.8 million meals were served to 87,500 Native American, Native Hawaiian, and Native Alaskan elderly. Every day, more than 16,000 meal sites operate in all fifty states.

Meal delivery programs have been developed by community nonprofit organizations and health and social service agencies, such as hospitals, churches, and nursing homes. In some locations, meals are delivered from congregate meal sites. Most home-delivered meals programs are funded through the Older Americans Act. Meals are delivered by volunteers, who often pay their own transportation costs, or by paid drivers. Programs operate on weekdays only and deliver a hot meal at noon. About half of all programs deliver additional cold or frozen meals on Friday to provide for the weekend, but only 22% of programs offer a cold supper meal.[69] No program provides meals on all days or for all meals of the day.

Older people can request meal delivery directly or can be referred by a family member, physician, visiting nurse, nutrition professional, or social worker. Programs receiving Title III-C funding require that recipients 1) are age sixty or over and 2) are unable to leave their homes because of disability or other extenuating circumstances. A two-person household may be in need of home-delivered meals if one person is so burdened caring for an

Title III-C
Statute of the Older Americans Act authorizing congregate and home-delivered meals for people sixty years of age and over.

STRATEGIES
FOR NUTRITION
EDUCATION

Nutrition Programs for the Elderly: Increasing Nutrient Density

Good nutrition plays a major role in keeping older people healthy and functioning. Many elderly Americans, however, are not eating as well as they should. For some, it may be a matter of not eating appropriate foods and, for others, of not eating at all. A government report estimated that as many as 1 million older people living in their own homes may be malnourished. (See text for a discussion of the factors that can lead to poor food intake in the elderly.) Both congregate and home-delivered meals funded by Title III-C of the Older Americans Act contribute significantly to the food intake of many older people in the community. Careful attention to both the quantity and nutrient density of the food provided may prevent the development of malnutrition in the older people dependent on these meals.

Current regulations require that all Title III-C meals conform to the Dietary Guidelines for Americans and that each meal provide one-third of the RDA. Based on the RDAs for men and women over age fifty, a meal providing about one-third of the day's energy needs should contain about 600 to 800 kcal. Although a diet containing no more than 30% fat is recommended for healthy adults, it is sometimes appropriate to allow a higher level of fat in Title III-C meals. Weight loss is a serious threat for older persons with chronic disease. Also, sauces and gravies help maintain temperature and moisture in foods that must be transported. Finally, for many elderly people the Title III-C meal at noon is their major meal of the day, justifying a higher level of all nutrients. All meals should be planned to maximize nutrient density. Some suggestions follow.

Main dish

Recipes including meat, fish, poultry, eggs, legumes, and peanut butter are good sources of protein, vitamin B_6, iron, and zinc; dishes made with cheese and milk supply protein, riboflavin, and calcium (if a dairy food is the major source of protein, iron and zinc will need to be supplied elsewhere in the meal).

Fruits and vegetables

Emphasize dark green and deep yellow vegetables and fruits, citrus, bananas, and potatoes to provide the carotenoids, vitamin B_6, ascorbic acid, folate, potassium, magnesium, and fiber.

Enriched or whole grains

Popular whole grains include whole-wheat bread, corn bread, and bran or oatmeal muffins; use whole-grain toppings on casseroles or fruit desserts to contribute important vitamins and minerals.

Dessert

Choose plain fruit or baked fruit, pudding, custard, ice cream or baked products made with whole grains, raisins, sweet potatoes, pumpkin, and bananas; these add protein, iron, calcium, carotenoids, and other vitamins and minerals.

Milk

Offer low-fat milk or buttermilk to increase consumption; nonfat dry milk or cheese can be used to fortify soups, sauces, or mashed potatoes.

All nutrition programs are expected to ensure that their meals meet nutritional guidelines. Unfortunately, many programs do not have a nutritionist or dietitian to develop their menus or monitor food safety, meal costs, and overall food quality. If meals are to include the highest appropriate level of nutrients possible, the input of nutrition professionals is essential.

Rhodes, S.S., ed. 1991. *Effective meal planning for the elderly nutrition program.* Chicago: American Dietetic Association.
U.S. Department of Health and Human Services. 1994. *Food and nutrition for life: Malnutrition and older Americans.* Report by the assistant secretary for aging. Administration on Aging. Washington, DC.

How Can We Learn More About the Nutritional Care of Older People in Our Community?

Tripp, F. 1997. The use of dietary supplements in the elderly: Current issues and recommendations. *J Am Diet Assoc* 97:S181.

Do active, community-living elderly people need dietary supplements? This article offers guidelines on when to recommend dietary supplements to older clients and when supplements are unnecessary or inappropriate.

Tepper, B.J., and R.M. Nayga. 1998. Awareness of the link between bone disease and calcium intake is associated with higher dietary calcium intake in women aged 50 years and older: Results of the 1991 CSFII-DHKS. *J Am Diet Assoc* 98:196.

What is an effective strategy for encouraging older people to increase their intakes of the nutrients that are important for health and well-being? The research study of Dr. Tepper and Dr. Nayga gives some background as to how older people can be motivated to increase their intakes of calcium.

Dornelas, E.A., J. Wylie-Rosett, and C. Swencionis. 1998. The DIET study: Long-term outcomes of a cognitive-behavioral weight-control intervention in independent-living elders. *J Am Diet Assoc* 98:1276.

Can a weight control intervention program bring about long-term changes in cardiovascular risk in overweight elderly people? Dr. Dornelas and her co-authors describe their intervention program with older people that emphasized positive lifestyle changes continued over a three-year follow-up period.

Evans, W.J., and D. Cyr-Campbell. 1997. Nutrition, exercise and healthy aging. *J Am Diet Assoc* 97:632.

How will a walking program or a strength training program help older people stay healthy and fit? These authors explain how physical activity affects skeletal muscle and describe a walking program that can be recommended to older people who want to stay active.

Jenson, G.L. et al. 1997. Nutrition risk screening characteristics of rural older persons: Relation to functional limitations and health care charges. *Am J Clin Nutr* 66:819.

What are some tools to assess nutritional intake and functional disability that can be used to identify older people at high risk for malnutrition? These researchers tested several sets of questions used as part of the Nutrition Screening Initiative. Their findings will help target programs to meet the needs of older people who require assistance with food shopping, food preparation, or personal care. Dr. Jensen and his co-authors also explain how nutrition problems and the need for assistance with the activities of daily living are related to the health care costs of older people.

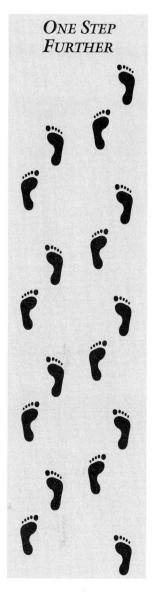

ONE STEP FURTHER

invalid spouse that he or she has little time or energy to prepare adequate meals. Implementation of the **diagnosis-related group (DRG)** guidelines has resulted in the earlier release of patients from medical facilities and a dramatic increase in requests for home-delivered meals. Unfortunately, the need for home-delivered meals exceeds the available resources to the extent that 41% of programs have waiting lists and the average time on a waiting list is two to three months.[68]

Diagnosis-related group (DRG)
U.S. government cost-containment management classification system for designating Medicare payments based on diagnosis categories, disease, or procedure.

Nutrition Standards for Meals Programs

Meals provided with Title III-C funds are expected to supply one-third of the RDA for people over age fifty. If two or three meals are provided, the total for the day should equal 67% or 100% of the RDA, respectively, thereby allowing some flexibility within individual meals. Limited funding and lack of professionally trained staff make it impractical to provide meals modified to meet the dietary requirements of particular chronic diseases. However, the meal served to all is likely to be acceptable for diabetics or for those who must limit their fat intake if portion size is controlled, skim milk is available, and fruit is offered as an alternative to a high-calorie dessert. Limiting the use of salt in meal preparation benefits all participants. Because weight loss is a serious threat to many older people, menus containing up to 35%

CASE STUDY

The Needs of an Elderly Woman Living Alone

Miss Evans has just celebrated her eightieth birthday. She is 65 inches tall, weighs 158 pounds, and has no major health problems other than arthritis. She uses aspirin regularly for pain. Miss Evans lives in a subsidized high-rise apartment complex for senior citizens with a small efficiency kitchen. She has a two-unit range top, small oven, and small refrigerator but very limited storage space for frozen or shelf-stable items. She prepares all her own meals and eats alone. She usually has toast and coffee for breakfast and either a bowl of cereal or a peanut butter sandwich for lunch. She does not drink any milk except with her cereal but is fond of cheese. She makes a lot of stews, often buying chicken when it is on sale. She likes all fruits and vegetables but uses mostly canned items, because they are cheaper than fresh. The amount of money she can spend for food is very limited. She likes whole-wheat bread, although her favorite brand is higher in cost than other breads. Miss Evans had been shopping about twice a week at a supermarket located about one mile from her apartment, traveling by bus. Since a recent fall, she is afraid to ride the bus alone, and now her nephew shops for her once every two weeks. In between, she buys necessary items at a convenience store about one city block from her apartment, but the prices there are much higher. She has been feeling very tired lately and has lost her appetite, although she has well-fitting dentures and is able to eat anything she wishes. She weighs herself every week and has noticed that she lost 5 pounds over the past month.

Questions for analysis
1. What are the socioeconomic or lifestyle factors that influence Miss Evans' food intake?
2. What are the physiologic factors that may influence her food intake?
3. Which nutrients appear to be lacking in her dietary pattern?
4. What would you recommend to improve her food intake?
5. What are some food programs that would assist Miss Evans in remaining independent?

---

of total kilocalories as fat are generally appropriate.[70] Suggestions for maximizing the nutrient density of congregate and home-delivered meals can be found in the box on p. 381.

Nutrition Program Evaluation

Success in targeting those at highest risk. A national evaluation conducted between 1993 and 1995[68,71] looked at the overall impact of congregate and home-delivered meals on the nutrition and well-being of the recipients. The results indicated that the program served a large proportion of elderly at high nutritional risk. In the United States, the average age of the population group age sixty and over is about seventy-two, whereas the average age of congregate meal participants is seventy-six, and the average age of home-delivered meal recipients is seventy-eight. Although only 15% of all older people have incomes at or below the poverty line, nearly one-half of home-delivered meal recipients are at the poverty line.[68]

Meeting nutrient needs. Program participants referred to above received a substantial proportion of their daily nutrient intake from the meal received at noon.[71] Overall, congregate participants obtain 44% of their total kilocalories for the day and 47–50% of their protein, zinc, and vitamins A, D, E, and B_{12}. They received 40% of their daily thiamin, folate, and iron from the congregate meal. Home-delivered meal participants eat less food than congregate participants but receive 47% of their daily nutrient total from the noon meal, although only 39% of their total kilocalories. Percentages of particular vitamins and minerals are similar to those for the congregate meal. Nutrition program participants consume better diets on days that include a congregate or home-delivered meal and consume better diets than nonparticipants similar in age and socioeconomic background.

Nevertheless, nutrients falling below the RDA or adequate intake for all participants are vitamins E and B$_6$, calcium, magnesium, and zinc. Energy intakes also fall below recommended levels.[71] Intakes of energy and important nutrients could be raised to recommended levels if additional meals were provided.

Summary

The number of people age sixty and older is increasing faster than that of any other segment of the population. Normal aging and the effects of chronic disease bring about changes in major organ systems, with less efficient cardiac, renal, and gastrointestinal function. Loss of skeletal muscle contributes to the decline in resting energy metabolism and protein reserves. These physiologic changes influence the energy and nutrient requirements of the elderly adult. At this time, the nutrient needs of both healthy and physically impaired older people are poorly understood. The current RDAs for those above age fifty have been extrapolated from the recommendations for younger adults, and studies conducted with older populations are urgently needed. Existing evidence suggests that the present recommendations for protein and vitamins B$_6$ and B$_{12}$ are too low to meet the needs of older adults. New adequate intakes for calcium and vitamin D may offer some protection against bone loss; however, the intakes of most older people do not approach these levels. The major influence on dietary quality in the elderly is total energy intake. Social isolation, poverty, physical disability, and gastrointestinal side effects of prescription and over-the-counter drugs reduce food intake. Inappropriate use of alcohol or psychotropic drugs negatively affects nutrient intake and utilization. Community nutrition programs funded by the Older Americans Act that provide congregate and home-delivered meals make positive contributions to the nutritional status and general well-being of the older population.

Review Questions

1. What factors have led to the significant increase in life expectancy at birth that has occurred since 1900? Why has life expectancy at age sixty-five not changed to the same extent over this period?
2. Describe several physiologic changes that occur with normal aging. What is a nutritional implication of each?
3. What are some limitations of the current dietary recommendations for older people? How do the RDAs and adequate intakes for people over age fifty differ from those for younger adults?
4. What are the major components of the energy requirement? How and why do they change with aging? What are the problems associated with low energy intake?
5. The requirements for protein, vitamin B$_6$, vitamin B$_{12}$, vitamin D, and calcium appear to increase in older adults. What evidence supports this idea? What foods would you recommend to ensure appropriate intake and utilization of these nutrients?
6. Explain the difference between osteoporosis and osteomalacia. What are the physiologic and dietary factors that are associated with the development of osteoporosis?
7. Describe the mechanisms by which prescription and over-the-counter drugs can adversely affect nutritional status. Describe two addictive behaviors that occur in older people. What circumstances might lead to these behaviors? What are the potential benefits and hazards of vitamin and mineral supplements for older people?
8. How do age, energy intake, sex, physical disability, poverty, household size, and ethnic group influence nutrient intake in older people? Which groups are most vulnerable to inadequate intakes?
9. Describe several types of community programs that serve older people. What levels of nutrients are provided by each?
10. You receive a telephone call from a woman who is concerned about the food intake and nutritional status of her elderly mother. What screening tool could you use to assess the mother's nutritional risk? What questions would you ask? What programs might you suggest if her nutrient intake is not adequate?

APPENDIX

A

PHYSICAL GROWTH
NCHS PERCENTILES

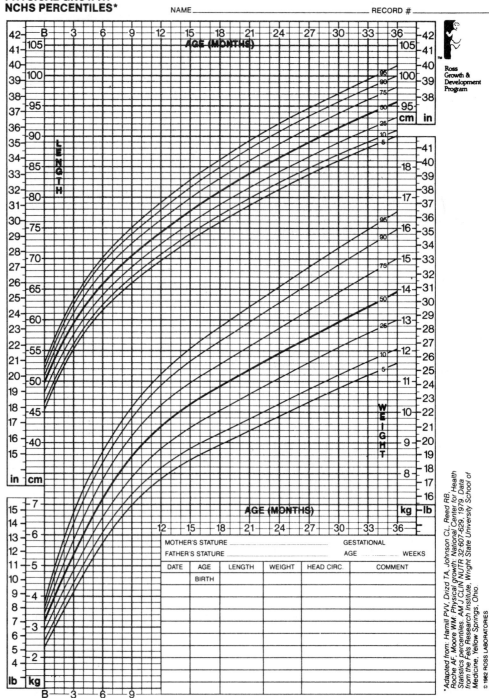

GIRLS: BIRTH TO 36 MONTHS
PHYSICAL GROWTH
NCHS PERCENTILES*

NAME _____ RECORD # _____

*Adapted from: Hamill PVV, Drizd TA, Johnson CL, Reed RB, Roche AF, Moore WM: Physical growth: National Center for Health Statistics percentiles. AM J CLIN NUTR 32:607-629, 1979. Data from the Fels Research Institute, Wright State University School of Medicine, Yellow Springs, Ohio.

BOYS: BIRTH TO 36 MONTHS
PHYSICAL GROWTH
NCHS PERCENTILES*

NAME _____   RECORD # _____

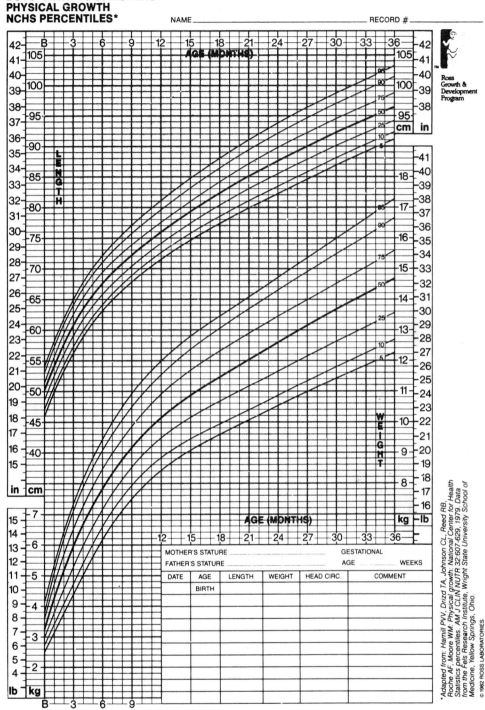

*Adapted from: Hamill PVV, Drizd TA, Johnson CL, Reed RB
Roche AF, Moore WM: Physical growth: National Center for Health
Statistics percentiles. AM J CLIN NUTR 32:607-629, 1979. Data
from the Fels Research Institute, Wright State University School of
Medicine, Yellow Springs, Ohio.

© 1982 ROSS LABORATORIES

Ross
Growth &
Development
Program

MOTHER'S STATURE _____ GESTATIONAL
FATHER'S STATURE _____ AGE _____ WEEKS

DATE	AGE	LENGTH	WEIGHT	HEAD CIRC.	COMMENT
	BIRTH				

GIRLS: BIRTH TO 36 MONTHS
PHYSICAL GROWTH
NCHS PERCENTILES*

NAME _____   RECORD # _____

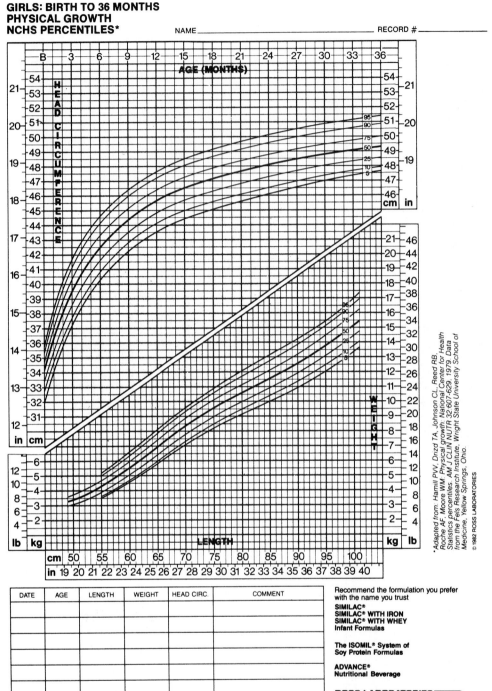

Recommend the formulation you prefer
with the name you trust

SIMILAC®
SIMILAC® WITH IRON
SIMILAC® WITH WHEY
Infant Formulas

The ISOMIL® System of
Soy Protein Formulas

ADVANCE®
Nutritional Beverage

ROSS LABORATORIES
COLUMBUS, OHIO 43216
Division of Abbott Laboratories, USA

G106/JUNE 1983   LITHO IN USA

*Adapted from: Hamill PVV, Drizd TA, Johnson CL, Reed RB, Roche AF, Moore WM. Physical growth: National Center for Health Statistics percentiles. AM J CLIN NUTR 32:607-629, 1979. Data from the Fels Research Institute, Wright State University School of Medicine, Yellow Springs, Ohio.

© 1982 ROSS LABORATORIES

BOYS: BIRTH TO 36 MONTHS
PHYSICAL GROWTH
NCHS PERCENTILES*

NAME _____ RECORD # _____

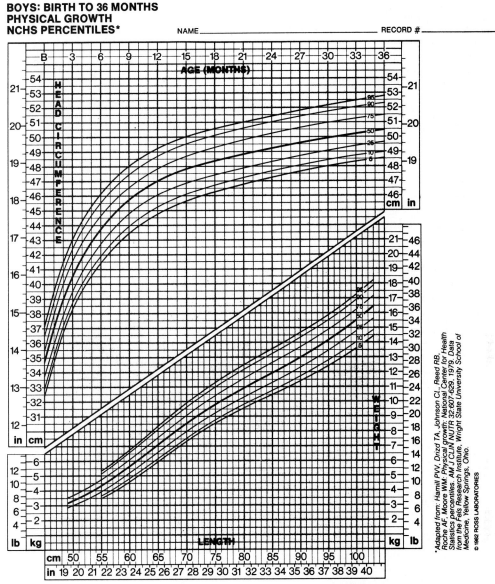

*Adapted from: Hamill PVV, Drizd TA, Johnson CL, Reed RB, Roche AF, Moore WM: Physical growth: National Center for Health Statistics percentiles. AM J CLIN NUTR 32:607-629, 1979. Data from the Fels Research Institute, Wright State University School of Medicine, Yellow Springs, Ohio.

© 1982 ROSS LABORATORIES

DATE	AGE	LENGTH	WEIGHT	HEAD CIRC.	COMMENT

Recommend the formulation you prefer
with the name you trust

SIMILAC®
SIMILAC® WITH IRON
SIMILAC® WITH WHEY
Infant Formulas

The **ISOMIL®** System of
Soy Protein Formulas

ADVANCE®
Nutritional Beverage

ROSS LABORATORIES
COLUMBUS, OHIO 43216
Division of Abbott Laboratories, USA

G105/JUNE 1983   LITHO IN USA

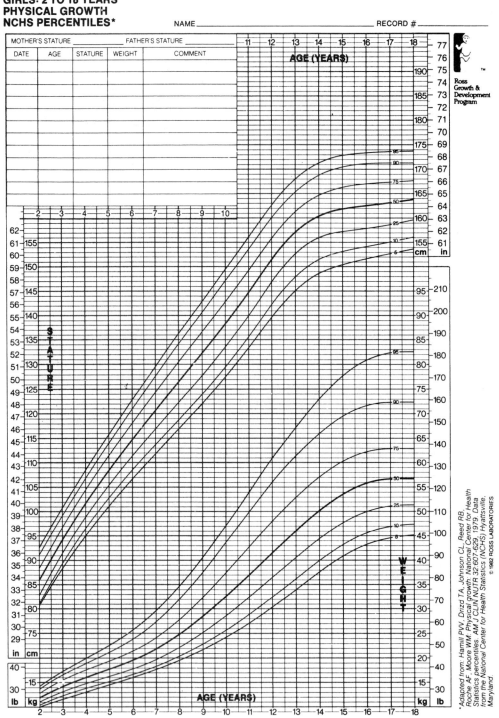

BOYS: 2 TO 18 YEARS
PHYSICAL GROWTH
NCHS PERCENTILES*

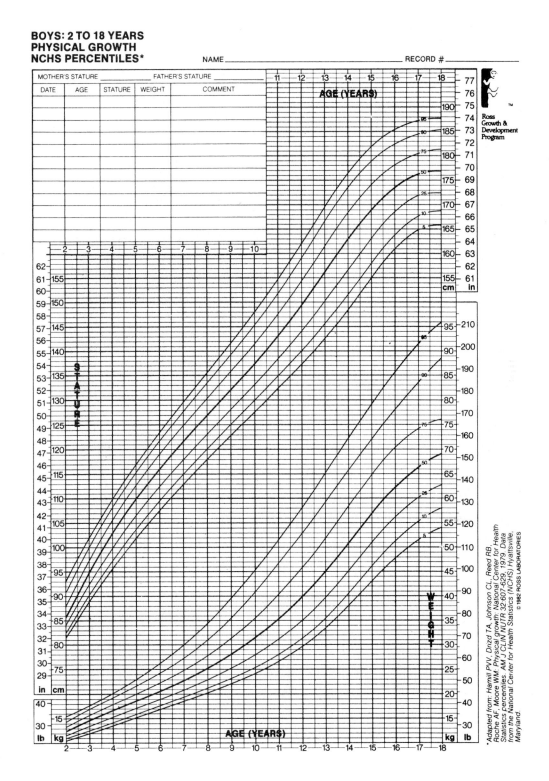

NAME _____   RECORD # _____

* Adapted from: Hamill PVV, Drizd T.A. Johnson CL, Reed RB, Roche AF, Moore WM. Physical growth: National Center for Health Statistics percentiles. AM J CLIN NUTR 32:607-629, 1979. Data from the National Center for Health Statistics (NCHS) Hyattsville, Maryland.
© 1982 ROSS LABORATORIES

Ross
Growth &
Development
Program

GIRLS: PREPUBESCENT PHYSICAL GROWTH NCHS PERCENTILES*

NAME _____ RECORD # _____

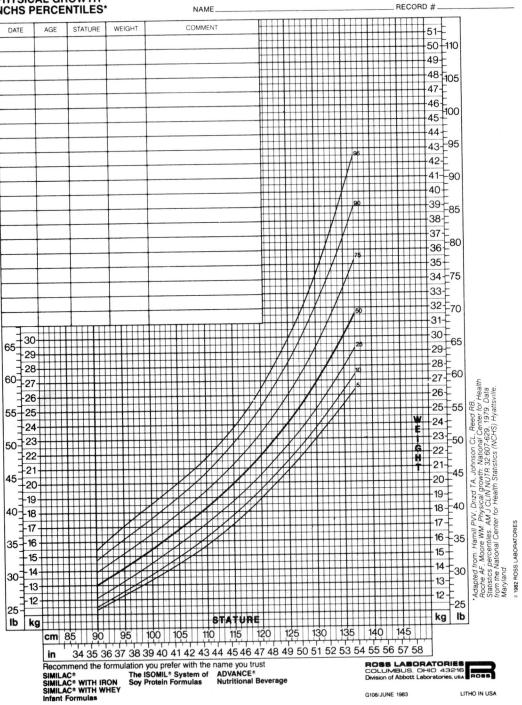

Adapted from: Hamill PVV, Drizd TA, Johnson CL, Reed RB, Roche AF, Moore WM. Physical growth: National Center for Health Statistics percentiles. AM J CLIN NUTR 32:607-629, 1979. Data from the National Center for Health Statistics (NCHS), Hyattsville, Maryland

© 1982 ROSS LABORATORIES

Recommend the formulation you prefer with the name you trust

SIMILAC®
SIMILAC® WITH IRON
SIMILAC® WITH WHEY
Infant Formulas

The ISOMIL® System of
Soy Protein Formulas

ADVANCE®
Nutritional Beverage

ROSS LABORATORIES
COLUMBUS, OHIO 43216
Division of Abbott Laboratories, USA

G108/JUNE 1983   LITHO IN USA

**BOYS: PREPUBESCENT
PHYSICAL GROWTH
NCHS PERCENTILES***

NAME _____   RECORD # _____

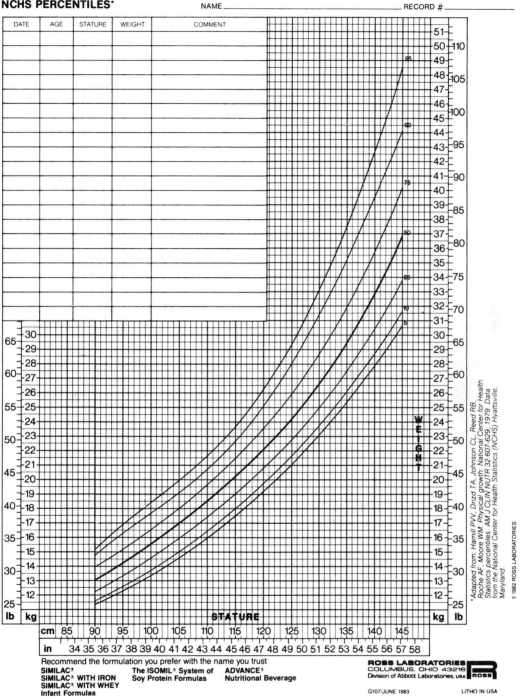

*Adapted from: Hamill PVV, Drizd TA, Johnson CL, Reed RB, Roche AF, Moore WM: Physical growth: National Center for Health Statistics percentiles. AM J CLIN NUTR 32:607-629, 1979. Data from the National Center for Health Statistics (NCHS) Hyattsville, Maryland.

© 1982 ROSS LABORATORIES

Recommend the formulation you prefer with the name you trust

**SIMILAC®
SIMILAC® WITH IRON
SIMILAC® WITH WHEY
Infant Formulas**

**The ISOMIL® System of
Soy Protein Formulas**

**ADVANCE®
Nutritional Beverage**

ROSS LABORATORIES
COLUMBUS, OHIO 43216
Division of Abbott Laboratories, USA   **ROSS**

G107/JUNE 1983   LITHO IN USA

WEIGHT-HEIGHT OF YOUTH TWELVE TO SEVENTEEN YEARS OF AGE

Weight–Height of Youths at Twelve Years (kg/cm)

Sex and Height	n	N	$\overline{X}$	s	$s_{\overline{x}}$	5th	10th	25th	50th	75th	90th	95th
Males												
Under 130 cm	5	15	*	*	*	*	*	*	*	*	*	*
130.0–134.9 cm	4	8	*	*	*	*	*	*	*	*	*	*
135.0–139.9 cm	34	111	32.50	3.741	0.727	26.6	27.6	30.2	31.6	34.7	37.7	39.4
140.0–144.9 cm	80	241	34.28	3.635	0.601	28.1	30.0	31.8	34.1	36.5	38.6	40.7
145.0–149.9 cm	123	386	39.27	6.243	0.615	32.1	33.2	35.7	38.2	40.9	46.1	52.5
150.0–154.9 cm	156	513	42.90	6.314	0.480	34.9	36.1	38.2	42.1	46.0	51.6	56.3
155.0–159.9 cm	135	432	47.35	7.551	0.769	38.3	39.4	41.9	46.2	50.5	57.4	61.9
160.0–164.9 cm	65	201	50.82	8.735	1.388	42.1	42.7	44.9	48.4	56.0	61.1	67.1
165.0–169.9 cm	29	88	55.75	8.811	2.031	43.3	46.4	49.0	54.4	59.9	68.3	76.6
170.0–174.9 cm	8	21	62.37	4.503	1.993	54.0	58.1	60.1	61.0	66.0	69.1	69.5
175.0–179.9 cm	3	10	*	*	*	*	*	*	*	*	*	*
180.0–184.9 cm	1	2	*	*	*	*	*	*	*	*	*	*
185.0–189.9 cm	—	—	—	—	—	—	—	—	—	—	—	—
190.0–194.9 cm	—	—	—	—	—	—	—	—	—	—	—	—
195.0 cm and over	—	—	—	—	—	—	—	—	—	—	—	—
Females												
Under 130 cm	3	10	*	*	*	*	*	*	*	*	*	*
130.0–134.9 cm	12	44	29.41	3.372	0.914	25.0	25.0	26.4	28.9	32.1	34.1	34.2
135.0–139.9 cm	32	116	38.30	7.314	1.194	28.8	30.6	33.3	36.8	41.4	49.2	55.1
140.0–144.9 cm	72	258	39.78	6.205	0.975	31.8	32.8	35.5	38.5	42.8	48.3	50.6
145.0–149.9 cm	147	517	44.00	7.421	0.677	34.4	35.8	38.9	42.8	47.4	52.9	57.4
150.0–154.9 cm	144	525	48.74	8.369	0.714	37.9	39.2	43.0	46.8	53.8	60.7	63.5
155.0–159.9 cm	95	336	53.06	8.010	0.658	42.5	43.9	47.2	51.1	57.2	65.6	69.6
160.0–164.9 cm	31	117	54.89	7.022	1.384	43.9	47.1	50.4	53.1	59.7	64.5	71.3
165.0–169.9 cm	11	42	63.66	14.501	6.214	48.7	50.1	50.8	56.7	82.2	86.0	86.1
170.0–174.9 cm	—	—	—	—	—	—	—	—	—	—	—	—
175.0–179.9 cm	—	—	—	—	—	—	—	—	—	—	—	—
180.0–184.9 cm	—	—	—	—	—	—	—	—	—	—	—	—
185.0–189.9 cm	—	—	—	—	—	—	—	—	—	—	—	—
190.0–194.9 cm	—	—	—	—	—	—	—	—	—	—	—	—
195.0 cm and over	—	—	—	—	—	—	—	—	—	—	—	—

Percentiles

From National Center for Health Statistics. 1973. *Height and weight of youths 12–17 years, United States.* In *Vital and health statistics*, series 11, no. 124, Health Services and Mental Health Administration, Washington, DC: U.S. Government Printing Office.

n: sample size; *N*: estimated number of youths in population in thousands; $\overline{X}$: mean; *s*: standard deviation; $s_{\overline{x}}$: standard error of the mean

Weight-Height of Youth at Thirteen Years (kg/cm)

Sex and Height	n	N	$\bar{X}$	s	$s_{\bar{x}}$	5th	10th	25th	50th	75th	90th	95th
Males												
Under 130 cm	—	—	—	—	—	—	—	—	—	—	—	—
130.0–134.9 cm	2	5	*	*	*	*	*	*	*	*	*	*
135.0–139.9 cm	6	25	32.62	5.624	7.716	27.2	27.6	28.9	31.0	34.9	43.1	43.2
140.0–144.9 cm	18	56	36.54	5.852	1.607	30.0	30.5	32.1	36.1	39.2	41.7	53.2
145.0–149.9 cm	65	204	39.03	5.270	0.662	32.4	33.9	36.1	37.9	41.2	44.5	46.4
150.0–154.9 cm	99	312	42.58	6.724	0.865	34.8	36.2	37.9	41.0	45.5	49.4	61.0
155.0–159.9 cm	131	421	47.27	7.482	0.717	37.8	39.2	41.7	45.8	51.1	58.7	61.7
160.0–164.9 cm	125	393	53.01	9.324	0.916	41.5	43.7	46.9	50.4	58.2	64.4	72.5
165.0–169.9 cm	91	285	55.92	8.560	0.833	46.3	47.5	49.3	53.6	59.4	69.0	75.0
170.0–174.9 cm	63	215	62.01	10.362	1.033	51.2	51.6	53.7	60.1	67.0	76.0	85.0
175.0–179.9 cm	19	68	67.92	12.085	3.428	56.3	57.9	60.1	63.3	70.3	88.3	89.0
180.0–184.9 cm	5	15	*	*	*	*	*	*	*	*	*	*
185.0–189.9 cm	—	—	—	—	—	—	—	—	—	—	—	—
190.0–194.9 cm	—	—	—	—	—	—	—	—	—	—	—	—
195.0 cm and over	—	—	—	—	—	—	—	—	—	—	—	—
Females												
Under 130 cm	—	—	—	—	—	—	—	—	—	—	—	—
130.0–134.9 cm	1	3	*	*	*	*	*	*	*	*	*	*
135.0–139.9 cm	—	—	—	—	—	—	—	—	—	—	—	—
140.0–144.9 cm	15	51	37.13	7.317	2.259	26.6	27.5	30.5	36.7	40.1	44.5	56.1
145.0–149.9 cm	47	165	42.23	6.880	0.888	34.7	35.6	38.2	40.5	44.2	53.6	57.6
150.0–154.9 cm	98	329	44.32	7.029	0.787	35.6	36.5	39.2	42.9	47.3	53.7	57.9
155.0–159.9 cm	152	499	49.75	8.757	0.699	39.1	39.9	43.8	48.4	53.8	61.0	65.9
160.0–164.9 cm	156	515	53.16	8.399	0.522	41.2	43.9	47.7	52.2	57.0	63.8	68.5
165.0–169.9 cm	86	284	58.17	9.125	0.921	46.2	47.4	52.2	58.1	61.5	69.3	76.2
170.0–174.9 cm	24	87	58.11	13.209	2.343	46.2	47.1	48.4	52.9	65.3	68.6	96.8
175.0–179.9 cm	3	10	*	*	*	*	*	*	*	*	*	*
180.0–184.0 cm	—	—	—	—	—	—	—	—	—	—	—	—
185.0–189.9 cm	—	—	—	—	—	—	—	—	—	—	—	—
190.0–194.9 cm	—	—	—	—	—	—	—	—	—	—	—	—
195.0 cm and over	—	—	—	—	—	—	—	—	—	—	—	—

Weight-Height of Youth at Fourteen Years (kg/cm)

Sex and Height	n	N	$\bar{X}$	s	$s_{\bar{x}}$	Percentiles						
						5th	10th	25th	50th	75th	90th	95th
Males												
Under 130 cm	—	—	—	—	—	—	—	—	—	—	—	—
130.0–134.9 cm	2	7	*	*	*	*	*	*	*	*	*	*
135.0–139.9 cm	3	13	*	*	*	*	*	*	*	*	*	*
140.0–144.9 cm	11	42	40.51	1.829	0.644	36.9	38.6	39.6	40.6	42.0	42.5	42.7
145.0–149.9 cm	45	135	43.63	6.277	1.182	36.2	37.0	39.0	41.4	48.0	51.7	55.3
150.0–154.9 cm	83	261	47.42	7.822	0.872	37.7	38.7	41.8	46.1	51.2	58.0	62.7
155.0–159.9 cm	96	299	52.28	6.785	0.584	42.5	44.0	47.5	52.1	56.3	61.5	65.1
160.0–164.9 cm	134	432	58.07	9.416	1.054	47.7	49.3	51.6	55.4	62.3	70.6	75.7
165.0–169.9 cm	144	435	62.37	11.516	1.095	49.7	51.0	55.0	59.4	65.6	79.2	86.3
170.0–174.9 cm	71	228	65.54	9.704	1.306	50.9	55.1	58.5	64.7	69.9	74.5	84.0
175.0–179.9 cm	25	81	72.44	13.014	2.298	59.6	60.0	65.1	69.4	77.0	83.0	94.3
180.0–184.9 cm	3	9	*	*	*	*	*	*	*	*	*	*
185.0–189.0 cm	1	3	*	*	*	*	*	*	*	*	*	*
190.0–194.9 cm	—	—	—	—	—	—	—	—	—	—	—	—
195.0 cm and over	—	—	—	—	—	—	—	—	—	—	—	—
Females												
Under 130 cm	—	—	—	—	—	—	—	—	—	—	—	—
130.0–134.9 cm	1	2	*	*	*	*	*	*	*	*	*	*
135.0–139.9 cm	2	6	*	*	*	*	*	*	*	*	*	*
140.0–144.9 cm	6	18	*	*	*	*	*	*	*	*	*	*
145.0–149.9 cm	17	52	42.00	5.879	1.683	32.0	35.3	36.3	42.3	47.5	49.5	51.1
150.0–154.9 cm	64	196	48.26	6.797	0.926	37.7	39.2	42.5	47.9	53.3	55.9	58.8
155.0–159.9 cm	157	508	51.35	7.705	0.520	42.1	43.4	46.3	49.6	55.6	62.2	64.3
160.0–164.9 cm	186	603	54.59	8.810	0.707	43.0	45.0	48.4	53.0	59.7	66.7	70.7
165.0–169.9 cm	114	372	58.46	10.185	0.955	45.9	47.5	52.1	56.8	61.8	70.5	76.4
170.0–174.9 cm	36	121	64.37	15.821	2.814	49.2	52.1	56.2	59.8	70.5	72.9	99.4
175.0–179.9 cm	7	28	61.33	5.496	2.620	51.7	52.0	57.7	59.8	64.6	70.2	70.6
180.0–184.9 cm	2	7	*	*	*	*	*	*	*	*	*	*
185.0–189.9 cm	—	—	—	—	—	—	—	—	—	—	—	—
190.0–194.9 cm	—	—	—	—	—	—	—	—	—	—	—	—
195.0 cm and over	—	—	—	—	—	—	—	—	—	—	—	—

Weight-Height of Youth at Fifteen Years (kg/cm)

Sex and Height	n	N	$\overline{X}$	s	$s_{\overline{x}}$	5th	10th	25th	50th	75th	90th	95th
Males												
Under 130 cm	—	—	—	—	—	—	—	—	—	—	—	—
130.0–134.9 cm	—	—	—	—	—	—	—	—	—	—	—	—
135.0–139.9 cm	—	—	—	—	—	—	—	—	—	—	—	—
140.0–144.9 cm	1	2	*	*	*	*	*	*	*	*	*	*
145.0–149.9 cm	10	30	45.72	8.582	3.550	35.7	39.2	42.6	44.7	46.0	48.7	76.1
150.0–154.9 cm	34	99	52.81	10.552	1.695	40.3	43.1	46.7	49.2	56.7	69.6	76.3
155.0–159.9 cm	71	206	53.01	8.417	0.986	42.7	44.1	46.9	51.5	56.3	65.3	68.8
160.0–164.9 cm	132	404	57.72	8.503	0.819	48.0	48.8	53.1	56.4	61.3	67.1	73.3
165.0–169.9 cm	176	574	62.88	8.464	0.633	51.6	53.4	56.7	61.9	67.2	72.9	78.1
170.0–174.9 cm	118	374	65.80	9.457	1.045	53.1	55.6	59.7	64.3	69.5	80.2	89.2
175.0–179.9 cm	51	144	72.00	11.928	1.724	54.6	60.3	64.4	70.2	68.4	84.4	96.6
180.0–184.9 cm	14	48	74.21	15.035	5.200	58.3	58.5	62.9	70.7	84.6	92.4	110.8
185.0–189.9 cm	6	15	83.39	16.431	10.332	66.4	66.7	69.6	73.8	103.0	105.7	106.2
190.0–194.9 cm	—	—	—	—	—	—	—	—	—	—	—	—
195.0 cm and over	—	—	—	—	—	—	—	—	—	—	—	—
Females												
Under 130 cm	—	—	—	—	—	—	—	—	—	—	—	—
130.0–134.9 cm	—	—	—	—	—	—	—	—	—	—	—	—
135.0–139.9 cm	—	—	—	—	—	—	—	—	—	—	—	—
140.0–144.9 cm	2	5	*	*	*	*	*	*	*	*	*	*
145.0–149.9 cm	15	51	47.91	7.875	3.623	36.0	39.4	42.1	45.4	52.7	55.7	66.3
150.0–154.9 cm	69	242	49.69	8.895	1.190	39.1	40.6	44.3	48.1	52.8	60.5	68.3
155.0–159.9 cm	111	400	51.52	8.473	0.934	41.4	43.5	46.3	50.8	55.1	59.8	65.2
160.0–164.9 cm	137	509	57.03	10.828	0.875	45.1	47.3	50.2	55.0	60.2	71.7	77.7
165.0–169.9 cm	109	398	60.71	10.357	1.053	47.5	49.3	55.1	58.4	65.7	74.1	81.0
170.0–174.9 cm	49	188	65.27	10.730	1.880	49.7	53.6	57.2	61.2	71.6	85.3	86.4
175.0–179.9 cm	7	23	63.30	8.872	4.807	49.7	49.9	53.8	62.4	71.1	71.9	79.2
180.0–184.9 cm	3	26	*	*	*	*	*	*	*	*	*	*
185.0–189.9 cm	1	3	*	*	*	*	*	*	*	*	*	*
190.0–194.9 cm	—	—	—	—	—	—	—	—	—	—	—	—
195.0 cm and over	—	—	—	—	—	—	—	—	—	—	—	—

Weight-Height of Youth at Sixteen Years (kg/cm)

Sex and Height	n	N	$\overline{X}$	s	$s_{\bar{x}}$	Percentiles						
						5th	10th	25th	50th	75th	90th	95th
Males												
Under 130 cm	—	—	—	—	—	—	—	—	—	—	—	—
130.0–134.9 cm	—	—	—	—	—	—	—	—	—	—	—	—
135.0–139.9 cm	—	—	—	—	—	—	—	—	—	—	—	—
140.0–144.9 cm	1	1	*	*	*	*	*	*	*	*	*	*
145.0–149.9 cm	4	12	*	*	*	*	*	*	*	*	*	*
150.0–154.9 cm	11	33	49.89	7.323	3.572	42.0	42.2	44.7	46.8	54.4	59.8	67.2
155.0–159.9 cm	32	108	53.09	6.459	1.273	44.2	44.9	48.2	51.4	58.0	60.9	66.1
160.0–164.9 cm	87	275	59.39	9.178	0.981	48.5	49.8	52.7	58.0	63.9	69.3	75.9
165.0–169.9 cm	166	552	62.66	7.556	0.629	51.6	53.8	57.5	61.6	67.1	73.1	78.0
170.0–174.9 cm	149	511	67.33	9.018	0.856	56.3	58.2	61.0	65.4	72.5	80.1	83.8
175.0–179.9 cm	72	227	72.38	12.485	1.993	58.3	59.3	64.4	68.9	76.5	90.2	96.9
180.0–184.9 cm	29	95	81.06	14.268	3.265	63.7	66.6	69.7	78.4	90.3	97.0	111.4
185.0–189.9 cm	30	10	*	*	*	*	*	*	*	*	*	*
190.0–194.9 cm	2	7	*	*	*	*	*	*	*	*	*	*
195.0 cm and over	—	—	—	—	—	—	—	—	—	—	—	—
Females												
Under 130 cm	—	—	—	—	—	—	—	—	—	—	—	—
130.0–134.9 cm	—	—	—	—	—	—	—	—	—	—	—	—
135.0–139.9 cm	—	—	—	—	—	—	—	—	—	—	—	—
140.0–144.9 cm	2	5	*	*	*	*	*	*	*	*	*	*
145.0–149.9 cm	10	33	52.58	8.198	3.191	43.9	44.1	44.9	51.0	54.5	72.0	72.1
150.0–154.9 cm	57	178	51.79	10.457	1.053	41.4	42.0	45.8	48.9	54.1	61.5	83.3
155.0–159.9 cm	117	354	53.20	7.766	0.734	44.0	45.6	48.4	51.6	56.4	61.9	69.0
160.0–164.9 cm	160	547	57.71	11.129	1.246	46.1	47.3	51.5	55.5	61.2	69.5	75.1
165.0–169.9 cm	122	450	61.72	11.998	0.802	47.1	48.8	53.3	59.1	67.3	78.7	86.7
170.0–174.9 cm	53	170	63.61	8.734	1.126	52.9	53.8	58.1	62.1	66.8	73.8	84.2
175.0–179.9 cm	14	45	72.55	15.012	5.224	58.6	58.8	61.7	65.9	80.6	99.1	105.5
180.0–184.9 cm	1	2	*	*	*	*	*	*	*	*	*	*
185.0–189.9 cm	—	—	—	—	—	—	—	—	—	—	—	—
190.0–194.9 cm	—	—	—	—	—	—	—	—	—	—	—	—
195.0 cm and over	—	—	—	—	—	—	—	—	—	—	—	—

Weight-Height of Youth at Seventeen Years (kg/cm)

Sex and Height	n	N	$\overline{X}$	s	$s_{\overline{x}}$	5th	10th	25th	50th	75th	90th	95th
Males												
Under 130 cm	—	—	—	—	—	—	—	—	—	—	—	—
130.0–134.9 cm	—	—	—	—	—	—	—	—	—	—	—	—
135.0–139.9 cm	—	—	—	—	—	—	—	—	—	—	—	—
140.0–144.9 cm	—	—	—	—	—	—	—	—	—	—	—	—
145.0–149.9 cm	1	3	*	*	*	*	*	*	*	*	*	*
150.0–154.9 cm	11	39	54.63	9.397	3.414	43.8	46.4	48.2	49.7	57.8	69.9	73.2
155.0–159.9 cm	25	81	57.75	6.503	1.355	49.7	51.1	52.5	56.9	61.6	70.1	70.8
160.0–164.9 cm	63	248	62.57	8.344	1.224	50.2	53.2	56.4	61.5	66.9	72.7	77.3
165.0–169.9 cm	115	396	67.06	11.163	0.704	53.3	55.5	59.5	64.6	71.9	80.9	91.6
170.0–174.9 cm	151	537	68.37	9.907	0.831	56.9	58.9	61.5	66.5	73.6	79.4	88.4
175.0–179.9 cm	80	297	73.31	12.454	1.335	59.6	61.0	65.1	71.2	78.4	91.8	102.7
180.0–184.9 cm	36	133	76.03	9.171	1.301	62.4	66.3	70.5	75.3	80.8	90.3	92.9
185.0–189.9 cm	7	25	81.40	10.985	7.588	62.9	62.9	67.8	87.3	90.3	90.6	90.6
190.0–194.9 cm	—	—	*	*	*	*	*	*	*	*	*	*
195.0 cm and over	—	—	—	—	—	—	—	—	—	—	—	—
Females												
Under 130 cm	—	—	—	—	—	—	—	—	—	—	—	—
130.0–134.9 cm	—	—	—	—	—	—	—	—	—	—	—	—
135.0–139.9 cm	—	—	—	—	—	—	—	—	—	—	—	—
140.0–144.9 cm	2	5	*	*	*	*	*	*	*	*	*	*
145.0–149.9 cm	8	26	43.49	3.939	1.604	38.6	38.8	40.1	45.1	45.7	51.1	51.2
150.0–154.9 cm	43	151	49.96	6.508	0.827	41.6	42.3	44.6	48.9	53.5	59.2	64.1
155.0–159.9 cm	103	385	54.71	9.903	0.775	44.4	45.5	48.7	53.2	57.7	61.6	76.2
160.0–164.9 cm	133	506	57.79	10.620	1.028	46.8	48.0	50.2	55.4	61.5	72.3	82.3
165.0–169.9 cm	116	433	60.63	10.117	1.182	47.9	50.3	55.1	59.3	65.1	69.4	71.6
170.0–174.9 cm	51	186	62.18	9.132	1.407	50.6	52.9	55.5	60.2	65.7	76.1	82.7
175.0–179.9 cm	12	47	65.76	8.405	2.229	54.9	56.7	60.1	61.7	75.2	75.9	83.0
180.0–184.9 cm	1	2	*	*	*	*	*	*	*	*	*	*
185.0–189.9 cm	—	—	—	—	—	—	—	—	—	—	—	—
190.0–194.9 cm	—	—	—	—	—	—	—	—	—	—	—	—
195.0 cm and over	—	—	—	—	—	—	—	—	—	—	—	—

Weight-Height of Youth at Twelve Years (lb/in)

| | | | | | | Percentiles | | | | | | |
Sex and Height	n	N	$\overline{X}$	s	$s_{\overline{x}}$	5th	10th	25th	50th	75th	90th	95th
Males												
Under 51.18 in	5	15	*	*	*	*	*	*	*	*	*	*
51.18–53.15 in	4	8	*	*	*	*	*	*	*	*	*	*
53.15–55.12 in	34	111	71.65	8.248	1.603	54.6	60.8	66.6	69.7	76.5	83.1	86.9
55.12–57.09 in	80	241	75.57	8.014	1.325	61.9	66.1	70.1	75.2	80.5	85.1	89.7
57.09–59.06 in	123	386	86.58	13.764	1.356	70.8	73.2	78.7	84.2	90.2	101.6	115.7
59.06–61.02 in	156	513	94.58	13.920	1.058	76.9	79.6	84.2	92.8	101.4	113.8	124.1
61.02–62.99 in	135	433	104.39	16.647	1.695	84.4	86.9	92.4	101.9	111.3	126.5	136.5
62.99–64.96 in	65	201	112.04	19.257	3.060	92.8	94.1	99.0	106.7	123.5	134.7	147.9
64.96–66.93 in	29	88	122.91	19.425	4.478	95.5	102.3	108.0	119.9	132.1	150.6	168.9
66.93–68.90 in	8	21	137.50	9.927	4.394	119.0	128.1	132.5	134.5	145.5	152.3	153.2
68.90–70.87 in	3	10	*	*	*	*	*	*	*	*	*	*
70.87–72.83 in	1	2	*	*	*	—	—	—	—	—	—	—
72.83–74.80 in	—	—	—	—	—	—	—	—	—	—	—	—
74.80–76.77 in	—	—	—	—	—	—	—	—	—	—	—	—
76.77 in and over	—	—	—	—	—	—	—	—	—	—	—	—
Females												
Under 51.18 in	—	—	—	—	—	—	—	—	—	—	—	—
51.18–53.15 in	3	10	*	*	*	*	*	*	*	*	*	*
53.15–55.12 in	12	44	64.84	7.434	2.015	55.1	55.1	58.2	63.7	70.8	75.2	75.4
55.12–57.09 in	32	116	84.44	16.125	2.632	63.5	67.5	73.4	81.1	91.3	108.5	121.5
57.09–59.06 in	72	258	87.70	13.680	2.150	70.1	72.3	78.3	78.9	94.4	106.5	111.6
59.06–61.02 in	147	517	97.00	16.361	1.493	75.8	78.9	85.8	94.4	104.5	116.6	126.5
61.02–62.99 in	144	525	107.45	18.451	1.574	83.6	86.4	94.8	103.2	118.6	133.8	140.0
62.99–64.96 in	95	336	117.00	17.659	1.451	93.7	96.8	104.1	112.7	126.1	144.6	153.4
64.96–66.93 in	31	117	121.01	15.481	3.051	96.8	103.8	111.1	117.1	131.6	142.2	157.2
66.93–68.90 in	11	42	140.35	31.969	13.700	107.4	110.5	112.0	125.0	181.2	189.6	189.8
68.90–70.87 in	—	—	—	—	—	—	—	—	—	—	—	—
70.87–72.83 in	—	—	—	—	—	—	—	—	—	—	—	—
72.83–74.80 in	—	—	—	—	—	—	—	—	—	—	—	—
74.80–76.77 in	—	—	—	—	—	—	—	—	—	—	—	—
76.77 in and over	—	—	—	—	—	—	—	—	—	—	—	—

Weight-Height of Youth at Thirteen Years (lb/in)

Sex and Height	n	N	$\overline{X}$	s	$s_{\overline{x}}$	Percentiles						
						5th	10th	25th	50th	75th	90th	95th
Males												
Under 51.18 in	—	—	—	—	—	—	—	—	—	—	—	—
51.18–53.15 in	2	5	*	*	*	*	*	*	*	*	*	*
53.15–55.12 in	8	25	71.91	12.399	17.011	60.0	60.8	63.7	68.3	76.9	95.0	95.2
55.12–57.09 in	18	56	80.56	12.902	3.543	66.1	67.2	70.8	79.6	86.4	91.9	117.3
57.09–59.06 in	65	204	86.05	11.618	1.460	71.4	74.7	79.6	83.6	90.8	98.1	102.3
59.06–61.02 in	99	312	93.87	14.824	1.907	76.7	79.8	83.6	90.4	100.3	108.9	134.5
61.02–62.99 in	131	421	104.21	16.495	1.581	83.3	86.4	91.9	101.0	112.7	129.4	136.0
62.99–64.96 in	125	393	116.87	20.556	2.019	91.5	96.3	103.4	111.1	128.3	142.0	159.8
64.96–66.93 in	91	285	123.28	18.872	1.837	102.1	104.7	108.7	118.2	131.0	152.1	165.3
66.93–68.90 in	63	215	136.71	22.844	2.277	112.9	113.8	118.4	132.5	147.7	167.6	187.4
68.90–70.87 in	19	68	149.72	26.643	7.557	124.1	127.6	132.5	139.6	155.0	194.7	196.2
70.87–72.83 in	5	15	*	*	*	*	*	*	*	*	*	*
72.83–74.80 in	—	—	—	—	—	—	—	—	—	—	—	—
74.80–76.77 in	—	—	—	—	—	—	—	—	—	—	—	—
76.77 in and over	—	—	—	—	—	—	—	—	—	—	—	—
Females												
Under 51.18 in	—	—	—	—	—	—	—	—	—	—	—	—
51.18–53.15 in	1	3	*	*	*	*	*	*	*	*	*	*
53.15–55.12 in	—	—	—	—	—	—	—	—	—	—	—	—
55.12–57.09 in	15	51	81.86	16.131	4.980	58.6	60.6	67.2	80.9	88.4	98.1	123.7
57.09–59.06 in	47	165	93.10	15.168	1.958	76.5	78.5	84.2	89.3	97.4	118.2	127.0
59.06–61.02 in	98	329	97.71	15.496	1.735	78.7	80.5	86.4	94.6	104.3	118.4	127.6
61.02–62.99 in	152	499	109.68	19.306	1.541	86.2	88.0	96.6	106.7	118.6	134.5	145.3
62.99–64.96 in	156	515	117.20	18.517	1.151	90.8	96.8	105.2	115.1	125.7	140.7	151.0
64.96–66.93 in	86	284	128.24	20.117	2.031	101.9	104.5	115.1	128.1	135.6	152.8	168.0
66.93–68.90 in	24	87	128.11	29.121	5.165	101.9	103.8	106.7	116.6	144.0	151.2	213.4
68.90–70.87 in	3	10	*	*	*	*	*	*	*	*	*	*
70.87–72.83 in	—	—	—	—	—	—	—	—	—	—	—	—
72.83–74.80 in	—	—	—	—	—	—	—	—	—	—	—	—
74.80–76.77 in	—	—	—	—	—	—	—	—	—	—	—	—
76.77 in and over	—	—	—	—	—	—	—	—	—	—	—	—

Weight-Height of Youth at Fourteen Years (lb/in)

									Percentiles				
Sex and Height	n	N	$\bar{X}$	s	$s_{\bar{x}}$	5th	10th	25th	50th	75th	90th	95th
Males												
Under 51.18 in	—	—	—	—	—	—	—	—	—	—	—	—
51.18–53.15 in	—	—	—	—	—	—	—	—	—	—	—	—
53.15–55.12 in	2	7	*	*	*	*	*	*	*	*	*	*
55.12–57.09 in	3	13	*	*	*	*	*	*	*	*	*	*
57.09–59.06 in	11	42	89.31	4.032	1.420	81.4	85.1	87.3	89.5	92.6	93.7	94.1
59.06–61.02 in	45	135	96.19	13.838	2.606	79.8	81.6	86.0	91.3	106.8	114.0	121.9
61.02–62.99 in	83	261	104.54	17.245	1.922	83.1	85.3	92.2	101.6	112.9	127.9	138.2
62.99–64.96 in	96	299	115.26	14.958	1.288	93.7	97.0	104.7	114.9	124.1	135.6	143.5
64.96–66.93 in	134	432	128.02	20.759	2.324	105.2	108.7	113.8	122.1	137.4	155.6	166.9
66.93–68.90 in	144	435	137.50	25.388	2.414	109.6	112.4	121.3	131.0	145.0	165.2	185.2
68.90–70.87 in	71	228	144.49	21.394	2.879	112.2	121.5	129.0	142.6	154.1	174.1	190.3
70.87–72.83 in	25	81	159.70	28.691	5.066	131.4	132.3	143.5	153.0	170.9	183.0	207.9
72.83–74.80 in	3	9	*	*	*	*	*	*	*	*	*	*
74.80–76.77 in	1	3	*	*	*	*	*	*	*	*	*	*
76.77 in and over	—	—	—	—	—	—	—	—	—	—	—	—
Females												
Under 51.18 in	—	—	—	—	—	—	—	—	—	—	—	—
51.18–53.15 in	—	—	—	—	—	—	—	—	—	—	—	—
53.15–55.12 in	1	2	*	*	*	*	*	*	*	*	*	*
55.12–57.09 in	2	6	*	*	*	*	*	*	*	*	*	*
57.09–59.06 in	17	52	92.59	12.961	3.710	70.5	77.8	80.0	93.3	104.7	109.1	112.7
59.06–61.02 in	64	196	106.40	14.985	2.042	83.1	86.4	93.7	105.6	117.5	123.2	129.6
61.02–62.99 in	157	508	113.21	16.987	1.146	90.8	95.7	102.1	109.3	122.6	137.1	141.8
62.99–64.96 in	186	603	120.35	19.423	1.559	94.8	99.2	106.7	116.8	131.6	147.0	155.0
64.96–66.93 in	114	372	128.88	24.454	2.105	101.2	104.7	114.9	125.2	136.2	155.4	168.4
66.93–68.90 in	36	121	141.91	34.879	6.204	108.5	114.9	123.9	131.8	155.4	160.7	219.1
68.90–70.87 in	7	28	135.21	12.117	5.776	114.0	114.6	127.2	131.8	142.4	154.8	155.6
70.87–72.83 in	2	7	*	*	*	*	*	*	*	*	*	*
73.83–74.80 in	—	—	—	—	—	—	—	—	—	—	—	—
74.80–76.77 in	—	—	—	—	—	—	—	—	—	—	—	—
76.77 in and over	—	—	—	—	—	—	—	—	—	—	—	—

Weight-Height of Youth at Fifteen Years (lb/in)

Sex and Height	n	N	$\bar{X}$	s	$s_{\bar{x}}$	5th	10th	25th	50th	75th	90th	95th
									Percentiles			
Males												
Under 51.18 in	—	—	—	—	—	—	—	—	—	—	—	—
51.18–53.15 in	—	—	—	—	—	—	—	—	—	—	—	—
53.15–55.12 in	—	—	—	—	—	—	—	—	—	—	—	—
55.12–57.09 in	1	2	*	*	*	*	*	*	*	*	*	*
57.09–59.06 in	10	30	100.80	18.920	7.826	78.7	86.4	93.9	98.5	101.4	107.4	167.8
59.06–61.02 in	34	99	116.43	23.263	3.737	88.8	95.0	103.0	108.5	125.0	153.4	168.2
61.02–62.99 in	71	206	116.87	18.556	2.174	94.1	97.2	103.4	113.5	124.1	144.0	151.7
62.99–64.96 in	132	404	127.25	18.746	1.806	105.8	107.6	117.1	124.3	135.1	147.9	161.6
64.96–66.93 in	176	574	138.63	18.660	1.396	113.8	117.7	125.0	136.5	148.2	160.7	172.2
66.93–68.90 in	118	374	146.06	20.849	2.304	117.1	122.6	131.6	141.8	153.2	176.8	196.7
68.90–70.87 in	51	144	158.73	26.297	3.801	120.4	132.9	142.0	154.8	172.8	186.1	213.0
70.87–72.83 in	14	48	163.61	33.147	11.464	128.5	129.0	138.7	155.9	186.5	203.7	244.3
72.83–74.80 in	6	15	183.84	36.224	22.778	146.4	147.0	153.4	162.7	227.1	233.0	234.1
74.80–76.77 in	—	—	—	—	—	—	—	—	—	—	—	—
76.77 in and over	—	—	—	—	—	—	—	—	—	—	—	—
Females												
Under 51.18 in	—	—	—	—	—	—	—	—	—	—	—	—
51.18–53.15 in	—	—	—	—	—	—	—	—	—	—	—	—
53.15–55.12 in	2	5	*	*	*	*	*	*	*	*	*	*
55.12–57.09 in	15	51	105.62	17.361	7.987	79.4	86.9	92.8	100.1	116.2	122.8	146.2
57.09–59.06 in	69	242	109.55	19.610	2.624	86.2	89.5	97.7	106.0	116.4	133.4	150.6
59.06–61.02 in	111	400	113.58	18.680	2.059	91.3	95.9	102.1	121.0	121.5	131.8	143.7
61.02–62.99 in	137	509	125.73	23.872	1.929	99.4	104.3	110.7	121.3	132.7	158.1	171.3
62.99–64.96 in	109	398	133.84	22.833	2.322	104.7	108.7	121.5	128.8	144.8	163.4	178.6
64.96–66.93 in	49	188	143.90	23.656	4.145	109.6	118.2	126.1	134.9	157.9	188.1	190.5
66.93–68.90 in	7	23	139.55	19.559	10.598	109.6	110.0	118.6	137.6	156.1	158.5	174.6
68.90–70.87 in	3	26	*	*	*	*	*	*	*	*	*	*
70.87–72.83 in	1	3	*	*	*	*	*	*	*	*	*	*
72.83–74.80 in	—	—	—	—	—	—	—	—	—	—	—	—
74.80–76.77 in	—	—	—	—	—	—	—	—	—	—	—	—
76.77 in and over	—	—	—	—	—	—	—	—	—	—	—	—

Weight–Height of Youth at Sixteen Years (lb/in)

Sex and Height	n	N	$\bar{X}$	s	$s_{\bar{x}}$	Percentiles						
						5th	10th	25th	50th	75th	90th	95th
Males												
Under 51.18 in	—	—	—	—	—	—	—	—	—	—	—	—
51.18–53.15 in	—	—	—	—	—	—	—	—	—	—	—	—
53.15–55.12 in	—	—	—	—	—	—	—	—	—	—	—	—
55.12–57.09 in	1	1	*	*	*	*	*	*	*	*	*	*
57.09–59.06 in	4	12	*	*	*	*	*	*	*	*	*	*
59.06–61.02 in	11	33	109.99	16.145	7.875	92.6	93.0	98.5	103.2	119.9	131.8	148.2
61.02–62.99 in	32	108	117.04	14.240	2.807	97.4	99.0	106.3	113.3	127.9	134.3	145.7
62.99–64.96 in	87	275	130.93	20.234	2.163	106.9	109.8	116.2	127.9	140.9	152.8	167.3
64.96–66.93 in	166	552	138.14	16.658	1.387	113.8	118.6	126.8	135.8	147.9	161.2	172.0
66.93–68.90 in	149	511	148.44	19.881	1.887	124.1	128.3	134.5	144.2	159.8	176.6	184.7
68.90–70.87 in	72	227	159.57	27.525	4.394	128.5	130.7	142.0	151.9	168.7	198.9	213.6
70.87–72.83 in	29	95	178.71	31.456	7.198	140.4	146.8	153.7	172.8	199.1	213.8	245.6
72.83–74.80 in	3	10	*	*	*	*	*	*	*	*	*	*
74.80–76.77 in	2	7	*	*	*	*	*	*	*	*	*	*
76.77 in and over	—	—	—	—	—	—	—	—	—	—	—	—
Females												
Under 51.18 in	—	—	—	—	—	—	—	—	—	—	—	—
51.18–53.15 in	—	—	—	—	—	—	—	—	—	—	—	—
53.15–55.12 in	—	—	—	—	—	—	—	—	—	—	—	—
55.12–57.09 in	2	5	*	*	*	*	*	*	*	*	*	*
57.09–59.06 in	10	33	115.92	18.074	7.035	96.8	97.2	99.0	112.4	120.2	158.7	158.9
59.06–61.02 in	57	178	114.18	23.054	2.322	91.3	92.6	101.0	107.8	119.3	135.6	183.6
61.02–62.99 in	117	354	117.29	17.121	1.618	97.0	100.5	106.7	113.8	124.3	136.5	152.1
62.99–64.96 in	160	547	127.23	24.535	2.747	101.6	104.3	113.5	122.4	134.9	153.2	165.6
64.96–66.93 in	122	450	136.07	26.451	1.768	103.8	107.6	117.5	130.3	148.4	173.5	191.1
66.93–68.90 in	53	170	140.24	19.255	2.482	116.6	118.6	128.1	136.9	147.3	173.7	185.6
68.90–70.87 in	14	45	159.95	33.096	11.517	129.2	129.6	136.0	145.3	177.7	218.5	232.6
70.87–72.83 in	1	2	*	*	*	*	*	*	*	*	*	*
72.83–74.80 in	—	—	—	—	—	—	—	—	—	—	—	—
74.80–76.77 in	—	—	—	—	—	—	—	—	—	—	—	—
76.77 in and over	—	—	—	—	—	—	—	—	—	—	—	—

Weight-Height of Youth at Seventeen Years (lb/in)

Sex and Height	n	N	$\bar{X}$	s	$s_{\bar{x}}$	5th	10th	25th	50th	75th	90th	95th
Males												
Under 51.18 in	—	—	—	—	—	—	—	—	—	—	—	—
51.18–53.15 in	—	—	—	—	—	—	—	—	—	—	—	—
53.15–55.12 in	—	—	—	—	—	—	—	—	—	—	—	—
55.12–57.09 in	—	—	—	—	—	—	—	—	—	—	—	—
57.09–59.06 in	1	3	*	*	*	*	*	*	*	*	*	*
59.06–61.02 in	11	39	120.44	20.717	7.527	96.6	102.3	106.3	109.6	127.4	154.1	161.4
61.02–62.99 in	25	81	127.32	14.337	2.987	109.6	112.7	115.7	125.4	135.8	154.5	156.1
62.99–64.96 in	63	248	137.94	18.395	2.699	110.7	117.3	124.3	135.6	147.5	160.3	170.4
64.96–66.93 in	115	396	147.84	24.610	1.552	117.5	122.4	131.2	142.4	158.5	178.4	202.2
66.93–68.90 in	151	537	150.73	21.841	1.832	125.4	129.9	135.6	146.6	162.3	175.0	194.9
68.90–70.87 in	80	297	161.62	27.456	2.943	131.4	134.5	143.5	157.0	172.8	202.4	226.4
70.87–72.83 in	36	133	167.62	20.219	2.868	137.6	146.2	155.4	166.0	178.1	199.1	204.8
72.83–74.80 in	7	25	179.46	24.218	16.729	138.7	138.7	149.5	192.5	199.1	199.7	199.7
74.80–76.77 in	—	—	—	—	—	—	—	—	—	—	—	—
76.77 in and over	—	—	—	—	—	—	—	—	—	—	—	—
Females												
Under 51.18 in	—	—	—	—	—	—	—	—	—	—	—	—
51.18–53.15 in	—	—	—	—	—	—	—	—	—	—	—	—
53.15–55.12 in	2	5	*	*	*	*	*	*	*	*	*	*
55.12–57.09 in	8	26	95.88	8.684	3.536	85.1	85.5	88.4	99.4	100.8	112.7	112.9
57.09–59.06 in	43	151	110.14	14.348	1.823	91.7	93.3	98.3	107.8	117.9	130.5	141.3
59.06–61.02 in	103	385	120.61	21.832	1.709	97.9	100.3	107.4	117.3	127.2	135.8	168.0
61.02–62.99 in	133	506	127.41	23.413	2.266	103.2	105.8	110.7	122.1	127.2	159.4	181.4
62.99–64.96 in	116	433	133.67	22.304	2.606	105.8	110.9	121.5	130.7	143.5	153.0	157.9
64.96–66.93 in	51	186	137.08	20.133	3.102	111.6	116.6	122.4	132.7	144.8	167.8	182.3
66.93–68.90 in	12	47	14.98	18.530	4.914	121.0	125.0	132.5	136.0	165.8	167.3	183.0
68.90–70.87 in	1	2	*	*	*	*	*	*	*	*	*	*
70.87–72.83 in	—	—	—	—	—	—	—	—	—	—	—	—
72.83–74.80 in	—	—	—	—	—	—	—	—	—	—	—	—
74.80–76.77 in	—	—	—	—	—	—	—	—	—	—	—	—
76.77 in and over	—	—	—	—	—	—	—	—	—	—	—	—

Percentiles

ANDRES AGE-SPECIFIC WEIGHT-HEIGHT TABLE FOR ADULTS AND THE ELDERLY*

Height (ft–in)	Weight Range for Men and Women by Age (Years) in Pounds[†]				
	25	35	45	55	65
4–10	84–111	92–119	99–127	107–135	115–142
4–11	87–115	95–123	103–131	111–139	119–147
5–0	90–119	98–127	106–135	114–143	123–152
5–1	93–123	101–131	110–140	118–148	127–157
5–2	96–127	105–136	113–144	122–153	131–163
5–3	99–131	108–140	117–149	126–158	135–168
5–4	102–135	112–145	121–154	130–163	140–173
5–5	106–140	115–149	125–159	134–168	144–179
5–6	109–144	119–154	129–164	138–174	148–184
5–7	112–148	122–159	133–169	143–179	153–190
5–8	116–153	126–163	137–174	147–184	158–196
5–9	119–157	130–168	141–179	151–190	162–201
5–10	122–162	134–173	145–184	156–195	167–207
5–11	126–167	137–178	149–190	160–201	172–213
6–0	129–171	141–183	153–195	165–207	177–219
6–1	133–176	145–188	157–200	169–213	182–225
6–2	137–181	149–194	162–206	174–219	187–232
6–3	141–186	153–199	166–212	179–225	192–238
6–4	144–191	157–205	171–218	184–231	197–244

*Values in this table are in pounds for height without shoes and weight without clothes. To convert inches to centimeters, multiply by 2.54; to convert pounds to kilograms, multiply by 0.455.
[†]Data from Andres, R. Baltimore, MD: Gerontology Research Center, National Institute of Aging.

Age (Years)	Females						Males					
	5th	25th	50th	75th	95th		5th	25th	50th	75th	95th	
1	13.8	14.8	15.6	16.4	17.7		14.2	15.0	15.9	17.0	18.3	
2	14.2	15.2	16.0	16.7	18.4		14.1	15.3	16.2	17.0	18.5	
3	14.3	15.8	16.7	17.5	18.9		15.0	16.0	16.7	17.5	19.0	
4	14.9	16.0	16.9	17.7	19.1		14.9	16.2	17.1	18.0	19.2	
5	15.3	16.5	17.5	18.5	21.1		15.3	16.7	17.5	18.5	20.4	
6	15.6	17.0	17.6	18.7	21.1		15.5	16.7	17.9	18.8	22.8	
7	16.4	17.4	18.3	19.9	23.1		16.2	17.7	18.7	20.1	23.0	
8	16.8	18.3	19.5	21.4	26.1		16.2	17.7	19.0	20.2	24.5	
9	17.8	19.4	21.1	22.4	26.0		17.5	18.7	20.0	21.7	25.7	
10	17.4	19.3	21.0	22.8	26.5		18.1	19.6	21.0	23.1	27.4	
11	18.5	20.8	22.4	24.8	30.3		18.6	20.2	22.3	24.4	28.0	
12	19.4	21.6	23.7	25.6	29.4		19.3	21.4	23.2	25.4	30.3	
13	20.2	22.3	24.3	27.1	33.8		19.4	22.8	24.7	26.3	30.1	
14	21.4	23.7	25.2	27.2	32.2		22.0	23.7	25.3	28.3	32.3	
15	20.8	23.9	25.4	27.9	32.2		22.2	24.4	26.4	28.4	32.0	
16	21.8	24.1	25.8	28.3	33.4		24.4	26.2	27.8	30.3	34.3	
17	22.0	24.1	26.4	29.5	35.0		24.6	26.7	28.5	30.8	34.7	
18	22.2	24.1	25.8	28.1	32.5		24.5	27.6	29.7	32.1	37.9	
19–25	21.1	24.7	26.5	29.0	34.5		26.2	28.8	30.8	33.1	37.2	
25–35	23.3	25.6	27.7	30.4	36.8		27.1	30.0	31.9	34.2	37.5	
35–45	24.1	26.7	29.0	31.7	37.8		27.8	30.5	32.6	34.5	37.4	
45–55	24.2	27.4	29.9	32.8	38.4		26.7	30.1	32.2	34.2	37.6	
55–65	24.3	28.0	30.3	33.5	38.5		25.8	29.6	31.7	33.6	36.9	
65–75	24.0	27.4	29.9	32.6	37.3		24.8	28.5	30.7	32.5	35.5	

Data derived from the Health and Nutrition Examination Survey data of 1971–1974, using same population samples as those of the National Center for Health Statistics (NCHS) growth percentiles for children. Adapted from Frisancho, A.R. 1981. New norms of upper limb fat and muscle areas for assessment of nutritional status. *Am J Clin Nutr* 34:2540.

E

TRICEPS SKINFOLD PERCENTILES (MM)

Age (Years)	Females					Males				
	5th	25th	50th	75th	95th	5th	25th	50th	75th	95th
1	6	8	10	12	16	6	8	10	12	16
2	6	9	10	12	16	6	8	10	12	15
3	7	9	11	12	15	6	8	10	11	15
4	7	8	10	12	16	6	8	9	11	14
5	6	8	10	12	18	6	8	9	11	15
6	6	8	10	12	16	5	7	8	10	16
7	6	9	11	13	18	5	7	9	12	17
8	6	9	12	15	24	5	7	8	10	16
9	8	10	13	16	22	6	7	10	13	18
10	7	10	12	17	27	6	8	10	14	21
11	7	10	13	18	28	6	8	11	16	24
12	8	11	14	18	27	6	8	11	14	28
13	8	12	15	21	30	5	7	10	14	26
14	9	13	16	21	28	4	7	9	14	24
15	8	12	17	21	32	4	6	8	11	24
16	10	15	18	22	31	4	6	8	12	22
17	10	13	19	24	37	5	6	8	12	19
18	10	15	18	22	30	4	6	9	13	24
19–25	10	14	18	24	34	4	7	10	15	22
25–35	10	16	21	27	37	5	8	12	16	24
35–45	12	18	23	29	38	5	8	12	16	23
45–55	12	20	25	30	40	6	8	12	15	25
55–65	12	20	25	31	38	5	8	11	14	22
65–75	12	18	24	29	36	4	8	11	15	22

Data derived from the Health and Nutrition Examination Survey data of 1971–1974, using same population samples as those of the National Center for Health Statistics (NCHS) growth percentiles for children. Adapted from Frisancho, A.R. 1981. New norms of upper limb fat and muscle areas for assessment of nutritional status. *Am J Clin Nutr* 34:2540.

MID-UPPER-ARM MUSCLE CIRCUMFERENCE PERCENTILES (CM)

Age (Years)	Females					Males				
	5th	25th	50th	75th	95th	5th	25th	50th	75th	95th
1	10.5	11.7	12.4	13.9	14.3	11.0	11.9	12.7	13.5	14.7
2	11.1	11.9	12.6	13.3	14.7	11.1	12.2	13.0	14.0	15.0
3	11.3	12.4	13.2	14.0	15.2	11.7	13.1	13.7	14.3	15.3
4	11.5	12.8	13.8	14.4	15.7	12.3	13.3	14.1	14.8	15.9
5	12.5	13.4	14.2	15.1	16.5	12.8	14.0	14.7	15.4	16.9
6	13.0	13.8	14.5	15.4	17.1	13.1	14.2	15.1	16.1	17.7
7	12.9	14.2	15.1	16.0	17.6	13.7	15.1	16.0	16.8	19.0
8	13.8	15.1	16.0	17.1	19.4	14.0	15.4	16.2	17.0	18.7
9	14.7	15.8	16.7	18.0	19.8	15.1	16.1	17.0	18.3	20.2
10	14.8	15.9	17.0	18.0	19.7	15.6	16.6	18.0	19.1	22.1
11	15.0	17.1	18.1	19.6	22.3	15.9	17.3	18.3	19.5	23.0
12	16.2	18.0	19.1	20.1	22.0	16.7	18.2	19.5	21.0	24.1
13	16.9	18.3	19.8	21.1	24.0	17.2	19.6	21.1	22.6	24.5
14	17.4	19.0	20.1	21.6	24.7	18.9	21.2	22.3	24.0	26.4
15	17.5	18.9	20.2	21.5	24.4	19.9	21.8	23.7	25.4	27.2
16	17.0	19.0	20.2	21.6	24.9	21.3	23.4	24.9	26.9	29.6
17	17.5	19.4	20.5	22.1	25.7	22.4	24.5	25.8	27.3	31.2
18	17.4	19.1	20.2	21.5	24.5	22.6	25.2	26.4	28.3	32.4
19–25	17.9	19.5	20.7	22.1	24.9	23.8	25.7	27.3	28.9	32.1
25–35	18.3	19.9	21.2	22.8	26.4	24.3	26.4	27.9	29.8	32.6
35–45	18.6	20.5	21.8	23.6	27.2	24.7	26.9	28.6	30.2	32.7
45–55	18.7	20.6	22.0	23.8	27.4	23.9	26.5	28.1	30.0	32.6
55–65	18.7	20.9	22.5	24.4	28.0	23.6	26.0	27.8	29.5	32.0
65–75	18.5	20.8	22.5	24.4	27.9	22.3	25.1	26.8	28.4	30.6

Values derived by formula calculation. Data derived from the Health and Nutrition Examination Survey data of 1971–1974, using same population samples as those of the National Center for Health Statistics (NCHS) growth percentiles for children. Adapted from Frisancho, A.R. 1981. New norms of upper limb fat and muscle areas for assessment of nutritional status. *Am J Clin Nutr* 34:2540.

APPENDIX

G

CLINICAL SIGNS AND SYMPTOMS OF VARIOUS NUTRIENT DEFICIENCIES

Areas of Examination	Signs/Symptoms	Potential Nutrient Deficiencies
Hair	Alopecia	Zinc, essential fatty acids
	Easy pluckability	Protein, essential fatty acids
Eyes	Lackluster	Protein, zinc
	"Corkscrew"	Vitamin C, vitamin A
	Decreased pigmentation	Protein, copper
	Xerosis of conjunctiva	Vitamin A
	Corneal vascularization	Riboflavin
	Keratomalacia	Vitamin A
	Bitot's spots	Vitamin A
Gastrointestinal tract	Nausea, vomiting	Pyridoxine
	Diarrhea	Zinc, niacin
	Stomatitis	Pyridoxine, riboflavin, iron
	Cheilosis	Pyridoxine, iron
	Glossitis	Pyridoxine, zinc, niacin, folate, vitamin B$_{12}$
	Magenta tongue	Riboflavin
	Swollen, bleeding gums	Vitamin C
	Fissured tongue	Niacin
	Hepatomegaly	Protein
Skin	Dry and scaling	Vitamin A, essential fatty acids, zinc
	Petechiae, ecchymoses	Vitamin C, vitamin K
Skin—cont'd	Follicular hyperkeratosis	Vitamin A, essential fatty acids
	Nasolabial seborrhea	Niacin, pyridoxine, riboflavin
	Bilateral dermatitis	Niacin, zinc
	Subcutaneous fat loss	Kilocalories
	Muscle wastage	Kilocalories, protein
	Edema	Protein
Extremities	Osteomalacia, bone pain, rickets	Vitamin D
	Arthralgia	Vitamin C
Hematologic	Anemia	Vitamin B$_{12}$, iron, folate, copper, vitamin E, vitamin K
	Leukopenia, neutropenia	Copper
	Low prothrombin, prolonged clotting time	Vitamin K
Neurologic	Disorientation	Niacin, thiamin
	Confabulation	Thiamin
	Neuropathy	Thiamin, pyridoxine, chromium
	Paresthesia	Thiamin, pyridoxine, vitamin B$_{12}$
Cardiovascular	Congestive heart failure, cardiomegaly, tachycardia	Thiamin
	Cardiomyopathy	Selenium

From Ross Laboratories

H

Normal Biochemical Levels for Nutrients and Test Measurements

Biochemical Indicators of Good Nutrition Status

Nutrients or Measurements	Tests	Normal or Acceptable Levels	
		Men	Women
Iron	Hemoglobin (g/100 ml)	≥14.0	≥12.0
	Infants (under 2 years)	≥10.0	≥10.0
	Children (6–12 years)	≥11.5	≥11.5
	Pregnancy (2nd trimester)		≥11.0
	(3rd trimester)		≥10.5
Protein	Serum albumin (g/100 ml)	≥3.5	≥3.5
Normal lipid metabolism	Serum cholesterol (mg/100 ml)	<200	<200
	Serum triglyceride (mg/100 ml)	<250	<250
Normal carbohydrate metabolism	Serum glucose (mg/100 ml)	75–110	75–110
Sodium	Serum sodium (mEq/L)	130–150	130–155
Potassium	Serum potassium (mEq/L)	3.5–5.3	3.5–5.3
Vitamin A	Plasma vitamin A (µg/100 ml)	>20	>20
Vitamin C	Serum vitamin C (mg/100 ml)	≥0.3	≥0.3
Riboflavin	Erythrocyte glutathione peroxidase (% stimulation of activity by added riboflavin cofactor)	<20	<20
Vitamin B_6	Tryptophan load test—increase in excretion of xanthurenic acid (mg/day)	<25	<25
Folate	Serum folate (nanogram/ml)	>6.0	>6.0
Thiamin	Urinary thiamin (µg/g creatinine)	>65	>65
Zinc	Plasma zinc (µg/100 ml)	80–115	80–115

Some information obtained from Roe, D.A. 1976. *Drug-induced nutritional deficiencies.* Westport, CT: AVI Press; and Sauberlich, H.E., H.H. Skala, and R.P. Dowdy. 1974. *Laboratory tests for the assessment of nutritional status.* Cleveland: CRC Press.

RECOMMENDED NUTRIENT INTAKES FOR CANADIANS

Age	Sex	Energy (kcal)	Thiamin (mg)	Riboflavin (mg)	Niacin NE	n-3 PUFA (g)	n-6 PUFA (g)
0–4 months	Both	600	0.3	0.3	4	0.5	3
5–12 months	Both	900	0.4	0.5	7	0.5	3
1 year	Both	1100	0.5	0.6	8	0.6	4
2–3 years	Both	1300	0.6	0.7	9	0.7	4
4–6 years	Both	1800	0.7	0.9	13	1.0	6
7–9 years	M	2200	0.9	1.1	16	1.2	7
	F	1900	0.8	1.0	14	1.0	6
10–12 years	M	2500	1.0	1.3	18	1.4	8
	F	2200	0.9	1.1	16	1.2	7
13–15 years	M	2800	1.1	1.4	20	1.5	9
	F	2200	0.9	1.1	16	1.2	7
16–18 years	M	3200	1.3	1.6	23	1.8	11
	F	2100	0.8	1.1	15	1.2	7
19–24 years	M	3000	1.2	1.5	22	1.6	10
	F	2100	0.8	1.1	15	1.2	7
25–49 years	M	2700	1.1	1.4	19	1.5	9
	F	1900	0.8	1.0	14	1.1	7
50–74 years	M	2300	0.9	1.2	16	1.3	8
	F	1800	0.8*	1.0*	14*	1.1*	7*
75+ years	M	2000	0.8	1.0	14	1.1	7
	F†	1700	0.8*	1.0*	14*	1.1*	7*
Pregnancy (addition)							
1st trimester		100	0.1	0.1	0.11	0.05	0.3
2nd trimester		300	0.1	0.3	0.22	0.16	0.9
3rd trimester		300	0.1	0.3	0.22	0.16	0.9
Lactation (additional)		450	0.2	0.4	0.33	0.25	1.5

From Scientific Review Committee. 1990. *Nutrition recommendations.* Ottawa: Health and Welfare.
NE: niacin equivalents; PUFA: polyunsaturated fatty acids
*Level below which intake should not fall
†Assumes moderate physical activity

Summary Examples of Recommended Nutrient Intake Based on Age and Body Weight Expressed as Daily Rates

Age	Sex	Weight (kg)	Protein (g)	Vitamin A RE	Vitamin D (µg)	Vitamin E (mg)	Vitamin C (mg)	Folate (µg)	Vitamin B_{12} (µg)	Calcium (mg)	Phosphorus (mg)	Magnesium (mg)	Iron (mg)	Iodine (µg)	Zinc (mg)
0–4 months	Both	6	12*	400	10.0	3	20	25	0.3	250†	150	20	0.3‡	30	2‡
5–12 months	Both	9	12	400	10.0	3	20	40	0.4	400	200	32	7	40	3
1 year	Both	11	13	400	10.0	3	20	40	0.5	500	300	40	6	55	4
2–3 years	Both	14	16	400	5.0	4	20	50	0.6	550	350	50	6	65	4
4–6 years	Both	18	19	500	5.0	5	25	70	0.8	600	400	65	8	85	5
7–9 years	M	25	26	700	2.5	7	25	90	1.0	700	500	100	8	110	7
	F	25	26	700	2.5	6	25	90	1.0	700	500	100	8	95	7
10–12 years	M	34	34	800	2.5	8	25	120	1.0	900	700	130	8	125	9
	F	36	36	800	2.5	7	25	130	1.0	1,100	800	135	8	110	9
13–15 years	M	50	49	900	2.5	9	30	175	1.0	1,100	900	185	10	160	12
	F	48	46	800	2.5	7	30	170	1.0	1,000	850	180	13	160	9
16–18 years	M	62	58	1,000	2.5	10	40§	220	1.0	900	1,000	230	10	160	12
	F	53	47	800	2.5	7	30§	190	1.0	700	850	200	12	160	9
19–24 years	M	71	61	1,000	2.5	10	40§	220	1.0	800	1,000	240	9	160	12
	F	58	50	800	2.5	7	30§	180	1.0	700	850	200	13	160	9
25–49 years	M	74	64	1,000	2.5	9	40§	230	1.0	800	1,000	250	9	160	12
	F	59	51	800	2.5	6	30§	185	1.0	700	850	200	13	160	9
50–74 years	M	73	63	1,000	5.0	7	40§	230	1.0	800	1,000	250	9	160	12
	F	63	54	800	5.0	6	30§	195	1.0	800	850	210	8	160	9
75+ years	M	69	59	1,000	5.0	6	40§	215	1.0	800	1,000	230	9	160	12
	F	64	55	800	5.0	5	30§	200	1.0	800	850	210	8	160	9
Pregnancy (additional)															
1st trimester			5	0	2.5	2	0	200	1.2	500	200	15	0	25	6
2nd trimester			20	0	2.5	2	10	200	1.2	500	200	45	5	25	6
3rd trimester			24	0	2.5	2	10	200	1.2	500	200	45	10	25	6
Lactation (additional)			20	400	2.5	3	25	100	0.2	500	200	65	0	50	6

From Scientific Review Committee. 1990. *Nutrition recommendations*. Ottawa: Health and Welfare.

RE: retinol equivalents

*Protein is assumed to be from breast milk and must be adjusted for infant formula.

†Infant formula with high phosphorus should contain 375 mg of calcium.

‡Breast milk is assumed to be the source of the mineral.

§Smokers should increase vitamin C by 50%.

J

FOOD GUIDE: EXCHANGE LISTS FOR MEAL PLANNING (1986 REVISION)

The *exchange system of dietary control,* developed by two professional organizations—the American Dietetic Association and the American Diabetes Association—is based on a simple grouping of common foods according to generally equivalent nutritional values. This system may be used for any situation requiring caloric and food value control.

The foods are divided into six basic groups (with subgroups), called the "exchange lists." Each food item within a group or subgroup contains about the same food value as other food items in that group, allowing for exchange within groups, thus providing for variety in foods choices as well as food value control. Hence, the term *food exchanges* is sometimes used to refer to food choices or servings. The total number of "exchanges" per day depends on individual nutritional needs, based on normal nutrition standards. Although there is some variation in the composition of foods within the exchange groups, for simplicity the following values for carbohydrate, protein, fat, and kilocalories are used.

Exchange Lists

Food Groups	Carbohydrate (g)	Protein (g)	Fat (g)	Kcal
Starch/bread	15	3	Trace	80
Meat				
Lean	—	7	3	55
Medium-fat	—	7	5	75
High-fat	—	7	8	100
Vegetable	5	2	—	25
Fruit	15	—	—	60
Milk				
Skim	12	8	Trace	90
Low-fat	12	8	5	120
Whole	12	8	8	150
Fat	—	—	5	45

List 1: Starch/Bread List

Whole-grain foods have about 2 g fiber per serving. Foods containing 3 g fiber per serving or more are marked with the symbol *.

Cereals/grains/pasta

*Bran cereals, concentrated	⅓ cup
*Bran cereals, flaked (such as Bran Buds, All Bran)	½ cup
Bulgur (cooked)	½ cup
Cooked cereals	½ cup
Cornmeal (dry)	2½ tbsp
Grapenuts	3 tbsp
Grits (cooked)	½ cup
Other ready-to-eat unsweetened cereals	¾ cup
Pasta (cooked)	½ cup
Puffed cereal	1½ cup
Rice, white or brown (cooked)	⅓ cup
Shredded Wheat	½ cup
*Wheat germ	3 tbsp

Dried beans/peas/lentils

*Beans and peas (cooked, such as kidney, white, split, black-eyed)	⅓ cup
*Lentils (cooked)	⅓ cup
*Baked beans	¼ cup

Starchy vegetables

*Corn	½ cup
*Corn on cob, 6 in long	1
*Lima beans	½ cup
*Peas, green (fresh, frozen, or canned)	½ cup
*Plantain	½ cup
Potato, baked	1 small (3 oz)
Potato, mashed	½ cup
Squash, winter (acorn, butternut)	¾ cup
Yam, sweet potato, plain	⅓ cup

Bread

Bagel	½ (1 oz)
Bread sticks, crisp (4 in long × ½ in)	2 (⅔ oz)
Croutons, low-fat	1 cup
English muffin	½
Frankfurter bun or hamburger bun	½ (1 oz)
Pita (6 in across)	½
Plain roll, small	1 (1 oz)
Raisin, unfrosted	1 slice (1 oz)
*Rye, pumpernickel	1 slice (1 oz)
Tortilla, 6 in across	1
White (including French, Italian)	1 slice (1 oz)
Whole-wheat	1 slice (1 oz)

Crackers/snacks

Animal crackers	8
Graham crackers (2½ in square)	3
Matzoth	¾ oz
Melba toast	5 slices
Oyster crackers	24
Popcorn (popped, no fat added)	3 cups
Pretzels	¾ oz
Rye crisp (2 in × 3½ in)	4
Saltine-type crackers	6
Whole-wheat crackers, no fat added (crisp breads, such as Finn, Kavli, Wasa)	2–4 slices (¾ oz)

Starch foods prepared with fat (count as 1 starch/bread serving + 1 fat)

Biscuit (2½ in across)	1
Chow mein noodles	½ cup
Corn bread (2-in cube)	1 (2 oz)
Cracker, round butter type	6
French fried potatoes (2 to 3½ in long)	10 (1½ oz)
Muffin, plain, small	1
Pancake (4 in across)	2
Stuffing, bread (prepared)	¼ cup
Taco shell (6 in across)	2
Waffle (4½-in square)	1
Whole-wheat crackers, fat added (such as Triscuits)	4–6 (1 oz)

List 2: Meat and Meat Substitutes List

To reduce fat intake, choose items mainly from the lean and medium-fat groups, using more fish and poultry (with skin removed) as meat choices and trimming fat from all meats. Items having 400 mg sodium or more per exchange are marked with the symbol **. None of the items on this list contributes fiber to the diet. One exchange is equal to the amount listed for each item. In the case of meat, for example, a serving may be 2–3 exchanges (2–3 oz).

Lean meat and substitutes

Beef	USDA Good or Choice grades of lean beef, such as round, sirloin, and flank steak; tenderloin; and chipped beef**	1 oz
Pork	Lean pork, such as fresh ham; canned, cured, or boiled ham**; Canadian bacon**; tenderloin	1 oz

Veal	All cuts except for veal cutlets (ground or cubed)	1 oz
Poultry	Chicken, turkey, Cornish hen (without skin)	1 oz
Fish	All fresh and frozen fish	1 oz
	Crab, lobster, scallops, shrimp, clams (fresh or canned in water**)	2 oz
	Oysters	6 medium
	Tuna** (canned in water)	$\frac{1}{4}$ cup
	Herring (uncreamed or smoked)	1 oz
	Sardines (canned)	2 medium
Wild game	Venison, rabbit, squirrel	1 oz
	Pheasant, duck, goose (without skin)	1 oz
Cheese	Any cottage cheese	$\frac{1}{4}$ cup
	Grated parmesan	2 tbsp
	Diet cheeses** (less than 55 kcal/oz)	1 oz
Other	95% fat-free luncheon meat	1 oz slice
	Egg whites	3 whites
	Egg substitutes (less than 55 kcal/$\frac{1}{4}$ cup)	$\frac{1}{4}$ cup

Medium-fat meat and substitutes

Beef	Ground beef, roast (rib, chuck, rump), steak (cubed, porterhouse, T-bone), and meatloaf (most beef products are in this category)	1 oz
Pork	Chops, loin roast, Boston butt, cutlets (most pork products fall into this category)	1 oz
Lamb	Chops, leg, and roast (most lamb products fall into this category)	1 oz
Veal	Cutlet (ground or cubes, unbreaded)	1 oz
Poultry	Chicken (with skin), domestic duck or goose (well-drained of fat), ground turkey	1 oz
Fish	Tuna** (canned in oil and drained)	$\frac{1}{4}$ cup
	Salmon** (canned)	$\frac{1}{4}$ cup
Cheese	Skim or part-skim cheeses, such as	
	Ricotta	$\frac{1}{4}$ cup
	Mozzarella	1 oz
	Diet cheeses** (56–80 kcal/oz)	1 oz
Other	86% fat-free luncheon meat**	1 oz
	Egg (high in cholesterol, limit to 3/week)	1
	Egg substitutes (56–80 kcal per $\frac{1}{4}$ cup)	$\frac{1}{4}$ cup
	Tofu ($2\frac{1}{2} \times 2\frac{3}{4} \times 1$ in)	4 oz
	Liver, heart, kidney, sweetbreads (high in cholesterol, limit use)	1 oz

High-fat meat and substitutes (these items are high in saturated fat, cholesterol, and kilocalories; limit to 3 times/week)

Beef	USDA Prime cuts, ribs; corned beef**	1 oz
Pork	Spareribs, ground pork, pork sausage**	1 oz
Lamb	Ground lamb patties	1 oz
Fish	Any fried fish product	1 oz
Cheese	Regular cheeses**, such as American, Blue, Swiss	1 oz
Other	Luncheon meat**, such as bologna, salami, pimento loaf	1 oz slice
	Sausage**, such as Polish, Italian	1 oz
	Knockwurst, smoked	1 oz
	Bratwurst**	1 oz
	Frankfurter** (turkey or chicken)	1 frank (10/lb)
	Frankfurter** (beef, pork, or combination) (count as 1 high-fat meat + 1 fat)	1 frank (10/lb)
	Peanut butter	1 tbsp

List 3: Vegetable List

Unless otherwise noted, one vegetable exchange is 1 cup raw vegetable or $\frac{1}{2}$ cup cooked vegetable or vegetable juice. Vegetables containing 400 mg sodium or more per serving are marked with the symbol **. Fresh and frozen vegetables have less added salt. Canned vegetables contain more salt, but rinsing helps remove much of it. In general, vegetables contain 2–3 g dietary fiber per serving. Starchy vegetables are found in the Starch/Bread List. Other free vegetables are in the Free Foods list.

Artichoke ($\frac{1}{2}$ medium)	Mushrooms, cooked
Asparagus	Okra
Beans (green, wax, Italian)	Onions
Bean sprouts	Pea pods
Beets	Peppers (green)
Broccoli	Rutabaga
Brussels sprouts	Sauerkraut**
Cabbage	Spinach
Carrots	Summer squash (crookneck)
Cauliflower	Tomato (1 large)
Eggplant	Tomato/vegetable juice
Greens (collard, mustard, turnip)	Turnips
Kohlrabi	Water chestnuts
Leeks	Zucchini

List 4: Fruit List

Fruits containing 3 g dietary fiber or more per serving are marked with the symbol *. Portions are usual serving sizes of commonly eaten fruits.

Fresh, unsweetened frozen, and unsweetened canned fruit

Apple (raw, 2 in across)	1
Applesauce (unsweetened)	$\frac{1}{2}$ cup
Apricots (medium, raw)	4
Apricots (canned)	$\frac{1}{2}$ cup or 4 halves
Banana (9 in long)	$\frac{1}{2}$
*Blackberries (raw)	$\frac{3}{4}$ cup
*Blueberries (raw	$\frac{3}{4}$ cup
Canteloupe (5 in across)	$\frac{1}{3}$
Canteloupe (cubes)	1 cup
Cherries (large, raw)	12
Cherries (canned)	$\frac{1}{2}$ cup
Figs (raw, 2 in across)	2
Fruit cocktail (canned)	$\frac{1}{2}$ cup
Grapefruit (medium)	$\frac{1}{2}$
Grapefruit (segments)	$\frac{3}{4}$ cup
Grapes (small)	15
Honeydew melon (medium)	$\frac{1}{8}$
Honeydew melon (cubes)	1 cup
Kiwi fruit (large)	1
Mandarin oranges (segments)	$\frac{3}{4}$ cup
Mango (small)	$\frac{1}{2}$
*Nectarine ($1\frac{1}{2}$ in across)	1
Orange ($2\frac{1}{2}$ in across)	1
Papaya (small cubes or balls)	1 cup
Peach ($2\frac{3}{4}$ in across)	1
Peach (slices)	$\frac{3}{4}$ cup
Peaches (canned)	$\frac{1}{2}$ cup or 2 halves
Pear	$\frac{1}{2}$ large or 1 small
Pears (canned)	$\frac{1}{2}$ cup or 2 halves
Persimmon (medium, native)	2
Pineapple (raw, cubes)	$\frac{3}{4}$ cup
Plum (raw, 2 in across)	2
*Pomegranate	$\frac{1}{2}$
*Raspberries (raw)	1 cup
*Strawberries (raw, whole)	$1\frac{1}{4}$ cups
Tangerine ($2\frac{1}{2}$ in across)	2
Watermelon (cubes or balls)	$1\frac{1}{4}$ cup

Dried fruit

*Apples	4 rings
*Apricots	7 halves
Dates	$2\frac{1}{2}$ medium

*Figs	1½
*Prunes	3 medium
Raisins	2 tbsp

Fruit juice

Apple juice or cider	½ cup
Cranberry juice cocktail	⅓ cup
Grapefruit juice	⅓ cup
Grape juice	⅓ cup
Orange juice	½ cup
Pineapple juice	½ cup
Prune juice	⅓ cup

List 5: Milk List

Milk may be used alone or in combination with other foods. See the Combination Foods list.

Skim and very lowfat milk

Skim or nonfat milk	1 cup
½% milk	1 cup
1% milk	1 cup
Low-fat buttermilk	1 cup
Evaporated skim milk	½ cup
Dry nonfat milk	⅓ cup
Plain nonfat yogurt	8 oz

Low-fat milk

2% milk	1 cup
Plain low-fat yogurt (with added nonfat milk solids)	8 oz

Whole milk (more than 3¼% butterfat; limit use)

Whole milk	1 cup
Evaporated whole milk	½ cup
Whole plain yogurt	8 oz

List 6: Fat List

Measure carefully; use mainly unsaturated fats. Sodium content varies widely, so check labels.

Unsaturated fats

Avocado	⅛ medium
Margarine	1 tsp
Margarine, diet	1 tbsp
Mayonnaise	1 tsp
Mayonnaise, reduced kcal	1 tbsp
Nuts and seeds	
Almonds, dry roasted	6 whole
Cashews, dry roasted	1 tbsp
Pecans	2 whole
Peanuts	20 small or 10 large
Walnuts	2 whole
Other nuts	1 tbsp
Seeds, pine nuts, sunflower (shelled)	1 tbsp
Pumpkin seeds	1 tsp
Oil (corn, cottonseed, safflower, soybean, sunflower, olive, peanut)	1 tsp
Olives	10 small or 5 large
Salad dressing, mayonnaise type	2 tsp
Salad dressing, mayonnaise type, low kcal	1 tbsp
Salad dressing (all varieties)	1 tbsp
Salad dressing, low-kcal	2 tbsp
(2 tbsp low-calorie salad dressing is a free food)	

Saturated fats

Bacon	1 slice
Butter	1 tsp
Chitterlings	$\frac{1}{2}$ oz
Coconut, shredded	2 tbsp
Coffee whitener, liquid	2 tbsp
Coffee whitener, powder	4 tsp
Cream (light, coffee, table)	2 tbsp
Cream, sour	2 tbsp
Cream (heavy, whipping)	1 tbsp
Cream cheese	1 tbsp
Salt pork	$\frac{1}{4}$ oz

Free Foods

Any food or drink containing less than 20 kcal/serving is "free." If a serving size is given, 2–3 servings per day are sufficient. Higher fiber* or sodium** foods are indicated. Use *nonstick pan spray* for cooking as desired.

Drinks

Bouillon** or broth, fat-free	
Bouillon, low-sodium	
Carbonated drinks, sugar-free	
Carbonated water	
Club soda	
Cocoa powder, unsweetened	1 tbsp
Coffee/tea	
Drink mixes, sugar-free	
Tonic water, sugar-free	

Condiments

Catsup	1 tbsp
Horseradish	
Mustard	
Pickles,** dill, unsweetened	
Salad dressing, low-kcal	2 tbsp
Taco sauce	1 tbsp
Vinegar	

Seasonings

Basil (fresh)
Celery seeds
Cinnamon
Chili powder
Chives
Curry
Dill
Flavoring extracts (vanilla, almond,
   walnut, butter)
Garlic, fresh and powdered
Herbs, spices
Hot pepper sauce and flakes
Lemon, juice and zest (outer skin)
Lemon pepper
Lime, juice and zest
Mint, fresh leaves
Onion powder
Oregano
Paprika
Parsley
Pepper
Pimento
Soy sauce**
Soy sauce, low sodium—"lite"

Wine, used in cooking	$\frac{1}{4}$ cup

Worcestershire sauce

Fruits

Cranberries, unsweetened	$\frac{1}{2}$ cup
Rhubarb, unsweetened	$\frac{1}{2}$ cup

Vegetables

Cabbage
Celery
*Chinese cabbage
Cucumber
Green onion
Hot peppers
Mushrooms
Radishes
*Zucchini

Salad greens

Endive
Escarole
Lettuce
Romaine
Spinach

Sweet substitutes

Candy, hard, sugar-free	
Gelatin dessert, sugar-free	
Gum, sugar-free	
Jam/jelly, sugar-free	2 tsp
Pancake syrup, sugar-free	1–2 tbsp
Sugar substitutes (saccharin, aspartame)	
Whipped topping	2 tbsp

Combination Foods

Check the *American Dietetic Association/American Diabetes Association Family Cookbooks* and the *American Diabetes Association Holiday Cookbook* for many recipes and much information, including combination foods.

Foods	Amount	Exchanges
Casserole, homemade	1 cup (8 oz)	2 starch, 2 medium-fat meat, 1 fat
Cheese pizza,** thin crust	¼ of 10 in	2 starch, 1 medium-fat meat, 1 fat
*Chili beans**	1 cup (8 oz)	2 starch, 2 medium-fat meat, 2 fat
*Chow mein** (without noodles or rice)	2 cups	1 starch, 2 vegetables, 2 lean meat
Macaroni and cheese**	1 cup	2 starch, 1 medium-fat meat, 2 fat
Spaghetti and meatballs (canned)	1 cup	2 starch, 1 medium-fat meat, 1 fat
Sugar-free pudding (made with skim milk)	½ cup	1 starch

Soups

*Bean**	1 cup	1 starch, 1 vegetable, 1 lean meat
Chunky, all varieties**	10¾ oz can	1 starch, 1 vegetable, 1 medium-fat meat
Cream** (made with water)	1 cup	1 starch, 1 fat
Vegetable** or broth**	1 cup	1 starch

Beans used as a meat substitute

*Dried beans, peas, lentils (cooked)	1 cup	2 starch, 1 lean meat

Foods for Occasional Use

Foods	Amount	Exchanges
Angel food cake	¹⁄₁₂ cake	2 starch
Plain cake, no icing	¹⁄₁₂ cake or 3 in square	2 starch, 2 fat
Cookies	2 small (¾ in across)	1 starch, 1 fat
Frozen fruit yogurt	⅓ cup	1 starch
Gingersnaps	3	1 starch
Granola	¼ cup	1 starch, 1 fat
Granola bars	1 small	1 starch, 1 fat
Ice cream, any flavor	½ cup	1 starch, 2 fat
Ice milk, any flavor	½ cup	1 starch, 1 fat
Sherbet, any flavor	¼ cup	1 starch
Snack chips,** all varieties	1 oz	1 starch, 2 fat
Vanilla wafers	6 small	1 starch, 1 fat

DIETARY FIBER AND KILOCALORIE VALUES FOR SELECTED FOODS

Foods	Serving	Dietary fiber (g)	Kcal
Breads and cereals			
All Bran	1/3 cup	8.5	70
Bran (100%)	1/2 cup	8.4	75
Bran Buds	1/3 cup	7.9	75
Corn Bran	2/3 cup	5.4	100
Bran Chex	2/3 cup	4.6	90
Cracklin' Oat Bran	1/3 cup	4.3	110
Bran Flakes	3/4 cup	4.0	90
Air-popped popcorn	1 cup	2.5	25
Oatmeal	1 cup	2.2	144
Grapenuts	1/4 cup	1.4	100
Whole-wheat bread	1 slice	1.4	60
Legumes, cooked			
Kidney beans	1/2 cup	7.3	110
Lima beans	1/2 cup	4.5	130
Vegetables, cooked			
Green peas	1/2 cup	3.6	55
Corn	1/2 cup	2.9	70
Parsnip	1/2 cup	2.7	50
Potato, with skin	1 medium	2.5	95
Brussels sprouts	1/2 cup	2.3	30
Carrots	1/2 cup	2.3	25
Broccoli	1/2 cup	2.2	20
Beans, green	1/2 cup	1.6	15
Tomato, chopped	1/2 cup	1.5	17
Cabbage, red and white	1/2 cup	1.4	15
Kale	1/2 cup	1.4	20
Cauliflower	1/2 cup	1.1	15
Lettuce (fresh)	1 cup	0.8	7
Fruits			
Apple	1 medium	3.5	80
Raisins	1/4 cup	3.1	110
Prunes, dried	3	3.0	60
Strawberries	1 cup	3.0	45
Orange	1 medium	2.6	60
Banana	1 medium	2.4	105
Blueberries	1/2 cup	2.0	40
Dates, dried	3	1.9	70
Peach	1 medium	1.9	35
Apricot, fresh	3 medium	1.8	50
Grapefruit	1/2 cup	1.6	40
Apricot, dried	5 halves	1.4	40
Cherries	10	1.2	50
Pineapple	1/2 cup	1.1	40

Adapted from Lanza, E., and R.R. Butrum. 1986. A critical review of food fiber analysis and data. *J Am Diet Assoc* 86:732.

EXERCISE LEVELS WITH AGE, NUTRITION, FLUID, AND HEALTH ASSESSMENT GUIDELINES

Definitions	Examples (Not Inclusive)	Recommended Ages
1. *Routine:* The duration of the activity is less than twenty minutes, and it may or may not reach 60% of maximum heartbeat rate.	Recess play, casual walking, recreational noncontinual sport (e.g., T-ball, volleyball)	Minimum activity level for any age
2. *Health fitness:* 60% to 80% of maximum heartbeat rate is achieved for greater than twenty minutes at least three times per week for a minimum of six months. The activity should involve muscular strength and flexibility.	Brisk walking, jogging, running, cycling, hiking, swimming, dancing	Preferred level for any age
3. *Competitive sports:* An activity less than or equal to six months that consists of team involvement, preseason training, and competing either as a team member or individually at an intramural or interschool level.	Swimming, gymnastics, diving, volleyball, wrestling, sprinting, relay, football, soccer, basketball, tennis, field hockey, cross-country	Junior high age and above
3a. *Competitive less than six months:* Short endurance—intense activity that lasts for twenty minutes or less	As above under #3	Junior high age and above
3b. *Competitive less than six months:* Long endurance—activity, intense or nonintense, that lasts for longer than twenty minutes	As above under #3	High school age and above
4. *Competitive sports:* Longer than six months; same as competitive above but usually involved at a personal level other than school	Same as #3 but may include state or national competition	High school age and above
4a. *Competitive six months:* Short endurance—same as above	As above under #4	
4b. *Competitive six months:* Long endurance—same as above	As above under #4	
5. *Performing:* An activity that requires dedicated practice (several times a week) to perform with a group or individually; a routine lasting anywhere from five minutes to one hour (or longer) in competition or performance	Ballet, dance, or gymnastics	Junior high age and above as determined by a physician
6. *Marching band:* Involvement with a band that competes or performs in marching or choreographed performance; includes preseason training as well as competition or performance	High school marching or competing bands	Junior high age and above
7. *Seasonal:* Intramural involvement with a team or an individual activity not based heavily on winning but just participation; practice required; may or may not last longer than twenty minutes three or more times a week, but activity is not sustained longer than two or three months.	Soccer, softball, swimming lessons	All ages

Nutrition Comments	Fluid Intake	Recommended Health Assessment
Normal nutrition for age from the basic food groups	Normal for age	Yearly routine exam from a pediatrician or physician for all children
Normal nutrition for age from the basic food groups; if desired weight for height, possibly more calories	Good hydration, especially in adverse weather; normal requirements for age plus replacement of lost fluid from activity	Yearly routine exam from a pediatrician or physician for all children; education from a physician or health professional on healthy practices (diet, fluid, injury prevention, warm-up and cool-down techniques, etc.); immediate attention from an appropriate health professional for an injury or insult
Nutrition assessment, recommendations, and education, preferably from a registered dietitian, for an individual's season intake to achieve weight and body composition for the sport; recommendations depend on type of activity, duration, and intensity	Preevent, event, and postevent (or prepractice and postpractice) hydration; good hydration at other times Electrolyte replacement needed if heavy sweating occurs or in adverse weather conditions	Preparticipation assessment by a health team consisting of a physician, a dietitian, a nurse or nurse practitioner, and possibly a physical therapist; examination as well as education given to students; immediate attention from an appropriate health professional for any injury or insult during the sports season
2 g protein/kg for growing athletes 1 g protein/kg for mature athletes May need carbohydrate during the event if long in duration (>4 hr); modified carbohydrate loading (normal diet; intense exercise 7–4 days before, high-carbohydrate diet 3–1 days before) no more than 2–3 times per year	Electrolyte replacement needs assessed and replacement given if necessary	
Same as #3	Same as #3	As in previous years; important that a physician determine that the maturation age of the participant is appropriate for the sport
Nutrition assessment, recommendations, and education provided, preferably by a registered dietitian due to the usually restricted intake to achieve desired weight for performance	Normal hydration and replacement of lost fluids from practice or performance	Preparticipation assessment by a physician, a dietitian, and possibly an orthopedist or a physical therapist; injury attention as in competitive sports
Nutrition assessment, recommendations, and education, preferably from a registered dietitian in a group setting, or individually if necessary	As in #3a, #3b	Same as in #2 or #3a, #3b; nutrition attention by a registered dietitian if the participant is less than 85% or greater than 120% of desired weight for height
As in #2	As in #3a, #3b	Preparticipation assessment by a pediatrician or physician, as in #2; nutrition attention by a registered dietitian if the participant is less than 85% or greater than 120% of desired weight for height

GLOSSARY

Abscissa (L *ab,* from; *scindere,* to cut) Usually the horizontal X line used as a base of reference in graphing relative data. When suitable values are assigned to both of the two lines of the graph—the horizontal X axis, or ordinates, and the bisecting vertical Y axis, or abscissas—corresponding data with reference to the other can be plotted.

Acetaldehyde Chemical compound, intermediate metabolic product in the breakdown of alcohol by liver enzymes.

Achlorhydria (L *a-,* negative; *chlorhydria,* hydrochloric acid) Absence or reduced amounts of hydrochloric acid in the gastric secretions.

Acne (Gr *achne,* chaff) Common inflammation *(acne vulgaris)* of the pilosebaceous (L *pilus,* hair; *sebum,* suet; thick semifluid secretion composed of fat and epithelial cell debris) glands of the skin, mainly on the face, chest, and back. Precise cause unknown but suggested factors include hormones, stress, heredity, and bacteria; usually self-limiting after the physiologic stress of puberty.

Acrocyanosis (Gr *akron,* extremity; *kyanos,* blue) Condition characterized by cyanotic discoloration, coldness, and sweating of the extremities, especially the hands, caused by arterial spasm that is usually precipitated by cold or emotional stress.

Acronym (Gr *acros,* topmost, foremost; *-onym,* word, name) Word or name formed from the initial letters or groups of letters of words in a set series.

Addiction (L *addictio,* a giving over, surrender, being enslaved to) State of being enslaved to an undesirable practice that is physically or psychologically habit-forming to the extent that its cessation causes severe trauma.

Adenoidal pad (Gr *adenos,* gland; *eidos,* form) Normal lymphoid tissue in the nasopharynx of children.

Adenosine triphosphate (ATP) High-energy compound formed in the cell, called the "energy currency" of the cell due to the binding of energy in its high-energy phosphate bonds for release for cell work as these bonds are split.

Adipocytes (L *adipis,* fat; *kytos,* hollow vessel, cell) Fat cells.

Adipose tissue (L *adipis,* fat, lard) Loose connective tissue in which fat cells (adipocytes) accumulate and are stored.

Affective goal Communication goal related to processes of feelings and desires, attitudes and values.

Alopecia (Gr *alopekia,* disease in which hair falls out) Baldness; absence of hair from skin areas of the body where it normally is present.

Alveoli (L *alveus,* hollow) Small, sac-like formations; thin-walled chambers in the lungs surrounded by networks of capillaries through whose walls exchange of carbon dioxide and oxygen takes place.

Alzheimer-type senile dementia (ATSD) Type of senile dementia first described by German physician Alois Alzheimer (1864–1915); progressive, irreversible degenerative changes in the brain, resulting in loss of neuromuscular function and mental capacity.

Amenorrhea (Gr *a-,* negative; *men,* month; *rhoia,* flow) Absence of menses. Nutritional amenorrhea results from extreme weight loss and malnutrition, as in eating disorders, such as anorexia nervosa.

Amino acids (*amino,* the monovalent chemical group-NH2) Carriers of the essential element nitrogen; structural units of protein, specific amino acids being linked in specific sequence by peptide chains to form specific proteins.

Amylase (Gr *amylon,* starch; *-ase,* enzyme suffix) Group name for enzymes that act on starch to render successively smaller and smaller molecules of dextrins and maltose—for example, salivary amylase (ptyalin) and pancreatic amylase (amylopsin). The generic group name amylase is now more widely used for any starch-splitting enzyme.

Anabolic steroids (Gr *anabole,* a building or construction) Synthetic derivatives of testosterone, the male sex hormone, having pronounced anabolic (tissue-building) properties; drugs used in clinical medicine to promote growth and repair of tissues in debilitating illness. Widespread illegal abuse by some athletes and body builders harms their health.

Anabolism Metabolic process by which body tissues are built.

Anemia (Gr *a-,* negative; *haima,* blood) Blood condition marked by a decrease in number of circulating red blood cells, hemoglobin, or both.

Anorexia (Gr *a, orexis* not appetite) Loss of appetite.

Anorexia nervosa (Gr *anorektos,* without appetite; L *nervosa,* nervous or emotional disorder) Severe psychophysiologic eating disorder, usually seen in girls and young women, in which the person does not lack appetite, as the label would indicate, but is psychologically unable to eat and refuses food, becoming extremely emaciated; a form of self-starvation.

Antagonist (Gr *antagonisma,* struggle) Agent that has an opposite, conflicting, or inhibiting action to another substance.

Antepartum (L *anto,* before; *partum,* parting, a separate part) Period of gestation before onset of maternal labor and birth of the infant.

Anthropometry (Gr *anthropos,* man, human; *metron,* measure) Science and procedures that deal with measurement of the size, weight, and proportional dimensions of the human body.

Antibodies Immune system components, specific immunoglobulins, especially secretory IgA in the bowel and upper respiratory mucosa that destroy invading antigens.

Antidiuretic hormone (ADH) Hormone secreted by the posterior pituitary gland in response to body stress. It acts on the distal tubules of the kidney's nephrons to cause water reabsorption and thus protect vital body water; also called *vasopressin.*

Antigen (antibody + Gr *gennan,* to produce) Any disease agent, such as toxins, bacteria, viruses, and other foreign substances, whose presence stimulates the production of antibodies of the immune system to combat and destroy them.

Antioxidant (Gr *anti-,* against; *oxys,* keen) Substance that inhibits oxidation of polyunsaturated fatty acids and formation of free radicals in the cells.

Antirachitic (Gr *anti-,* against; *rachitis,* a spinal disorder) Agent that is therapeutically effective against rickets, a nutritional deficiency disease affecting childhood bone development, in which vitamin D is lacking.

Aorta Main large trunk blood vessel from the heart, leading down the center of the body through the chest and upper abdomen from which the systemic arterial blood system proceeds.

Apgar score Scale developed by American anesthesiologist Virginia Apgar (1909–1974), by which an infant's condition is defined at one minute and five minutes after birth by scoring the heart rate, respiratory effort, muscle tone, reflex irritability, and color.

Apocrine (Gr *apokrinesthai,* to be secreted) Type of glandular secretion in which the end portion of the secreting cell is removed with the secretory product.

Areola (L *areola,* area, space) Pigmented area surrounding the nipple of the human breast.

Ascorbic acid Chemical name for vitamin C, based on its antiscorbutic function in prevention of the deficiency disease scurvy.

Atherosclerosis (Gr *athere,* gruel; *skleros,* hard) Condition characterized by gradual formation, beginning in childhood in genetically predisposed individuals, of fatty, cheese-like streaks that develop into hardened plaques in the intima, or inner lining, of major blood vessels, such as coronary arteries, eventually in adulthood cutting off blood supply to the tissue served by the vessel; the underlying pathology of coronary heart disease.

Atherosclerotic lesions Characteristic lesions, called athromas; the fatty, raised streaks and plaques that signal atherosclerosis, the underlying cardiovascular disease associated with elevated levels of serum lipids, especially cholesterol, and related risk factors, such as smoking, obesity, and hypertension.

Atrophic gastritis Chronic inflammation of the stomach, causing damage to the mucosal lining and reduced secretion of hydrochloric acid and in some cases intrinsic factor; loss of intrinsic factor and the inability to absorb vitamin B_{12} leads to pernicious anemia.

Autonomy (Gr *autos,* self; *nomos,* law) State of functioning independently; self-determination.

Axis (L *axis,* axle, central line) One of two coordinates used as a frame of reference between values in graphing data; usually the vertical Y axis, also called ordinate axis.

Barbiturate (Saint Barbara, drug discovered on day of the saint, 1864) Drug used to reduce anxiety or induce sleep; sometimes used to treat disorders causing convulsions.

Basal oxygen consumption Amount of oxygen intake to meet basal metabolic needs; a means of measuring basal metabolic rate (BMR). Comparative metabolic measures in current use are derived by formula calculation using individual factors of weight, height, age, and sex: basal energy expenditure (BEE) and resting energy expenditure (REE).

Basic four food groups A simple general food guide issued by the U.S. Department of Agriculture, using a grouping of commonly used foods and agricultural products for planning a day's balanced meals: breads/cereals, vegetables/fruits, milk and dairy products, and meat, with recent suggested food item revisions to reduce fats and sugars.

Behavioral goal Communication goal related to processes of changing behavior.

Bile (L *bilis,* bile) Fluid secreted by the liver and transported to the gallbladder for concentration and storage; released into duodenum on entry of fat to facilitate enzymatic fat digestion by acting as an emulsifying agent.

Bioavailability Amount of a nutrient ingested in food that is absorbed and thus available to the body for metabolic use.

Blastocyst (Gr *blastos,* germ; *kystis,* sac, bladder) Stage in the development of the embryo in which the cells are arranged in a single layer to form a hollow sphere.

Body compartment The collective quantity of a particular vital substance in the body—for example, the mineral compartment, composed mainly of the skeletal bone mass.

Body composition The relative sizes of the four body compartments that make up the physical body—lean body mass, fat, water, and mineral mass.

Body mass index Calculated assessment of body mass based on weight and height: BMI = weight (kg) divided by height $(m)^2$.

Botulism Serious, often fatal, form of food poisoning from ingesting food contaminated with the powerful toxins of the bacterium *Clostridium botulinum.* The toxin blocks transmission of neural impulses at the nerve terminals, causing gradual paralysis and death when affecting respiratory muscles. Most cases result from eating carelessly home-canned food, so that all such foods should be boiled at least ten minutes before eating. Cases reported in infants have been related to eating spore-containing honey, so honey should not be fed to infants.

Bradycardia (Gr *bradys,* slow; *kardia,* heart) Slow heartbeat, evidenced by slowing of the pulse rate to less than 60 beats/min.

Brush border Vast array of microvilli covering each villus on the absorptive surface of the small intestine, holding nutrients ready for absorption within an unstirred layer of water and facilitating their absorption with a greatly expanded surface area. So named because they appear like the bristles of a brush when viewed with an electron microscope.

Buffering capacity Function of the body's main buffer system, composed of two balancing partners, an acid partner (carbonic acid) and a base partner (sodium bicarbonate), which act together to buffer or neutralize any incoming acid or base to maintain the necessary degree of acidity and alkalinity in the body fluids that is compatible with life and health.

Bulimia nervosa (L *bous,* ox; *limos,* hunger; *nervosa,* nervous or emotional condition) Psychophysiologic eating disorder, seen mainly in girls and young women, marked by alternate gorging on large amounts of food and self-induced vomiting and purging with laxatives; weight usually remains fairly stable at a normal amount.

Cachexia (Gr *kakos,* bad, ill; *hexia,* habit) Profound and grave state of body disorder and deterioration, as seen in cases of advanced malignant disease or starvation, causing gross body weight loss to cadaverous proportions as a result of disorder metabolism.

Calcitonin (L *calx,* lime, calcium; *tonus,* balance) Polypeptide hormone secreted by the thyroid gland in response to hypercalcemia, which lowers both calcium and phosphate in the blood.

Calcitriol Activated hormone form of vitamin D $[1,25(OH)_2D_3]$—1,25,dihydroxycholecalciferol.

Candida albicans (L *candidus,* glowing white) Most frequent agent of *candidiasis,* a yeast-like fungus infecting moist tissue areas of the body, involving skin, vaginal, and oral mucosa.

Carbohydrate fuel Basic organic carbon compound in food (starches and sugars), which is the primary and most efficient form of body fuel for energy, especially for building body muscles.

Carboxypeptidase (L *carbo-,* coal, carbon—fundamental element in all organic compounds) Chemical group *carboxyl*—COOH—at the end of the carbon chain identifies the compound as an organic acid. The end of this term, *-peptidase,* indicates a protein-splitting enzyme, which together with the first part means that this is an enzyme that acts on the peptide bond of the terminal amino acid having a free-end carboxyl group.

Cardiac output Total amount of blood pumped by the heart per minute.

Carnitine Naturally occurring amino acid $(C_7H_{15}NO_3)$ formed from methionine and lysine, required for transport of long-chain fatty acids across the mitochondrial membrane, where they are oxidized as fuel substrate for metabolic energy.

Carotenemia Condition associated with excess intake or impaired metabolism of carotenoid pigments, especially beta-carotene, resulting in excess carotene in the blood, sometimes to the extent of producing a yellowing of the skin resembling jaundice.

Carotenoids Red and yellow pigments chemically similar to and including carotene, found in dark green and yellow vegetables and fruits.

Casein hydrolysate formula Infant formula with a base of hydrolyzed casein, major milk protein, produced by partially breaking down the casein of cow's milk into smaller peptide fragments, making a product that is more easily digested.

Catabolism Metabolic process by which body tissue is broken down.

Catalyst (Gr *katalysis,* dissolution) Substance, such as enzymes and their component trace elements, that controls specific cell metabolism reactions but is not changed or consumed itself in the reaction as are the specific substrates on which it works.

Cathartic (Gr *katharsis,* cleansing) Substance used to empty the bowel; a laxative.

Celiac disease (Gr *koilia,* belly) Malabsorption diarrheal disease of intestinal mucosa caused by an abnormal reaction to gluten in certain grains such as wheat; infantile form marked by extreme wasting, growth retardation, and celiac crisis.

Cephalopelvic disproportion (Gr *kephale,* head; *pyelos,* an oblong trough, pelvis) Relationship of fetal head to size of the maternal pelvis.

Cerebral hemorrhage Rupture of an artery in the brain; cerebrovascular accident (CVA), stroke.

Cheilosis (Gr *cheilos,* lip) General symptom of tissue inflammation and breakdown, producing swelling and reddening of the lips, a chapped appearance, and fissures at the corners of the mouth; associated with general malnutrition, especially a deficiency of riboflavin.

Cholecalciferol Chemical name for vitamin D in its inactive dietary form (D_3). Formerly measured in terms of International Units (IU), a concept based on the "biologic activity" of a vitamin as measured in rats according to its ability to forestall the development of a disease associated with a deficiency of that vitamin. Now, instead, vitamin recommendations are given in direct quantity (mg or μg) needed for health based on current population studies. In the case of vitamin D, 10 μg as cholecalciferol equals 400 IU. When the inactive cholecalciferol is consumed, it is activated first in the liver and then completed in the kidney to its active vitamin D hormone form, *calcitriol* (1,25-dihydroxycholecalciferol $[1,25(OH)_2D_3]$). Additional amounts of D_3 are generated by the effect of sunlight on 7-dehydrocholesterol in the skin, a precursor cholesterol compound.

Chronic diseases (Gr *chronos,* time) Diseases of aging or long duration.

Chronologic age Age of an individual based on the number of years lived, compared, for example, with *biologic age,* the relative age of a person based on physiologic capacity and measurements.

Chymotrypsin (Gr *chymos,* chyme; creamy, gruel-like material produced by gastric digestion of food) One of the protein-splitting and milk-curdling pancreatic enzymes, activated in the intestine from precursor chymotrypsinogen; breaks peptide linkages of the amino acids phenylalanine and tyrosine.

Cineradiographs (Gr *cine-,* kinesis, movement; L *radius,* ray; Gr *graphein,* to write) Fluoroscopic motion film records of internal structures and functions.

Citric acid cycle Final energy production pathway in the cell mitochondria that transforms the ultimate fuel acetyl CoA from carbohydrate and fat, capturing this energy in the cell's metabolic enzyme cycle production of high-energy phosphate bonds of ATP.

Clinical care process   Interactive process between health care professional and client of planning personal health care through five phases of assessing and collecting data, analyzing findings, planning care according to a written individual plan, implementing the plan, and evaluating and recording results.

Cobalamin   Chemical name for vitamin B_{12}, from its structure as a complex red crystalline compound of high molecular weight, with a single cobalt atom at its core. Its food sources are of animal origin, but the ultimate source is from colonies of synthesizing microorganisms inhabiting the gastrointestinal tract of herbiverous animals.

Coefficient of variation   Change or effect produced by the variation in certain factors, or the ratio between two different quantities.

Coenzyme factors   Major metabolic role of the micronutrients, vitamins, and minerals as essential partners with cell enzymes in a variety of reactions in both energy and protein metabolism.

Cognitive goal   (L *cognito*, to know) Communication goal related to the process of knowing and learning; mental processes of thinking and remembering.

Colostrum   (L *colostrum*, bee sting swelling and secretions) Thin, yellowish, milky liquid; mother's initial breast secretion before and immediately after birth of her baby; rich in immune factors and nutrition, especially protein and minerals; foremilk.

Communication   Process of giving or interchanging information, thoughts, or feelings by speaking, writing, signing, discussing, listening, responding.

Community care process   Program planning to meet defined community health needs through assessment procedures, objectives, program plan, and evaluation.

Complement   Series of enzymatic proteins that interact with an antigen-antibody complex to promote phagocyte activity or destroy other cells; component of the body's immune system.

Complementary amino acids   Combinations of amino acids from a variety of combined protein foods that complete one another according to their relative amounts of individual amino acids in order to meet growth requirements for the nine essential amino acids that the body does not sufficiently synthesize.

Complete protein   Protein food containing all of the essential amino acids; animal food sources are milk, cheese, meat, eggs. Plant proteins alone are incomplete, but complementary combinations may be planned to make a complete protein mix, as a vegetarian would do.

Complex carbohydrates   Main dietary carbohydrates; the polysaccharide starch in various foods, such as legumes, grains, breads, pasta, cereals, and potatoes.

Condom   (L *condus*, a receptacle) Penile sheath serving not only as a barrier method of contraception but also as a means of preventing the spread of sexually transmitted diseases.

Congregate meals   Group meals for older adults, served in a social setting in the community and funded by Title III-C of the Older Americans Act.

Constipation   (L *constipation*, a crowding together) Infrequent, sometimes difficult passage of feces; condition is often a source of anxiety to elderly persons and may be perceived more in mental attitude than in physiologic reality; sometimes called "irritable bowel."

Corpus luteum   (Gr *corpus*, body; *luteum*, yellow) Mass of estrogen and progesterone secretory cells; produced monthly from the ovarian follicle in the postovulation phase of the female sexual cycle.

Cortical bone   (Gr *corticis*, bark, shell) Long bones of the body extremities with heavy outer cortex layer, giving strength to body movements.

Corticosteroid   (L *corticis*, bark, shell) Any of the steroids affecting carbohydrate, fat, and protein metabolism that are produced in the outer region (cortex) of the adrenal glands in response to stimulus of the adrenocorticotropic hormone (ACTH) from the pituitary gland, or any of their synthetic derivatives. These compounds include *glucocorticoids* affecting glucose metabolism and *mineralocorticoids* affecting electrolyte (Na^+) concentration and hence fluid-electrolyte balance.

Counseling   Dynamic process of communication that is client-centered; the counselor's role is to guide the client to identify problems and priorities and to set goals and possible solutions.

Crohn's disease   Inflammatory disease first described by New York physician Bernard Crohn (born 1884), involving any part of the gastrointestinal tract but commonly affecting the lower small intestine and colon.

Cushing's syndrome   Condition first described by Boston surgeon Harvey Cushing (1869–1939), due to hypersecretion of adrenocorticotropic hormone (ACTH) or excessive intake of glucocorticoids; characterized by rapidly developing fat deposits of face, neck, and trunk, giving an enlarged and rounded "moon-face" or cushingoid appearance.

Cytoplasm   (Gr *kytos*, hollow vessel; *plasma*, anything formed or molded) Protoplasm of the cell outside the nucleus, a continuous, gel-like aqueous solution in which the cell organelles are suspended; site of major cell metabolism.

Deamination   Process by which the nitrogen radical (NH_2) is split off from amino acids, important in maintaining nitrogen balance.

Decubitus ulcer   Bedsore caused by prolonged pressure on the skin and tissues covering a bony area; occurs in elderly people who are confined to bed or immobilized.

Dementia   (L *de* + *mens*, mind) Progressive organic mental disorder causing changes in personality, disorientation, deterioration in intellectual function, and loss of memory and judgment; dementia caused by drug overdose, electrolyte or fluid imbalance, or insulin shock is reversed on treatment; dementia caused by injury or degenerative changes in brain tissue is not reversible.

De novo   (L *anew*, from the beginning) To make a new product from the beginning with the principal components; akin to "from scratch," as in cooking.

Dental caries   (L *caries*, "rottenness") Molecular decay or death of hard tissue; disease of the calcified tissues of the teeth resulting from action of microorganisms on carbohydrate, producing acid erosion of the tooth surface; characterized by disintegration of hard outer enamel, followed by breakdown of softer inner dentin material, leaving cavities and exposed soft tissue.

Dentin (L *dens*, tooth) Chief substance of the tooth; surrounds the innermost tooth pulp and is covered by the enamel of the crown and the cementum on the roots.

Depot fat Body fat stored in adipose tissue.

Desquamation (L *de-*, from; *squama*, scale) Shedding of epithelial tissue, mainly from the skin and oral mucosa, in scales or small sheets.

Diagnosis-related groups (DRGs) U.S. government cost-containment management classification scheme for predesignation of Medicare payments based on specific diagnosis categories of disease.

Dietary fiber Nondigestible form of carbohydrate; of nutritional importance in gastrointestinal disease, such as diverticulosis, and in management of serum lipid and glucose levels in risk reduction related to chronic conditions, such as heart disease and diabetes.

Dietary Guidelines for Americans Diet and health guidelines for planning a healthy diet and reducing disease risks.

Diuresis (Gr *diourein*, to urinate) Increased excretion of urine.

Diuretics (Gr *diouretikos*, promoting urine) Drugs that stimulate urination.

Docosahexaenoic acid (DHA) (Gr *docosa*, 22; *hexa*, 6) Long-chain polyunsaturated omega-3 fatty acid, having a 22-carbon chain with 6 double bonds; a metabolic product of omega-3 eicosapentaenoic (*eicosa*, 20; *penta*, 5)—EPA, long-chain fatty acid with 20 carbon atoms and 5 double bonds. Both are found in fatty fish. The body also synthesizes both EPA and DHA from the essential fatty acid linoleic and its product, linolenic acid.

Dysgeusia (Gr *dys*, bad; *geusis*, taste) Abnormally perverted sense of taste, or bad taste in the mouth.

Ectoderm (Gr *ektos*, outside; *derma*, skin) Outermost of the three primary cell layers of the embryo.

Edema (Gr *oidema*, swelling) Unusual accumulation of fluid in the intercellular tissue spaces of the body.

Edentulous (L *e-*, without; *dens*, tooth) Absence of natural teeth.

Eicosapentaenoic acid (EPA) (Gr *eicosa*, 20; *penta*, 5) Long-chain polyunsaturated fatty acid composed of a chain of 20 carbon atoms with 5 double (unsaturated) bonds; one of the omega-3 fatty acids found in fatty fish and fish oils.

18:2 fatty acid Naming system for fatty acids according to structure: carbon chain length and number of double (unsaturated) bonds. Thus, an 18:2 fatty acid has a long chain of 18 carbon atoms with 2 double bonds. This is the chemical shorthand for linoleic acid, the essential fatty acid.

Electrolyte (Gr *electron*, amber [which emits electricity when rubbed]; *lytos*, soluble) Chemical element or compound that in solution dissociates as ions carrying a positive or negative charge—for example, H^+, Na^+, K^+, Ca^{++}, Mg^{++}, and Cl^-, HCO^-_3, HOP^-_4, SO^-_4. Electrolytes constitute a major force controlling fluid balances within the body through their concentrations and shifts

from one place to another to restore and maintain balance—*homeostasis*.

Elemental formula Infant formula produced with elemental, ready-to-be-absorbed components of free amino acids and carbohydrate as simple sugars.

Enamel Very hard white surface substance that covers and protects the soft inner dentin of a tooth.

Endoderm (Gr *endon*, within; *derma*, skin) Innermost of the three primary embryonic cell layers.

Endometrium (Gr *endon*, within; *metra*, uterus) Inner mucous membrane of the uterus.

Endoplasmic reticulum (Gr *endon*, within; *plassein*, to form; L *rete*, net) Protoplasmic network in cells of flattened double membrane sheets; important metabolic cell organelles, some with rough surfaces bearing ribosomes for protein synthesis and other smooth surfaces synthesizing fatty acids.

Energy (Gr *energeia*, energy) Power to overcome resistance, to do work.

Energy balance Physiologic aspect of weight management, based on balance between energy intake in food and energy output in physical activity and internal metabolic work.

Energy intake Energy value of the three energy-yielding macronutrients in food—carbohydrate, fat, and protein—measured in kilocalories; abbreviated kcalories or kcal.

Enmeshed To catch, as in a net, and entangle; intertwined family relationships that capture and diminish individual autonomy or self-regard.

Epidemiology (Gr *epidemois*, prevalent; *-ology*, study) Study of factors determining the frequency, distribution, and strength of diseases in population groups.

Epiglottis (Gr *epi-*, on; *glottis*, vocal apparatus of the larynx) Lid-like, cartilaginous structure overhanging the entrance to the larynx and preventing food from entering the larynx and trachea while swallowing.

Epipharynx (Gr *epi-*, on; *pharynx*, throat) Nasopharynx, which lies above the level of the soft palate.

Episiotomy (Gr *epision*, pubic region; *tome*, a cutting) Surgical incision into the peritoneum and vagina for obstetrical purposes.

Epithelium (Gr *epi-*, on, upon, over; *thele*, nipple) Covering tissue of internal and external surfaces of the body, including linings of vessels and other small cavities.

Erythrocyte (Gr *erythro-*, red; *cyte*, hollow vessel) Red blood cell.

Erythropoiesis (Gr *erythros*, red; *poiesis*, making) Production of erythrocytes, red blood cells.

Essential amino acid Any one of nine amino acids that the body cannot synthesize at all or in sufficient amounts to meet body needs so it must be supplied by the diet, hence a *dietary* essential for these nine specific amino acids: histidine, isoleucine, leucine, lysine, methionine, phenylalanine, threonine, tryptophan, and valine.

Esterification Chemical process of converting an acid into an *ester*, catalyzed by the enzyme *esterase*. An ester is any compound formed from an alcohol and an acid by removal of water—for example, cholesterol esterification by attaching a fatty acid to the sterol base.

Estrogen Generic group name for the ovarian hormones—beta-estradiol (the most potent), estrone, and estriol, which develop and maintain the female sexual organs and stimulate bone growth.

Ethanol Chemical name for beverage alcohol.

Evaluation Process of determining the value of an educational or a clinical program in terms of its initial identified objectives.

Extracellular fluid (ECF) Total body water compartment composed of the collective water outside of cells.

Extracellular water Alternate term for collective body water or fluids outside of cells.

Ferrous sulfate Iron fortification compound in infant formulas used as needed to prevent anemia.

Flatulence (L *flatus,* a blowing) Excessive formation and expulsion of gases in the gastrointestinal tract.

Follicle (L *follis,* leather bag) Sac-like secretory cavity encasing an ovum and nourishing its growth.

Food abuse Misuse and excessive eating of food as a reflection of underlying personal needs or problems, rather than in normal amount and nature as an essential part of good health and enjoyment.

Food exchange lists (groups) Meal-planning food guide of six food exchange lists, with indicated portion sizes and equivalent food values for each item in a group; thus, items may be exchanged within each group to maintain both variety and food values. The six food groups are bread/cereal, vegetable, fruit, milk, meat, and fat. Easily used for nutrient and energy calculations for management of diabetes and weight.

Food frequency questionnaire (FFQ) Tool for collecting nutrition information about food habits. Consists of a comprehensive list of foods and a scale for checking frequency of use over a period of time.

Food guide Model for planning and evaluating a daily diet.

Food record Three- to seven-day record of all food consumed, detailed with portion sizes, amounts, and preparation methods or recipes, for nutrition analysis as part of a total nutritional assessment process for planning nutrition care and education or as an ongoing tool for monitoring nutrition therapy.

Fortified cereal Cereal food products enriched by additions of minerals, such as iron and zinc, and vitamins, such as thiamin, riboflavin, niacin, folate, B_6, and B_{12}.

Free radical Unstable, high-energy cell molecule with an unpaired electron that causes oxidation reactions in unsaturated fatty acids and may act as a carcinogen.

Frontal bossing (ME *boce,* lump, growth) Rounded protuberance of the forehead. In general terms, a boss is a knob-like, rounded protuberance on the body or a body organ.

Functional disability Disability that interferes with activities of daily living, such as bathing, dressing, shopping, preparing meals, eating.

Galactosemia Rare genetic disease in newborns caused by a missing enzyme (galactose-1-phosphate uridyltransferase-G-1-PUT) required for conversion of galactose to glucose for metabolic use in the body. Untreated, galactose (from lactose) accumulates in the blood, causing extensive tissue damage and potential death. Normal growth and development now follow mandatory newborn screening and immediate initiation of a galactose-free diet with a special soy-based formula.

Gastrectomy Surgical removal of all or part of the stomach.

Gastric (Gr *gaster,* stomach) Pertaining to the stomach.

Gastric pH (Gr *gaster,* stomach; *pH,* power of the hydrogen ion—H^+) Chemical symbol relating to H^+ concentration or activity in a solution; expressed numerically as the negative logarithm of H^+ concentration: pH 7.0 is neutral—above it, alkalinity increases and below it, acidity increases. The hydrochloric acid (HCl) gastric secretions maintain a gastric pH of about 2.0.

Generativity (L *generatio,* generation) Dynamic psychosocial process of renewing a society's values from one generation to the next.

Gerontology Study of aging, including biologic, physiologic, psychologic, and sociologic aspects. Contrast with *geriatrics,* which is the medical specialty dealing with chronic disease, as well as physical health, in older adults.

Gestation (L *gestare,* to bear) Intrauterine fetal growth period (forty weeks) from conception to birth.

Gestational age Period of embryonic-fetal growth and development from ovum fertilization to birth, varying from preterm development of a premature infant to a full-term, mature newborn.

Gingivitis (L *gingiva,* "gum of the mouth") Inflammation of the gum tissue surrounding the base of the teeth.

Glomerular filtration rate Measure of the amount of blood filtered by the cup-like glomerulus at the head of each kidney nephron, per unit of time (ml/min).

Gluconeogensis (Gr *gleukos,* sweetness; *neos,* new; *gennan,* to produce) Production of glucose from keto-acid carbon skeleton from deaminated amino acids and the glycerol portion of fatty acids.

Glucose Simple sugar, basic refined body fuel, circulated in the blood to cells for energy production.

Glycogen Briefly stored form of carbohydrate in the liver and muscle tissues, available for energy fuel during brief fasting periods of sleep; built up in larger storage amounts by high-starch meals prior to endurance athletic events for sustained energy.

Glycogen loading Practice among athletes in endurance events of increasing intake of complex carbohydrates days before an event to increase glycogen storage for energy reserve fuel during the event.

Glycolysis Initial energy production enzyme pathway outside the mitochondria, by which 6-carbon glucose is changed to active 3-carbon fragments of acetyl CoA, the fuel ready for final energy production in the mitochondria to the high-energy phosphate compound adenosine triphosphate (ATP).

Goitrogens Natural substances in certain foods, such as soybeans, that cause hypothyroidism and a compensatory enlargement of the thyroid gland, producing symptoms of iodine-deficiency goiter; effect diminished by adequate heating of the soy meal and adding iodine supplementation.

Golgi apparatus Complex, cup-like structure of membranes with associated vesicles, first described by Italian Nobel prize–winning histologist Camillo Golgi (1843–1926); site for synthesis of numerous carbohydrate metabolic products, such as lactose, glycoproteins, and mucopolysaccharides.

Granulosa cells Cells surrounding the primitive ovarian follicle and forming its outer layer and the mature ovary.

Grazing Informal descriptive label for eating pattern of frequent, small snacks throughout the day rather than more formal regular meals. Term taken from animal pattern of constant eating in a pastureland.

Growth acceleration Period of increased speed of growth at different points of childhood development.

Growth channel Progressive, regular growth pattern of children, guided along individual genetically controlled channels, influenced by nutritional and health status.

Growth deceleration Period of decreased speed of growth at different points of childhood development.

Growth grid Chart indicating weight-height growth rates of infants and children by percentiles of a representative population, on which an individual child's growth may be plotted for comparison and monitoring over time.

Growth velocity (L *velocitas,* speed) Rapidity of motion or movement; rate of childhood growth over normal periods of development, as compared with a population standard.

Guaiac test Laboratory test for occult (unseen) blood in the stool.

Gynecologic age (Gr *gynaikos,* women) Length of time from onset of menses to present time of conception.

Hematocrit (Gr *haima,* blood; *krinein,* to separate) Volume percentage of red blood cells in whole blood, showing ratio of RBC volume to total blood volume, normally about 35% in women; abbreviated HCT.

Heme iron Dietary iron from animal sources, from heme portion of hemoglobin in red blood cells. More easily absorbed and transported in the body than nonheme iron from plant sources but supplying the smaller portion of the body's total dietary iron intake.

Hemochromatosis (Gr *haima,* blood; *chroma,* color) Disorder of iron metabolism characterized by excess iron deposits in the tissues, especially the liver and pancreas; results from iron overload from prolonged use of iron supplements or from transfusions.

Hemoglobin (Gr *haima,* blood; L *globus,* a ball) Oxygen-carrying pigment in red blood cells; a conjugated protein containing 4 heme groups combined with iron and 4 long polypeptide chains forming the protein globin, named for its ball-like form; made by the developing RBC in bone marrow.

Hemolytic anemia (Gr *haima,* blood; *lysis,* dissolution) Anemia (reduced number of red blood cells) caused by breakdown of red blood cells and loss of their hemoglobin.

Hemorrhoids (Gr *haima,* blood; *rhoia,* to flow) Enlarged veins in the mucous membranes inside or outside of the rectum; cause pain, itching, discomfort, and bleeding.

Heterozygote (Gr *hetero,* other; *zygotos,* yoked together) An individual possessing different *alleles* (gene forms occupying corresponding chromosome sites) in regard to a given character trait.

Hirsutism (L *hirsutus,* shaggy hair) Condition marked by abundant and excessive hair; abnormal hairiness, especially an adult male pattern of body hair distribution in women.

Homeostasis (Gr *homoios,* like, unchanging; *stasis,* standing, steady) Life-sustaining, relative dynamic equilibrium within the body's internal environment; a biochemical and physiologic balance achieved through the constant operation of numerous interrelated homeostatic mechanisms.

Homogenization (Gr *homos,* same; *genos,* kind) Process of forming a permanent emulsion by breaking up fat portion into fine globules and dispersing them equally throughout the milk for uniform quality.

Hydrocephalus (Gr *hydro-,* water; *kephale,* head) Condition characterized by enlargement of the cranium caused by abnormal accumulation of fluid.

Hydrolysis (Gr *hydro-,* water; *lysis,* dissolution) Process by which a chemical compound is split into other, simpler compounds by taking up the elements of water, as in the manufacture of infant formulas to produce easier-to-digest derivatives of the main protein, casein, in the cow's milk base; process occurs naturally in digestion.

Hydroscopic (Gr *hydro-,* water; *skopein,* to measure or examine) Possessing tendency to take up and hold water readily.

Hydroxyapatite Inorganic compound of calcium, phosphate, and hydroxide found in the matrix of bones and teeth, giving rigidity and strength to the structure.

Hypercalcemia Elevated level of calcium in the blood.

Hyperinsulinemia (Gr *hyper* + L *insula,* island) Excessively high level of insulin in the blood.

Hyperlipidemia (Gr *hyper,* above; *lipos,* fat; *haemia,* blood) General term for elevated concentrations of any or all of the lipids in the blood plasma.

Hypernatremic dehydration Abnormally high sodium ion (Na^+) concentration in the extracellular fluid, due to water loss or restriction, drawing cell water to restore osmotic balance, causing dangerous cell dehydration. Compare with *hyponatremia.*

Hyperplasia (Gr *hyper,* above; *plasis,* formation) Enlargement of tissue due to a process of rapidly increasing cell number. Compare with *hypertrophy.*

Hypertrophy (Gr *hyper,* above; *trophe,* nutrition) Enlargement of an organ or a part due to the process of increasing cell size.

Hyperventilation (Gr *hyper,* above; L *ventilatio,* ventilation) Increased respiration with larger intake and consequent oxygen–carbon dioxide exchange in the lungs above the normal amount.

Hypogeusia (Gr *hypo-,* under; *geusis,* taste; *aisthesis,* perception) Abnormally diminished acuteness of the sense of taste.

Hyponatremia Abnormally low levels of sodium (Na^+) in the blood; can be easily caused by excess water intake to point of water intoxication, with resulting dilution of the major electrolyte (Na^+) in extracellular circulating fluids.

Hypothalamus (Gr *hypo-*, under; *thalamos*, inner chamber) Small gland adjacent to the pituitary in the midbasal brain area; serves as a collection and dispatching center for information about the internal well-being of the body, using much of this neuroendocrine information to stimulate and control many widespread important pituitary hormones.

Hypovolemia (Gr *hypo-*, under; ME *volume*, volume; Gr *haima*, blood) Low blood volume.

Ideal weight Optimal weight for an individual of a given height, sex, or age in relation to personal health.

Immunoglobulins (L *immunis*, free, exempt; *globulus*, globule, ball) Special components of the body's immune system; proteins synthesized by lymphocytes and plasma cells that have specific antibody activity.

Infant mortality Number of infant deaths during the first year of life (one month to one year) per 1,000 live births.

Insensible water loss Daily water loss through the skin and respiration, so named because a person is not aware of it. An additional, smaller amount is lost in normal perspiration, the amount varying with the surrounding temperature.

Interpolation (L *interpolare*, to make new) Process of injecting new interpretation or application of data to expand meaning or use, as in deriving data from one age group and applying it to another.

Intracellular water Collective body water or fluids inside of cells; in body composition measures a large portion assigned to total lean body mass, a vital component in cell metabolism.

Intubation Passage of a tube into a body hole—specifically, the insertion of a breathing tube through the mouth or nose into the trachea to ensure a patent airway for the delivery of an anesthetic gas or oxygen.

Involution (L *involutio*, in, into; *volvere*, to roll) Process of rolling or turning inward, shrinking an organ to its normal size, like the uterus after childbirth.

Ions (Gr *ion*, wanderer) Activated form of certain minerals, such as sodium (Na^+), potassium (K^+), and chloride Cl^-), that carry an electrical charge and perform a variety of essential metabolic tasks.

Iron absorption Degree of iron absorption, relativity small at best, depends on its acid reduction, either by accompanying food such as orange juice or by the gastric HCl secretions, from the ferric form (Fe^{+++}) in foods to the ferrous form (Fe^{++}) required for absorption. After absorption (about 30% of the total intake), it is oxidized back to the ferric form required for incorporation in body metabolism.

Isomaltase (Gr *isos*, equal; L *maltum*, grain) Enzyme of the intestinal mucosa that splits isomaltose, an *isomer* of maltose (an isomer is a compound like another compound capable of behaving in a similar manner), a digestive product of starch in grains.

Juxtaglomerular apparatus (L *juxta*, near; *glomus*, ball) Complex of special cells located near or adjoining the cuplike glomerulus at the head of each kidney nephron; responsible for sensing the level of sodium in the blood.

Ketones Class of organic compounds, including three keto-acid basis that occur as intermediate products of fat metabolism: acetoacetate, hydroxybutyrate, and acetone; excess production, as in the initial stages of starvation from burning body fat for energy fuel, leads to ketoacidosis, which if continued uncontrolled can bring coma and death.

Kilocalorie (kcalorie, kcal) Unit of measure for energy produced in the body by the energy-yielding macronutrients carbohydrate, fat, and protein.

Kwashiorkor Classic protein-deficiency disease, frequently encountered in children in developing countries but also seen in developed countries, such as the United States, in poverty areas and in metabolically stressed and debilitated hospitalized patients.

Kyphosis (Gr *kyphos*, hunchbacked) Abnormal outward curvature of the upper back resulting from age-related bone loss from the vertebrae.

Lactation (L *lactare*, to suckle) Process of milk production and secretion in the mammary glands.

Lactiferous ducts (L *lac*, milk; *ferre*, to bear; *ducere*, to lead or draw) Vessels conducting milk from producing cells to storage and release areas of the breast; tube or passage for secretions.

Lactobacillus bifidus (L *bifidus*) Predominant fermentative lactobacillus in the intestinal flora of breast-fed infants.

Lactoferrin (L *lac*, milk; *ferrum*, iron) Iron-binding protein found in human milk.

Lactoperoxidase Enzyme found in human milk that catalyzes the oxidation of organic substrate, including harmful microorganisms, thereby protecting the infant.

Lacunae (L *lacuna*, small pit or hollow cavity) Blood spaces of the placenta in which the fetal villi are found.

Lanolin (L *lana*, wool) Fatty substance extracted from wool, used in ointments and salves.

Larynx (Gr *larynx*, upper part of windpipe) Structure of muscle and cartilage lined with mucous membrane, connected to top part of the trachea and to the pharynx; essential sphincter muscle guarding the entrance to the trachea and functioning secondarily as the organ of the voice.

Laws of thermodynamics (Gr *therme*, heat; *dynamis*, power) Basic three laws of physics relating to heat-energy balance: (1) energy-like matter is neither created nor destroyed, only constantly transformed and recycled, thus conserving energy in any process; (2) there is always an increase in *entropy* (Gr *entrope*, a turning inward), a measure of the part of heat or other energy form in a system that is not available to perform work (thus entropy increases in all natural [spontaneous and irreversible] processes); and (3) absolute zero in energy balance is unattainable.

Lean body mass Collective fat-free mass of body composition; most metabolically active portion of body tissues.

Life expectancy Average remaining years a person of a given age may expect to live, based on statistical population averages.

Lifestyle Unique pattern of living, which, depending on its form, can be negative or positive in its health result.

Linear growth (L *linearis,* a line) Linear measure of growing body length; height.

Linoleic acid Ultimate essential fatty acid for humans.

Lipase (Gr *lipos,* fat; *-ase,* as, ending indicating an enzyme, attached to a stem that indicates the substrate on which it works) Group name for enzymes that work on lipids (fats), splitting fatty acids from the glycerol base.

Lipids Chemical group name for fats and fat-related compounds, such as cholesterol, lipoproteins, and phospholipids; general group name for organic substances of a fatty nature, including fats, oils, waxes, and related compounds.

Lipolysis (Gr *lipos,* fat; *lysis,* dissolution) Breakdown of fat; fat digestion.

Lobule (L *lobus,* lobe, a well-defined area) Small lobe, one of the primary divisions of a larger lobe; smaller branching vessels or subdivisions that make up a lobe of the mammary gland.

Locus of control (L *locus,* place, site) Perceived control center over one's life.

Longitudinal study Study of persons or populations over a long period of time to measure effects of specific factors on the aging process and incidence and course of disease.

Long-term care Medical, personal, or homemaking services provided within an institution or in the community for older adults who are no longer able to care for their own needs.

Low birth weight Birth weight less than 2,500 g (5.4 lb); very low birth weight, less than 1,500 g (3.2 lb).

Lymphoblasts (L *lympha,* water; Gr *blastos,* germ) Immature stage of the mature lymphocyte.

Lymphocytes Mature leukocytes, special lymphoid white blood cells, T cells and B cells, major components of the body's immune system; found in human milk.

Lymphoid tissue (L *lympha,* water) Tissue related to the body system of lymphatic fluids; body tissues giving rise to lymphocytes of the immune system, such as intestinal mucosa and lymph gland.

Lyophilization (Gr *lyein,* to dissolve; *philein,* to love, having an affinity for a stable solution) Process of rapid freezing and dehydration of a frozen product under high vacuum to stabilize or preserve a biologic substance.

Lysozyme (Gr *lysis,* dissolution; *zyme,* leaven) Crystalline basic enzyme in many body fluids, such as saliva, tears, and human milk; an antibacterial agent.

Macronutrients (Gr *makros,* large; L *nutriens,* nourishment) Group name for the three large energy-yielding nutrients—carbohydrate, fat, and protein—all organic compounds of large molecular size.

Macrophage (Gr *makros,* large; *phagein,* to eat) Large phagocytes, cells of the immune system that engulf and consume microorganisms, other cells, or foreign particles and interact with T cells and B cells to produce inflammatory process and antibodies.

Major minerals Minerals that occur in relatively large quantities in the body and hence have greater dietary requirements.

Maltase Enzyme acting on the disaccharide maltose, from starch breakdown, into its two component monosaccharides, two units of glucose.

Mammalian Any vertebrate animal belonging to the class *Mammalia,* or humans, who give birth to live young and nourish them with milk from the female mammary glands.

Mammary glands (Gr *mamme,* mother's milk) Milk-producing glands in females of all mammalian species, humans and animals, who are distinguished from all other life by bearing live young and producing milk to nourish them.

Marsupial (L *marsupium,* a pouch) Member of the animal class of mammals who bear undeveloped young, which they carry in an abdominal pouch and nourish with their milk until development is complete; includes such animals as kangaroos and koala bears.

Mastitis (Gr *mastos,* breast; *-itis,* inflammation) Breast infection; inflammation of the mammary gland.

Maturation (L *maturus,* mature) Process or stage of attaining one's full physical, psychosocial, and mental development. Individual genetic potential guides physical and mental development, which in turn bears the imprint of environmental, psychosocial, and cultural influence.

Mean Mathematical term for the average numerical value of a group of numbers.

Median (L *medianus,* middle) Middle value in a distribution of numbers, with half of the values falling above and half falling below.

Megaloblastic anemia (Gr *mega,* great size; *blastos,* embryo, germ) Anemia due to faulty production of abnormally large, immature red blood cells, due to a deficiency of vitamin B_{12} and folate.

Menarche (Gr *men,* month; *arche,* beginning) Onset of menses.

Menopause (Gr *meno-,* month; *pausis,* cessation) Cessation of menses, occurring in North American women at approximately fifty years of age.

Menses Monthly menstrual periods.

Menstruation Monthly discharge of blood and mucosal tissue from the nonpregnant uterus; final phase of the female sexual cycle.

Mesoderm (Gr *mesos,* middle; *derma,* skin) Intermediate layer of embryonic cells developing between the ectoderm (outer layer) and endoderm (inner layer).

Metabolic acidosis Abnormal rise in acid partner of the carbonic acid–base bicarbonate buffer system by excess of organic acids, which displace part of the base bicarbonate in the buffer system and cause the H^+ concentration (acidity) to rise.

Metabolic activity Sum of biochemical actions and reactions in the body that build and maintain tissue, regulate body functions, and require a constant energy source. The most metabolically active tissue is the lean body mass.

Metabolism (Gr *metaballein,* to change) Sum of all the biochemical and physiologic processes by which the body grows and maintains itself (anabolism) and breaks down and reshapes tissue (catabolism), transforming energy to do its work.

Micelle (L *micella*, small body) Microscopic colloid particle of fat and bile formed in the small intestine for initial stage of fat absorption.

Microcephaly (Gr *mikros*, small; *kephate*, head) Small size of the head in relation to the rest of the body.

Micronutrients (Gr *mikros*, small; L *nutriens*, nourishing) Group name for the nonenergy-yielding nutrients, the vitamins, organic compounds of small molecular size, and minerals, single inert elements; essential coenzyme factors in metabolism and tissue structure.

Microphthalmia (Gr *micro*, small; *ophthalmos*, eye) Abnormal smallness of one or both eyes.

Mid-upper-arm muscle circumference (MAMC) Indirect measure of the body's skeletal muscle mass based on mid-arm circumference (MAC) and triceps skinfold (TSF): MAMC (cm) = MAC (cm) − [0.314 × TSF (mm)].

Milieu (Fr *milieux*, surroundings) Environment, social or physical; an important concept in nutrition, referring to both external sociophysical setting and internal biochemical environments, and interacting balances between them.

Milliosmoles (mOsm/L) Osmole (Gr *osme*, small), standard unit of osmotic pressure; equal to the gram molecular weight of solute divided by the number of particles (ions) into which a substance dissociates in solution. Thus, milliosmole is a much smaller unit of measure of osmotic pressure—1/1,000 of an osmole, equal to 1/1,000 gram molecular weight of a substance divided by the number of ions into which a substance dissociates in 1 liter (L) of solution. *Osmolality* refers to this concentration of solutes per unit of solvent.

Mineral compartment Smallest part of the body composition, found mainly in the skeletal bone mass.

Mitochondria (Gr *mitos*, thread; *chondrion*, granule) Cells' "powerhouse"; small, elongated organelles located in the cell cytoplasm; principal site of energy generation (ATP synthesis); contains enzymes of the final energy cycle (citric acid cycle) and cell respiration, as well as ribonucleic acid (RNA) and deoxyribonucleic acid (DNA) for some synthesis of protein.

Mortality rate Total number of deaths in a specific category divided by the total number of deaths in the total population.

Morula (L *morus*, mulberry) Solid mass of cells resembling a mulberry, formed by cleavage of a fertilized ovum.

Motivation Forces that affect individual, goal-directed behavior toward satisfying needs or achieving personal goals.

Multigravida (L *multus*, many; *gravida*, pregnant) Woman who has had two or more pregnancies.

Multiparous (L *multus*, many, much; *parere*, to bring forth) Women who have had two or more pregnancies resulting in live births.

Myelin (Gr *myelos*, marrow) High lipid-to-protein substance-forming sheath to insulate and protect neuron axons and facilitate their neuromuscular impulses.

Myocardial infarction (MI) (Gr *mys*, muscle; *Kardia*, heart; L *infarcire*, to stuff it) Death of heart muscle tissue resulting from blockage of blood flow to or through the coronary arteries, usually caused by fatty plaques and blood clot formation from their tissue irritation to the surrounding blood vessel, effectively "stuffing" the vessel at that point and cutting off blood supply to the heart muscle tissue served by the vessel. This event is commonly called a heart attack.

Myocardium (Gr *mys*, muscle; *kardia*, heart) Heart muscle; middle and thickest layer of heart wall.

Myoepithelial cells (Gr *mys*, muscle; *epi-*, on; *thele*, nipple) Tissue composed of contractile epithelial cells surrounding the alveoli and duct system of the lactating breast.

Nanogram (abbreviated ng) (Gr *nano-*, dwarf) One-billionth gram; also called millimicrogram.

Nanomole (abbreviated nmole) (Gr *nanos*, dwarf; *molekul*, molecule) Metric system unit for measuring very small amounts. Prefix *nano-* used in naming very small amounts to indicate one-billionth of the unit with which it is combined. *Mole* is chemical term for the molecular weight of a substance expressed in grams—gram molecular weight.

Narcissism Self-love; from Narcissus, a character in Greek mythology who saw his image mirrored in a pool of water and fell in love with his own reflection.

Necrotizing enterocolitis (Gr *nekrosis*, deadness; *enterion*, intestine) Infectious, tissue-destroying intestinal disease of the small intestine and colon; acute inflammation of intestinal mucosa.

Negative nitrogen balance Situation in which the amount of nitrogen consumed is less than the amount of nitrogen lost through all excretory routes, resulting in a net loss of body nitrogen.

Neonatal (Gr *neos*, new; L *natus*, born) Period surrounding birth; especially the first four weeks after birth, when the infant is called a neonate.

Neonatal mortality Number of newborn deaths during the neonatal period (birth to one month postpartum) per 1,000 live births.

Neonate Newborn infant; term usually refers to the first four weeks of life.

Nephron Functional unit of the kidneys, constantly filtering the blood, selectively reabsorbing its components as needed to maintain normal blood values, and excreting the remainder in a concentrated urine. At birth, each kidney has about a million of these minute units, far more than actually needed.

Neuromotor (Gr *neuron*, nerve; L *motorium*, movement center) Movement involving nerve impulses to muscles.

Neurotransmitter (Gr *neuron*, nerve; L *trans*, through, across; *missio*, sending) Large group of forty chemical substances, including compounds as diverse as acetylcholine, various hormones, and several amino acids, that function as essential synaptic transmitters, chemical messengers for sending (or inhibiting) nerve impulses across synapses of connecting nerve endings.

Niacin equivalent (NE) Current international measure for recommended amounts of B vitamin niacin that accounts for both the preformed vitamin and the amino acid precursor tryptophan, from which the vitamin can be synthesized. Thus, 1 NE equals 1 g niacin or 60 mg dietary tryptophan.

Nitrogen balance   Metabolic balance between nitrogen intake in dietary protein and output in urinary nitrogen compounds, such as urea and creatinine. For every 6.25 g dietary protein consumed, 1 g nitrogen is excreted.

Nonheme iron   Larger portion of dietary iron, including all the plant food sources and 60% of the animal food sources, that lacks the more easily absorbed and bioavailable heme iron in the remaining 40% of the animal food sources that contain hemoglobin residues of iron-containing heme.

Normochromic   Normal red blood cell color.

Normocytic   Normal cell size.

Nulliparity   (L *nullus*, none; *parere*, to bring forth) Reproductive status of a woman who has never borne a viable child.

Nutrient density   Protein, vitamin, or mineral content of a food expressed in relation to its energy (caloric) content.

Nutritional assessment   (L *nutritio*, nourishment; *assessare*, to assess, to estimate property or income value for purposes of taxation) Process of determining individual or group nutritional status as a basis for identifying needs and goals and planning personal health care or community programs to meet these identified goals.

Nutritional status   (L *status*, condition, situation) Condition of an individual's body tissues and health, especially as related to the nutrients that are essential to the structure, function, and maintenance of body tissues.

Nutrition care plan   Person-centered care plan, based on nutritional assessment data and evaluation, for individual nutritional care and education to promote health and prevent or treat disease.

Nutrition education   Process of helping individuals obtain the knowledge, skills, and motivation needed to make appropriate food choices for positive health throughout life.

Nutrition environment   (L *nutritio*, nourishment; Fr *environner*, to surround, encircle) The sum of substances, materials, and processes involved in taking in food and nutrients and assimilating and using them for body health and strength.

Nutrition label   Food product label providing nutrition information concerning nutrient and energy values per designated size portion.

Obligatory nitrogen loss   Lowest level of nitrogen excretion that can be reached by an individual despite all body conservation mechanisms.

Odd-numbered carbon-chain fatty acids   Most fatty acid carbon chains in the human diet are even-numbered, broken down by beta oxidation, successively clipping off 2-carbon fragments of *acetyl-CoA* to feed into the final energy production pathway, the citric acid cycle. A few odd-numbered ones do exist, however. When they occur, they go through the same beta-oxidation process, clipping off 2-carbon fragments until the final 3-carbon residue remains, *proprionyl-CoA,* which is also an intermediate

metabolic product of the essential amino acid threonine. These 3-carbon fragments from both sources are converted to *succinyl-CoA,* a 4-carbon compound in the citric acid cycle, so they feed into the final energy production cycle at this point.

Oligosaccharides   (Gr *oligos*, little; *saccharide*, sugar) Intermediate products of polysaccharide carbohydrate breakdown, containing a small number (from four to ten) of single sugar units of the monosaccharide glucose.

Omega-3 fatty acids   Group of long-chain, polyunsaturated fatty acids having important precursor roles in producing highly active, hormone-like substances, the *eicosanoids,* involved in critical metabolic activities, such as vascular muscle tone and blood clotting.

Omnivorous   (L *omnia*, all; *vovare*, to eat) Eating all kinds of foods, from both animal and plant sources.

Organohalides   (Gr *organon*, organ; Chem *halides*, compounds of fluorine, chlorine, bromine, or iodine) Chemical compounds used as pesticides or in industrial processes—for example, DDT and PCBs.

Orofacial muscles   (L *os, oris*, mouth) Adjoining muscles of the mouth and face.

Osmolality   (Gr *osmos*, impulsion through a membrane) Property of a solution that depends on the concentration of the particles (solutes) in solution per unit of solvent base; measured as milliosmoles per liter (mOsm/L).

Osteoarthritis   (Gr *osteon* + *arthron*, joint; *-itis*, inflammation) Form of arthritis in which joints undergo degenerative changes, resulting in stiffness, pain, and swelling; arthritis in the hip, knee, or spine can result in some degree of disability.

Osteomalacia   (Gr *osteon*, bone; *malakia*, softness) Condition marked by softening of the bones due to impaired mineralization with excess accumulation of osteoid (immature young bone matrix that has not had mineralization to harden it); results from deficiency of vitamin D and calcium.

Osteoporosis   (Gr *osteon*, bone; *poros*, passage, pore) Abnormal thinning of bone, producing a porous, fragile, lattice-like bone tissue of enlarged spaces, prone to fracture or deformity.

Ovulation   Monthly process in female sexual cycle of secreting a mature ovum for transport through the fallopian tubes to the uterus.

Ovum   (L *ovum*, egg) Female reproductive cell (egg) capable of fertilization and development into a new organism.

Oxalic acid   Compound in a variety of foods, including green, leafy vegetables; corn; soy products such as tofu; and wheat germ; that binds calcium in the food mix and hinders its absorption.

Oxyhemoglobin   Hemoglobin with bound oxygen for transport by the red blood cells from the lungs to the body tissue cells for vital metabolic work.

Oxytocin   (Gr *oxys*, sharp, sour; *tokos*, birth) Pituitary hormone causing uterine contractions and milk ejection.

Palate   (L *palatum*, palate) Partition separating the nasal and oral cavities, with a hard, bony front section and a soft, fleshy back section.

Palmar grasp   Early grasp of the young infant; clasping an object in the palm and wrapping the whole hand around it.

Paraprofessional   (Gr *para-*, alongside) Nonprofessional person, often from the community being served and thus having valuable insights concerning needs, who is trained to assist the professional community or clinical nutrition specialist in carrying out a nutrition program.

Parenteral nutrition   (Gr *para*, beyond, beside; *enteron*, intestine) Nourishment received not through the gastrointestinal tract but, rather, by an alternate route, such as injection into a vein; intravenous feeding of elemental nutrients.

Parietal cells   (L *parietes*, wall) Cells lining the stomach that secrete hydrochloric acid; chief cells.

Parity   (L *parere*, to bring forth, produce) Number of pregnancies a woman has had producing viable offspring.

Parkinson's disease   Neurologic disorder, described by English physician James Parkinson (1755–1824), characterized by tremor, muscular rigidity, and abnormally decreased motor function and ability, affecting mobility.

Parturition   (L *parturitio*, to give birth) Act or process of childbirth; maternal labor and delivery.

Pattern for daily food choices   Expanded accompaniment to dietary guidelines to apply them to practical meal planning.

Percentile   (L *per*, through; *centrum*, a hundred, "by the hundred") Rate or proportion per hundred; statistical term indicating status of a value in relation to 100 equal parts of a series of values in order of their measurable magnitude. For example, a value at the 60th percentile means that 60% of all the values in the distribution of the population studies lie at or below the 60th percentile, 40% above it.

Perinatal mortality   (Gr *peri-*, around; L *natus*, born) Infant deaths in the perinatal period, shortly before and after birth, approximately from weeks twenty to twenty-eight of gestation to one to four weeks postpartum, per 1,000 live births.

Periodontal disease   (Gr *peri*, around + *odove*, tooth) Inflammation and breakdown of the tissues and ligaments that surround the tooth and hold it in place; periodontal disease is often the cause of tooth loss in older people.

Peristalsis   (Gr *peri*, around; *stalsia*, contraction) Wave-like progression of alternate contraction and relaxation of the muscle fibers of the gastrointestinal tract.

Pernicious anemia   Chronic macrocytic anemia occurring most commonly after age forty; caused by absence of the intrinsic factor normally present in the gastric juices and necessary for the absorption of cobalamin (B_{12}); controlled by intramuscular injections of vitamin B_{12}.

pH   Power of the hydrogen ion (H^+), a measure indicating degree of acidity or alkalinity of solutions. A pH of 7.0 indicates neutrality, with numbers above it indicating increasing alkalinity and those below increasing acidity.

Phagocytosis   (Gr *phagein*, to eat; *-cyte*, hollow vessel, anything that contains or covers) The engulfing of microorganisms, other cells, or foreign particles by phagocytes.

Pharynx   (Gr *pharynx*, throat) Muscular, membranous passage between the mouth and the posterior nasal passages and the larynx and esophagus.

Phenylketonuria (PKU)   Genetic disease caused by a missing enzyme, phenylalanine hydroxylase, required for the metabolic conversion of the essential amino acid phenylalanine to the amino acid tyrosine. Untreated, profound mental retardation occurs. Normal growth and development now follow current mandatory newborn screening and immediate initiation of a low phenylalanine diet with special "low-phe" formula, such as Lofenalac.

Physiologic age   Rate of biologic maturation in individual adolescents, which varies widely and accounts, far more than does chronologic age, for wide and changing differences in their metabolic rates, nutritional needs, and food requirements.

Phytic acid   Compound in certain grains, such as wheat, that binds calcium and hinders its absorption.

Pincer grasp   Later digital grasp of the older infant, usually picking up smaller objects with a precise grip between thumb and forefinger.

Pinocytosis   (Gr *pinein*, to drink; *kytos*, cell) Uptake of fluid nutrient material by a living cell by means of incupping and invagination of the cell membrane, which closes off and forms free cell vacuoles.

Placebo   (L *placere*, to please) Inactive substance or preparation used in controlled drug or nutrient studies to determine the efficacy of an agent under study.

Placenta   (L *placentas*, a flat cake) Characteristic organ of mammals during pregnancy joining mother and offspring, providing supportive nourishment and endocrine secretions for embryonic-fetal development and growth.

Polymer   (Gr *poly-*, many; *meros*, part) Large compound formed by chains of simpler repeating molecules—for example, the glucose polymer oligosaccharide.

Postpartum   (L *post*, after; *partum*, separate part) Period following childbirth or delivery.

Postprandial   Following a meal.

Poverty line   Minimum income required to provide the basic necessities of food, clothing, and shelter for an individual or a family as determined by a U.S. government agency.

Precursor   Substance from which another substance is produced.

Preeclampsia   (Gr *pre-*, before; *eklampein*, to shine forth) Abnormal condition of late pregnancy marked by rather sudden hypertension and increased edema, usually accompanied by proteinuria; may progress to eclampsia, with convulsions and coma; better prevented by good prenatal care and optimal nutrition throughout the pregnancy.

Preterm milk   Milk produced by mothers of premature infants.

Preventive approach   Positive health care that seeks to identify and reduce risk factors for disease.

Primigravida   (L *prima*, first; *gravida*, pregnant) Woman pregnant for the first time.

Primiparous   (L *prima*, first; *parere*, to bring forth) State of a woman bearing or having borne only one child.

Primordial follicle Primitive ovarian follicle (*follis,* a leather bag), formed during fetal life; a sac- or pouch-like cavity, a small secretory sac or gland; an ovarian follicle, ovum surrounded by specialized epithelial cells.

Primordial ova (L *primordia,* the beginning; *ovum,* egg) Primitive ova cells produced in large life-supply numbers in the female fetal ovaries before birth.

Progesterone Ovarian hormone that regulates secretory function of the mucosal linings of the uterus and fallopian tubes and stimulates development of milk-producing structures of the breast.

Prolactin (Gr *pro-,* before; L *lac,* milk) Hormone of the anterior pituitary gland that stimulates and maintains lactation in postpartum mothers.

Prophylactic (Gr *prophylassein,* to keep guard before) Preventive treatment to avoid disease—for example, vitamin K for newborns to prevent the formerly widespread hemorrhagic disease of newborns, since they are born with a sterile gastrointestinal tract and lack the microorganisms that synthesize vitamin K.

Proprietary (L *proprietarius,* owner) Referring to commercial products, such as infant formulas and medical items, that are designed, manufactured, and sold for profit only by the owner of the patent, formula, brand name, or trademark associated with the product.

Prostaglandins Highly active, hormone-like, eicosanoid substances produced from essential fatty acid precursors and acting locally in various body tissues with many physiologic effects.

Protein turnover Metabolic process in the body by which proteins are being constantly synthesized, broken down, and the resulting amino acids resynthesized into new proteins.

Proteolytic (Gr *protos,* first, protein; *lysis,* dissolution) Protein splitting by a series of enzymes through hydrolysis of the peptide bonds into smaller peptides and amino acids.

Prothrombin (Gr *pro-,* before; *thrombos,* clot) Blood-clotting factor (number II), synthesized in the liver from glutamic acid and CO_2, catalyzed by vitamin K.

Protocol (Gr *protokollon,* leaf or tag attached to a rolled papyrus manuscript containing notes as to its contents) Set of governing rules; plan and procedures for carrying out a scientific study or a person's treatment regimen.

Psychotropic (Gr *psyche* + *trepein,* to turn) To exert an effect on the mind, altering behavior, mental activity, or emotional experience.

Pubertal development Rapid physical growth and sexual development of puberty.

Pyridoxine Chemical name for vitamin B_6, derived from its ring-like structure. In its active form, pyridoxal phosphate, it acts as a coenzyme factor in many types of transamination and decarboxylation reactions in amino acid metabolism.

Radioimmunoassay (L *radius,* ray; *immunis,* free, exempt; *assay,* examine, analyze) Technique using radioactive labeling of the material being studied, for measuring minute quantities of antigen or antibody, hormones, certain drugs, and other substances.

Recommended Dietary Allowances (RDAs) Nutrient and energy standards for healthy population groups in the United States by age and sex, updated every four to five years by expert committees of scientists to reflect current research and issued by the National Research Council of the National Institutes of Health.

Renal solute load Collective number and concentration of solute particles in solution, carried by the blood to the kidney nephrons for excretion in the urine, usually nitrogenous products from protein metabolism, and the electrolytes Na^+, K^+, Cl^-, and HPO_4^{--}.

Requirement Amount of a nutrient that, when fed to a human or an animal, will prevent the appearance of deficiency symptoms and maintain health.

Resorption (L *resorbere,* to swallow again) Process by which bone is lost; the mineral crystals are dissolved, and the protein matrix is broken down and removed.

Resting energy expenditure (REE) Energy expended by a person at rest in a neutral surrounding temperature, neither hot nor cold; similar to other measures of energy needs, such as the classic test of basal metabolic rate (BMR) and the calculated basal energy expenditure (BEE). The three values are often used interchangeably.

Retinol Chemical name for vitamin A derived from its function relating to the retina of the eye and light-dark adaptation. Daily RDA standards are stated in retinol equivalents (RE) to account for sources of the preformed vitamin A and its precursor provitamin A, beta-carotene.

Retinol equivalent (RE) Unit of measure for dietary sources of vitamin A, both preformed vitamin, retinol, and the precursor provitamin, beta-carotene. 1 RE = μg retinol or 6 μg beta-carotene.

Reverse peristalsis (Gr *peri-,* around; *stalsis,* contraction) Wave-like contractions of longitudinal and circular muscles of the gastrointestinal tract that normally propel the food mass forward but may act in reverse in upper GI tract of young infants, causing easy spitting-up of milk.

Salicylates Compound salts of salicylic acid, found in certain plants and in drugs such as common aspirin (acetylsalicylic acid—ASA).

Senescence (L *senescere,* to grow old) Normal process or condition of growing old.

Senile dementia of the Alzheimer type (SDAT) Type of senile dementia first described by German physician Alois Alzheimer (1864–1915); causes progressive, irreversible degenerative changes in the brain, resulting in loss of neuromuscular function and mental capacity.

Sexual maturity ratings Scale defining stages of sexual maturation during puberty.

Simple carbohydrates The monosaccharides glucose, fructose, and galactose and the disaccharides sucrose, maltose, and lactose.

Skeletal muscle Muscles attached to skeletal bones for control of body movements; major component of lean body mass.

Sociodemographic Relating to the characteristic social and cultural values, geographic distribution, and physical environments of persons and populations.

Solutes (Gr *solvere,* to dissolve) Particles of a substance in solution; a solution consists of solutes and a dissolving medium (solvent), usually a liquid.

Stereotype Oversimplified and generalized conception or image held by persons and groups that have distorted or unreal meaning but influences attitudes and behavior of those holding such views.

Stress Sum of biologic reactions to adverse stimuli, physical, mental, or emotional, internal or external, that disturbs the state of homeostasis and sense of well-being.

Sucrase Intestinal enzyme that splits the disaccharide sucrose into its two component monosaccharides, glucose and fructose.

Supine Lying on the back.

Tactile (L *tactio,* to touch) Sense of touching, perception by the touch.

Tannic acid Compound of certain plants, such as tea leaves, giving an astringent taste and having astringent properties, which promote local tissue healing; an herbal remedy.

Tetany (Gr *teinein,* to stretch) Condition caused by decrease in ionized serum calcium, marked by intermittent spastic muscle contractions and muscular pain; manifest by characteristic carpopedal spasm of the arm muscles, causing flexion of the wrist and thumb with extension of the fingers, called *Trousseau's sign.* A so-called milk tetany has been reported in young infants fed undiluted cow's milk, due to the greater ratio of phosphorus to calcium in cow's milk than in human milk, and these infants could not clear the phosphate load, which then accumulated in the blood and caused a compensatory decrease in the serum calcium, resulting in the typical muscular spasms of tetany.

Tidal volume Amount of gases, oxygen, and carbon dioxide passing into and out of the lungs in each respiratory cycle.

Title III-C Statute of the Older Americans Act, authorizing congregate and home-delivered meals for people age sixty and over.

Tocopherol (Gr *tokos,* childbirth; *pherein,* to carry) Chemical name for vitamin E, so named by early investigators because their initial work with rats indicated a reproductive function, which did not turn out later to be the case with humans, in whom it functions as a strong antioxidant to preserve structural membranes, such as cell walls.

Tonsils (L *tonsilla,* tonsil) Small, rounded masses of lymphoid tissue in the roof and posterior wall of the nasopharynx.

Trabeculae (L *trabs,* a little beam) Small bones at the ends of long bones at joints, such as wrist, vertebrae, and hips.

Trabecular bone General term for small mesh-work of bones at ends of long bones forming attached joints and part of the connecting network between vertebrae.

Trace elements Minerals that occur in small amounts or traces in the body and hence are required in very small amounts.

Tretinoin Form of retinoic acid, a vitamin A derivative, used as a drug in the medical treatment of chronic acne as a topical keralytic agent (Gr *keras,* horn; *lysis,* dissolution).

Keratin is a hard protein; it is the principal constituent of skin, hair, nails, and scar tissue.

Triglyceride Chemical name for fat, indicating structure: attachment of three fatty acids to a glycerol base. A neutral fat, synthesized from carbohydrate, stored in adipose tissue. It releases free fatty acids into the blood when hydrolyzed by enzymes.

Trophoblast (Gr *trophe,* nutrition; *blastos,* embryo, germ) Extraembryonic ectodermal tissue on the surface of the cleaving, fertilized ovum that is responsible for contact with the maternal circulation and supply of nutrients to the embryo.

Trypsin (Gr *trypein,* to rub; *pepsis,* digestion) Protein-splitting enzyme formed in the intestines by action of enterokinase on the inactive precursor trypsinogen.

Trypsin inhibitor Natural substance in raw soybeans that is responsible for a toxin in the bean. Fortunately, this substance is destroyed by heat and rendered inactive.

Ulnar deviation Turning and articulation of the *ulna* (inner and larger bone of the forearm on the side opposite the thumb) with the wrist joint to accomplish coordinated movement of the wrist and hand.

U.S. dietary guidelines A set of seven statements to guide food choices that reflects current health promotion and disease prevention national health objectives.

U.S. RDA Condensed food-labeling version of the regular National Research Council's Recommended Dietary Allowances, not to be confused with the regular NRC standards. This U.S. RDA, set up by the FDA in 1974 to replace the old minimum daily requirements (MDA), was compiled at the time from the 1968 regular RDAs, using the highest value within age/sex categories. Cost of label changing prevents updating with revised RDA editions, causing confusion to consumers.

Vascular spaces Spaces within fluid vessels in the body, blood vessels, and lymph vessels; contain body fluids in transit, a greater amount in blood and remainder in the interconnecting lymphatic system.

Vasodilation (L *vas,* vessel; *dilatare,* to spread out) Expansion or stretching of a blood vessel.

Vasopressin Hormone formed in the hypothalamus and stored in the posterior pituitary gland. Stimulates muscle contraction of capillaries and arterioles to maintain blood pressure and acts on the epithelial cells of the distal tubule of the nephron to cause water reabsorption, producing a concentrated urine and preventing water loss. Thus, it is also called the antidiuretic hormone (ADH).

Vegan diet Strict vegetarian diet allowing no animal protein; requires careful food combinations of incomplete plant proteins to complement one another and achieve an overall adequacy of essential amino acids for growth needs.

Venipuncture Technique in which a vein is punctured through the skin by a sharp, rigid stylet or cannula carrying a flexible plastic catheter or by a steel needle attached to a syringe or catheter.

Venous stasis (L *venosus,* vein; Gr *stasis,* standing still) Stoppage, or decreased flow, of blood in the veins draining an organ, causing engorgement of the affected vessels and tissues.

Vesicle (L *vesica,* bladder) Small bladder or sac containing liquid; secretory transport sacs that move out into the cell cytoplasm to aid metabolism.

Visceral organs (L *viscus,* large body organ) Large internal organs of the body, located in the chest and abdomen.

Vital capacity Volume of air moved in and out of the lungs with each breath. The residual volume is the amount of air remaining in the lungs after the person has exhaled.

Vitamin Nonenergy-yielding micronutrient that is required in very small amounts for specific metabolic tasks but that cannot be synthesized by the body so must be supplied in the diet.

Water intoxication Abnormal increase in the amount of water in the body; sodium concentration of body fluids is lowered, causing confusion, stupor, seizures, and harmful effects on the central nervous system.

Wellness approach Approach to health care that promotes the planning of a healthy, positive lifestyle for maintaining physical and mental well-being.

Whey Thin liquid of milk remaining after the curd—containing the major protein, casein—and the cream have been removed; contains other milk proteins, lactalbumin and lactoferrin.

Xerostomia (Gr *xeros,* dry; *stoma,* mouth) Dryness of the mouth from lack of normal secretions.

REFERENCES

CHAPTER ONE

1. American Dietetic Association. 1997. Position of the American Dietetic Association: Health implications of dietary fiber. *JADA* 97:1157.
2. U.S. Department of Agriculture. 1995. *Dietary Guidelines for Americans,* 4th ed. Washington DC: U.S. Government Printing Office.
3. Underwood, B.A. 1998. Micronutrient malnutrition. *Nutr Today* 33:121.
4. Williams, S.R. 1998. *Basic nutrition and diet therapy,* 11th ed. St. Louis: Times Mirror.
5. Worthington-Roberts, B., and S.R. Williams. 1997. *Nutrition in pregnancy and lactation,* 6th ed. Dubuque, IA: Brown & Benchmark.
6. Trahms, C., and P. Pipes. 1997. *Nutrition in infancy and childhood,* 6th ed. Dubuque, IA: Brown & Benchmark.
7. Mahan, L.K., and J.M. Rees. 1984. *Nutrition in adolescence.* St. Louis: Mosby.
8. Schlenker, E.D. 1997. *Nutrition in aging,* 2d ed. Dubuque, IA: Brown & Benchmark.
9. Truswell, A.S. 1998. Practical and realistic approaches to healthier diet modifications. *Am J Clin Nutr* 67 (suppl):583S.
10. Crane, N.T., V.S. Hubbard, and C.J. Lewis. 1998. National nutrition objectives and the Dietary Guidelines for Americans. *Nutr Today* 33:49.
11. Crane, N.T., V.S. Hubbard, and C.J. Lewis. 1998. Food pyramids. *Nutr Today* (entire issue #5) 33:183–216.
12. Food and Nutrition Board, National Academy of Sciences: National Research Council. *Recommended Dietary Allowances,* 10th ed. Washington, DC.
13. Sims, L.S. 1996. Uses of Recommended Dietary Allowances: A commentary. *JADA* 96:659.
14. Sims, L.S. 1996. Revisiting dietary allowances and requirements. *Nutr Rev* 54:246.
15. Kant, A.K. 1996. Indexes of diet quality: A review. *JADA* 96:785.
16. Kant, A.K. 1998. Translating the science behind Dietary Reference Intakes. *JADA* 98:756.
17. Yates, A.A., S.A. Schlinker, and C.W. Suitor. 1998. Dietary Reference Intakes: The new basis for recommendations for calcium and related nutrients, B vitamins and choline. *JADA* 98:699.
18. Pennington, J.A.T., and V.S. Hubbard. 1997. Derivation of daily values used for nutrition labeling. *JADA* 97:1407.
19. Hathcock, J.N. Vitamins and minerals: Efficacy and safety. *Am J Clin Nutr* 66:427.
20. Nesheim, M.C. 1998. Regulation of dietary supplements. *Nutr Today* 33:62.
21. Geiger, C.J. 1998. Health claims: History, current regulatory status, and consumer research. *J Am Diet Assoc* 98:1312.

CHAPTER TWO

1. Posthauer, M.E. et al. 1994. ADA's definitions for nutrition screening and nutrition assessment. *J Am Diet Assoc* 94(8):838.
2. Orphanido, C. et al. 1994. Accuracy of subcutaneous fat measurement: Comparison of skinfold calipers, ultrasound, and computed tomography. *J Am Diet Assoc.* 94(8):855.
3. Crawford, P.B. et al. Comparative advantage of 3-day food records over 24-hour recall and 5-day food frequency validated by observations of 9- and 10-year-old girls.
4. Achterberg, C. et al. 1994. How to put the Food Guide Pyramid into practice. *J Am Diet Assoc* 94(9):1030.
5. Peters, J.R. et al. 1994. The Eating Pattern Assessment Tool: A simple instrument for assessing dietary fat and cholesterol intake. *J Am Diet Assoc* 94(9):1008.
6. Institute of Medicine, Food and Nutrition Board, National Academy of Science. 1990. *Nutrition during pregnancy.* Washington, DC: National Academy Press.

CHAPTER THREE

1. Worthington-Roberts, B., and S.R. Williams. 1997. *Nutrition in pregnancy and lactation,* 6th ed. Dubuque, IA: WCB/McGraw-Hill.
2. Giroud, A. 1973. Nutritional requirements of the embryo. *World Rev Nutr Diet* 18:195.
3. Hytten, F.E., and I. Leitch. 1971. *The physiology of human pregnancy,* 2nd ed. Oxford: Blackwell Scientific Publications.
4. Brown, J.F., and R.B. Toma. 1986. Taste changes during pregnancy. *Am J Clin Nutr* 43:414.

CHAPTER FOUR

1. Worthington-Roberts, B., and S.R. Williams. 1997. *Nutrition in pregnancy and lactation,* 6th ed. Dubuque, IA: WCB/McGraw-Hill.
2. Committee on Maternal Nutrition, Food and Nutrition Board, National Research Council. 1973. *Maternal nutrition and the course of pregnancy.* Washington, DC: National Academy of Sciences.
3. Christakis, G., ed. 1973. Maternal nutrition assessment. *Am J Public Health* 63(Suppl): 1.
4. Committee on Maternal Nutrition, Food and Nutrition Board, National Research Council. 1973. *Nutritional supplementation and the outcome of pregnancy.* Washington, DC: National Academy of Sciences.
5. Select Panel for the Promotion of Child Health, U.S. Department of Health and Human Services. 1981. *Better health for our children: A national strategy,* vols. 1–3, Pub. No. (PHS) 79-55071. Washington, DC: U.S. Government Printing Office.

6. Task Force on Nutrition. 1978. *Assessment of maternal nutrition*. Chicago: American College of Obstetricians and Gynecologists.

7. Committee on Nutrition of the Mother and Preschool Child. 1981. *Nutrition services in perinatal care*. Washington, DC: National Academy Press.

8. Institute of Medicine, National Academy of Sciences. 1990. *Nutrition during pregnancy: Weight gain and nutrient supplements*. Washington, DC: National Academy Press.

9. Owen, A.L., and G.M. Owen. 1997. Twenty years of WIC: A review of some effects of the program. *J Am Diet Assoc* 97:777–82.

10. Brown, H.L., K. Watkins, and A.K. Hiett. 1996. The impact of Women, Infants, and Children Food Supplement Program on birth outcome. *Am J Obstet General* 174:1279–83.

11. Disbrow, D.D. 1987. The economic cost of nutrition service for a low income prenatal population. I. Direct costs. *J Pediatr Perinatal Nutr* 1:35–40.

12. Disbrow, D.D. 1988. The economic costs of nutrition service for a low income prenatal population: Indirect and intangible costs. *J Pediatr Perinatal Nutr*, 2:17–21.

13. Splett, P.L. et al. 1987. Prenatal nutrition services: A cost analysis. *J Am Diet Assoc* 87:204–8.

14. Mathematics Policy Research Inc. 1990. *The savings in Medicaid costs for newborns and their mothers from prenatal participation in the WIC program*. Washington, DC: USDA, Food and Nutrition Services.

15. Buescher, P.A. et al. 1993. Prenatal WIC participation can reduce low birth weight and newborn medical costs: A cost:benefit analysis of WIC participation in North Carolina. *J Am Diet Assoc* 93:163–66.

16. Culpepper, J.B. 1990. Preconception care: Risk reduction and health promotion. *JAMA* 264:1147.

17. Winick, M. 1970. Fetal malnutrition. *Clin Obstet Gynecol* 13:526.

18. Thomson, A.M. et al. 1968. The assessment of fetal growth. *J Obstet Gynaecol Br Commonw* 75:903.

19. Naeye, P.L. 1979. Causes of fetal and neonatal mortality by race in a selected U.S. population. *Am J Public Health* 69:857.

20. Edwards, L.E. et al. 1979. Pregnancy in the underweight woman: Course, outcome, and growth patterns of the infant. *Am J Obstet Gynecol* 135:297.

21. Hickey, C.A., S.P. Cliver, S.F. McNeal, and R.L. Goldenberg. 1997. Low pregravid body mass index as a risk factor for preterm birth: Variation by ethnic group. *Obstet Gynecol* 89:206.

22. Shepard, M.I. et al. 1986. Proportional weight gain and complications of pregnancy, labor, and delivery in healthy women of normal prepregnant status. *Am J Obstet Gynecol* 155:947.

23. Bianco, A.T., S.W. Silen, Y. Davis, S. Lopez, R. Lapinski, and C.J. Lockwood. 1998. Pregnancy outcome and weight gain recommendations for the morbidly obese woman. *Obstet Gynecol* 91:97.

24. Primrose, T., and A. Higgins. 1971. A study of human antepartum nutrition. *J Reprod Med* 7:257.

25. Higgins, A.C. et al. 1989. Impact of the Higgins Nutrition Intervention Program on birth weight: A within mother analysis. *J Am Diet Assoc* 89:1097.

26. Clements, D.E. 1988. The nutrition intervention project for underweight pregnant women. *Clin Nutr* 7:205.

27. Bruce L., and J. Tsabo. 1989. Nutrition intervention program in a prenatal clinic. *Obstet Gynecol* 74:310.

28. Orstead, C. et al. 1985. Efficacy of prenatal nutrition counseling: Weight gain, infant birthweight, and cost effectiveness. *J Am Diet Assoc* 85:40.

29. Rush, D. 1986. *The National WIC Evaluation: An evaluation of the Special Supplemental Food Program for Women, Infants, and Children*, vols. I and II. Research Triangle Park, NC: Research Triangle Institute and New York State Research Foundation for Mental Hygiene.

30. Food and Nutrition Board, National Research Council, National Academy of Sciences. 1989. *Recommended dietary allowances*, 10th ed. Washington, DC: National Academy Press.

31. Durnin, J.V.G.A. 1987. Energy requirements of pregnancy: An integration of the longitudinal data from the five-country study. *Lancet* 2:1131.

32. Giroud, A. 1973. Nutritional requirements of the embryo. *World Rev Nutr Diet* 18:195.

33. Lechtig, A. et al. 1975. Effect of food supplementation during pregnancy on birth weight. *Pediatrics* 56:508.

34. National Academy of Sciences, Institute of Medicine. 1990. Nutrition during pregnancy: Weight gain and nutrient supplements. Washington DC: National Academy Press.

35. Czeizel, A.E. 1995. Folic acid in the prevention of neural tube defects. *J Pediatr Gastroent Nutr* 20:4–16.

36. MRC Vitamin Study Research Group. 1991. Prevention of neural tube defects: Results of the Medical Research Council Vitamin Study. *Lancet* 338:131–37.

37. Czeizel, E.A., and I. Dudas. 1992. Prevention of the first occurrence of neural-tube defects by periconceptional vitamin supplementation. *N Engl J Med* 327:1832.

38. Bunduki, V., M. Dommergues, J. Zittoun, J. Marquet, F. Muller, and Y. Dumez. 1995. Maternal-fetal folate status and neural tube defects: A case-control study. *Biol Neonate* 67:154.

39. Mills, J.L., J.M. McPartin, P.N. Kirke et al. 1995. Homocysteine metabolism in pregnancies complicated by neural tube defects. *Lancet* 345:149.

40. Molloy, A.M., S. Daly, J.L. Mills et al. 1997. Thermolabile variant of 5, 10-methylenetetrahydrofolate reductase associated with low red-cell folates: Implications for folate intake recommendations. *Lancet* 349:1591.

41. Shaw, G.M. et al. 1995. Risks of orofacial clefts in children born to women using multivitamins containing folic acid periconceptionally. *Lancet* 346:393–96.

42. Li, D. et al. 1995. Periconceptional multivitamin use in relation to the risk of congenital urinary tract anomalies. *Epidemiol* 6:212–18.

43. Czeizel, A.E. 1995. Congenital abnormalities are preventable. *Epidemiol* 6:205–6.

44. MMWR. 1997. Knowledge and use of folic acid by women of childbearing age—United States, 1997. *JAMA* 278:892.

45. Vutyavanich, T., S. Wongtra-ngan, and R. Ruangsri. 1995. Pyridoxine for nausea and vomiting of pregnancy: A randomized, double-blind, placebo-controlled trial. *Am J Obstet Gynecol* 173:881–84.

46. Rothman, K.J. et al. 1995. Teratogenicity of high vitamin A intake. *N Engl J Med* 333:1369–73.

47. Mills, J.L., J.L. Simpson, G.C. Cunningham, et al. 1997. Vitamin A and birth defects. *Am J Obstet Gynecol* 177:31.

48. Jick, S.S., B.Z. Teris, and H. Jick. 1993. First trimester topical tretinoin and congenital disorders. *Lancet* 341:1181–82.

49. Institute of Medicine. 1990. *Nutrition during pregnancy: Weight gain and nutrient supplements.* Washington, DC: National Academy of Sciences.

50. Ritchie, L.D., E.B. Fung, and B.P. Halloran. 1998. A longitudinal study of calcium homeostasis during human pregnancy and lactation and after resumption of menses. *Am J Clin Nutr* 67:693.

51. Carrolli, G. et al. 1994. Calcium supplementation during pregnancy: A systematic review of randomized trials. *Brit J Obstet Gynecol* 101:753–58.

52. Bucher, H.C. et al. 1996. Effect of calcium supplementation on pregnancy-induced hypertension and preeclampsia. A meta-analysis of randomized controlled trials. *JAMA* 275:1113–17.

52a. Levine, R.J., J.C. Hauth, L.B. Curet, et al. 1997. Trial of calcium to prevent preeclampsia. *N Engl J Med* 337:69.

53. DeCherney, A.H., and B. Koos. 1997. Obstetrics and gynecology. *JAMA* 277:1878–79.

54. Dahle, L.O. et al. 1995. The effect of oral magnesium substitution on pregnancy-induced leg cramps. *Am J Obstet Gynecol* 173:175–80.

55. Hetzel, B. 1994. Iodine deficiency and fetal brain damage. *N Engl J Med* 331:1770.

56. Konde, M., Y. Ingenbleek, B. Sylla, and S. Diallo. 1994. Goitrous endemic in Guinea. *Lancet* 344:1675.

57. Knuist, M., G.J. Bonsel, H.A. Zondervan, and P.E. Treffers. 1998. Low sodium and pregnancy-induced hypertension: A multicentre randomised controlled trial. *Br J Obstet Gynaecol* 105:430.

58. van Buul, B., E. Steegers, H.W. Jongsma et al. 1995. Dietary sodium restriction in the prophylaxis of hypertensive disorders of pregnancy: Effects on the intake of other nutrients. *Am J Clin Nutr* 62:49.

CHAPTER FIVE

1. Worthington-Roberts, B., and S.R. Williams. 1997. *Nutrition in pregnancy and lactation,* 6th ed. Dubuque, IA: WCB/McGraw-Hill.

2. Horner, R.D. et al. 1991. Pica practices of pregnant women. *J Am Diet Assoc* 91:34.

3. National Research Council, Food and Nutrition Board. 1982. *Alternative dietary practices and nutritional abuses in pregnancy.* Washington, DC: National Academy of Sciences.

4. Lackey, C.J. 1982. *Pica—Pregnancy etiological mystery.* In *Alternative dietary practices and nutritional abuses in pregnancy.* Washington, DC: National Academy of Sciences.

5. Rainville, A.J. 1998. Pica practices of pregnant women are associated with lower maternal hemoglobin level at delivery. *J Am Diet Assoc* 98:293.

6. Streissguth, A.P. 1994. A long-term perspective of FAS. *Alcohol Health & Res World* 18:74.

7. Michaelis, E.K., and M.L. Michaelis. 1994. Cellular and molecular bases of alcohol's teratogenic effects. *Alcohol Health & Res World* 18:17.

8. Phillips, D.K., G.I. Henderson, and S. Schenker. 1989. Pathogenesis of fetal alcohol syndrome. *Alcohol Health & Res World* 13:219.

9. Cordero, J.F., R.L. Floyd, M.L. Martin et al. 1994. Tracking the prevalence of FAS. *Alcohol Health & Res World* 18:82.

10. Dufour, M.C., G.D. Williams, K.E. Campbell, and S.S. Aitken. 1994. Knowledge of FAS and the risks of heavy drinking during pregnancy, 1985 and 1990. *Alcohol Health & Res World* 18:86.

11. Chang, G., L. Wilkins-Haug, S. Berman et al. 1998. Alcohol use and pregnancy: Improving identification. *Obstet Gynecol* 91:892.

12. Ebrahim, S.H., E.T. Luman, R.L. Floyd et al. 1998. Alcohol consumption by pregnant women in the United States 1988–1995. *Obstet Gynecol* 92:187.

13. Cicero, T.J. 1994. Effects of paternal exposure to alcohol on offspring development. *Alcohol Health & Res World* 18:37.

14. Collins, T.F.N. et al. 1980. *A comprehensive study of the teratogenic potential of caffeine in rats when given by oral intubation.* Washington, DC: Data Acquisition and Monitoring Division, Environmental Data and Information Services, National Oceanic and Atmospheric Administration.

15. Nehlig, A., and G. Debry. 1994. Potential teratogenic and neurodevelopmental consequences of coffee and caffeine exposure: A review of human and animal data. *Neurotoxicol Teratol* 16:531.

16. Pastore, L.M., and D.A. Savitz. 1995. Case-control study of caffeinated beverages and preterm delivery. *Am J Epid* 141:61.

17. Infante-Rivard, C., A. Fernandez, R. Gauthier et al. 1993. Fetal loss associated with caffeine intake before and during pregnancy. *JAMA* 270:2940.

18. Mills, J.L., L.B. Holmes, J.H. Aarons et al. 1993. Moderate caffeine use and the risk of spontaneous abortion and intrauterine retardation. *JAMA* 269:593.

19. Nygard, O., H. Refsum, P.M. Ueland, et al. 1997. Coffee consumption and plasma total homocysteine: The Hordaland Homocysteine Study. *Am J Clin Nutr* 65:136.

20. Davidson, P.W., G.J. Myers, C. Cox et al. 1998. Effects of prenatal and postnatal methylmercury exposure from fish consumption on neurodevelopment. *JAMA* 280:701.

21. Clapp, J.F. 1990. The course of labor after endurance exercise during pregnancy. *Am J Obstet Gynecol* 163:1799.

22. Clapp, J.F. 1989. The effects of maternal exercise on early pregnancy outcome. *Am J Obstet Gynecol* 161:1453.

23. Clapp, J.F., and S. Dickstein. 1984. Endurance exercise and pregnancy outcome. *Med Sci Sports Exer* 16:556.

24. Clapp, J.F., and K.D. Little. 1995. Effect of recreational exercise on pregnancy weight gain and subcutaneous fat deposition. *Med Sci Sports Exercise* 27:170.
25. Clapp, J.F., and K.D. Little. 1995. The interaction between regular exercise and selected aspects of women's health. *Am J Obstet Gynecol* 173:2.
26. Clapp, J.F. 1996. Morphometric and neurodevelopmental outcome at age five years of the offspring of women who continued to exercise regularly throughout pregnancy. *J Pediatr* 129:856.
27. Monthly Vital Statistics Report 43(#5 suppl), October 25, 1994. Advance Report of Final Natality Statistics, 1992.
28. Scholl, T.O., M.L. Hediger, J.G. Ances et al. 1988. Growth during early teenage pregnancies. *Lancet* 1:701.
29. Scholl, T.O., and M.L. Hediger. 1993. A review of the epidemiology of nutrition and adolescent pregnancy and its effect on the fetus. *J Am Coll Nutr* 12:101.
30. Scholl, T.O., M.L. Hediger, C.E. Cronk, and J.L. Schall. 1993. Maternal growth during pregnancy and lactation. *Horm Res* 39S:59.
31. Stevens-Simon, C., E.R. McAnarney, and K.I. Roghmann. 1993. Adolescent gestational weight gain and birth weight. *Pediatrics* 92:805.
32. Institute of Medicine. National Academy of Sciences. 1990. *Nutrition during pregnancy: Weight gain and nutrient supplements.* Washington DC, National Academy Press.
33. McAnarney, E.R., and Stevens-Simon, C. 1993. First, do no harm. *Am J Dis Child* 147:983.
34. McAnarney, E.R., and R.A. Lawrence. 1993. Day care and teenage mothers: Nurturing the mother-child dyad. *Pediatrics* 91:202.

CHAPTER SIX

1. Worthington-Roberts, B., and S.R. Williams 1997. Nutrition in pregnancy and lactation, 6th ed. Dubuque, IA: WCB/McGraw-Hill.
2. Shaul, D.M.B. 1962. The composition of milk from wild animals. *Int Year Zoo Book* 4:333.
3. Institute of Medicine, National Academy of Sciences. 1991. *Nutrition during lactation.* Washington, DC: National Academy Press.
4. Hartmann, P.E. et al. 1982. Studies on breastfeeding and reproduction in women in Western Australia—A review. *Birth Fam J* 8:215.
5. Lovelady, C.A. et al. 1990. Lactation performance of exercising women. *Am J Clin Nutr* 52:103.
6. Lawrence, R.A. 1994. *Breastfeeding: A guide for the medical profession,* 4th ed. St. Louis: Mosby.
7. Lindblad, B.S., and R.J. Rahimtoola. 1974. A pilot study of the quality of human milk in a lower socioeconomic group in Karachi, Pakistan. *Acta Paediatr Scand* 63:125.
8. Chavalittamrong, B. et al. 1981. Protein and amino acids of breast milk from Thai mothers. *Am J Clin Nutr* 34:1126.
9. Sturman, J.A. 1988. Taurine in development. *J Nutr* 118:1169.
10. Simopoulos, A.P. 1988. α-3 fatty acids in growth and development and in health and disease. *Nutr Today* 23:10.
11. Carroll, J.E. et al. 1987. Carnitine deficiency revisited. *J Nutr* 117:1501.
12. Heitlinger, L.A. et al. 1983. Mammary amylase: A possible alternate pathway of carbohydrate digestion in infancy. *Pediatr Res* 17:15.
13. McMillan, J.A. et al. 1976. Iron sufficiency in breast-fed infants and the availability of iron from human milk. *Pediatrics* 58:686.
14. McMillan, J.A. et al. 1977. Iron absorption from human milk, simulated human milk and proprietary formulas. *Pediatrics* 60:896.
15. Garry, P.J. et al. 1981. Iron absorption from human milk and formula with and without iron supplementation. *Pediatr Res* 15:822.
16. Pisacane, A., B. Vizia, A. Valiante, et al. 1995. Iron status of breast-fed infants. *J Pediatr* 127:429.
17. Casey, C.E. et al. 1981. Availability of zinc: Loading tests with human milk, cow's milk and infant formulas. *Pediatrics* 68:394.
18. Specker, B.L. et al. Calcium kinetics in lactating women with low and high calcium intakes. *Am J Clin Nutr* 59:593.
19. Laskey, M.A., A. Prentice, L.A. Hanratty et al. 1998. Bone changes after 3 months of lactation: Influence of calcium intake, breast-milk output, and vitamin D–receptor genotype. *Am J Clin Nutr* 67:685.
20. Allen, L. 1998. Women's dietary calcium requirements are not increased by pregnancy or lactation. *Am J Clin Nutr* 67:591.
21. Sowers, M., D. Zhang, B.W. Hollis, et al. 1998. Role of calciotropic hormones in calcium mobilization of lactation. *Am J Clin Nutr* 67:284.
22. Krebs, N.F., C.J. Reidinger, A.D. Robertson, and M. Brenner. 1997. Bone mineral density changes during lactation: Maternal dietary and biochemical correlates. *Am J Clin Nutr* 65:1738.
23. Prentice, A., L. Jarjou, T. Cole, et al. 1995. Calcium requirements of lactating mothers. *Am J Clin Nutr* 62:58.
24. Hollis, B.W. et al. 1982. *The effects of oral vitamin D supplementation and ultraviolet phototherapy on the antirachitic sterol content of human milk.* American Society of Bone and Mineral Research Annual Meeting (abstract).
25. Greer, F.R. et al. 1981. Bone mineral content and serum 25-hydroxyvitamin D concentration in breastfed infants with and without supplemental vitamin D. *J Pediatr* 98:696.
26. Greer, F.R. et al. 1982. Bone mineral content and serum 25-hydroxyvitamin D concentrations in breastfed infants with and without supplemental vitamin D: One year follow-up. *J Pediatr* 100:919.
27. Ozsoylu, S., and A. Hasanoglu. 1982. Vitamin D supplementation in breast-fed infants. *J Pediatr* 100:1000.
28. Finberg, L. 1981. Human milk feeding and vitamin D supplementation—1981. *J Pediatr* 99:228.
29. Bachrach, S. et al., 1979. An outbreak of vitamin D deficiency rickets in a susceptible population. *Pediatrics* 64:871.
30. Edidin, D.V. et al. 1980. Resurgence of nutritional rickets associated with breastfeeding and special dietary practices. *Pediatrics* 65:232.

31. Brownick, S.K., and K.R. Rettig. Rickets caused by vitamin D deficiency in breastfed infants in Southern United States. *Am J Dis Child* 145:127.

32. Feldman, K.W. 1990. Nutritional rickets. *J Am Fam Pract* 42:1311.

33. Byerly, L.O., and A. Kirksey. 1985. Effects of different levels of vitamin C intake on the vitamin C concentration in human milk and the vitamin C intakes of breast-fed infants. *Am J Clin Nutr* 41:665.

34. Felice, J.H., and A. Kirksey. 1981. Effects of vitamin B_6 deficiency during lactation on the vitamin B_6 content of milk, liver, and muscle of rats. *J Nutr* 111:610.

35. Borschel, M.W., and A. Kirksey. 1983. Relationship of plasma pyridoxal phosphate levels to vitamin B_6 intakes during the first six months. *Fed Proc* 42:1331.

36. Sandberg, D.P. et al. 1981. The content, binding, and forms of vitamin B_{12} in milk. *Am J Clin Nutr* 34:1717.

37. Specker, B.L. et al. 1990. Vitamin B_{12}: Low milk concentrations are related to low serum concentrations in vegetarian women and to methylmalonic aciduria in their infants. *Am J Clin Nutr* 52:1073.

38. Kuhn, T. et al. 1991. Maternal vegan diet causing a serious infantile neurological disorder due to vitamin B_{12} deficiency. *Eur J Pediatr* 150:205.

39. Beerens, H. et al. 1980. Influence of breastfeeding on the bifid flora of the newborn intestine. *Am J Clin Nutr* 33:2434.

40. Reid, B. et al. 1980. Prostaglandins in human milk. *Pediatrics* 66:870.

41. Miranda, R. et al. 1983. Effect of maternal nutritional status on immunological substances in human colostrum and milk. *Am J Clin Nutr* 37:632.

42. American Academy of Pediatrics, Committee on Drugs. 1994. The transfer of drugs and other chemicals into human breast milk. *Pediatrics* 93:137.

43. Jacobson, J.L. 1989. Determinants of polychlorinated biphenyls (PCBs), polybrominated biphenyls (PBBs), and dichlorodiphenyl trichloroethane (DDT) levels in the sera of young children. *Am J Public Health* 79:1401.

44. Savage, E.P. et al. 1981. National study of chlorinated hydrocarbon insecticide residues in human milk, USA. *Am J Epidemiol* 113:413.

45. Rogan, W.G., A. Bagniewska, and T. Damstra. 1980. Pollutants in breast milk. *N Engl J Med* 302:1450.

46. Le Guennec, J.C., and B. Billon. 1987. Delay in caffeine elimination in breast-fed infants. *Pediatrics* 79:264.

47. Binkiewicz, A. et al. 1978. Pseudo-Cushing syndrome caused by alcohol in breast milk. *J Pediatr* 93:965.

48. Little, R.E. et al. 1989. Maternal alcohol use during breastfeeding and infant mental and motor development at one year. *N Engl J Med* 321:425.

49. Seitzer, V., and F. Benjamin. 1990. Breastfeeding and the potential for human immunodeficiency virus transmission. *Obstet Gynecol* 75:713.

50. Belec, L. et al. 1990. Antibodies of human immunodeficiency virus in breast milk of healthy, sero-positive women. *Pediatrics* 85:1022.

51. Davis, M.K. 1990. The role of human milk in human immunodeficiency virus infection. In *Breastfeeding, nutrition, infection and infant growth in developed and emerging countries,* ed. S.A Atkinson et al. St. Johns, Newfoundland, Canada: ARTS Biomedical Publishing and Distributing.

52. Mehta, N.R., and K.N.S. Subramanian. 1990. Human milk banking: Current concepts. *Indian J Pediatr* 57:361.

53. Mackey, A.D., M.F. Picciano, D.C. Mitchell, and H. Smiciklas-Wright. 1998. Self-selected diets of lactating women often fail to meet dietary recommendations. *J Am Diet Assoc* 98:297.

54. English, R.M., and N.E. Hitchcock. 1968. Nutrient intakes during pregnancy, lactation, and after the cessation of lactation in a group of Australian women. *Br J Nutr* 22:615.

55. Butte, N.F. et al. 1983. Maternal energy balance during lactation. *Fed Proc* 42:922.

56. Manning-Dalton, C. and L.H. Allen. 1983. The effects of lactation on energy and protein consumption, postpartum weight change and body composition of well nourished North American women. *Nutr Res* 32:293.

57. Potter, S. et al. 1991. Does infant feeding method influence maternal postpartum weight loss? *J Am Diet Assoc* 91(4):441.

CHAPTER SEVEN

1. American Dietetic Association. 1997. Position of the American Dietetic Association: Promotion of breast-feeding. *J Am Diet Assoc* 97:662.

2. Garza, C., and E.A. Frongillo. 1998. Infant feeding recommendations. *Am J Clin Nutr* 67:815.

3. Cunningham, A.S., D.B. Jelliffe, and E.F.P. Jelliffe. 1991. Breast-feeding and health in the 1980s: A global epidemiologic review. *J Pediatr* 118:659.

4. Popkin, B.M. et al. 1990. Breastfeeding and diarrheal morbidity. *Pediatrics* 86:874.

5. DeZoysa, I., M. Rea, and J. Martines. 1991. Why promote breastfeeding in diarrheal disease control programmes? *Health Policy Plan* 6:371.

6. Broadbent, J.B., and H.A. Sampson. 1988. Food hypersensitivity and atopic dermatitis. *Pediatr Allergic Dis* 35:1115.

7. Worthington-Roberts, B., and S.R. Williams. Nutrition in pregnancy and lactation, 6th ed. Dubuque, IA: WCB/McGraw-Hill.

8. Lucas, A. 1992. Breast milk and subsequent intelligence quotient in children born preterm. *Lancet* 339:261.

9. Maki, M. 1987. Changing pattern of childhood coeliac disease in Finland. *Acta Paediatr Scand* 77:408.

10. Bradley, M.W. 1986. Breast feeding and necrotizing enterocolitis. *Indiana Med* 10:859.

11. Davis, M. et al. 1988. Infant feeding and childhood cancer. *Lancet* 2:365.

12. Agras, W. et al. 1987. Does a vigorous feeding style influence early development of adiposity? *J Pediatr* 110:799.

13. Virden, S.F. 1988. The relationship between infant feeding method and maternal role adjustment. *J Nurse Midwifery* 33:31.

14. Montague, A. 1971. *Touching.* New York: Harper & Row.

15. Petrakis, N. et al. 1987. Influence of pregnancy and lactation on serum and breast fluid estrogen levels: Implications for breast cancer risk. *Int J Cancer* 40:587.

16. American Academy of Pediatrics. 1994. Practice parameter: Management of hyperbilirubinemia in the healthy term newborn. *Pediatrics* 94(4):558–65.

17. Schneider, A.P. 1987. Risk factor for ovarian cancer. *N Engl J Med* 317:508.

18. Jackson, R.L. 1988. Ecological breastfeeding and child spacing. *Clin Pediatr* 27:373.

19. Rickitt, C.W. 1986. A study in nipple care. *Midwives Chron* 99:131, 132.

20. American Dietetic Association. 1997. Position of the ADA: Promotion of breastfeeding. *J Am Diet Assoc.* 97:662.

21. Gielen, A.C. et al. 1991. Maternal employment during early postpartum period: Effects on initiation and continuance of breast-feeding. *Pediatrics* 87:298.

22. Kurinu, N. et al. 1989. Does maternal employment affect breast-feeding? *Am J Public Health* 79:1247.

23. American Academy of Pediatrics, Committee on Nutrition. 1981. Nutrition and lactation. *Pediatrics* 68:435.

24. American Academy of Pediatrics. 1982. The promotion of breast-feeding. *Pediatrics* 69:654.

25. Lawrence, R.A. 1995. Early discharge alert. *Pediatrics* 96(5):966–67.

26. Williams, B.C., and C.A. Miller. 1992. Preventive health care for young children: Findings from a 10-country study and directions for United States policy. *Pediatrics* 89:983.

27. Minchin, M. 1985. *Breastfeeding matters: What we need to know about infant feeding.* Sydney, Australia: Alma.

28. Minchin, M. 1986. *Food for thought: A parents' guide to food intolerance,* 2d ed. Sydney, Australia: Alma.

29. Hill, P.D., and J. Aldag. 1991. Potential indicators of insufficient milk supply syndrome. *Res Nurs Health* 14:11.

30. Grekas, D., and A. Tourkantonis. 1986. Serum and human milk IgA and zinc concentrations after successful renal transplantation. *Biol Res Preg* 7: 118.

31. Hawkins, L.M. et al. 1987. Predictors of duration of breastfeeding in low-income women. *Birth* 14:204.

32. Royal College of Midwives. 1991. *Successful breast-feeding,* 2d ed. Edinburgh, Scotland: Churchill Livingstone.

33. Rosier, W. 1988. Cool cabbage compresses. *Breast-feeding Rev.* 11:28.

34. Kaufmann, R., and B. Foxman. 1991. Mastitis among lactating women: Occurrence and risk factors. *Soc Sci Med* 33:701.

35. Williamson, M.T., and P.K. Murti. 1996. Effects of storage, time, temperature, and composition of container on biologic components of human milk. *J Hum Lact* 12(1):31.

36. Meier, P. 1988. Bottle and breast-feeding: Effects of transcutaneous oxygen pressure and temperature in preterm infants. *Nurs Res* 37:36.

37. Weatherly-White, R.C.A. et al. 1987. Early repair and breast-feeding for infants with cleft lip. *Plast Reconstr Surg* 79:879.

38. Bowles, B.C., and B.P. Williamson. 1989. Pregnancy and lactation following anorexia and bulimia. *J Obstet Gynecol Neonatal Nurs* 19:243.

39. Brinch, M., T. Isager, and K. Tolstrup. 1988. Anorexia nervosa and motherhood: Reproduction pattern and mothering behavior of 50 women. *Acta Paediatr Scand* 77:611.

40. Carey, W.B. 1981. Letter to the editor. *Am J Dis Child* 135:973.

41. Frantz, K.B., and P.M. Fleiss. 1980. Ineffective suckling as a frequent cause of failure to thrive in the totally breast-fed infant. In *Human milk: Its biological and social value.* ed. S. Freier and A.I. Eidelman. Amsterdam: Excerpta Medica.

CHAPTER EIGHT

1. Dobbing, J. 1973. Nutrition and the developing brain. *Lancet* 1:48.

2. Smith, D.W., W. Truog, J.E. Rogers et al. 1976. Shifting linear growth during infancy: Illustration of genetic factors in growth from fetal life through infancy. *J Pediatr* 89:225–30.

3. Goldenberg, R.L., S.P. Cliver, G.R. Cutter et al. 1991. Black-white differences in newborn anthropometric measurements. *Obstet Gynecol* 78:782–88.

4. Robson, J.R., F.A. Larkin, J.H. Bursick, and K.P. Perri. 1975. Growth standards for infants and children: A cross-sectional study. *Pediatrics* 56:1014–20.

5. Dewey, K.G., M.J. Heinig, L.A. Nommsen, J.M. Peerson, and B. Lonnerdal. 1992. Growth of breast-fed and formula-fed infants from 0 to 18 months: The DARLING Study. *Pediatrics* 89:1035–41.

6. Hamosh, M. 1996. Digestion in the newborn. *Clin Perinatol* 23(2):191–209.

7. Hernell, O.B.L. 1994. Human milk bile salt-stimulated lipase: Functional and molecular aspects. *J Pediatr* 125:S56–S61.

8. Ziegler, E.E., and S.J. Fomon. 1989. Potential renal solute load of infant formulas. *J Nutr* 119:1785–88.

9. Food and Nutrition Board, Subcommittee on the Tenth Edition of the RDAs. 1989. *Recommended Dietary Allowances,* 10th ed. Washington, DC: National Academy Press.

10. Butte, N.F. 1996. Energy requirements of infants. *Eur J Clin Nutr* 50Suppl1:S24–36.

11. Fomon, S.J. 1993. *Nutrition of normal infants.* St. Louis: Mosby-Year Book.

12. American Academy of Pediatrics. 1998. *Pediatric nutrition handbook,* 4th ed. American Academy of Pediatrics. Elk Grove Village, IL.

13. Committee on Nutrition AAP. 1976. Commentary on breastfeeding and infant formulas, including proposed standards for formulas. *Pediatrics* 57:278–85.

14. Michaelsen, K.F., and M.H. Jorgensen. 1995. Dietary fat content and energy density during infancy and childhood; the effect on energy intake and growth. *Eur J Clin Nutr* 49:467–83.

15. Lucas, A., R. Morley, T.J. Cole, G. Lister, and C. Leeson Payne. 1992. Breast milk and subsequent intelligence quotient in children born preterm. *Lancet* 339:261–64.

16. Lanting, C.I., V. Fidler, M. Huisman, B.C. Touwen, and E.R. Boersma. 1994. Neurological differences between 9-year-old children fed breast-milk or formula-milk as babies. 344:1319–22.

17. Fergusson, D.M., and L.J. Horwood. 1994. Early solid food diet and eczema in childhood: A 10-year longitudinal study. *Pediatr Allergy Immunol* 5:44–47.

18. 1994. Long chain polyunsaturated fatty acids in neonatal nutrition. *J Am Coll Nutr* 13:546–48.

19. Keating, J.P., G.J. Schears, and P.R. Dodge. 1991. Oral water intoxication in infants. An American epidemic. *Am J Dis Child* 145:985–90.

20. Food and Nutrition Board IOM. 1998. Dietary Reference Intakes for thiamin, riboflavin, niacin, vitamin B_6, folate, vitamin B_{12}, pantothenic acid, biotin, and choline. Washington, DC: National Academy Press.

21. Food and Nutrition Board IOM. 1998. Dietary Reference Intakes for calcium, phosphorus, magnesium, vitamin D, and fluoride. Washington, DC: National Academy Press.

22. Abrams, S.A., J. Wen, and J.E. Stuff. 1997. Absorption of calcium, zinc, and iron from breast milk by five- to seven-month-old infants. *Pediatr Res* 41:384–90.

23. Wheeler, R.E., and R.T. Hall. 1996. Feeding of premature infant formula after hospital discharge of infants weighing less than 1800 grams at birth. *J Perinatol* 16:111–16.

24. Calvo, E.B., A.C. Galindo, and N.B. Aspres. 1992. Iron status in exclusively breast-fed infants. *Pediatrics* 90:375–79.

25. Pisacane, A., B. De Vizia, A. Valiante et al. 1995. Iron status in breast-fed infants. *J Pediatr* 127:429–31.

26. Davidsson, L. 1994. Minerals and trace elements in infant nutrition. *Acta Paediatr Suppl* 83:38–42.

27. Levy, S.M., M.C. Kiritsy, and J.J. Warren. 1995. Sources of fluoride intake in children. *J Public Health Dent* 55:39–52.

28. Schuman, A.J. 1995. How much fluoride is too much? *Contemporary Pediatrics* 12:65–74.

29. Hathcock, J.N., D.G. Hattan, M.Y. Jenkins, J.T. McDonald, P.R. Sundaresan, and V.L. Wilkening. 1990. Evaluation of vitamin A toxicity. *Am J Clin Nutr* 52:183–202.

30. Sills, I.N., K.A. Skuza, M.N. Horlick, M.S. Schwartz, and R. Rapaport. 1994. Vitamin D deficiency rickets. Reports of its demise are exaggerated. *Clin Pediatr* (Phila.) 33:491–93.

31. McMillan, D.D. 1996. Administration of vitamin K to newborns: Implications and recommendations. *CMAJ* 154:347–49.

32. Gesell, A., and F.L. Ilg. 1937. *Feeding behaviors of infants.* Philadelphia: J.B. Lippincott.

33. Guo, S.M., A.F. Roche, S.J. Fomon et al. 1991. Reference data on gains in weight and length during the first two years of life. *J Pediatr* 119:355–62.

34. Hallberg, L., L. Rossander-Hulten, M. Brune, and A. Gleerup. 1992. Bioavailability in man of iron in human milk and cow's milk in relation to their calcium contents. *Pediatr Res* 31:524–27.

35. Hurrell, R.F., L. Davidsson, M. Reddy, P. Kastenmayer, and J.D. Cook. 1998. A comparison of iron absorption in adults and infants consuming identical infant formulas. *Br J Nutr* 79:31–36.

36. Fomon, S.J., E.E. Ziegler, and R.R. Rogers et al. 1989. Iron absorption from infant foods. *Pediatr Res* 26:250–54.

37. Barnard, K. 1994. *Caregiver/parent-child interaction feeding manual.* University of Washington School of Nursing. Seattle: NCAST.

CHAPTER NINE

1. American Academy of Pediatrics, Work Group on Breastfeeding. 1998. Breastfeeding and the use of human milk. *Pediatrics* 101:31–36.

2. American Academy of Pediatrics Committee on Nutrition. 1998. Soy protein–based formulas: Recommendations for use in infant feeding. *Pediatrics* 101:148–53.

3. American Academy of Pediatrics. 1998. *Pediatric nutrition handbook,* 4th ed. American Academy of Pediatrics, Elk Grove Village, IL.

4. Food and Drug Administration. 1985. Rules and Regulations. *Nutrient requirements for infant formulas.* Federal Register 36, 23553-23556. 21 CFR Part 107.

5. Fabius, R.J., R.J. Merritt, P.M. Fleiss, and J.M. Ashley. 1981. Malnutrition associated with a formula of barley water, corn syrup, and whole milk. *Am J Dis Child* 135:615–17.

6. Sinatra, F.R., and R.J. Merritt. 1981. Iatrogenic kwashiorkor in infants. *Am J Dis Child* 135:21–23.

7. Keating, J.P., G.J. Schears, and P.R. Dodge. 1991. Oral water intoxication in infants. An American epidemic. *Am J Dis Child* 145:985–90.

8. Lucas, A., S. Lockton, and P.S. Davies. 1992. Randomised trial of a ready-to-feed compared with powdered formula. *Arch Dis Child* 67:935–39.

9. Birenbaum, E., E. Shahar, M. Aladjem, and M. Brish. 1981. Neonatal hypernatremic dehydration due to excessively concentrated prepared milk formula. *Clin Pediatr* (Phila.) 20:627–29.

10. Illingworth, R.S., and J. Lister. 1964. The critical or sensitive period with special reference to certain feeding problems in infants and children. *J Pediatr* 65:839.

11. Lawrence, R. 1995. The clinician's role in teaching proper infant feeding techniques. *J Pediatr* 126:S112–17.

12. Tully, S.B., Y. Bar Haim, and R.L. Bradley. 1995. Abnormal tympanography after supine bottle feeding. *J Pediatr* 126:S105–11.

13. Skuse, D. 1993. Identification and management of problem eaters. *Arch Dis Child* 69:604–8.

14. Hill, A.S., S. Bishop, and M.H. Malloy. 1995. Introduction of solid foods to African American and Anglo American low-birth-weight and full-term infants. *ABNF J* 6:118–14.

15. Shulman, R.J., N. Gannon, and P.J. Reeds. 1995. Cereal feeding and its impact on the nitrogen economy of the infant. *Am J Clin Nutr* 62:969–72.

16. Forsyth, J.S., S.A. Ogston, A. Clark, C.D. Florey, and P.W. Howie. 1993. Relation between early introduction of solid food to infants and their weight and illnesses during the first two years of life. *BMJ* 306:1572–76.

17. Orenstein, S.R., T.M. Shalaby, and P.E. Putnam. 1992. Thickened feedings as a cause of increased coughing when

used as therapy for gastroesophageal reflux in infants. *J Pediatr* 121:913–15.

18. Zeiger, R.S., and S. Heller. 1995. The development and prediction of atopy in high-risk children: Follow-up at age seven years in a prospective randomized study of combined maternal and infant food allergen avoidance. *J Allergy Clin Immunol* 95:1179–90.

19. Scott, F.W., J.M. Norris, and H. Kolb. 1996. Milk and Type I diabetes: Examining the evidence and broadening the focus. *Diabetes Care* 19:379–83.

20. Agostoni, C., E. Riva, and M. Giovannini. 1995. Dietary fiber in weaning foods of young children. *Pediatrics* 96:1002–5.

21. Balon, A.J. 1997. Management of infantile colic. *Am Fam Physician* 55:235–42, 2456.

22. Clyne, P.S., and A.J. Kulczycki. 1991. Human breast milk contains bovine IgG. Relationship to infant colic? *Pediatrics* 87:439–44.

23. Hill, D.J., I.L. Hudson, L.J. Sheffield, M.J. Shelton, S. Menahem, and C.S. Hosking. 1995. A low allergen diet is a significant intervention in infantile colic: Results of a community-based study. *J Allergy Clin Immunol* 96:886–92.

24. Bergstrom, E., O. Hernell, L.A. Persson, and B. Vessby. 1995. Serum lipid values in adolescents are related to family history, infant feeding, and physical growth. *Atherosclerosis* 117:1–13.

25. Kramer, M.S., R.G. Barr, D.G. Leduc, C. Boisjoly, L. McVey White, and I.B. Pless. 1985. Determinants of weight and adiposity in the first year of life. *J Pediatr* 106:10–14.

CHAPTER TEN

1. Jones, K.L. 1997. *Smith's recognizable patterns of human malformations,* 5th ed. Philadelphia: W.B. Saunders.

2. Smith, D.W. 1977. *Growth and its disorders.* Philadelphia: W.B. Saunders.

3. Ryan, A.S. et al. 1990. An evaluation of the association between socioeconomic status and the growth of Mexican American children: Data from the Hispanic Health and Nutrition Examination Survey (HHANES 1982-1984). *Am J Clin Nutr* 51:944S.

4. Yip, R. et al. 1992. Improving growth status of Asian refugee children in the United States. *JAMA* 267:937.

5. National Center for Health Statistics: NCHS growth charts, 1976. *Monthly Vital Statistics Report,* vol. 25, no. 3, suppl (HRA) 76-1120. Rockville, MD: Health Resources Administration.

6. Trahms, C.M., and P.L. Pipes. 1997. *Nutrition in infancy and childhood.* Dubuque, IA: McGraw-Hill.

7. Scott, B.J. et al. 1992. Growth assessment in children: A review. *Top Clin Nutr* 8:5.

8. Daniels, S.R. et al. 1997. The utility of body mass index as a measure of body fatness in children and adolescents: Differences by race and gender. *Pediatrics* 99:804.

9. Pietrobelli, A., M.S. Faith, D.B. Allison, D. Gallagher, G. Chiumello, and S.B. Heymsfield. 1998. Body mass index as a measure of adiposity among children and adolescents: A validation study. *J of Peds* 132:204.

10. Food and Nutrition Board, National Research Council. 1989. *Recommended dietary allowances.* 10th ed. Washington, DC: National Academy of Sciences.

11. Pellet, P.L. 1990. Food energy requirements in humans. *Am J Clin Nutr* 51:711.

12. Birch, L.L. et al. 1991. The variability of young children's energy intake. *N Engl J Med* 324:232.

13. Ashworth, A., and D.J. Millward. 1986. Catch-up growth in children. *Nutr Rev* 44:157.

14. Pellet, P.L. 1990. Protein requirements in humans. *Am J Clin Nutr* 51:723.

15. Sabate, J. et al. 1990. Anthropometric parameters of school children with different lifestyles. *Am J Dis Child* 144:1159.

16. Prentice, A. 1995. Calcium requirements of children. *Nutr Rev* 53:37.

17. Schlage, C., and B. Wortberg. 1972. Zinc in the diet of healthy preschool and school children. *Acta Paediatr Scand* 61:421.

18. Walravens, P.A. et al. 1989. Zinc supplementation in infants with a nutritional pattern of failure to thrive: A double-blind, controlled study. *Pediatrics* 83:1089.

19. Looker, A.C., P.R. Dallman, M.D. Carroll, E.W. Gunter, and C.L. Johnson. 1997. Prevalence of iron deficiency in the United States. *JAMA* 277:973.

20. Freeman, V.E., J. Mulder, M.A. van't Hof, H.M.V. Hoey, and M.J. Gibney. 1998. A longitudinal study of iron status in children at 12, 24 and 36 months. *Public Health Nutr* 1:93.

21. Lozoff, B. et al. 1991. Long-term developmental outcome of infants and iron deficiency. *N Engl J Med* 325:687.

22. Stephenson, L. 1995. Possible new developments in community control of iron-deficiency anemia. *Nutr Rev* 53:23.

23. Lobosco, R.M. 1994. A commentary on domestic hunger: A problem we can solve. *Top Clin Nutr* 9:8–12.

24. Zive, M.M. et al. 1995. Vitamin and mineral intakes of Anglo-American and Mexican-American preschoolers. *J Am Diet Assoc* 95:329.

25. Murphy, S.P. et al. 1990. An evaluation of food group intakes by Mexican-American children. *J Am Diet Assoc* 90:388.

26. Jackson, M.Y. 1993. Height, weight and body mass index of American Indian school children 1990–91. *J Am Diet Assoc* 93:1136.

27. DuRousseau, P.C. et al. 1991. Children in foster care: Are they at nutritional risk? *J Am Diet Assoc* 91:83.

28. Fierman, A.H. et al. 1991. Growth delay in homeless children. *Pediatrics* 88:918.

29. Taylor, M.L., and S.A. Koblinsky. 1993. Dietary intake and growth status of young homeless children. *J Am Diet Assoc* 93:464.

30. Drake, M.A. 1991. Dietary adequacy of children residing in temporary shelters. *J Am Diet Assoc* 91:A-77.

31. Kleinman, R.E., J.M. Murphy, M. Little, M. Pagano et al. 1998. Hunger in children in the United States: Potential behavioral and emotional correlates. *Pediatrics* 101:e3.

32. Barnes, L.A., ed. 1998. *Pediatric nutrition handbook.* Elk Grove Village, Ill: Committee on Nutrition, American Academy of Pediatrics.

33. Beauchamp, G.K., and B.J. Cowart. 1985. Congenital and experimental factors in the development of human flavor preferences. *Appetite* 6:357.

34. Cowart, B.J., and G.K. Beauchamp. 1986. The importance of sensory content in young children's acceptance of salty tastes. *Child Dev* 57:1034.

35. Falciglia, G.E., and P.A. Norton. 1994. Evidence for a genetic influence on preference for some foods. *J Am Diet Assoc* 4:154.

36. Anliker, J.A. et al. 1991. Children's food preferences and genetic sensitivity to the bitter taste of 6-n-propylthiouracil (PROP). *Am J Clin Nutr* 54:16.

37. Swanson-Rudd, J. et al. 1982. Nutrition orientations of working mothers in the North Central Region. *J Nutr Educ* 14:132.

38. Phillips, D.E., M.A. Bass, and E. Yetley. 1980. Use of food and nutrition knowledge by mothers of preschool children. *J Nutr Educ* 10:73.

39. Burroughs, M.L., and R.D. Terry. 1992. Parents' perspectives toward their children's eating behavior. *Top Clin Nutr* 8:45.

40. DeWalt, K.M. 1990. The use of itemized register tapes for analysis of household food acquisition patterns prompted by children. *J Am Diet Assoc* 90:559.

41. Kirk, M.C., and A.H. Gillespie. 1990. Factors affecting food choices of working mothers with young families. *J Nutr Educ* 22:161.

42. Stanek, K. et al. 1990. Diet quality and the eating environment of preschool children. *J Am Diet Assoc* 90:1582.

43. Birch, L.L. et al. 1981. Mother-child interaction patterns and the degree of fatness in children. *J Nutr Educ* 12:17.

44. Birch, L.L. et al. 1981. The influence of social-affective context on the formation of children's food preferences. *J Nutr Educ* 13:115.

45. Birch, L.L. et al. 1984. Eating as a "means" activity in contingency: Effect on young children's food preferences. *Child Dev* 55:431.

46. Birch, L.L., and M. Deysher. 1986. Caloric compensation and sensory specific satiety: Evidence for self regulation of food intake by young children. *Appetite* 7:323.

47. Birch, L.L., and J.O. Fisher. 1998. Development of eating behaviors among children and adolescents. *Pediatrics* 101:S539.

48. Klesges, R.C. et al. 1991. Parental influence on food selection in young children and its relationship to childhood obesity. *Am J Clin Nutr* 53:859.

49. Story, M., and J.E. Brown. 1987. Do young children instinctively know what to eat? The studies of Clara Davis revisited. *N Engl J Med* 316:103.

50. Sylvester, G.P. et al. 1995. Children's television and nutrition: Friends or foes? *Nutr Today* 30:6.

51. Anderson, R.E., C.J. Crespo, S.J. Bartlett, L.J. Cheskin, and M. Pratt. 1998. Relationship of physical activity and television watching with body weight and level of fatness among children: Results of the Third National Health and Nutrition Examination Survey. *JAMA* 279:938.

52. Dietz, W.H., and S.L. Gortmaker. 1985. Do we fatten our children at the television set? Obesity and television viewing in children and adolescents. *Pediatrics* 75:807.

53. Kotz, K., and M. Story. 1994. Food advertisements during children's Saturday morning television programming: Are they consistent with dietary recommendations? *J Am Diet Assoc* 94:1296.

54. Taras, H.L. et al. 1989. Television's influence on children's diet and physical activity. *J Dev Behav Pediatr* 10:176.

55. Beal, V.A. 1961. Dietary intake of individuals followed through infancy and childhood. *Am J Public Health* 51:1107.

56. Eppright, E.S. et al. 1970. The North Central Regional Study of diets of preschool children. III. Frequency of eating. *J Home Econ* 62:407.

57. Hertzler, A.A. 1989. Preschoolers' food handling skills-motor development. *J Nutr Educ* 21:100B.

58. 1996. Position of the American Dietetic Association: Child and adolescent food and nutrition programs. *J Amer Diet Assoc* 96:913.

59. Sherry, B. et al. 1992. Short, thin or obese? Comparing growth indexes of children from high- and low-poverty areas. *J Am Diet Assoc* 92:1092–95.

60. Pugliese, M.M. et al. 1987. Parental health beliefs as a cause of non-organic failure to thrive. *Pediatrics* 80:175.

61. Lifshitz, F., and N. Moses. 1989. Growth failure. *Am J Dis Child* 143:537.

62. Wolfe, W.S., and C. Campbell. 1993. Food pattern, diet quality, and related characteristics of schoolchildren in New York State. *J Am Diet Assoc* 93:1280.

63. McPherson, R.S. et al. 1990. Intake and food sources of dietary fat among school children in the Woodlands, Texas. *Pediatrics* 86:520.

64. Pollitt, E.L. et al. 1981. Brief fasting stress and cognition in children. *Am J Clin Nutr* 34:1526.

65. Nicklas, T.A. et al. 1993. Breakfast consumption affects adequacy of total daily intake in children. *J Am Diet Assoc* 93:886–91.

66. Briggs, M. et al. 1994. Nutrient standard menu planning in child nutrition programs. *Top Clin Nutr* 9:37.

67. Trioano, R.P., and K.M. Flegal. 1998. Overweight children and adolescents: Description, epidemiology, and demographics. *Pediatrics* 101:S497.

68. Ogden, C.L., R.P. Troiano, R.R. Briefel et al. 1997. Prevalence of overweight among preschool children in the United States, 1971 through 1994. *Pediatrics* 99:e1.

69. Mei, Z., K.S. Scanlon, L.M. Grummer-Strawn et al. 1998. Increasing prevalence of overweight among US low-income preschool children: The Centers for Disease Control and Prevention Nutrition Surveillance, 1983–1995. *Pediatrics* 101:e12.

70. Lissau, I., and T.I.A. Sorensen. 1994. Parental neglect during childhood and increased risk of obesity in young adulthood. *Lancet* 343:324.

71. Barlow, S.E., and W.H. Dietz. 1998. Obesity evaluation and treatment: Expert committee recommendations. *Pediatrics* 102:e29.

72. Dietz, W.H. 1998. Health consequences of obesity in youth: Childhood prediction of adult disease. *Pediatrics* 101:S518.

73. Gustafson-Larson, A.M., and R.D. Terry. 1992. Weight-related behaviors and concerns of fourth grade children. *J Am Diet Assoc* 92:818–22.

74. Wilkins, S.C., O.W. Kendrick, K.R. Stitt, N. Stinette, and V.A. Hammaralund. 1998. Family functioning is related to overweight children. *J Amer Diet Assoc* 98:572.

75. Hertzler, A.A. 1981. Obesity impact of the family. *J Am Diet Assoc* 75:525.

76. 1989. *Oral health of United States children: The national survey of dental caries in US school children (1986–1987)*, NIH Pub. No. 89-2247. Bethesda, MD: U.S. Department of Health and Human Services.

77. Tucker, A.W., and R. Touger-Decker. 1994. Improving nutrition and oral health of minority urban children: A model university/community program. *Top Clin Nutr* 9:49.

78. Gustafson, B.E. et al. 1954. The Vipeholm dental caries study: The effect of different levels of carbohydrate intake on dental caries in 436 individuals observed for five years. *Acta Odontal Scand* 11:232.

79. White-Graves, M.V., and M.R. Schiller. 1986. History of foods in the caries process. *J Am Diet Assoc* 86:241.

80. Clancy, K.L. et al. 1977. Snack food intakes of adolescents and caries development. *J Dent Res* 56:568.

81. Kaplan, B.J. et al. 1989. Dietary replacement in preschool hyperactive boys. *Pediatrics* 83:7.

82. Printz, R.J. et al. 1980. Dietary correlates of hyperactive behavior in children. *J Consult Clin Psychol* 48:760.

83. Lester, M.B. et al. 1982. Refined carbohydrate intake, hair cadmium levels, and cognitive function in children, *Nutrition and Behavior* 1:3.

84. Berenson, G.S. et al. 1979. Serum high density lipoprotein and its relationship to cardiovascular disease risk

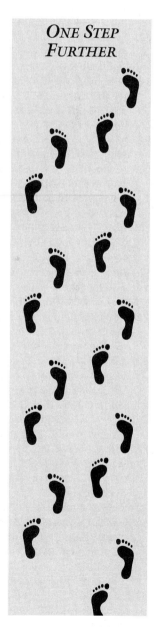

ONE STEP FURTHER

Resources to Learn More About Childhood Nutrition

- Position papers and handbooks have been published to address the critical need for appropriate meal service in child care centers and educational programs. The components of nutrition education, appropriate food to provide needed nutrients, and a supportive physical and emotional environment are endorsed to protect and promote children's health and well-being.
- Several useful handbooks address the complex issues of child health.
- An increasingly multicultural population requires that all health care providers have knowledge and skills in understanding the foodways of people in the United States.

1992. *Building for the future: Nutrition guidance for the child nutrition programs.* U.S. Department of Agriculture, Food and Nutrition Service, FNS-279.

Edelstein, S. 1992. *Nutrition and meal planning in child-care programs: A practical guide.* Chicago, IL: The American Dietetic Association.

1998. Carol Parkman Williams, ed. *Pediatric Manual of Clinical Dietetics,* Chicago, IL: The American Dietetic Association.

1995. Position of ADA, SNE, and ASFSA: School-based nutrition programs and services. *J Am Diet Assoc* 95:367.

Position paper of the American Dietetic Association. 1996. Child and adolescent food and nutrition programs. *J Am Diet Assoc* 96:913.

1993. Nutrition standards in child care programs: Technical support paper. *J Am Diet Assoc* 93:334.

1991. *Healthy children 2000: National health promotion and disease prevention objectives related to mothers, infants, children, adolescents and youth.* Department of Health and Human Services, Public Health Service, Health Resources and Service Administration, Maternal and Child Health Bureau.

Sharbaugh, C.O., ed. 1991. *Call to action: Better nutrition for mothers, children and families.* Washington, D.C. National Center for Education in Maternal and Child Health.

Green, M., ed. 1998. *Bright futures: Guidelines for health supervision of infants, children, and adolescents.* Arlington, VA: National Center for Education in Maternal and Child Health.

Bronner, Y. et al. 1994. African-American/soul foodways and nutrition counseling. *Top Clin Nutr* 9:20–27.

Bronner, Y. 1994. Cultural sensitivity and nutrition counseling. *Top Clin Nutr* 9:13–19.

Eliades, D.C., and C.W. Suitor. 1994. *Celebrating diversity: Approaching families through their food.* Arlington, VA: National Center for Education in Maternal and Child Health.

Lynch, E.W., and M.J. Johnson. 1994. *Developing cross-cultural competence: A guide for working with young children and their families.* Baltimore: Brookes.

Randall-David, E. 1989. *Strategies for working with culturally diverse communities and clients,* Bethesda, MD: Association for the Care of Children's Health.

Rodriguez, J. 1994. Diet, nutrition, and the Hispanic client. *Top Clin Nutr* 9:28–39.

Wu-Jung, C.J. 1994. Understanding food habits of Chinese Americans. *Top Clin Nutr* 9:40–44.

factor variables in children—The Bogalusa Heart Study. *Lipids* 14:91.

85. Enos, W.F. et al. 1952. Coronary disease among United States soldiers killed in action in Korea. *JAMA* 152:1090.

86. McNamara, J.J. et al. 1971. Coronary artery disease in combat casualties in Vietnam. *JAMA* 216:1185.

87. Department of Health and Human Services, National Heart, Lung, and Blood Institute, The National Cholesterol Education Program. 1990. *Report of the expert panel on population strategies for blood cholesterol reduction,* DHHS Pub. No. (NIH) 90-3046. Washington, DC: U.S. Government Printing Office.

88. Department of Health and Human Services, National Heart, Lung, and Blood Institute, The National Cholesterol Education Program. 1991. *Report of the expert panel on blood cholesterol levels in children and adolescents,* NIH Pub. No. 91-2732. Bethesda, MD.

89. American Academy of Pediatrics, Committee on Nutrition. 1989. Indications for cholesterol testing in children. *Pediatrics* 83:141.

90. National Academy of Sciences, National Research Council, Food and Nutrition Board. 1989. *Diet and health, implications for reducing chronic disease risk.* Washington, DC: National Academy Press.

91. U.S. Department of Health and Human Services, Public Health Services. 1990. *Healthy People 2000, national health promotion and disease prevention objectives,* DHHS Pub. No. (PHS) 91-50212. Washington, DC: U.S. Government Printing Office.

92. ADA Reports. 1991. Timely statement on NCEP report on children and adolescents. *J Am Diet Assoc* 91(8):983.

93. National Cholesterol Education Program (NCEP). 1992. Report of the expert panel on blood cholesterol in children and adolescents. *Pediatrics* 89:575.

94. Statement on Cholesterol, Committee on Nutrition, American Academy of Pediatrics. 1992. *Pediatrics* 90:469.

95. Department of Health and Human Services, Public Health Administration, Health Resources and Service Administration, Maternal and Child Health Bureau. 1991. *Healthy children 2000: National health promotion and disease prevention objectives related to mothers, infants, children, adolescents, and youth.* Jones and Bartlett Publishers, Boston, MA.

Chapter Eleven

1. Tanner, J.M. 1978. *Fetus into man: Physical growth from conception to maturity.* Cambridge: Harvard University Press.

2. Newman, B., and P. Newman. 1986. *Adolescent development.* Columbus, OH: Merrill Press.

3. Spear, B.A. 1996. Adolescent growth and development. In *Adolescent nutrition: Assessment and management,* ed. V.I. Rickert. New York: Chapman and Hall, pp.3–24.

4. Gong, E., and F.T. Heald. 1998. Diet nutrition and adolescence. In *Modern nutrition in health and disease,* 7th ed., ed. M. Shils and V.R. Young. Philadelphia: Lea and Febiger.

5. Gong, E.J., and B.A. Spear. 1988. Adolescent growth and development: Implications for nutritional needs. *J Nutr Educ* 20:273.

6. Hurwitz, S. 1995. Acne treatment for the '90's. August *Contemporary Pediatrics.*

7. Thompson, P. et al. 1986. Zinc status and sexual development in adolescent girls. *J Am Diet Assoc* 86:892.

8. Wait, B., R. Blair, and L.J. Roberts. 1969. Energy intake of well-nourished children and adolescents. *Am J Clin Nutr* 22:1383.

9. Wait, B. 1973. Protein intake of well-nourished children and adolescents. *Am J Clin Nutr* 26(12): 1303–10.

10. Johnson, R.K., D.G. Johnson, M.Q. Wang, H. Smiciklas-Wright, and H. Guthrie. 1994. Characterizing nutrient intakes of adolescents by sociodemographic factors. *J Adol Health* 15:149.

11. Yates, A.M., S.A. Schlicker, and C.W. Suitor. 1998. Dietary Reference Intakes: The new basis of recommendations for calcium and related nutrients, B vitamins and choline. *J Am Dietetic Assoc* 98:699–706.

12. National Institutes of Health, Consensus Development Conference Statement, *Optimal calcium intake,* Bethesda, MD, June 6–8, 1994.

13. Alaimo, K. et al. 1994. *Dietary intake of vitamins, minerals and fiber of persons ages 2 months and over in the United States: Third National Health and Nutrition Examination Survey. Phase 1, 1988–91. Advance data from vital and health statistics, No. 258.* Hyattsville, MD: National Center for Health Statistics.

14. Albertson, A.M., R.C. Tobelmann, and M. Leonard. 1997. Estimated dietary calcium intake and food sources for adolescent females: 1980–92. *J Adol Health Care* 20:20–26.

15. Jacobson, M.F. 1998. *Liquid candy: How soft drinks are harming Americans' health.* Washington, DC: Center for Science in the Public Interest.

16. Dallmon, P.R. 1989. Iron deficiency: Does it matter? *J Int Med* 226:367–72.

17. Centers for Disease Control. 1998. Recommendations to prevent and control iron deficiency in the United States. April *MMWR*

18. Witschi, J.C. et al. 1990. Sources of fat, fatty acids and cholesterol in the diets of adolescents. *J Am Diet Assoc* 90:1429.

19. Read, M.H. et al. 1988. Adolescent compliance with dietary guidelines: Health and education implications. *Adolescence* 23:567.

20. Bigler-Doughter, S., and M.R. Jenkins. 1987. Adolescent snacks: Nutrient density and nutritional contribution to total intake. *J Am Diet Assoc* 87:1678.

21. Portnoy, B., and G.M. Christenson. 1989. Cancer knowledge and related practices: Results from the National Adolescent Student Health Survey. *J School Health* 59:218.

22. Story, M., and M.D. Resnick. 1986. Adolescents' views on food and nutrition. *J Nutr Educ* 18:188.

23. Chapman, G., and Maclean, H. 1993. *"Junk food" and "healthy food": Meanings of food in adolescent women's culture.* J Nutr Ed 25:108.

24. 1994. *Spotlight on research: Heart memo, special edition.* Bethesda, MD: Office of Prevention, Education and

Control, National Heart, Lung and Blood Institute, Public Health Service, National Institutes of Health.

25. Berenson, G.S., S.R. Srinivasan, and B. Weihang. 1998. Precursors of cardiovascular risk in young adults from a biracial (black-white) population: The Bogalusa Heart Study. In *Adolescent nutritional disorders: Prevention and treatment,* ed. M.S. Jacobson, J.M. Rees, N.H. Golden, and C.E. Irwin. New York: The New York Academy of Science.

26. National Cholesterol Education Program (NCEP). September 1991. *Report of the expert panel on blood cholesterol levels in children and adolescents.* NIH Publication No. 91-2732. Washington, D.C.: National Heart, Lung and Blood Institute, Public Health Service.

27. 1997. *Bright futures in practice:* Oral Health, Maternal Child Health Bureau, Department of Health Resources and Service Administration.

28. Farrow, J.A. 1990. Adolescent chemical dependency. In ed. J.A. Farrow Adolescent medicine. *Medical Clin North Am* 74:1265.

29. Farrow, J.A. et al. 1987. Health, developmental and nutritional status of adolescent alcohol and marijuana abusers. *Pediatrics* 79:218.

30. Story, M., P. Van Zyl Yrok. 1987. Nutritional status of Native American adolescent substance users. *J Am Diet Assoc* 87:1680.

31. Must, A., G.E. Dallal, and W.H. Dietz. 1991. Reference data for obesity: 85th and 95th percentiles of body mass index (wt/ht$_2$) and triceps skinfold thickness. *Am J Clin Nutr* 53:839.

32. Must, A., G.E. Dallal, and W.H. Dietz. 1991. Reference data for obesity: 85th and 95th percentiles of body mass index (wt/ht$_2$)—A correction. *Am J Clin Nutr* 54:773.

33. WHO. 1995. *Physical status: The use and interpretation of anthropometry.* Report of a WHO Expert Committee. World Health Organization Technical Report Series 854:1–452.

34. Steen, S.N. 1998. Nutrition for the school-age child athlete. In *Nutrition for sports and exercise,* ed. J.R. Berning and S. Nelson-Steen. Gaithersburg, MD: Aspen.

35. Spear, B.A., D.R. Jennings, R. Keith, and R. Feinstein. 1994. Sports nutrition for the adolescent athlete. UAB Press. Birmingham, AL.

36. Maughan, R.J., and S.M. Shirreffs. 1998. Dehydration, rehydration and exercise in the heat. *International Journal of Sports Medicine* 19(supp2):S89–S168.

37. Burke, E.R. 1998. Nutritional ergogenic aids. In *Nutrition for sports and exercise,* ed. J.R. Berning and S. Nelson-Steen. Gaithersburg, MD: Aspen.

38. Colgan, M. 1998. Androstenedione. In *Muscular development.* Internet.

CHAPTER TWELVE

1. Neumark-Sztainer, D. 1991. The weight to eat: A high school program for the promotion of healthy eating habits and a positive body image.

2. Story, M., and M. Resnick. 1986. Adolescents' views on food and nutrition. *J Nutr Educ* 18:188–92.

3. Albertson, A.M., R. Tobelmann, and L. Marquart. 1997. Estimated dietary calcium intake and food sources for adolescent females: 1980–92. *J Adolesc Health* 20:20–26.

4. Eck, L.H., and C. Hackett-Renner. 1992. Calcium intake in youth: Sex, age, and racial differences in NHANES II. *Prev Med* 21:473–82.

5. French, S.A., M. Story, and C.L. Perry. 1995. Self-esteem and obesity in children and adolescents: A literature review. *Obes Res* 3:479–90.

6. Neumark-Sztainer, D., M. Story, S. French, P. Hannan, M. Resnick, and R.W. Blum. 1997. Psychosocial concerns and health-compromising behaviors among overweight and non-overweight adolescents. *Obes Res* 5:237–49.

7. Neumark-Sztainer, D., M. Story, L. Faibish, J. Ohlson, and M. Adamiak. 1998. Issues of self-image among overweight African American and Caucasian girls. *J Nutr Educ.* In press.

8. American Psychiatric Association. 1994. *Diagnostic and statistical manual of mental disorders,* 4th ed. *(DSM-IV).* Washington, DC: American Psychiatric Press.

9. Nylander, I. 1971. The feeling of being fat and dieting in a school population: An epidemiological investigation. *Acta Socio-Medica Scand* 1:17–26.

10. Lucas, A.R., C.M. Beard, W.M. O'Fallon, and L.T. Kurland. 1991. 50-year trends in the incidence of anorexia nervosa in Rochester, Minnesota: A population-based study. *Am J Psychiatry* 148:917–22.

11. Stein, D.M. 1991. The prevalence of bulimia: A review of the empirical research. *J Nutr Educ* 23:205–13.

12. Story, M., S. French, M. Resnick, and R. Blum. 1995. Ethnic/racial and socioeconomic differences in dieting behaviors and body image perceptions in adolescents. *Int J Eat Disord* 18:173–79.

13. Fisher, M., N.H. Golden, D.K. Katzman, R.E. Kreipe, J. Rees, J. Schebendach, G. Sigman, S. Ammerman, and H.M. Hoberman. 1995. Eating disorders in adolescents: A background paper. *J Adolesc Health* 16:420–37.

14. Serdula, M.K., E. Collins, D.F. Williamson, R.F. Anda, E. Pamuk, and T.E. Byers. 1993. Weight control practices of US adolescent and adults. *Ann Intern Med* 119:667–71.

15. Neumark-Sztainer, D., and M. Story. 1998. Dieting and binge eating among adolescents: What do they really mean? *J Am Diet Assoc* 98:446–50.

16. Neumark-Sztainer, D., M. Story, L.B. Dixon, M. Resnick, and R. Blum. 1997. Correlates of inadequate consumption of dairy products among adolescents. *J Nutr Ed* 29:12–20.

17. Story, M., and I. Alton. 1996. Adolescent nutrition: Current trends and critical issues. *Top Clin Nutr* 11:56–69.

18. Kreipe, R.E., and G.B. Forbes. 1990. Osteoporosis: A "new morbidity" for dieting female adolescents? *Pediatrics* 86:478–80.

19. Spitzer, R., S. Yanovski, T. Wadden, R. Wing, M. Marcus, A. Stunkard, M. Devlin, D. Hasin, and R.L. Horne. 1993. Binge eating disorder: Its further validation in a multisite study. *Int J Eat Disord* 13:137–53.

20. Must, A., G.E. Dallal, and W.H. Dietz. 1991. Reference data for obesity: 85th and 95th percentiles of body mass index (wt/ht^2) and tricep skinfold thickness. *Am J Clin Nutr* 53:839–46.

21. Must, A., G.E. Dallal, and W.H. Dietz. 1991. Reference data for obesity: 85th and 95th percentiles of body mass index (wt/ht²)—A correction. *Am J Clin Nutr* 54:773.

22. Himes, J.H., and W.H. Dietz. 1994. Guidelines for overweight in adolescent preventive services: Recommendations from an expert committee. *Am J Clin Nutr* 59:307–16.

23. Gortmaker, S.L., W.H. Dietz, A.M. Sobol, and C.A. Wehler. 1987. Increasing pediatric obesity in the United States. *Am J Dis Child* 141:531–40.

24. Troiano, R.P., K.M. Flegal, R.J. Kuczmarski, S.M. Campbell, and C.L. Johnson. 1995. Overweight prevalence and trends for children and adolescents. *Arch Pediatr Adolesc Med* 149:1085–91.

25. 1997. Update: Prevalence of overweight among children, adolescents, and adults—United States, 1988–1994. *MMWR* 46:199–202.

26. Szmulker, G. 1985. The epidemiology of anorexia nervosa and bulimia. *J Psychiatr Res* 19:143–53.

27. Patton, G.C., and M.B. King. 1991. Epidemiological study of eating disorders: Time for a change of emphasis [editorial]. *Psychol Med* 21:287–91.

28. Neumark-Sztainer, D., M. Story, M. Resnick, and R.W. Blum. In press. Adolescent nutrition: Lessons learned from the Minnesota Adolescent Health Survey. *J Am Diet Assoc*.

29. Rosen, L.W., D.B. McKeag, D.O. Hough, and V. Curley. 1986. Pathogenic weight-control behavior in female athletes. *The Physician and Sports Medicine* 14:79–86.

30. Dummer, G.M., L.W. Rosen, W.W. Heusner, P. Roberts, and J.E. Counsilman. 1987. Pathogenic weight-control behaviors of young competitive swimmers. *Physician Sportsmed* 15:75–84.

31. Smith, A. 1996. The female athlete triad: Causes, diagnosis and treatment. *Physician Sportsmed* 24:67–86.

32. Johnson, M.D. 1994. Disordered eating in active and athletic women. *Clin Sports Med* 13:355–69.

33. Rucinski, A. 1989. Relationship of body image and dietary intake of competitive ice skaters. *J Am Diet Assoc* 89:98–100.

34. Pope, H.G., Jr., D.L. Katz, and J.I. Hudson. 1993. Anorexia nervosa and "reverse anorexia" among 108 male bodybuilders. *Compr Psychiatry* 34:406–9.

35. Joy, E., N. Clark, M. Ireland, J. Matire, A. Nattiv, and S. Varechok. 1997. Team management of the female athlete triad: Part 2: Optimal treatment and prevention tactics. *Physician Sportsmed* 25:55–69.

36. Nattiv, A., R. Agostini, B. Drinkwater, and K.K. Yeager. 1994. The female athlete triad. The interrelatedness of disordered eating, amenorrhea, and osteoporosis. *Clin Sports Med* 13:405–18.

37. Neumark-Sztainer, D., M. Story, M. Resnick, and R.W. Blum. 1997. Adolescent vegetarians: A behavioral profile of a school-based population in Minnesota. *Arch Pediatr Adolesc Med* 151:833–38.

38. Neumark-Sztainer, D., M. Story, M. Resnick, A. Garwick, and R.W. Blum. 1995. Body dissatisfaction and unhealthy weight-control practices among adolescents with and without chronic illness: A population-based study. *Arch Pediatr Adoles Med* 149:1330–35.

39. Neumark-Sztainer, D., M. Story, N. Falkner, T. Beuhring, and M. Resnick. In press. Disordered eating among adolescents with chronic illness: Exploring the role of family and other social factors. *Arch Pediatr Adolesc Med*.

40. Everill, J., and G. Waller. 1995. Reported sexual abuse and eating psychopathology: A review of the evidence for a causal link. *Int J Eat Disord* 18:1–11.

41. Rorty, M., J. Yager, and E. Rossotto. 1995. Aspects of childhood physical punishment and family environment correlates of bulimia nervosa. *Child Abuse Neglect* 19:659–67.

42. Wonderlich, S., R. Wilsnack, S. Wisnack, and T.R. Harris. 1996. Childhood sexual abuse and bulimic behavior in a nationally representative sample. *Am J Public Health* 86:1082–86.

43. French, S.A., M. Story, B. Downes, M.D. Resnick, and R.W. Blum. 1995. Frequent dieting among adolescents: Psychosocial and health behavior correlates. *Am J Public Health* 85:695–701.

44. Neumark-Sztainer, D SM, P. Hannan, T. Beuhring, and M. Resnick. 1999. Disordered eating among adolescents: Associations with sexual/physical abuse and other familial/psychosocial factors. *Health Psychology*.

45. Bandura, A. 1977. *Social learning theory*. Englewood Cliffs, NJ: Prentice Hall.

46. Bandura, A. 1986. *Social foundations of thought and action: A social cognitive theory*. Englewood Cliffs, NJ: Prentice Hall.

47. Neumark-Sztainer, D., R. Butler, and H. Palti. 1996. Personal and socio-environmental predictors of disordered eating among adolescent females. *J Nutr Educ* 28:195–201.

48. Rosen, D., and D. Neumark-Sztainer. In press. Eating disturbances among adolescents: Options for primary prevention. *J Adolesc Health*

49. Silverman, J.A. 1983. Richard Morton, 1637–1698. Limner of anorexia nervosa: His life and times. A tercentenary essay. *JAMA* 250:2830–32.

50. Woodside, D.B. 1995. A review of anorexia nervosa and bulimia nervosa. *Current Problems Pediatr* 25:67–89.

51. Mott, A., and D. Lumsden. 1994. *Understanding eating disorders*. Washington, DC: Tayler & Francis.

52. Johnson, C., and M. Connors. 1987. *The etiology and treatment of bulimia nervosa: A biopsychosocial perspective*. New York: Basic Books.

53. Kaplan, A., and P. Garfinkel. 1993. *Medical issues and eating disorders*. New York: Brunner/Mazel.

54. Yates, A. 1992. Biologic considerations in the etiology of eating disorders. *Pediatr Ann* 21:739–44.

55. Garfinkel, P., and D. Garner. 1982. *Anorexia nervosa: A multidimensional perspective*. New York: Brunner/Mazel.

56. de Castro, J.M. 1987. Circadian rhythms of the spontaneous meal pattern, macronutrient intake, and mood of humans. *Physiol Behav* 40:437–46.

57. Goodwin, G.M., C.G. Fairburn, and P.J. Cowen. 1987. Dieting changes serotonergic function in women, not men: Implications for the aetiology of anorexia nervosa? *Psychol Med* 17:839–42.

58. Holland, A.J., N. Sicotte, and J. Treasure. 1988. Anorexia nervosa: Evidence for a genetic basis. *J Psychosom Res* 32:561–71.

59. Holland, A.J., A. Hall, R. Murray, G.F. Russell, and A.H. Crisp. 1984. Anorexia nervosa: A study of 34 twin pairs and one set of triplets. *Br J Psychiatry* 145:414–19.

60. Fava, M., P.M. Copeland, U. Schweiger, and D.B. Herzog. 1989. Neurochemical abnormalities of anorexia nervosa and bulimia nervosa. *Am J Psychiatry* 146:963–71.

61. Jimerson, D.C., M.D. Lesem, A.P. Hegg, and T.D. Brewerton. 1990. Serotonin in human eating disorders. *Ann Ny Acad Sci* 600:532–44.

62. 1994. Eating disorders. *Harvard Mental Health Newsletter.* 14:1–5.

63. Bruch, H. 1985. Four decades of eating disorders. In *Handbook of psychotherapy for anorexia and bulimia.* ed. D. Garner and P. Garfinkel. New York: Garfield Press, pp. 7–18.

64. Powers, P.S. 1996. Initial assessment and early treatment options for anorexia nervosa and bulimia nervosa. *Psychiatr Clin North Am* 19:639–55.

65. Bruch, H. 1973. *Eating disorders.* New York: Basic Books.

66. Minuchin, S., B.L. Rosman, and L. Baker. 1978. *Psychosomatic families: Anorexia nervosa in context.* Cambridge, MA: Harvard University Press, pp. viii, 351.

67. Garner, D.M. 1993. Pathogenesis of anorexia nervosa. *Lancet* 341:1631–35.

68. Reiff, D., and K. Reiff. 1992. *Eating disorders: Nutrition therapy in the recovery process.* Gaithersberg, MD: Aspen.

69. Ponton, L.E. 1995. A review of eating disorders in adolescents. *Adolesc Psychiatry* 20:267–85.

70. American Psychiatric Association. 1993. Practice guidelines for eating disorders. *Am J Psychiatry* 150:212–20.

71. Zerbe, K.J. 1993. *The body betrayed: Women, eating disorders, and treatment.* Washington, DC: American Psychiatric Press, pp. xv; 447.

72. Bachrach, L.K., D.K. Katzman, I.F. Litt, D. Guido, and R. Marcus. 1991. Recovery from osteopenia in adolescent girls with anorexia nervosa. *J Clin Endocrinol Metab* 72:602–6.

73. Rock, C., and J. Curran-Celentano. 1996. Nutritional management of eating disorders. *Psychiatric Clinics North Am* 19:701–13.

74. Russell, G. 1979. Bulimia nervosa: An ominous variant of anorexia nervosa. *Psychol Med* 9:429–48.

75. Wrate, R. 1996. Getting to the cause of eating disorders. *Practitioner* 240:306–17.

76. Magrann, S. 1992. *Weight control and eating disorders.* San Marcos, CA: Nutrition Dimension.

77. Sobel, S. 1996. What's new in the treatment of anorexia nervosa and bulimia? *Medscape Women's Health* 1.

78. Kendler, K.S., C. MacLean, M. Neale, R. Kessler, A. Heath, and L. Eaves. 1991. The genetic epidemiology of bulimia nervosa [see comments]. *Am J Psychiatry* 148:1627–37.

79. Johnson, C., and K.L. Maddi. 1986. Factors that affect the onset of bulimia. *Sem Adolesc Med* 2:11–19.

80. Fluoxetine Bulimia Nervosa Collaborative Study Group. 1992. Fluoxetine in the treatment of bulimia nervosa. A multicenter, placebo-controlled, double-blind trial. *Arch Gen Psychiatry* 49:139–47.

81. Fairburn, C., M. Marcus, and G. Wilson. 1993. Cognitive-behavioral therapy for binge eating and bulimia nervosa: A comprehensive treatment manual. In *Binge eating: Nature, assessment, and treatment.* ed. C.G. Fairburn and G.T. Wilson. New York: Guilford Press.

82. Gannon, M.A., and J.E. Mitchell. 1986. Subjective evaluation of treatment methods by patients treated for bulimia. *J Am Diet Assoc* 86:520–21.

83. Pi-Sunyer, F.X. 1991. Health implications of obesity. *Am J Clin Nutr* 53:1595S–1603S.

84. Smoak, C.G., G.L. Burke, L.S. Webber, D.W. Harsha, S.R. Srinivasan 1987. Relation of obesity to clustering of cardiovascular disease risk factors in children and young adults. *Am J Epidemiol* 125:364–72.

85. Must, A., P. Jaques, G. Dallal, C. Bajema, and W. Dietz. 1992. Long-term morbidity and mortality of overweight adolescents: A follow-up of the Harvard growth study of 1922–1935. *N Engl J Med* 327:1350–54.

86. Levy, E., P. L., LePen, and A. Basdevant. 1995. The economic cost of obesity: The French situation. *Int J Obesity* 19:788–92.

87. Colditz, G. 1992. Economic costs of obesity. *Am J Clin Nutr* 55:503S–7S.

88. Segal, L., R. Carter, and P. Zimmet. 1994. The cost of obesity: The Australian perspective. *Pharmacoeconomics* 5:42–52.

89. Seidell, J., and I. Deerenberg. 1994. Obesity in Europe: Prevalence and consequences for use of medical care. *Pharmacoeconomics* 5:38–44.

90. Neumark-Sztainer, D., M. Story, and L. Faibisch. In press. Perceived stigmatization among overweight African American and Caucasian adolescent girls. *J Adolesc Health.*

91. Story, M., and D. Neumark-Sztainer. In press. Diet and adolescent behavior: Is there a relationship. *Adolesc Med State Art Rev.*

92. Neumark-Sztainer, D. 1995. Excessive weight preoccupation: Normative but not harmless. *Nutr Today* 30:68–74.

93. Jackson, M.Y., J.M. Proulx, and S. Pelican. 1991. Obesity prevention. *Am J Clin Nutr* 53:1625S–30S.

94. Crisp, A.H. 1988. Some possible approaches to prevention of eating and body weight/shape disorders, with particular reference to anorexia nervosa. *Int J Eat Disord* 7:1–17.

95. Levine, M., and L. Smolak. In press. The mass media and disordered eating: Implication for primary prevention. In *Primary prevention of eating disorders.* ed. G. Noordenbos and V. Vandereyecken. London: Athlone.

96. Shisslak, C.M., M. Crago, and M.E. Neal. 1990. Prevention of eating disorders among adolescents. *Am J Health Promot* 5:100–6.

97. Steiner-Adair, C. 1994. The politics of prevention. In *Feminist perspectives on eating disorders.* ed. P. Fallon, M.A. Katzman, and S.C. Wooley. 381–94.

98. Killen, J.D., C.B. Taylor, L.D. Hammer, I. Litt, D.M. Wilson, T. Rich, C. Hayward, B. Simmonds, H. Kraemer, and A. Varady. 1993. An attempt to modify unhealthful eating attitudes and weight regulation practices of young adolescent girls. *Int J Eat Disord* 13:369–84.

99. Neumark-Sztainer, D., R. Butler, and H. Palti. 1995. Eating disturbances among adolescent girls: Evaluation of a school-based primary prevention program. *J Nutr Ed* 27:24–31.

100. Neumark-Sztainer, D. 1996. School-based programs for preventing eating disturbances. *J Sch Health* 66:64–71.

CHAPTER THIRTEEN

1. United States Department of Health and Human Services. 1979. *Healthy people: the surgeon general's report on health promotion and disease prevention.* Washington, DC: U.S. Government Printing Office.
2. Saunders, R.P. 1988. What is health promotion?, *Health Educ Q* 19:14.
3. Holli, B.B., and R.J. Calabrese. 1991. Communication and education skills: The dietitian's guide, 2d ed. Philadelphia: Lea and Febiger.
4. Contento, I., and B.M. Murphy. 1990. Psycho-social factors differentiating people who reported making desirable changes in their diets from those who did not. *J Nutr Educ* 22:6.
5. Johnson, R.K. et al. 1994. Medical nutrition therapy and health care reform: Strategies of the American Dietetic Association. *Pers Applied Nutr* 2(1):3.
6. Kritchevsky, D. 1998. History of recommendations to the public about dietary fat. *J Nutr* 128(2-suppl):449S.
7. Yansk, L.R. et al: 1998. Hypertension among siblings of persons with premature coronary heart disease. *Hypertension* 32:123–28.
8. Yusuf, H.R. et al. 1998. Impact of multiple risk factor profiles on determining cardiovascular disease risk. *Preventive Med* 27:1.
9. Dallonville, J. et al. 1998. Cigarette smoking is associated with unhealthy patterns of nutrient intake: A meta-analysis. *J Nutr* 128.
10. Committee on Diet and Health, Food and Nutrition Board. 1989. Diet and health: Implications for reducing chronic disease risk. Washington, DC: National Academy Press.
11. United States Department of Health and Human Services. 1993. *Second report of the Expert Panel on Detection, Evaluation, and Treatment of High Blood Cholesterol in Adults,* NIH pub. no. 93-3095. Washington, DC: U.S. Government Printing Office.
12. Murphy, S.P. et al. 1992. Demographic and economic factors associated with dietary quality for adults in the 1987-88 Nationwide Food Consumption Survey. *J Am Diet Assoc* 92:1352.
13. United States Department of Health and Human Services. 1991. *Healthy people 2000: National health promotion and disease prevention objectives,* DHHS pub. no. (PHS) 91-50212. Washington, DC: U.S. Government Printing Office.
14. Kristal, A.R. et al. 1992. Long-term maintenance of a low-fat diet: Durability of fat-related dietary habits in the Women's Health Trial, *J Am Diet Assoc* 92:553.
15. Salonen, J.T. et al. 1992. High stored iron levels are associated with excess risk of myocardial infarction in eastern Finnish men. *Circulation* 86:803.
16. United States Department of Health and Human Services. 1993. *The fifth report of the Joint National Committee on Detection, Evaluation, and Treatment of High Blood Pressure,* NIH pub. no. 93-1088. Washington, DC: U.S. Government Printing Office.
17. Paffenbarger, R.S. et al. 1993. The association of changes in physical-activity level and other lifestyle characteristics with mortality among men. *N Engl J Med* 328:533.
18. Sandovik, L. et al. 1993. Physical fitness as a predictor of mortality among healthy, middle-aged Norwegian men. *N Engl J Med* 328:533.
19. DeBacquer, D. et al. 1998. Prognostic value of ischemic electrocardiographic findings for cardiovascular mortality in men and women. *J Am Cardiology* 9:680.
20. United States Department of Health and Human Services. 1989. *Reducing the health consequences of smoking, 25 years of progress: A report of the surgeon general,* DHHS pub. no. (CDC) 89-8411. Washington, DC: U.S. Government Printing Office.
21. 1994. Update: Study finds tobacco and poor diet to cause most deaths. *J Am Diet Assoc* 94:138.
22. United States Department of Health and Human Services. 1993. *Health United States 1992 and healthy people 2000 review,* DHHS Pub. no. (PHS) 93-1232. Washington, DC: U.S. Government Printing Office.
23. Williamson, D.F. et al. 1991. Smoking cessation and severity of weight gain in a national cohort. *N Engl J Med* 324, 739.
24. Pelican, S. et al. 1994. Nutrition services for alcohol/substance abuse clients: Indian Health Service's tribal survey. *J Am Diet Assoc* 94:835.
25. Speicher, C.E. 1993. The right test: A physician's guide to laboratory medicine, 2d ed. Philadelphia: W.B. Saunders.
26. Watson, R.R. et al. 1986. Identification of alcohol abuse and alcoholism with biological parameters. *Alcoholism: Clin Exp Res* 10:364.
27. Shattuck, D.K. 1994. Mindfulness and metaphor in relapse prevention: An interview with G. Alan Marlatt. *J Am Diet Assoc* 94:846.
28. Beckley-Barrett, L.M., and P.B. Mutch. 1990. Position of the American Dietetic Association: Nutrition intervention in treatment and recovery from chemical dependency. *J Am Diet Assoc* 90:1274.
29. Biery, J.R. et al. 1991. Alcohol craving in rehabilitation: Assessment of nutrition therapy. *J Am Diet Assoc* 91:463.
30. Lemberg, R., ed. 1992. *Controlling disorders with facts, advice, and resources.* Phoenix: Phoenix Oryx Press.
31. Steinberg, D. 1993. Antioxidant vitamins and coronary heart disease. *N Engl J Med* 328:1487.
32. Monsen, E. 1991. Reversing heart disease through diet, exercise, and stress management: An interview with Dean Ornish. *J Am Diet Assoc* 91:162.
33. Siani, A. et al. 1991. Increasing the dietary potassium intake reduces the need for antihypertensive medication. *Ann Intern Med* 115:753.
34. Kucznarski, R.J. et al. 1994. Increasing prevalence of overweight among US adults, the National Health and Examination Surveys, 1960 to 1991. *JAMA* 272:205.
35. Simopoulos, A.P., and T.B. Van Itallie. 1984. Body weight, health, and longevity. *Ann Intern Med* 100:285.
36. Launer, L.J. et al. 1994. Body mass index, weight change, and the risk of mobility disability in middle-aged and older women, the Epidemiologic Follow-up Study of NHANES I. *JAMA* 271:1093.

37. Kushner, R.F. 1993. Body weight and mortality. *Nutr Rev* 51:127.

38. D'Eramo-Melkus, M.G., and J.A. Hagen. 1991. Weight reduction interventions for persons with a chronic illness: Findings and factors for consideration. *J Am Diet Assoc* 91:1093.

39. Council of Scientific Affairs, American Medical Association. 1993. Diet and cancer: Where do matters stand? *Arch Intern Med* 153:5056.

40. American Cancer Society. 1996. Guidelines on diet, nutrition, and health. *Nation's Health* 26:23.

41. Foerster, S.B. et al. 1995. California's "5-a-day-for better health" campaign: An innovative population-based effort to effect large-scale dietary change. *Am J Prev Med* 11:124.

42. Greenwald, P. 1996. Chemoprevention of cancer. *Sci Am* 275:96.

43. Steinmetz, K.A., and J.D. Potter. 1996. Vegetables, fruit, and cancer prevention: A review. *J Am Diet Assoc* 96:1027.

44. Bloch, A.S., and C.A. Thomson. 1995. Position of The American Dietetic Association: Phytochemicals and functional foods. *J Am Diet Assoc* 95:493.

45. Dwyer, J. 1993. Dietary fiber and colorectal cancer risk. *Nutr Rev* 51:147.

46. Tinker, L.F. et al. 1994. Diabetes Care and Education, a practice group of The American Dietetic Association: Commentary and translation: 1994 nutrition recommendations for diabetes. *J Am Diet Assoc* 94:507.

47. Johnson, C.L. et al. 1993. Declining serum total cholesterol levels among US adults: The National Health and Nutrition Examination Surveys. *JAMA* 269:3002.

48. Croft, J.B. et al. 1994. Community intervention and trends in dietary fat consumption among black and white adults. *J Am Diet Assoc* 94:1284.

49. Kerber, B.A., ed. 1994. *How employers are saving through wellness and fitness programs,* 2d ed. Wall Township, NJ: American Business Publishing.

50. Baer, J.T. 1993. Improved plasma cholesterol levels in men after a nutrition education program at the worksite. *J Am Diet Assoc* 93:658.

51. Maiman, L.A. et al. 1994. Public cholesterol screening in the previously diagnosed, misuse of resources or beneficial function. *Am J Prev Med* 10:20.

52. Holloway, M. 1994. Trends in women's health: A global view. *Sci Am* 271:76.

53. Erikson, E. 1963. *Childhood and society.* New York: W.W. Norton.

54. Food and Nutrition Board, National Research Council. 1989. *Recommended Dietary Allowances,* 10th ed. Washington, DC: National Academy Press.

55. Anderson, J.J.B. 1990. Dietary calcium and bone mass through the life cycle. *Nutr Today* 25:9.

56. U.S. Department of Health and Human Services, U.S. Department of Agriculture, Joint Advisory Committee. 1995. *Dietary guidelines for Americans,* 4th ed. Washington, DC: U.S. Government Printing Office.

57. Hahn, N.I. 1995. Variety is still the spice of a healthful diet: A look at the proposed revisions for the 1995 Dietary Guidelines for Americans. *J Am Diet Assoc* 95:1096.

58. Guyton, A.C. 1996. *Textbook of medical physiology,* 9th ed. Philadelphia: W.B. Saunders.

59. Clarke, L.L. et al. 1998. Norplant selection and satisfaction among low-income women. *Am J Pub Health* 88:1175.

60. Eilers, G.M., and T.K. Swanson. 1994. Women's satisfaction with Norplant as compared with oral contraceptives. *J Fam Pract* 38:596.

61. Stunkard, A.J. et al. 1990. The body mass of twins who have been reared apart. *N Engl J Med* 322:1483.

62. Bouchard, C. et al. 1990. The response to long-term overfeeding in identical twins. *N Engl J Med* 322: 1483.

63. Williamsson, D.F. et al. 1990. The 10-year incidence of overweight and major weight gain in U.S. adults. *Arch Intern Med* 150:665.

64. Van Dale, D. et al. 1990. Weight maintenance and resting metabolic rate 18–40 months after a diet/exercise treatment. *Ind J Obesity* 14:347.

65. Golay, A. et al. 1990. Effect of central obesity on regulation of carbohydrate metabolism in obese patients with varying degrees of glucose toleration. *J Clin Endocrinal Metab* 71:1299.

66. Haffer, S.M. et al. 1990. Cardiovascular risk factors in confirmed prediabetic individuals. *JAMA* 263:2893.

CHAPTER FOURTEEN

1. US Senate Special Committee on Aging. 1990. *Aging America: Trends and projections (annotated),* Serial No. 101-J. Washington, DC: U.S. Government Printing Office.

2. Taeuber, C. 1992. *Sixty-five plus in America,* Curr Pop Reports P23-278. Washington, DC: U.S. Bureau of Census.

3. Shock, N.W. et al. 1984. *Normal human aging: The Baltimore Longitudinal Study of Aging,* NIH pub. no. 84-2450. Washington, DC: U.S. Government Printing Office.

4. National High Blood Pressure Education Program Working Group: 1994. National high blood pressure education program working group report on hypertension in the elderly. *Hypertension* 23:275.

5. Rolls, B.J., and P.A. Phillips. 1990. Aging and disturbances of thirst and fluid balance. *Nutr Rev* 48:137.

6. Russell, R.M. 1992. Changes in gastrointestinal function attributed to aging. *Am J Clin Nutr* 55:1203S.

7. Krasinski, S.D. et al. 1986. Fundic atrophic gastritis in an elderly population, effect on hemoglobin and several serum nutritional indicators. *J Am Geriatr Soc* 34:800.

8. Masoro, E.J. 1993. Dietary restriction and aging. *J Amer Geriatr Soc* 41:994.

9. Breslow, L., and N. Breslow. 1993. Health practices and disability: Some evidence from Alameda County. *Prev Med* 22:86.

10. Johnson, M.A. et al. 1992. Nutritional patterns of centenarians. *Int J Aging Hum Dev* 34(1):57.

11. Trichopoulou, A. et al. 1995. Diet and survival of elderly Greeks: A link to the past. *Am J Clin Nutr* 61:1346S.

12. Willett, W.C. et al. 1995. Weight, weight change, and coronary heart disease in women. *JAMA* 273:461.

13. Lee, I.M. et al. 1993. Body weight and mortality. A 27-year follow-up of middle-aged men. *JAMA* 270:2823.

14. Harris, T.B. et al. 1997. Carrying the burden of cardiovascular risk in old age: Associations of weight and weight change with prevalent cardiovascular disease, risk factors,

and health status in the Cardiovascular Health Study. *Am J Clin Nutr* 66:837.

15. Barker, D.J.P. 1996. The fetal origins of adult disease. *Nutr Today* 31(3):108.

16. Food and Nutrition Board. 1989. *Recommended Dietary Allowances*, 10th ed. Washington, DC: National Academy of Sciences.

17. Food and Nutrition Board. 1998. *Dietary Reference Intakes: Recommended levels for individual intake*. Washington, DC: National Academy of Sciences.

18. Blumberg, J. 1994. Nutrient requirements of the healthy elderly—Should there be specific RDAs. *Nutr Rev* 52:515.

19. Russell, R.M. 1997. New views on the RDAs for older adults. *J Am Diet Assoc* 97:515.

20. James, W.P.T., A. Ralph, and A. Ferro-Luzzi. 1989. Energy needs of the elderly: A new approach. In *Nutrition, aging, and the elderly, human nutrition, a comprehensive treatise*, vol. 6. ed. H.N. Munro and D.E. Danford. New York: Plenum Press.

21. Elahi, V.K. et al. 1983. A longitudinal study of nutritional intake in men. *J Gerontol* 38:162.

22. Evans, W.J., and D. Cyr-Campbell. 1997. Nutrition, exercise, and healthy aging. *J Am Diet Assoc* 97:632.

23. Roberts, S.B. et al. 1995. Influence of age on energy requirements. *Am J Clin Nutr* 62(suppl):1053S.

24. Sawaya, A.L. et al. 1995. Dietary energy requirements of young and older women determined by using the doubly labeled water method. *Am J Clin Nutr* 62:338.

25. Life Sciences Research Office, Federation of American Societies for Experimental Biology. 1995. *Third report on nutrition monitoring in the United States, Vol. I and II*. Washington, DC: U.S. Government Printing Office.

26. McGandy, R.B. et al. 1986. Nutritional status survey of healthy noninstitutionalized elderly: Nutrient intakes from three-day diet records and nutrient supplements. *Nutr Res* 6:785.

27. Young, V.R. 1990. Protein and amino acid metabolism with reference to aging and the elderly. In *Nutrition and aging*. ed. D.M. Prinsley and H.H. Sandstead. New York: Alan R. Liss.

28. Campbell, W.W. et al. 1994. Increased protein requirements in older people: New data and retrospective assessments. *Am J Clin Nutr* 60:501.

29. Castaneda, C. et al. 1995. Elderly women accommodate to a low-protein diet with losses of body cell mass, muscle function, and immune response. *Am J Clin Nutr* 62:30.

30. Krasinski, S.D. et al. 1989. Relationship of vitamin A and vitamin E intake to fasting plasma retinol, retinol-binding protein, retinyl esters, carotene, alpha tocopherol, and cholesterol among elderly people and young adults. *Am J Clin Nutr* 49:112.

31. Meydani, S.N. et al. 1997. Vitamin E supplementation and in vivo immune response in healthy elderly subjects. A randomized controlled trial. *JAMA* 277(17):1380.

32. Sano, M. et al. 1997. A controlled trial of selegiline, alphatocopherol, or both as treatment for Alzheimer's disease. *N Engl J Med* 336:1216.

33. Dawson-Hughes, B. et al. 1991. Effect of vitamin D supplementation on wintertime and overall bone loss in healthy postmenopausal women. *Ann Intern Med* 115:505.

34. Dawson-Hughes, B. et al. 1997. Effect of calcium and vitamin D supplementation on bone density in men and women 65 years of age or older. *N Eng J Med* 337:670.

35. Smidt, L.J. et al. 1991. Influence of thiamin supplementation on the health and general well-being of an elderly Irish population with marginal thiamin deficiency. *J Gerontol* 46:M16.

36. VanderJaqt, D.J., P.J. Garry, and H.N. Bhagavan. 1987. Ascorbic acid intake and plasma levels in healthy elderly people. *Am J Clin Nutr* 46:290.

37. Seddon, J.M. et al. 1994. Dietary carotenoids, vitamins A, C, and E, and advanced age-related macular degeneration. *JAMA* 272:1413.

38. Lindenbaum, J. et al. 1994. Prevalence of cobalamin deficiency in the Framingham elderly population. *Am J Clin Nutr* 60:2.

39. Fleming, D.J. et al. 1998. Dietary determinants of iron stores in a free living elderly population: The Framingham Heart Study. *Am J Clin Nutr* 67:722.

40. U.S. Department of Health and Human Services. 1994. *Optimal calcium intake: NIH consensus statement*. Bethesda, MD: National Institutes of Health.

41. Aloia, J.F. et al. 1994. Calcium supplementation with and without hormone replacement therapy to prevent postmenopausal bone loss. *Ann Intern Med* 120:97.

42. Gibson, R.S. et al. 1985. Dietary chromium and manganese intakes of a selected sample of Canadian elderly women. *Hum Nutr Appl Nutr* 39A:43.

43. Sandstead, H. et al. 1982. Zinc nutriture in the elderly in relation to taste acuity, immune response, and wound healing. *Am J Clin Nutr* 36:1046.

44. Goren, S., L.J. Siverstein, and N. Gonzales. 1993. A survey of food service managers of Washington State boarding homes for the elderly. *J Nutr Elderly* 12(3):27.

45. Shimokata, H. et al. 1991. Age as an independent determinant of glucose tolerance. *Diabetes* 40:44.

46. Recker, R.R. et al. 1995. Patient care of osteoporosis. *Clin Geriatr Med* 11(4):625.

47. Perry, H.M. et al. 1993. A preliminary report of vitamin D and calcium metabolism in older African Americans. *J Am Geriatr Soc* 41:6121.

48. Beard, J.L., M.H. Ashraf, and H. Smiciklas-Wright. 1994. Iron nutrition in the elderly. In *Handbook of nutrition in the aged*, 2d ed. ed. R.R. Watson. Boca Raton, FL: CRC Press.

49. Lindebaum, J. et al. 1988. Neuropsychiatric disorders caused by cobalamin deficiency in the absence of anemia or macrocytosis. *N Engl J Med* 318:1720.

50. Chrischilles, E.A. et al. 1992. Use of medications by persons 65 and over: Data from the established populations for epidemiologic studies of the elderly. *J Gerontol* 47(5):M137.

51. Roe, D.A. 1989. *Handbook on drug and nutrient interactions. A problem-oriented reference guide*, 4th ed. Chicago: American Dietetic Association.

52. Mares-Perlman, J.A. et al. 1993. Nutrient supplements contribute to the dietary intake of middle- and older-aged adult residents of Beaver Dam, Wisconsin. *J Nutr* 123:176.

53. Ranno, B.S., G.M. Wardlaw, and C.J. Geiger. 1988. What characterizes elderly women who overuse vitamin and mineral supplements? *J Am Diet Assoc* 88:347.

54. Hathcock, J. 1997. Vitamins and minerals: Efficacy and safety. *Am J Clin Nutr* 66(2):427.

55. Solomon, K. et al. 1993. Alcoholism and prescription drug abuse in the elderly: St. Louis University Grand Rounds. *J Am Geriatr Soc* 41:57.

56. Schafer, R.B., and P.M. Keith. Social-psychological factors in the dietary quality of married and single elderly. *J Am Diet Assoc* 81:30.

57. Schiffman, S.S. 1997. Taste and smell losses in normal aging and disease. *JAMA* 278:1357.

58. Davis, M.A. et al. 1990. Living arrangements and dietary quality of older U.S. adults. *J Am Diet Assoc* 90:1667.

59. Senauer, B., E. Asp, and J. Kinsey. 1991. *Food trends and the changing consumer.* St. Paul: Eagen Press.

60. Rubin, R.M., and M. Nieswindomy. 1994. Expenditure patterns of retired and nonretired persons. *Monthly Labor Rev* 117(4):10.

61. Posner, B.M. et al. 1993. Nutrition and health risks in the elderly: The Nutrition Screening Initiative. *Am J Public Health* 83:972.

62. U.S. General Accounting Office. 1992. *Elderly Americans. Health, housing and nutrition gaps between the poor and nonpoor.* Report to the Chairman, Select Committee on Aging, U.S. House of Representatives, GAO/PEMD 92-29. Washington, DC: U.S. Government Printing Office.

63. Bartholomew, A.M. et al. 1990. Food frequency intakes and sociodemographic factors of elderly Mexican-Americans and nonHispanic whites. *J Am Diet Assoc* 90:1693.

64. Kim, K.A. et al. 1993. Nutritional status of Chinese, Korean, and Japanese-American elderly. *J Am Diet Assoc* 93:1416.

65. Fanelli, M.T., and K.S. Stevenhagen. 1985. Characterizing consumption patterns by food frequency methods: Core foods and variety of foods in diets of older Americans. *J Am Diet Assoc* 85:1570.

66. Murphy, S.P., D.F. Everett, and C.M. Dresser. 1989. Food group consumption reported by the elderly during the NHANES I Epidemiologic Followup Study. *J Nutr Educ* 21:214.

67. White, J.V. et al. 1992. Nutrition Screening Initiative: Development and implementation of the public awareness checklist and screening tools. *J Am Diet Assoc* 92:163.

68. Ponza, M., J.C. Ohls, and B.F. Millen. 1996. *Serving elders at risk. The Older Americans Act Nutrition Programs: National evaluation of the Elderly Nutrition Program 1993–1995.* Executive summary. Princeton, NJ: Mathematica Policy Research.

69. Balsam, A.L. et al. 1992. Weekend home-delivered meals in elderly nutrition programs. *J Am Diet Assoc* 92:1125.

70. Rhodes, S.S., ed. 1991. *Effective menu planning for the elderly nutrition program.* Chicago: The American Dietetic Association.

71. Ponza, M. et al. 1996. *Serving elders at risk. The Older Americans Act Nutrition Programs: National evaluation of the Elderly Nutrition Program 1993–1995. Vol. I, Title III evaluation findings.* Princeton, NJ: Mathematica Policy Research. Available on the web site of the National Policy and Resource Center on Nutrition and Aging, Florida State University; access at *http://www.aoa.dhhs.gov/aoa/pages/nutreval.html*

INDEX

Median Heights and Weights and Recommended Energy Intake

Category	Age (years) or Condition	Weight (kg)	Weight (lb)	Height (cm)	Height (in)	REE[a] (kcal/day)	Multiples of REE	Average Energy Allowance (kcal)[b] Per kg	Average Energy Allowance (kcal)[b] Per day[c]
Infants	0.0–0.5	6	13	60	24	320		108	650
	0.5–1.0	9	20	71	28	500		98	850
Children	1–3	13	29	90	35	740		102	1,300
	4–6	20	44	112	44	950		90	1,800
	7–10	28	62	132	52	1,130		70	2,000
Males	11–14	45	99	157	62	1,440	1.70	55	2,500
	15–18	66	145	176	69	1,760	1.67	45	3,000
	19–24	72	160	177	70	1,780	1.67	40	2,900
	25–50	79	174	176	70	1,800	1.60	37	2,900
	51+	77	170	173	68	1,530	1.50	30	2,300
Females	11–14	46	101	157	62	1,310	1.67	47	2,200
	15–18	55	120	163	64	1,370	1.60	40	2,200
	19–24	58	128	164	65	1,350	1.60	38	2,200
	25–50	63	138	163	64	1,380	1.55	36	2,200
	51+	65	143	160	63	1,280	1.50	30	1,900
Pregnant	1st trimester								+0
	2nd trimester								+300
	3rd trimester								+300
Lactating	1st 6 months								+500
	2nd 6 months								+500

[a] Resting energy expenditure (REE); calculation based on FAO equations, then rounded
[b] In the range of light to moderate activity, the coefficient of variation is ±20%.
[c] Figure is rounded.